1694870

14-

1/77

DATE DUE

UPI SP........ PRINTED IN U.S.A.

D0966348

OBSTETRIC-
GYNECOLOGIC
TERMINOLOGY

with

SECTION ON NEONATOLOGY

and

GLOSSARY
OF CONGENITAL ANOMALIES

EDWARD C. HUGHES, M.D., FACOG

Editor-in-Chief

F. A. DAVIS COMPANY

Philadelphia

Dedicated to the younger generation of obstetricians and gynecologists, hoping that it may serve to encourage and challenge them to always strive for the increased knowledge and high standards of the Discipline which serve to protect the health and lives of women and infants.

Foreword

The standardization of terms and definitions is essential to communication and reporting in all branches of medicine. This is particularly true in certain aspects of obstetrics and gynecology, since vital statistics, such as those relating to birth and death, are involved. Although it is not easy to reach agreement on terminology, the present volume represents a major effort to achieve consistent, generally acceptable terms and definitions. The College Committee on Terminology, under the chairmanship of Edward C. Hughes, M.D., by whom the project was conceived and consistently directed, has worked long and patiently to produce this book. The work of the Committee has been supported by a grant from the Children's Bureau, now designated as the Maternal and Child Health Service of the Health Services and Mental Health Administration.

It is recognized that, at this time, it is impossible to achieve agreement in regard to all of the definitions and terms commonly used. Nevertheless the Executive Board believes that the publication of this book and the discussions that are certain to follow will lead eventually to a generally accepted and standardized nomenclature in obstetrics and gynecology.

MICHAEL NEWTON, M.D., FACOG
Director, The American College of
Obstetricians and Gynecologists

Preface

The publication of the first edition of Obstetric and Gynecologic Terminology with a Glossary of Congenital Anomalies represents a desideratum for the discipline which heretofore has never been attempted. The purpose of this publication is to establish a universal language so that variability of definition, to which we are always subject, may be minimized. However utopian such a project may appear, its accomplishment may surely have some reflection in the comparability of medical teaching, statistical reporting in hospitals and among state, national, and international health agencies. The increasingly rapid expansion of scientific research and knowledge at the closing half of the 20th Century has brought an inevitable increase in new discoveries and in new terms which must be properly recorded and defined. Because utility was believed to be the principal intention of this publication, the aims of the Committee have been to sift the vast stores of available knowledge and render its essential parts accessible to all who read and practice the art and science of this discipline. The text is a scholarly contribution and is not intended to be taken as individual research.

A universal language is not only useful as a medium through which we can more accurately communicate ideas to one another, but it fulfills a more important function as it serves as an instrument of investigation by initiating new concepts and by improving the preciseness and accuracy of defined results. Advances in the use of computer technology for the recording and retrieving of essential information demand that medical terms be well defined in a standard manner in order that we may proceed along a series of premises to their logical conclusion by reasoning that is accurate and universally understandable.

In accumulating these terms and definitions, the Committee is indebted to many interested individuals, both within and outside the discipline. Before starting the adventure, the opinions of many obstetricians, gynecologists, statisticians, public health administrators, medical librarians, state and national health officials, and world-wide authorities from other related organizations and societies were obtained. Meetings were held with maternal welfare committees and state health officers and authorities around the world to obtain their support and suggestions. Questionnaires were sent to many individuals in the United States. A conference was held in Washington, D.C., called by Katherine Bain, M.D., at that time the Deputy Chief of the Children's Bureau, to discuss this project. Communications from many national and international organizations indicated that standardization of terms in this discipline was essential for medical education and accurate, comparable statistical reporting. Burgess Gordon, M.D., Editor of *Current Medical Terminology* and *Current Procedural Terminology* of the American Medical Association, allowed the Committee to extract all terms relating to gynecology and obstetrics from these publications as one of the beginning sources of material.

The Committee realized soon that it was necessary to obtain funds to complete the task and to seek assistance of individuals knowledgeable in medical terminology and research. An application was prepared by the Committee Chairman, approved by the Executive Board of The American College of Obstetricians and Gynecologists, and granted by the Children's Bureau, now designated as the Maternal and Child Health Service of the Health Services and Mental Health Administration. We are particularly grateful to Charles Gershenson, M.D., Winslow Tompkins, M.D., and Mrs. Gloria Wackernah for their assistance.

In completing this work, the Committee has winnowed the current literature, textbooks, dictionaries, and all other sources of reference for new terms and for new uses for old ones. The Committee deleted with caution some of the terms which have been entombed in medical literature and which have outlasted their significance in the scientific world. It has been our experience in preparing this volume that there is almost no end to new discoveries, new concepts, and new theories.

The Committee would be remiss in not acknowledging the motivating force of the late Robert A. Kimbrough, the first Director of The American College of Obstetricians and Gynecologists. His encouragement from the very beginning of the project stimulated the Committee to go forward in its effort to complete this edition. The Committee wishes to express its sincere appreciation to the various presidents of the College, their executive boards, and the Director, Michael Newton, M.D., for their encouragement and guidance. The Committee is indebted to Mr. Donald Richardson for his expertise in assisting in the preparation of the grant applications and the transactions with the publisher.

It is impossible to thank adequately all who have helped in the cooperative project of compiling this book, but the Committee is especially grateful for the support and encouragement of the dedicated physicians in this country and around the world who have sanctioned the work from the start.

As Chairman of the Committee, I wish to express my sincere gratitude to the Co-Chairman, Craig Muckle, M.D., and to all the members of the Committee, since without them the task could never have been completed. I also wish to express my appreciation to Miss Nancy Cochrane and Mr. John MacDonald, the medical editors, who have labored long and hard to complete the main text. Particular indebtedness is expressed to Mrs. Virginia King for her dedicated efforts in every phase of the preparation of the index and typing of the manuscript. We also wish to thank Mrs. Beverly Yevich for her extensive editorial counsel. The Committee wishes to thank the staff of the F. A. Davis Company and particularly Mr. Robert Craven and Mrs. Miriam Maritato for their patience and guidance.

EDWARD C. HUGHES, M.D., FACOG
Editor-in-Chief

Introduction

The purpose of this text is to gather together in one volume all terms related to obstetrics and gynecology. It is hoped that this effort will in some measure help to unravel the difficulties in communication and statistical reporting at the local, state, national, and international levels. The material has been arranged so the book can be used as a teaching manual for the three basic functions of medicine—education, research, and application.

The selection of the preferred terms from various fields of our discipline has been a difficult matter. We have secured the opinions of experts in the various fields of obstetrics and gynecology. Our group of consultants had two functions: to make sure that we had included basic current terms and to check the accuracy of the facts in the definitions themselves.

Although an effort has been made to eliminate rarely used eponyms as preferred terms, eponymic designations which are firmly entrenched in medical literature have been retained, as their elimination would serve no useful purpose.

Each section of the book is complete within itself. Terms within each section are listed alphabetically. The format for each entry is as follows: preferred term, definition, synonyms and eponyms, abbreviations. In the Genetics section the mode of inheritance precedes the synonyms, eponyms, and abbreviations.

We have incorporated an extensive index which lists all preferred terms and terms that appear within a definition, lists all synonyms in italics, and directs the reader to the page on which the definitions appear.

Major Consultants
and Contributors

GEORGE W. ANDERSON, M.D.
Associate Professor of Obstetrics & Gynecology
Tufts University School of Medicine at the Providence Lying-In Hospital
Providence, Rhode Island

VIRGINIA APGAR, M.D., M.P.H.
Vice-President of Medical Affairs
The National Foundation
White Plains, New York

N. S. ASSALI, M.D.
Professor of Obstetrics, Gynecology & Physiology
University of California
Los Angeles, California

ELEANOR BECHTOLD, M.D.
Assistant Professor of Pathology
State University of New York
Upstate Medical Center
Syracuse, New York

NESRIN BINGOL, M.D.
Assistant Professor of Pediatrics
Director of Genetics Laboratory
New York Medical College
Flower Fifth Avenue Hospital
Metropolitan Hospital Center
New York, New York

BENT BÖVING, M.D.
Professor of Obstetrics & Gynecology
Wayne State University
Detroit, Michigan

LEON C. CHESLEY, Ph.D.
Professor of Obstetrics & Gynecology
State University of New York
Downstate Medical Center
Brooklyn, New York

TIIU CSERMELY, Ph.D.
Research Associate
Department of Obstetrics & Gynecology
State University of New York
Upstate Medical Center
Syracuse, New York

ROBERT K. CURTISS, M.D.
Clinical Assistant Professor of Surgery (Proctology)
State University of New York
Upstate Medical Center
Syracuse, New York

LAURENCE M. DEMERS, Ph.D.
Research Fellow in Reproductive Endocrinology
Laboratory for Human Reproduction & Reproductive Biology
Harvard Medical School
Boston, Massachusetts

FRANK A. ELLIOTT, M.D.
Professor of Neurology
University of Pennsylvania
Philadelphia, Pennsylvania

EDUARD G. FRIEDRICH, JR., M.D.
Assistant Professor of Obstetrics & Gynecology
The Medical College of Wisconsin
Madison, Wisconsin

SPRAGUE H. GARDINER, M.D.
Professor of Obstetrics & Gynecology
University of Indiana
Indianapolis, Indiana

HERMAN L. GARDNER, M.D.
Clinical Professor of Obstetrics & Gynecology
Baylor University College of Medicine
Houston, Texas;
Clinical Professor of Gynecology
The University of Texas
Houston, Texas

LYTT GARDNER, M.D.
Professor of Pediatrics
State University of New York
Upstate Medical Center
Syracuse, New York

BURGESS L. GORDON, M.D.
Editor of *Current Medical Information and Terminology*
Visiting Professor of Medicine
Jefferson Medical College
Philadelphia, Pennsylvania

CHARLES M. GOSS, M.D.
Visiting Professor of Anatomy
George Washington University
School of Medicine
Washington, D. C.

RUSSELL GREENHALGH, M.D.
Clinical Instructor of Surgery
State University of New York
Upstate Medical Center;
Attending Surgeon, St. Joseph's Hospital
Syracuse, New York

SAUL B. GUSBERG, M.D., D.Sci.
(Medicine)
Professor and Chairman of Obstetrics
& Gynecology
Mount Sinai School of Medicine
New York, New York

ALICE GWYNN, A.B.
Medical Technologist
Crouse-Irving Memorial Hospital
Syracuse, New York

CHARLES A. GWYNN, M.D.
Clinical Professor Emeritus of Obstetrics & Gynecology
State University of New York
Upstate Medical Center
Syracuse, New York

ARTHUR T. HERTIG, M.D.
Professor of Pathology
Chief, Division of Pathobiology
New England Regional Primate Research Center
Harvard Medical School
Boston, Massachusetts

SHEILA A. HUNTER, M.Sc.
Worcester Foundation for Experimental
Biology
Shrewsbury, Massachusetts

ROBERT A. ISRAEL
Director, Division of Vital Statistics
National Center for Health Statistics
Health Services and Mental Health
Administration
Public Health Service
Washington, D. C.

ROSS JACOBS, Ph.D.
Assistant Professor of Obstetrics, Gynecology & Biochemistry
State University of New York
Upstate Medical Center
Syracuse, New York

OTTO LILIAN, M.D.
Professor and Chairman of Urology
State University of New York
Upstate Medical Center
Syracuse, New York

JULIA LOBOTSKY, M.S.
Worcester Foundation for Experimental Biology
Shrewsbury, Massachusetts

EUGENE L. LOZNER, M.D.
Professor of Medicine
State University of New York
Upstate Medical Center
Syracuse, New York

CHARLES P. McCARTNEY, M.D.
Professor of Obstetrics & Gynecology
University of Chicago
Chicago Lying-In Hospital
Chicago, Illinois

JOHN M. MORRIS, M.D.
John Slade Ely Professor of Gynecology
Yale University School of Medicine
New Haven, Connecticut

JOHN B. NETTLES, M.D.
Professor of Obstetrics & Gynecology
University of Oklahoma
School of Medicine
Oklahoma City, Oklahoma

ERNEST W. PAGE, M.D.
Professor and Chairman of Obstetrics
& Gynecology
University of California
San Francisco, California

PAUL G. PETERSON, M.D.
Clinical Assistant Professor of Obstetrics & Gynecology
University of Washington
Seattle, Washington

RAYMOND J. PIERI, M.D.
Clinical Professor Emeritus of Obstetrics & Gynecology
State University of New York
Upstate Medical Center
Syracuse, New York

JACK A. PRITCHARD, M.D.
Gillette Professor of Obstetrics & Gynecology
The University of Texas
Southwestern Medical School
Dallas, Texas

A. E. RAKOFF, M.D.
Professor of Obstetrics, Gynecology &
Medicine (Endocrinology)
Jefferson Medical College
Philadelphia, Pennsylvania

EDWARD C. REIFENSTEIN, JR., M.D.
Senior Associate Clinical Research Director
The Squibb Institute for Medical Research
New Brunswick, New Jersey

RALPH A. REIS, M.D.
Editor Emeritus "Obstetrics & Gynecology"
Chicago, Illinois

ALBERT J. SCHAEFER, M.D.
Professor of Pathology and Associate
Professor of Urology
State University of New York
Upstate Medical Center
Syracuse, New York

DAVID H. P. STREETEN, M.B., D.Phil.
Professor of Medicine
Head, Division of Endocrinology
State University of New York
Upstate Medical Center
Syracuse, New York

ROBERT TAUBER, M.D.
Associate Professor Emeritus of Obstetrics & Gynecology
University of Pennsylvania
School of Medicine
Philadelphia, Pennsylvania

ROBERT WESTLAKE, M.D.
Clinical Professor of Medicine
State University of New York
Upstate Medical Center
Syracuse, New York

MARY L. VOORHEES, M.D.
Professor of Pediatrics
State University of New York
Upstate Medical Center
Syracuse, New York

Contents

OBSTETRIC-GYNECOLOGIC
TERMINOLOGY

Section 1: *Anatomy*

Cells

CELL

A cell is a microscopic structure that is the living basis of all animal organisms. It is composed of a mass of protoplasm containing differentiated particles such as the mitochondria, Golgi apparatus, agranular reticulum, ribosomes, lysosomes, and a nucleus. Living cells are enclosed in a cell membrane, which allows many substances to enter and leave. A cell may vary in form and structure according to its function. Some cells are simple and lead an independent or quasi-independent existence. They are capable of reproduction and environmental adaptation. Other cells are highly differentiated, fixed in form and location, and incapable of reproduction, self-nutrition, or locomotion. The chromosomes, which are subnuclear particles, initiate metabolic activity within other subcellular particles in response to inherent mechanisms and to environmental feedback mechanisms.

ACINAR CELL

An acinar cell is a secretory cell that lines an acinus of an acinous gland.

ADIPOSE CELL

An adipose cell is a connective tissue cell distended with fat globules. The cytoplasm is compressed into a thin envelope with the nucleus at a point on the periphery.

AGRANULAR RETICULUM

The agranular reticulum is a system of canaliculi in the cytoplasm without associated ribosomes.

SYNONYM: *Endoplasmic Reticulum.*

ALPHA CELL

An alpha cell is a cell located in the anterior lobe of the pituitary gland or in the pancreas.

ALPHA CELL OF PANCREAS

The alpha cell of the pancreas is a cell in the islets of Langerhans believed to secrete glucagon.

SYNONYM: *Acidophil Cell of Pancreas.*

ALPHA CELL OF PITUITARY

The alpha cell of the pituitary is a cell of the anterior lobe of the pituitary gland whose cytoplasm stains with acid dyes.

SYNONYM: *Acidophil Cell of Pituitary.*

ALVEOLAR CELL

An alveolar cell is a thin epithelial cell that lines an alveolar space in the lung.

AMEBOID CELL

An ameboid cell is a cell having wandering movements with power of locomotion, (for example, leukocyte).

ANAPLASTIC CELL

An anaplastic cell is an abnormal cell that has undergone asynchronous differentiation of nucleus and cytoplasm. Often these cells have failed to develop differential characteristics and resemble embryonal cells in structure and reproductive activity.

BASAL CELLS

Basal cells are cells that originate from the deep layer of the transitional zone. They are small, round cells, four or five times larger than a leukocyte. Basal cells have a small amount of cytoplasm and relatively large nuclei.

SYNONYM: *Inner Basal Cells.*

BASOPHILIC GRANULES

Basophilic granules are granules in the cytoplasm of the cyanophilic cells that have an affinity for basic dyes.

BETA CELL OF PANCREAS

The beta cell of the pancreas is a cell in the islets of Langerhans that secretes insulin.

SYNONYM: *Basophil Cell of Pancreas.*

BETA CELL OF PITUITARY

The beta cell of the pituitary is a cyanophilic cell of the anterior lobe of the pituitary gland. It contains basophilic granules and is believed to secrete gonadoptropic hormones.

SYNONYM: *Basophil Cell of Pituitary.*

BLASTOMERE

A blastomere is any one of the cells produced by one of the early divisions of the zygote.

SYNONYM: *Cleavage Cell.*

BLOOD CELL

A blood cell is one of the formed elements of the blood—that is, a leukocyte or an erythrocyte.

CASTRATION CELL
A castration cell is an altered cyanophilic cell of the anterior lobe of the pituitary gland found after castration. It resembles a signet ring in shape.

SYNONYM: *Signet-Ring Cell.*

CELL MEMBRANE
The cell membrane is the protoplasmic boundary of animal cells. It is semipermeable and is a selective barrier through which substances enter and leave the cell.

SYNONYM: *Plasma Membrane.*

CHROMAFFIN CELL
A chromaffin cell is a cell found in the adrenal medulla and the paraganglia of the sympathetic nervous system, characteristically staining brownish yellow with chromic salts.

CHROMOPHOBE CELL
A chromophobe cell is a cell of the anterior lobe of the pituitary.

CILIATED CELL
A ciliated cell is a tall, broad cell that measures 35μ in height and 12μ in width. Its superior border measures 7 to 8μ in length. Each cell possesses 180 to 190 cilia. These cells are found in the endoderm, endosalpinx, and other tissues.

CLEAR CELL
A clear cell is one found in the deepest layer of the epidermis. It is thought to be derived from neuroectoderm and gives rise to a melanoblast of the skin.

COLUMNAR CELL
A columnar cell is an epithelial cell that is longer than it is broad.

CONNECTIVE TISSUE CELL
A connective tissue cell is any of the cells of varied form found in connective tissue.

CYANOPHILIC CELL
A cyanophilic cell is a cell containing basophilic granules.

CYANOPHILIC KARYOPYKNOTIC SUPERFICIAL CELL
A cyanophilic karyopyknotic superficial cell is a cell with a flat squame and a pyknotic nucleus. It usually stains basophilic.

SYNONYM: *Precornified Cell* (obsolete).

CYTOPLASM
Cytoplasm is the protoplasm of a cell exclusive of the nucleus. This substance contains organelles that are responsible for cell function—

namely, mitochondria, ribosomes, Golgi apparatus, agranular reticulum, and others.

CYTOPLASMIC VACUOLAR SYSTEM
The cytoplasmic vacuolar system is an intracellular membrane system composed of tubules, vesicles, and flattened sacs. The agranular reticulum, the nuclear envelope, and the Golgi apparatus are components, interconnected by permanent or temporary channels.

CYTOTROPHOBLAST
The cytotrophoblast is composed of giant, multinucleated cells. It forms the innermost of two layers covering the early chorionic villi. These cells ordinarily disappear before midpregnancy.
SYNONYM: *Langhans' Cell.*

DAUGHTER CELL
A daughter cell is a cell resulting from division of a mother cell.

DECIDUAL CELL
A decidual cell is an endometrial cell, polyhedral or ovoid, found in the endometrium of pregnancy.

DEEP INTERMEDIATE CELL
A deep intermediate cell is a cell with a slightly flattened oval squame and a vesicular nucleus. It usually stains basophilic.

DIFFERENTIATED CELL
A differentiated cell is one that has a different character or function from the surrounding cells or from the original cell type.

ELEMENTARY CELL
An elementary cell is one of the primitive embryonic cells from which all cells of the body are developed. It can be an undifferentiated cell of the adult with characteristics of a cell of the embryo.
SYNONYM: *Primary Embryonic Cell.*

ENDOTHELIAL CELL
An endothelial cell is one of the cells forming the lining of blood and lymph vessels, and the inner layer of the endocardium.

EOSINOPHIL
An eosinophil is a structure, cell, or histologic element readily stained by eosin. The term is most commonly used to designate an eosinophilic leukocyte.

EOSINOPHILIC CELL
An eosinophilic cell is a cell whose cytoplasm stains with acid dyes.

EOSINOPHILIC KARYOPYKNOTIC SUPERFICIAL CELL
An eosinophilic karyopyknotic superficial cell is a cell with a flat squame and pyknotic nucleus. It usually stains acidophilic.
SYNONYM: *Cornified Cell* (obsolete).

EPIDERMIC CELL
An epidermic cell is a cell of the epidermis.

EPITHELIAL CELL
An epithelial cell is one of many varieties of cells that form epithelium.

ERYTHROCYTE
An erythrocyte is a non-nucleated, agranular, circulating blood cell that contains hemoglobin for the purpose of accepting, transporting, and delivering oxygen.

FIBROBLASTIC CELL
A fibroblastic cell is a cell that produces collagen and elastic fibers and is generally flattened in shape with pale homogeneous protoplasm.

FOLLICULAR CELL
A follicular cell is one of the cells that line an ovarian follicle.
SYNONYM: *Follicular Epithelial Cell.*

FUSIFORM CELL
A fusiform cell is a spindle-shaped cell.

GAMETE
A gamete is a mature sex cell, either a secondary oocyte (macrogamete) or a spermatozoon (microgamete).

GERMINAL CELL
A germinal cell is one of the columnar cells that constitute the reproductive source of all epidermoid cells.

GIANT CELL
A giant cell is a large multinucleated cell, usually a macrophage (exception: syncytiotrophoblast).

GOBLET CELL
A goblet cell is an epithelial cell distended with mucin.
SYNONYM: *Mucous Cell.*

GOLGI APPARATUS
The Golgi apparatus is a network of fine tubules adjacent to the nucleus of a cell. It is associated with the intracellular formation of secretory products.

GRANULAR CELL
A granular cell is one of the cells in the granular layer of the dermis. It is a flattened cell that contains granules of eleiden.

GRANULAR RETICULUM
The granular reticulum is a system of canaliculi in the cytoplasm with associated ribosomes.
SYNONYM: *Ergastoplasm.*

GRANULOSA CELLS
Granulosa cells are cells surrounding the female germ cell after antrum formation. They form the cumulus oophorus and the lining of the follicle.

HILAR CELL
A hilar cell is an elongated, oval, polygonal cell with eosinophilic cytoplasm, normally present in the hilum of the ovary. Hilar cells are thought to be the homologues of the interstitial, or Leydig cells of the testis.
SYNONYMS: *Berger Cell, Hilus Cell, Sympathicotropic Cell.*

HOFBAUER CELL
A Hofbauer cell is a mononuclear, wandering phagocyte found in the stroma of the chorionic villi.

HYPERCHROMATIC CELL
A hyperchromatic cell is a cell resulting from asymmetric mitosis or one that has failed to undergo mitosis after replication of its deoxyribonucleic acid (DNA) complement. It contains more than the normal number of chromosomes.

HYPOCHROMATIC CELL
A hypochromatic cell is a cell resulting from asymmetric mitosis. The nucleus contains less than the normal number of chromosomes.

INDIFFERENT CELLS
Indifferent cells lie at the base of the normal tubal epithelium and apparently serve as progenitors of the epithelial and stromal element of the fallopian tube. These cells are metabolically more active than the other epithelial cells of the fallopian tubes.

INTERCALARY CELLS
Intercalary cells are long, slender cells possessing a long, rodlike nucleus. These cells are located between other cells of the tubal epithelium. The function of these cells is to form cytoplasmic material that is secreted into the fallopian tube for the nutrition of the ovum and sperm.
SYNONYM: *Peg Cells.*

INTERMEDIATE CELL
An intermediate cell is a cell with a flat squame and vesicular nucleus. It usually stains basophilic.
SYNONYM: *Deep Precornified Cell* (obsolete).

INTERPHASE CELL
An interphase cell is a cell that is not undergoing mitotic division.

Gap 1-Phase Cell
A gap 1-phase cell is a cell that is about to replicate deoxyribonucleic acid (DNA).

Gap S-Phase Cell
A gap S-phase cell is a cell that is in the process of deoxyribonucleic acid (DNA) replication.

Gap 2-Phase Cell
A gap 2-phase cell is a cell that has completed deoxyribonucleic acid (DNA) replication. There are several distinct cell populations in gap 2-phase. Some are committed to prompt mitosis; others remain dormant in the gap 2-phase for variable periods.

INTERSTITIAL CELL
An interstitial cell is a connective tissue cell located between the seminiferous tubules of the testis. These cells are believed to furnish the male sex hormone.
SYNONYM: *Leydig Cell.*

KARYOMICROSOME
A karyomicrosome is a minute particle or granule in the substance of the cell nucleus.
SYNONYM: *Nucleomicrosome.*

KARYOPLASM
The karyoplasm is the protoplasm of the cell nucleus.
SYNONYM: *Nuclear Sap.*

KARYOSOME
A karyosome is a chromatin filament in the interphase cell nucleus.

LEUKOCYTE
A leukocyte is any colorless, ameboid cell mass. The term is applied especially to one of the formed elements of the blood consisting of a colorless granular mass of protoplasm.

LUTEIN CELL
A lutein cell is one of the granulosa cells of the ovarian follicles that form the corpus luteum of the ovary.
SYNONYM: *Luteal Cell.*

LYMPHOCYTE
A lymphocyte is a type of white cell formed in lymphoid tissue.

LYSOSOME
A lysosome is any one of a class of membrane-bound cytoplasmic structures replete with hydrolytic enzymes and capable of autolytic processes that effect the dissolution of nucleic acids, proteins, and polysaccharides. Common pleomorphic forms of lysosome are phagosomes, microbodies, residual bodies, and multivesicular bodies.

Autophagic Vacuole
An autophagic vacuole is a subcellular structure appearing when the cell must utilize its own cytoplasm during episodes of starvation, anoxia, or degeneration. It has intrinsic lysosomal properties.

Microbody
A microbody is a pleomorphic form of lysosome possessing the same characteristics as lysosomes but smaller.

Multivesicular Body
A multivesicular body is a lysosomal form that has arisen through fusion of endocytic vesicles with components of the Golgi apparatus.

Phagosome
A phagosome is an endocytic vacuole formed as an invagination of the cell membrane during cellular ingestion of foreign materials. Phagosomes merge with lysosomes resulting in autodigestion of the engulfed material in the vacuoles.

Residual Body
A residual body is a lysosome that has conducted various digestive functions and now contains undigested fragments of lipoid debris.

MACROCYTE
A macrocyte is an abnormally large erythrocyte. The diameter is greater than 9μ or the volume is greater than 95 cu μ.

MACROPHAGE
A macrophage is a large mononuclear phagocyte.
SYNONYMS: *Histiocyte, Wandering Cell.*

MAST CELL
A mast cell is a connective tissue cell that contains coarse basophilic granules. It is believed to contain histamine, heparin, and lipoprotein lipase.

MEIOSIS
Meiosis is the process of germ cell division. Half of each pair of chromosomes is removed in preparation for postfertilization replacement with a corresponding chromosome from a gamete of the other sex. In the

female, the prophase of meiosis begins in fetal life and is not complete until penetration of the ovum by a spermatozoon. The first meiotic (maturation) division in the primary oocyte takes place at about the time of ovulation. It produces two cells, each with a haploid (23) number of chromosomes. One of the cells (secondary oocyte) receives all the cytoplasm and the other (first polar body) receives none. The chromosomes of the secondary oocyte, previously produced in mitotic division, now separate (equation division) and produce two cells, each having a haploid number of chromosomes. One cell (ootid) receives all the cytoplasm, and the other (second polar body) receives none. In the male, meiosis begins after puberty, and each primary spermatocyte gives rise to four functional sperm cells.

SYNONYM: *Maturation Division.*

MESENCHYMAL CELL

A mesenchymal cell is a fusiform or stellate cell located between the ectoderm and endoderm of the embryo.

MESOTHELIAL CELL

A mesothelial cell is one of the flat cells of mesothelium lining serous membranes.

MICROSOMES

Microsomes are subcellular artifacts of isolation composed of agranular reticulum with attached ribosomal granules.

MICROVILLUS

A microvillus is a submicroscopic projection of a cell membrane.

MITOCHONDRION

A mitochondrion is an organelle located in the cytoplasm. The mitochondria are responsible for the production of high-energy phosphates by oxidative phosphorylation.

SYNONYM: *Cytoplasmic Organelle.*

MITOSIS

Mitosis is a cell division. It provides identical numbers and types of chromosomes to all descendent cells.

MOTHER CELL

A mother cell is a cell that, by division, gives rise to two or more daughter cells.

MYOEPITHELIAL CELL

A myoepithelial cell is a cell that consists of a nucleus and many stringlike projections. These cells surround the alveoli and the portion of the mammary duct adjacent to the alveolus. They play an important part in the milk-ejection reflex.

SYNONYM: *Basket Cell.*

NONCILIATED CELL
A nonciliated cell is a cell that does not possess a cilium. These cells are found in the endosalpinx and other tissues.

NUCLEAR ENVELOPE
The nuclear envelope is an integral component of the cytoplasmic vacuolar system that provides continuity of the system from the nucleus to the agranular reticulum.
SYNONYM: *Nuclear Membrane.*

NUCLEOLUS
A nucleolus is a circumscribed structure. There may be one or several in a nucleus at any given time. It consists largely of acid, basic proteins, and ribonucleic acid (RNA).
SYNONYM: *Plasmosome.*

NUCLEUS
A nucleus is a differentiated mass of protoplasm surrounded by a membrane and located within a cell. The nucleus is made up of karyoplasm, chromosomes, organelles, and one or more nucleoli. The nucleus is the coordinating center of the cell's functional activity.

PAGET'S CELL
Paget's cell is a neoplastic malignant epithelial cell having a hyperchromatic nucleus and pale-staining cytoplasm. It is found in Paget's disease of the breast and vulva.

PARABASAL CELLS
The parabasal cells are cells that originate from the upper layer of the transitional zone. They are round cells having an increased amount of cytoplasm that stains a light blue with the Papanicolaou stain. The nuclei have fine chromatin material in their substances.
SYNONYM: *Outer Basal Cells.*

PERICYTE
A pericyte is a slender connective tissue cell in close relationship to the outside of the capillary wall.

PHAGOCYTE
A phagocyte is a cell that ingests microorganisms, cells, or foreign particles.

PIGMENT CELL
A pigment cell is generally a connective tissue cell that contains pigment granules.

PINOCYTE
A pinocyte is a cell, usually a macrophage, that engulfs plasma by means of pinocytosis.

PINOCYTOSIS
Pinocytosis is a process of engulfing plasma into the substance of the trophoblastic syncytium.

PLASMA CELL
A plasma cell is an ovoid cell with an eccentric nucleus and radiating particles of chromatin. The cytoplasm is strongly basophilic because of the abundant ribonucleic acid (RNA) in the agranular reticulum. It produces immunoglobulins.

PRICKLE CELL
A prickle cell is a cell of the stratum germinativum of the skin having numerous radiating processes or prickles (desmosomes).

PRIMORDIAL GERM CELL
A primordial germ cell is an undifferentiated sex cell possessing the potential of becoming either a male or female gamete. It is found only in the young embryo.

PYKNOSIS
Pyknosis is a term used to indicate degeneration of a nucleus. The changes are shrinkage of the nucleus and condensation of the chromatin to a solid structureless mass.
SYNONYM: *Karyopyknosis.*

RESERVE CELL
A reserve cell is the germinal cell of the endocervical epithelium.

RETICULAR CELL
A reticular cell is a stellate cell found in the cellular stroma of the lymph nodes, spleen, and bone marrow. It produces reticulin fibers.
SYNONYMS: *Fixed Macrophage, Primitive Reticulum Cell (Hemocytoblast), Hematopoietic Reticulum Cell.*

RIBOSOME
A ribosome is a submicroscopic cellular particle composed of protein and ribonucleic acid (RNA) and is considered the site of protein synthesis.

SEROUS CELL
A serous cell is one that produces a watery albuminoid secretion.

SERTOLI CELLS
Sertoli cells are cells in the testicular tubules in which the spermatids become embedded. They furnish nutrition to the developing spermatids.
SYNONYMS: *Sustentacular Cells, Nurse Cells, Foot Cells, Trophocytes.*

SQUAMOUS CELL
A squamous cell is a flat scalelike epithelial cell.

STELLATE CELL
A stellate cell is a star-shaped cell.

SYMPATHOCHROMAFFIN CELL
A sympathochromaffin cell is one of the cells in the embryo from which both sympathetic ganglia and chromaffin cells develop.

SYNCYTIOTROPHOBLAST
The syncytiotrophoblast is the outer layer of cells covering each chorionic villus and in contact with maternal blood or decidua.

SYNONYMS: *Plasmoditrophoblast, Syntrophoblast, Syncytial Trophoblast.*

THECA CELLS
Theca cells are cells that surround the granulosa cells and form the outer part of the wall of an ovarian follicle.

THECA-LUTEIN CELL
A theca-lutein cell is one of the cells of the corpus luteum derived from the theca interna.

TRANSITIONAL CELL
A transitional cell is any cell thought to represent a phase of development from one form to another.

UNDIFFERENTIATED CELL
An undifferentiated cell is a primitive cell that has not assumed the morphologic or functional characteristics of a mature cell—for example, cells found in a malignant neoplasm, or the germinal cells that replenish normal tissues.

Arteries

AORTA, ABDOMINAL

The abdominal aorta is a continuation of the thoracic aorta from the level of the inferior border of the 12th thoracic vertebra. The branches of the abdominal aorta may be divided into three sets: the visceral, parietal, and terminal.

SYNONYM: *Aorta Abdominalis* (NA).

AXILLARY ARTERY

The axillary artery is the continuation of the subclavian artery. It begins at the outer border of the first rib and ends at the lower border of the teres major muscle.

SYNONYM: *Arteria Axillaris* (NA).

BULBAR ARTERY OF VESTIBULE

The bulbar artery of the vestibule is a branch of the internal pudendal artery that passes through the inferior fascia of the urogenital diaphragm to supply the cavernous tissue of the vestibular bulb and the major vestibular gland.

SYNONYM: *Arteria Bulbi Vestibuli* (NA).

CERVICOVAGINAL ARTERY

The cervicovaginal artery is a large branch of the uterine artery that extends along the lateral aspect of the cervix and the vagina. It supplies the uterus, cervix, and upper vagina.

SYNONYM: *Arteria Cervicovaginalis* (NA).

CLITORAL ARTERY

The clitoral artery enters the deep compartment of the urogenital diaphragm and runs along the inferior ramus of the pubis in the substance of the deep transverse perineal muscle and the sphincter of the membranous urethra. It ends in four branches, which supply, chiefly, the erectile tissue of the superficial perineal compartment.

SYNONYM: *Arteria Corporis Cavernosorum* (NA).

Clitoral Artery, Deep

The deep clitoral artery pierces the fascial floor of the deep compartment just medial to the corpus cavernosum of the clitoris, which it enters.

SYNONYM: *Arteria Profunda Clitoridis* (NA).

15

Clitoral Artery, Dorsal

The dorsal clitoral artery leaves the deep perineal compartment just behind the transverse pelvic muscle and runs over the dorsum of the clitoris to the glans.

SYNONYM: *Arteria Dorsalis Clitoridis* (NA).

ENDOMETRIAL ARTERIES

The endometrial arteries consist of the endometrial coiled arteries and the endometrial basal arteries.

Endometrial Arteries, Basal

The endometrial basal arteries are branches of the radial arteries that supply the basalis layer of the endometrium. The basal arteries are not affected by hormonal influences. These arteries supply blood to the regenerating endometrium.

Endometrial Arteries, Coiled

The endometrial coiled arteries are essentially a continuation of the radial arteries. The coiled arteries supply the functional zone of the endometrium and are sensitive to the biphasic stimulation of the ovarian steroids. These arteries furnish the nutritional substances to the endometrial glands and stroma, and they exhibit a period of vasoconstriction creating ischemia in endometrial segments, tissue sloughing, and menstrual bleeding.

SYNONYM: *Endometrial Spiral Arterioles.*

EPIGASTRIC ARTERY, INFERIOR

The inferior epigastric artery arises from the external iliac artery immediately above the inguinal ligament. It courses upward, piercing the fascia transversalis and finally divides into numerous branches, which anastomose with the obturator arteries and, above the umbilicus, with the superior epigastric artery.

SYNONYMS: *Deep Epigastric Artery, Arteria Epigastrica Inferior* (NA).

FEMORAL ARTERY

The femoral artery is the continuation of the external iliac artery beginning at the inguinal ligament. Its branches are the external pudendal, superficial epigastric, superficial circumflex iliac, deep femoral, and descending genicular arteries. This artery terminates in the popliteal artery at the upper part of the popliteal space. It supplies the skin of the lower part of the abdomen and groin, external genitalia, inguinal lymph nodes, and medial, lateral, and anterior aspects of the thigh, femur, and knee joint.

SYNONYM: *Arteria Femoralis* (NA).

Femoral Artery, Deep

The deep femoral artery is a large vessel arising from the lateral and posterior part of the femoral artery, from 2 to 5 cm below the inguinal ligament.

SYNONYM: *Arteria Profunda Femoris* (NA).

Femoral Artery, Lateral Circumflex

The lateral circumflex femoral artery arises from the deep femoral artery. It supplies the hip joint muscles of the thigh and gluteal area.

SYNONYM: *Arteria Circumflexa Femoris Lateralis* (NA).

Femoral Artery, Medial Circumflex

The medial circumflex femoral artery arises from the deep femoral artery. It supplies the hip joint muscles of the thigh and gluteal area.

SYNONYM: *Arteria Circumflexa Femoris Medialis* (NA).

GLUTEAL ARTERY, INFERIOR

The inferior gluteal artery is a terminal branch of the internal iliac artery. It pierces the fascia in front of the piriformis muscle and leaves the pelvis through the greater sciatic foramen to supply the gluteus maximus and the muscles of the back of the thigh.

SYNONYM: *Arteria Glutea Inferior* (NA).

GLUTEAL ARTERY, SUPERIOR

The superior gluteal artery arises from the internal iliac artery and supplies the gluteal area. It anastomoses with the lateral sacral, inferior gluteal, internal pudendal, deep circumflex iliac, and lateral circumflex femoral arteries.

SYNONYM: *Arteria Glutea Superior* (NA).

ILIAC ARTERIES, COMMON

The common iliac arteries are divisions of the abdominal aorta, which bifurcates at the left side of the body of the fourth lumbar vertebra. They terminate opposite the lumbosacral articulation by dividing into the external iliac and internal iliac arteries. The right common iliac artery is crossed by the ovarian vessels, the ureter, and the sympathetic nerve fibers descending to the superior hypogastric plexus. In addition, the left common iliac artery is covered by the sigmoid colon and mesocolon and by the termination of the inferior mesenteric artery.

SYNONYM: *Arteria Iliaca Communis* (NA).

ILIAC ARTERY, DEEP CIRCUMFLEX

The deep circumflex iliac artery arises from the external iliac artery and supplies the muscles and skin of the lower abdomen, sartorius muscles, gluteal area, and tensor fascia lata.

SYNONYM: *Arteria Circumflexa Ilium Profunda* (NA).

ILIAC ARTERY, EXTERNAL

The external iliac artery is the larger and lateral subdivision of the common iliac artery. It extends downward along the superior border of the true pelvis to the lower margin of the inguinal ligament. It lies on the medial border of the psoas major muscle. It enters the thigh as the femoral artery, midway between the pubic symphysis and the anterior superior iliac spine.

SYNONYM: *Arteria Iliaca Externa* (NA).

ILIAC ARTERY, INTERNAL

The internal iliac artery is the medial terminal branch of the common iliac artery. It arises opposite the lumbosacral articulation and passes downward and backward to the upper border of the greater sciatic notch. It crosses the psoas major and piriformis muscles and the lumbosacral nerve trunk and then divides. The posterior division is the common stem of origin of three parietal branches: the iliolumbar, the lateral sacral, and the superior gluteal arteries. The anterior division of the internal iliac artery gives rise to parietal branches (the obturator, inferior gluteal, and internal pudendal) and visceral branches (the superior vesical, middle rectal, uterine, and vaginal).

SYNONYMS: *Hypogastric Artery, Arteria Iliaca Interna* (NA).

ILIAC ARTERY, SUPERFICIAL CIRCUMFLEX

The superficial circumflex iliac artery originates from the femoral artery and supplies the inguinal lymph nodes and integument in that area, the sartorius muscle, and the tensor fascia lata.

SYNONYM: *Arteria Circumflexa Ilium Superficialis* (NA).

LABIAL ARTERY, ANTERIOR

The anterior labial artery arises from the external pudendal artery and supplies the anterior portion of the labia majora.

SYNONYM: *Rami Labiales Anteriores Arteriae Pudendae Externae* (NA).

LABIAL ARTERY, POSTERIOR

The posterior labial artery arises from the internal pudendal artery and supplies the posterior portion of the labia majora.

SYNONYM: *Rami Labiales Posteriores Arteriae Pudendae Internae* (NA)

MYOMETRIAL ARCUATE ARTERIES

The myometrial arcuate arteries are branches of the uterine and ovarian arteries. They terminate in the myometrial radial arteries.

MYOMETRIAL RADIAL ARTERIES

The myometrial radial arteries are a continuation of the myometrial arcuate arteries. They penetrate the endometrium and divide into the larger endometrial coiled arteries and the smaller endometrial basal arteries.

OBTURATOR ARTERY

The obturator artery sometimes arises from the inferior epigastric artery or from the internal iliac artery. It accompanies the obturator nerve into the obturator canal. Its branches include iliac, vesical, pubic, and anterior and posterior terminal divisions that supply soft and bony structures inside and outside the anterior pelvic wall. These branches communicate with branches of the inferior epigastric artery and other offshoots of the external iliac artery.

SYNONYM: *Arteria Obturatoria* (NA).

OVARIAN ARTERIES

The ovarian arteries arise from the aorta just below the origin of the renal vessels. The ovarian arteries course obliquely downward and laterally over the psoas major muscle and the ureter. They enter the true pelvis by crossing the common iliac artery just before its bifurcation. The ovarian artery enters the broad ligament at the junction of its superior and lateral borders. Continuing beneath the fallopian tube, it enters the mesovarium to supply the ovary. In addition to broad anastomoses with the ovarian rami of the uterine arteries, branches extend to the ampullar and isthmic portion of the fallopian tube, the ureter, and the round ligament.

SYNONYM: *Arteria Ovarica* (NA).

PERINEAL ARTERY, SUPERFICIAL

The superficial perineal artery is a branch of the internal pudendal artery. It supplies the labia majora and minora.

SYNONYM: *Arteria Perinealis* (NA).

PUDENDAL ARTERY, DEEP EXTERNAL

The deep external pudendal artery is distributed to the labia, anastomosing with the superficial perineal artery.

SYNONYM: *Arteria Pudenda Externa Profunda.*

PUDENDAL ARTERY, INTERNAL

The internal pudendal artery enters the ischiorectal fossa through the lesser sciatic foramen. It lies in a fibrous canal (pudendal canal) formed by the fascia covering the obturator internus muscle. The branches of the internal pudendal artery include small branches to the gluteal region, the inferior rectal artery, the perineal artery, and the clitoral artery.

SYNONYMS: *Internal Pudic Artery, Arteria Pudenda Interna* (NA).

PUDENDAL ARTERY, SUPERFICIAL

The superficial pudendal artery arises from the femoral artery and supplies the skin of the lower part of the abdomen, skin of the clitoris, and labia majora.

SYNONYMS: *Superficial External Pudic Artery, Arteria Pudenda Externa Superficialis.*

RECTAL ARTERY, INFERIOR

The inferior rectal artery pierces the wall of the pudendal canal and passes medially through the ischiorectal fat to supply the anal canal, anus, and perineal area.

SYNONYMS: *Inferior Hemorrhoidal Artery, Arteria Rectalis Inferior* (NA).

RECTAL ARTERY, MIDDLE

The middle rectal artery is a branch of the internal iliac artery, which supplies the middle portion of the rectum and anastomoses with the superior and inferior rectal arteries.

SYNONYMS: *Middle Hemorrhoidal Artery, Arteria Rectalis Media* (NA).

RECTAL ARTERY, SUPERIOR

The superior rectal artery branches from the inferior mesenteric artery and descends into the pelvis between the layers of the sigmoid mesocolon. At the junction of the pelvic colon and rectum, it divides into two lateral and two posterior divisions, which anastomose with the middle rectal vessels of the internal iliac and the inferior rectal branches of the internal pudendal artery.

SYNONYMS: *Superior Hemorrhoidal Artery, Arteria Rectalis Superior* (NA).

ROUND LIGAMENT, ARTERY OF

The artery of the round ligament arises from the inferior epigastric artery and supplies the round ligament.

SYNONYM: *Arteria Ligamenti Teretis Uteri* (NA).

SACRAL ARTERY, INFERIOR LATERAL

The inferior lateral sacral artery arises from the internal iliac artery and supplies the contents of the sacral canal, muscles, and skin on the dorsal surface of the sacrum.

SYNONYM: *Arteria Sacralis Lateralis Inferior* (NA).

SACRAL ARTERY, MIDDLE

The middle sacral artery is a continuation of the aorta. It passes downward in the midline over the inferior surface of the fourth and fifth lumbar vertebrae, the sacrum, and coccyx. The middle sacral artery terminates in the glomus coccygeum, after giving off lumbar, lateral, sacral, and rectal branches. These branches anastomose with branches of the iliolumbar artery and supply muscular and bony structures of the posterior pelvic wall.

SYNONYM: *Arteria Sacralis Mediana* (NA).

SACRAL ARTERY, SUPERIOR LATERAL

The superior lateral sacral artery arises from the internal iliac artery and supplies the skin and muscles on the dorsal surface of the sacrum.

SYNONYM: *Arteria Sacralis Lateralis Superior* (NA).

SUBCLAVIAN ARTERY

The subclavian artery is one of two arteries, the left arising from the arch of the aorta and the right from the innominate artery behind the right sternoclavicular articulation. They are continuous with the axillary arteries.

SYNONYM: *Arteria Subclavia* (NA).

THORACIC ARTERY, INTERNAL

The internal thoracic artery is an artery that arises from the under surface of the first portion of the subclavian artery.

SYNONYMS: *Internal Mammary Artery, Arteria Thoracica Interna* (NA).

THORACIC ARTERY, LATERAL

The lateral thoracic artery is a branch of the axillary artery that follows the lower border of the pectoralis minor muscle to the side of the chest, supplying the pectoralis, and sends branches across the axilla to the axillary glands and subscapularis muscle. It anatomoses with the internal thoracic, subscapular, and intercostal arteries. It supplies an external mammary branch, which turns around the free edge of the pectoralis major muscle and supplies the breast.

SYNONYMS: *Long Thoracic Artery, Arteria Thoracica Lateralis* (NA).

THORACIC ARTERY, SUPERIOR

The superior thoracic artery is a small vessel that may arise from the thoracoacromial artery or may be absent. It runs forward and medially along the upper border of the pectoralis minor muscle. It passes between the pectoralis major and minor muscles to the side of the chest. It anastomoses with the internal thoracic and intercostal arteries.

SYNONYMS: *Highest Thoracic Artery, Arteria Thoracica Suprema* (NA).

URETHRAL ARTERY

The urethral artery is a branch of the internal pudendal artery. It runs medially toward the urethra and anastomoses with branches of the bulbar artery.

SYNONYM: *Arteria Urethralis* (NA).

UTERINE ARTERY

The uterine artery arises from the anterior division of the internal iliac artery, close to or in common with the middle rectal or vaginal artery. It courses slightly forward and medially on the superior fascia of the levator ani muscle to the lower margin of the broad ligament. After entering the broad ligament, the uterine artery is surrounded in the parametrium by the uterine veins and a condensed sheath of connective tissue. It arches over the ureter to the uterus. At the level of the isthmus, it gives off a descending cervical branch, which surrounds the cervix and anastomoses with branches of the vaginal artery. The uterine artery terminates in a tubal branch within the mesosalpinx, and an ovarian ramus that anastomoses with the ovarian artery in the mesovarium.

SYNONYM: *Arteria Uterina* (NA).

VAGINAL ARTERY

The vaginal artery arises from the internal iliac artery. It passes behind the ureter to the upper vagina, where it anastomoses with the descending branches of the uterine artery and internal pudendal artery and forms a network of vessels around the vagina. It supplies the mucous membrane of the vagina, the bulb of the vestibule, the fundus of the bladder, and the contiguous part of the rectum.

SYNONYM: *Arteria Vaginalis* (NA).

VESICAL ARTERIES

The vesical arteries course over the ureter, sending branches to it, and then anastomose over the lateral and superior surfaces and the base of the bladder with the branches of the opposite side.

Veins

AXILLARY VEIN
The axillary vein begins at the junction of the basilic and brachial veins near the lower border of the teres major muscle and ends at the outer border of the first rib.
SYNONYM: *Vena Axillaris* (NA).

BULBAR VEIN OF VESTIBULE
The bulbar vein of the vestibule is the vein draining the bulb of the vestibule. It terminates in the internal pudendal vein.
SYNONYM: *Vena Bulbi Vestibuli* (NA).

CLITORAL VEIN, DEEP DORSAL
The deep dorsal clitoral vein passes from the dorsum of the clitoris to join the vesical venous plexus.
SYNONYM: *Vena Dorsalis Clitoridis Profunda* (NA).

CLITORAL VEIN, SUPERFICIAL DORSAL
The superficial dorsal clitoral vein collects blood subcutaneously from the clitoris and drains into the external pudendal vein.
SYNONYM: *Venae Dorsales Clitoridis Superficiales* (NA).

EPIGASTRIC VEIN, INFERIOR
The inferior epigastric vein is a vein that accompanies the inferior epigastric artery and opens into the external iliac vein.
SYNONYMS: *Deep Epigastric Vein, Vena Epigastrica Inferior* (NA).

FEMORAL VEIN
The femoral vein accompanies the femoral artery through the upper two-thirds of the thigh. It joins the deep femoral vein about 4 cm below the inguinal ligament. Near its termination it is joined by the great saphenous vein.
SYNONYM: *Vena Femoralis* (NA).

FEMORAL VEIN, DEEP
The deep femoral vein receives tributaries corresponding to the perforating branches of the deep femoral artery. It joins the femoral artery in the femoral triangle along with the medial and lateral circumflex femoral veins.
SYNONYM: *Vena Profunda Femoris* (NA).

FEMORAL VEINS, LATERAL CIRCUMFLEX
The lateral circumflex femoral veins are the veins that accompany the lateral circumflex femoral artery.
SYNONYM: *Venae Circumflexae Femoris Laterales* (NA).

FEMORAL VEINS, MEDIAL CIRCUMFLEX
The medial circumflex femoral veins are the veins that parallel the medial circumflex femoral artery.
SYNONYM: *Venae Circumflexae Femoris Mediales* (NA).

GLUTEAL VEIN, INFERIOR
The inferior gluteal vein is one of the veins that accompanies the branches of the inferior gluteal artery. These unite at the sciatic foramen to form a common trunk that empties into the internal iliac vein.
SYNONYM: *Venae Gluteae Inferiores* (NA).

GLUTEAL VEIN, SUPERIOR
The superior gluteal vein is one of the veins that accompanies the superior gluteal artery. It enters the pelvis as two veins, which unite and empty into the internal iliac vein.
SYNONYM: *Venae Gluteae Superiores* (NA).

ILIAC VEIN, COMMON
The common iliac vein is formed by the union of the external and internal iliac veins at the brim of the pelvis. The right common iliac vein passes upward behind the internal iliac artery to the right of the body of the fifth lumbar vertebra, where it unites with its fellow of the opposite side to form the inferior vena cava.
SYNONYM: *Vena Iliaca Communis* (NA).

ILIAC VEIN, DEEP CIRCUMFLEX
The deep circumflex iliac vein corresponds to the deep circumflex iliac artery and joins the external iliac vein about 2 cm above the inguinal ligament.
SYNONYM: *Vena Circumflexa Ilium Profunda* (NA).

ILIAC VEIN, EXTERNAL
The external iliac vein is a direct continuation of the femoral vein. It begins behind the inguinal ligament and unites with the internal iliac to form the common iliac vein.
SYNONYM: *Vena Iliaca Externa* (NA).

ILIAC VEIN, INTERNAL
The internal iliac vein extends from the upper border of the great sciatic notch to the brim of the pelvis, where it joins the external iliac vein to form the common iliac vein. It drains most of the region supplied by the internal iliac artery.
SYNONYMS: *Hypogastric Vein, Vena Iliaca Interna* (NA).

ILIAC VEIN, SUPERFICIAL CIRCUMFLEX
The superficial circumflex iliac vein empties into the greater saphenous vein or into the femoral vein.

SYNONYM: *Vena Circumflexa Ilium Superficialis* (NA).

LABIAL VEINS, ANTERIOR
The anterior labial veins pass from the labia majora into the external pudendal vein.

SYNONYM: *Venae Labiales Anteriores* (NA).

LABIAL VEINS, POSTERIOR
The posterior labial veins pass from the labia majora into the internal pudendal vein.

SYNONYM: *Venae Labiales Posteriores* (NA).

OBTURATOR VEIN
The obturator vein is formed by the union of tributaries draining the hip and the muscles in the upper and back part of the thigh. It enters the pelvis by the obturator foramen and runs dorsad to empty into the internal iliac vein.

SYNONYM: *Venae Obturatoriae* (NA).

OVARIAN VEINS
The ovarian veins are two in number, the right and the left. They arise at the pampiniform plexus at the hilum of the ovary and open into the inferior vena cava on the right and into the renal vein on the left.

SYNONYM: *Vena Ovarica Sinistra* (NA), *Vena Ovarica Dextra* (NA).

PUDENDAL VEINS, EXTERNAL
The external pudendal veins empty into the great saphenous or directly into the femoral veins. They receive the subcutaneous dorsal vein of the clitoris and the anterior labial veins.

SYNONYM: *Venae Pudendae Externae* (NA).

PUDENDAL VEIN, INTERNAL
The internal pudendal vein is a branch of the internal iliac vein that accompanies the internal pudendal artery as a single or double vessel. It drains the perineum.

SYNONYM: *Vena Pudenda Interna* (NA).

RECTAL VEINS, INFERIOR
The inferior rectal veins are veins that pass to the internal pudendal vein from the venous plexus around the anal canal.

SYNONYMS: *Inferior Hemorrhoidal Veins, Venae Rectales Inferiores* (NA).

RECTAL VEINS, MIDDLE
The middle rectal veins are veins that pass from the rectal venous plexus to the internal iliac vein.

SYNONYMS: *Middle Hemorrhoidal Veins, Venae Rectales Mediae* (NA).

RECTAL VEIN, SUPERIOR

The superior rectal vein drains the greater part of the rectal venous plexus. It ascends between the layers of mesorectum to the brim of the pelvis, where it becomes the inferior mesenteric vein.

SYNONYMS: *Superior Hemorrhoidal Vein, Vena Rectalis Superior* (NA).

SACRAL VEINS, LATERAL

The lateral sacral veins are veins that accompany the corresponding arteries. They empty into the internal iliac vein on either side.

SYNONYM: *Venae Sacrales Laterales* (NA).

SACRAL VEIN, MIDDLE

The middle sacral vein is the vein accompanied by the middle sacral artery. It empties into the left common iliac vein.

SYNONYM: *Vena Sacralis Mediana* (NA).

SAPHENOUS VEIN, GREAT

The great saphenous vein is the longest vein in the body. It begins in the medial marginal vein of the dorsum of the foot and ends in the femoral vein about 3 cm below the inguinal ligament. It ascends in front of the tibial malleolus and along the medial side of the leg in relation with the saphenous nerve. The great saphenous vein runs upward behind the medial condyles of the tibia and femur, along the medial side of the thigh, and passing through the fossa ovalis, ends in the femoral vein. At the ankle, it receives branches from the sole of the foot through the medial marginal vein; in the leg, it anastomoses freely with the small saphenous vein, communicates with the anterior and posterior tibial veins, and receives many cutaneous veins. In the thigh, it communicates with the femoral vein and receives numerous tributaries. The tributaries from the medial and posterior parts of the thigh frequently unite to form a large *accessory saphenous vein,* which joins the main vein at a variable level. Near the fossa ovalis, it is joined by the superficial external pudendal veins. The *thoracoepigastric vein* runs along the lateral aspect of the trunk between the superficial epigastric vein and the lateral thoracic vein and establishes an important communication between the femoral and axillary veins.

SYNONYM: *Vena Saphena Magna* (NA).

SUBCLAVIAN VEIN

The subclavian vein is a continuation of the axillary vein. It extends from the outer border of the first rib to the sternal end of the clavicle.

SYNONYM: *Vena Subclavia* (NA).

THORACIC VEINS, INTERNAL

The internal thoracic veins accompany the lower half of the internal thoracic arteries.

SYNONYMS: *Internal Mammary Veins, Vena Mammaria Interna* (sing.),
Venae Thoracicae Internae (NA).

THORACIC VEIN, LATERAL

The lateral thoracic vein is a tributary of the axillary vein. It drains the lateral thoracic wall.

SYNONYMS: *Long Thoracic Vein, Vena Thoracica Lateralis* (NA).

UTERINE VEINS

The uterine veins are one or more veins that arise from the uterine plexus, pass through a part of the broad ligament and peritoneal fold, and empty into the internal iliac vein. These veins have no valves, frequently resulting in varicosities, especially in multiparas.

SYNONYM: *Venae Uterinae* (NA).

UTERINE VENULES

The uterine venules are venous channels of the endometrium that drain the surface epithelium and capillary networks.

VENA CAVA, INFERIOR

The inferior vena cava is a vein that receives blood from the lower extremities, the greater part of the pelvis, and the abdominal organs. It begins at the level of the fifth lumbar vertebra on the right side, pierces the diaphragm, passes through the anterior mediastinum, and empties into the posterior surface of the right atrium of the heart.

SYNONYM: *Vena Cava Inferior* (NA).

VENA CAVA, SUPERIOR

The superior vena cava is the venous trunk for the head, neck, upper extremities, and chest. It begins at the union of the two brachiocephalic veins, passes directly downward, and empties into the right atrium of the heart.

SYNONYM: *Vena Cava Superior* (NA).

VESICAL VEINS

The vesical veins drain the vesical plexus and follow the course of the vesical arteries. They terminate in the internal iliac veins.

SYNONYM: *Venae Vesicales* (NA).

Lymphatic Vessels

LYMPHATIC VESSELS

The lymphatic vessels are vessels that convey lymph. There are two types: the afferent and efferent.

SYNONYM: *Vasa Lymphatica* (NA).

LYMPHATIC VESSELS OF BLADDER

The lymphatic vessels of the bladder originate in two plexuses—intramuscular and extramuscular—for it is generally acknowledged that the mucous membrane is devoid of lymphatic vessels. The efferent vessels are arranged in two groups, one from the anterior and another from the posterior surface of the bladder. The vessels from the anterior surface pass to the external iliac lymph nodes. The vessels from the posterior surface pass to the internal, external, and common iliac lymph nodes; those draining the upper part of this surface traverse the lateral vesical lymph nodes.

LYMPHATIC VESSELS OF BREAST

The lymphatic vessels of the breast are separated into two planes—the superficial or subareolar plexus of lymphatic vessels and the deep or fascial plexus. Both originate in the interlobular spaces and in the walls of the mammary ducts. The superficial plexus collects lymph from the central parts of the gland, the skin, areola, and nipple, and it drains laterally toward the axilla. The drainage passes to the central axillary lymph nodes. From there, the drainage is to the subclavian lymph nodes at the apex of the axilla, where the axillary and subclavian veins join. The deep fascial plexus extends through the pectoral muscles to Rotter's nodes, and then to the subclavian lymph nodes. This is known as *Groszman's pathway*. The rest of the fascial plexus, for the most part, extends medially along the internal thoracic artery via the internal mammary lymph nodes to the anterior mediastinal lymph nodes. Other paths of lymphatic drainage proceed from the lower and medial portion of the breast. One of these is the paramammary route of Gerota, through the lymphatic vessels of the abdomen to the liver or subdiaphragmatic lymph nodes. Another is a cross-mammary pathway, via superficial lymphatic vessels to the opposite breast and opposite axilla. From the lower medial portion of the gland some lymphatic vessels of the fascial group drain, passing beneath the sternum, to the anterior mediastinal lymph nodes situated in front of the aorta.

LYMPHATIC VESSELS OF FALLOPIAN TUBE
The lymphatic vessels of the fallopian tube pass partly with the lymphatic vessels of the ovary and partly with those of the uterus.

LYMPHATIC VESSELS OF OVARY
The lymphatic vessels of the ovary ascend with the ovarian artery to the lateral and preaortic lymph nodes.

LYMPHATIC VESSELS OF PERINEUM AND EXTERNAL GENITALIA
The lymphatic vessels of the perineum and external genitalia follow the course of the external pudendal vessels; they end in the superficial inguinal and subinguinal lymph nodes. The lymphatic vessels of the clitoris terminate partly in the deep subinguinal lymph nodes and partly in the external iliac lymph nodes.

LYMPHATIC VESSELS OF RECTUM
The lymphatic vessels of the rectum traverse the pararectal glands and pass to those in the sigmoid mesocolon; the efferents of the latter terminate in the preaortic lymph nodes around the origin of the inferior mesenteric artery.

LYMPHATIC VESSELS OF URETER
The lymphatic vessels of the ureter run in different directions. Those from its upper portion end partly in the efferent lymphatic vessels of the kidney and partly in the lateral aortic lymph nodes. The lymphatic vessels from the portion immediately above the brim of the lesser pelvis are drained into the common iliac lymph nodes. The vessels from the intrapelvic portion of the tube either join the efferents from the bladder or end in the internal iliac lymph nodes.

LYMPHATIC VESSELS OF URETHRA
The lymphatic vessels of the urethra pass to the internal iliac lymph nodes.

LYMPHATIC VESSELS OF UTERUS
The lymphatic vessels of the uterus consist of two sets, superficial and deep. The superficial vessels are situated beneath the peritoneum, and the deep vessels are situated in the substance of the organ. The lymphatic vessels of the cervix run in three directions: transversely to the external iliac lymph nodes, posterolaterally to the internal iliac lymph nodes, and dorsad to the common iliac lymph nodes. Most of the lymphatic vessels of the corpus and fundus of the uterus pass lateral in the broad ligaments, and continue up with the ovarian lymphatic vessels to the lateral and preaortic lymph nodes. A few lymphatic vessels run to the external iliac lymph nodes, and one or two to the superficial inguinal lymph nodes. In the nongravid uterus, the lymphatic vessels are very small, but during gestation they are greatly enlarged.

LYMPHATIC VESSELS OF VAGINA

The lymphatic vessels of the vagina are carried in three directions: those of the upper part of the vagina to the external iliac lymph nodes, those of the middle part to the internal iliac lymph nodes, and those of the lower part to the common iliac lymph nodes. Small nodes are situated along the course of the vessels from the middle and lower parts. Some lymphatic vessels from the lower part of the vagina join those of the vulva and pass to the superficial inguinal lymph nodes. The lymphatic vessels of the vagina anastomose with those of the cervix, vulva, and rectum, but not with those of the bladder.

Lymph Nodes

LYMPH NODE

A lymph node is one of numerous round or oval nodules located along the course of lymphatic vessels. They vary greatly in size (1 to 25 mm in diameter). On one side, blood vessels enter and efferent lymphatic vessels emerge. Afferent lymphatic vessels enter a lymph node at many points on its periphery.

SYNONYM: *Nodus Lymphaticus* (NA).

AXILLARY LYMPH NODES, ANTERIOR

The anterior axillary lymph nodes are from four to six in number and lie along the border of the pectoralis minor muscles, adjacent to the lateral thoracic artery.

SYNONYMS: *Pectoral Lymph Nodes, Nodi Lymphatici Pectorales* (NA).

AXILLARY LYMPH NODES, CENTRAL

The central axillary lymph nodes lie along the course of the axillary vein.

SYNONYMS: *Intermediate Axillary Lymph Nodes, Midaxillary Lymph Nodes, Nodi Lymphatici Centrales* (NA).

AXILLARY LYMPH NODES, MEDIAL

The medial axillary lymph nodes lie at the apex of the axilla, where the axillary and subclavian veins join.

SYNONYMS: *Subclavian Lymph Nodes, Nodi Lymphatici Apicales* (NA).

CLOQUET'S LYMPH NODE

Cloquet's lymph node is one of the deep inguinal lymph nodes situated in the lateral part of the femoral ring.

SYNONYM: *Rosenmüller's Node.*

EPIGASTRIC LYMPH NODES

The epigastric lymph nodes are located along the side of the lower portion of the inferior epigastric vessels.

SYNONYM: *Nodi Lymphatici Epigastrici* (NA).

ILIAC LYMPH NODES, COMMON

The common iliac lymph nodes are situated along the course of the common iliac artery and drain the internal and external iliac lymph nodes. Their efferents pass to the lateral aortic lymph nodes.

SYNONYM: *Nodi Lymphatici Iliaci Communes* (NA).

ILIAC LYMPH NODES, EXTERNAL

The external iliac lymph nodes are located along the course of the external iliac artery and vein. Their principal efferents are derived from the superficial inguinal and deep inguinal lymph nodes, the deep lymphatic vessels of the abdominal wall below the umbilicus, the adductor region of the thigh, and the lymphatic vessels from the clitoris, urethra, prostate, fundus of the bladder, cervix uteri, and upper part of the vagina.

SYNONYM: *Nodi Lymphatici Iliaci Externi* (NA).

ILIAC LYMPH NODES, INTERNAL

The internal iliac lymph nodes are situated along the course and branches of the internal iliac artery and vein. They receive lymphatic vessels from all the pelvic viscera, the deeper parts of the perineum, buttock, and back of the thigh.

SYNONYMS: *Hypogastric Lymph Nodes, Nodi Lymphatici Iliaci Interni* (NA).

INGUINAL LYMPH NODES, DEEP

The deep inguinal lymph nodes are located under the fascia lata on the medial side of the femoral vein. They receive the deep lymphatic afferent trunks, the lymphatic vessels from the clitoris, and also some of the efferents from the superficial inguinal lymph nodes. They accompany the femoral vessels.

SYNONYM: *Nodi Lymphatici Inguinales Profundi* (NA).

INGUINAL LYMPH NODES, SUPERFICIAL

The superficial inguinal lymph nodes form a chain immediately below the inguinal ligament. They receive the afferent lymphatic vessels from the integument of the perineum, buttocks, and abdominal wall below the level of the umbilicus. The superficial inguinal lymph nodes are arbitrarily divided into a superior and inferior group by a horizontal line drawn through the middle of the fossa ovalis.

SYNONYM: *Nodi Lymphatici Inguinales Superficiales* (NA).

LUMBAR LYMPH NODES

The lumbar lymph nodes are numerous and consist of the right and left lateral aortic, preaortic, and retroaortic groups.

SYNONYMS: *Periaortic Lymph Nodes, Nodi Lymphatici Lumbales* (NA).

Lateral Aortic Lymph Nodes, Left

The left lateral aortic lymph nodes form a chain on the left side of the abdominal aorta in front of the origin of the psoas major muscle and the left crus of the diaphragm. The lymph nodes on either side receive the efferents of the common iliac lymph nodes; the lymphatic vessels from the ovary, fallopian tube, and body of the uterus; the lymphatic vessels from the kidney and adrenal lymph nodes; and the lymphatic vessels draining the lateral abdominal muscles and the accompanying lumbar veins. Most of the efferent

vessels to the lateral aortic lymph nodes converge to form the right
and left lumbar trunks, which join the cisterna chyli. Some efferent
vessels enter the preaortic and retroaortic lymph nodes, and others
pierce the crura of the diaphragm to drain the lower end of the
thoracic duct.

SYNONYM: *Paraaortic Lymph Nodes, Left.*

Lateral Aortic Lymph Nodes, Right

The right lateral aortic lymph nodes are situated partly in front
of the inferior vena cava, near the termination of the renal vein and
partly behind it on the origin of the psoas major muscle, and on
the right crus of the diaphragm.

SYNONYM: *Paraaortic Lymph Nodes, Right.*

Preaortic Lymph Nodes

The preaortic lymph nodes lie in front of the aorta, and are
divided into celiac, superior mesenteric, and inferior mesenteric
groups, arranged around the origins of the corresponding arteries.
They receive a few vessels from the lateral aortic lymph nodes, but
their principal efferents are derived from the viscera supplied by the
three arteries with which they are associated. Some of their efferents
pass to the retroaortic lymph nodes but most of them unite to form
the intestinal trunk, which enters the cisterna chyli.

Retroaortic Lymph Nodes

The retroaortic lymph nodes are situated below the cisterna chyli
on the bodies of the third and fourth lumbar vertebrae. They receive
lymphatic trunks from the lateral and preaortic lymph nodes; their
efferents end in the cisterna chyli.

MAMMARY LYMPH NODES, INTERNAL

The internal mammary lymph nodes are located at the anterior ends
of the intercostal spaces, by the side of the internal thoracic artery. They
derive afferents from the breast, from the deeper structures of the anterior
abdominal wall above the level of the umbilicus, from the upper surface
of the liver through a small group of lymph nodes that lie behind the
xiphoid process, and from the deeper parts of the anterior portion of the
thoracic wall. Their efferents usually unite to form a single trunk on
either side.

SYNONYMS: *Sternal Lymph Nodes, Nodi Lymphatici Parasternales*
(NA).

MEDIASTINAL LYMPH NODES, ANTERIOR

The anterior mediastinal lymph nodes are located in the superior
mediastinum, in relation to the great vessels. These nodes receive lymph
from the thymus, the pericardium, and the internal mammary lymph
nodes. Their efferent vessels join those of the tracheal lymph nodes to
form the bronchomediastinal trunks.

SYNONYM: *Nodi Lymphatici Mediastinales Anteriores* (NA).

NODE OF BIFURCATION

The node of bifurcation is a lymph node at the bifurcation of the right common iliac artery.

OBTURATOR LYMPH NODE

The obturator lymph node is sometimes found in the upper part of the obturator foramen.

ROTTER'S NODES

Rotter's nodes are lymph nodes situated beneath the pectoralis major muscle.

SACRAL LYMPH NODES

The sacral lymph nodes are placed in the concavity of the sacrum in relation to the middle and lateral sacral arteries. These lymph nodes receive lymphatic vessels from the rectum and posterior wall of the pelvis.

SYNONYM: *Nodi Lymphatici Sacrales* (NA).

Glands

GLAND

A gland is a secreting organ. The secretion may be poured out on a surface or into a cavity, or it may be secreted into the blood without appearing externally. The substance may contain enzymes or hormones, serve as a lubricant, or be purely excrementitious, removing waste and toxic material from the body.

SYNONYM: *Glandula* (NA).

ACCESSORY GLAND

An accessory gland is a small mass of glandular tissue detached from, but situated near, another gland.

ADRENAL GLAND

The adrenal gland is a flattened, roughly triangular gland situated on the upper pole of each kidney. It is a ductless gland that produces internal secretions: epinephrine and cortical steroid hormones.

SYNONYMS: *Suprarenal Gland, Glandula Suprarenalis* (NA).

Adrenal Cortex

The adrenal cortex is the cortical portion (outer layer) of the adrenal gland. It produces several steroid hormones, including hydrocortisone, corticosterone, and aldosterone.

SYNONYM: *Cortex* (NA).

ADRENAL GLAND, ACCESSORY

The accessory adrenal gland is one of several isolated masses of adrenal tissue sometimes found near the main gland.

SYNONYMS: *Accessory Suprarenal Gland, Glandula Suprarenalis Accessoria* (NA).

AREOLAR GLAND

The areolar gland is one of several cutaneous glands forming small, rounded projections from the surface of the areola of the breast.

SYNONYMS: *Montgomery's Gland, Glandulae Areolares* (NA).

BREAST

The breast is a modified sweat gland. Its size varies, but in most instances it extends from the second to the sixth rib and from the sternum to the anterior axillary line, with an axillary tail in the upper outer portion. The mammary tissue lies directly over the pectoralis major muscle and is separated from its outer fascia by a layer of adipose tissue. This layer is continuous with the fatty stroma of the gland itself. The breast is composed of the stroma and the parenchyma. The physiology of the breast is greatly affected by secretion of the anterior pituitary and by secretions from the follicles and corpus luteum of the ovary. Follicle-stimulating hormone (FSH), acting on the ovary, stimulates follicular growth and estrogen output, which in turn stimulates the growth of mammary ducts and periductal stroma. After ovulation, luteinizing hormone (LH) stimulates the formation of the corpus luteum and output of progesterone, which then stimulates the growth of the mammary lobules. The lactogenic hormone of the anterior pituitary acts directly on the mammary gland to initiate lactation. Once initiated, lactation is stimulated and maintained by the act of suckling through the *milk-ejection reflex,* which is mediated by oxytocin. During lactation, follicular ripening and ovulation are suppressed. Conversely, large doses of estrogen tend to inhibit breast secretion.

> SYNONYMS: *Mammary Gland, Mamma* (NA), *Glandula Mammaria* (NA).

CERVICAL GLAND

The cervical gland is a branched mucus-secreting gland of the cervical mucosa.

> SYNONYM: *Glandula Cervicales Uteri* (NA).

CIRCUMANAL GLAND

The circumanal gland is one of the large apocrine sweat glands surrounding the anus.

> SYNONYM: *Glandula Circumanalis* (NA).

ENDOCRINE GLANDS

The endocrine glands are ductless glands. These glands secrete hormones, which influence metabolism and other body processes.

> SYNONYMS: *Endocrinous Glands, Ductless Glands, Glandulae Sine Ductibus* (NA).

ENDOMETRIAL GLANDS

The endometrial glands are the secretory structures of the endometrium. In the immediate postmenstrual phase, they are straight, narrow, and collapsed. In the proliferative phase, they begin to grow. The epithelial cells of the glands are of the low columnar type. There is no evidence of secretory activity. During the secretory phase, the glands are larger and longer. The epithelial cells of the glands are secretory. Vacuolization occurs beneath the nuclei of these cells, pushing the nuclei to the mid-portion of the cells. Later in the same phase, vacuoles disappear and nuclei recede to the basal membrane. In the premenstrual phase, the epithelial cells of the glands are of the low columnar type and possess frayed edges. The glands are wide, tortuous, and filled with secretory material. The glands metabolize glucose and store glycogen in increasing amounts. The maximum storage and metabolism of glycogen occurs from the 17th to the 19th day of the cycle. This is followed by regression.

> SYNONYMS: *Uterine Glands, Glandulae Uterinae* (NA).

PANCREAS

The pancreas is a compound racemose gland 12.5 to 15 cm in length and weighing approximately 85 gm in the female and 90 gm in the male. The gland is composed of a broad portion designated as the head, and a main portion called the body, both being connected by a slight constriction, the neck. The gland is situated transversely across the posterior wall of the abdomen in the epigastric and left hypochondriac regions. The pancreas is both an external (exocrine) and internal (endocrine) structure, the former portion secreting several enyzmes that aid in the digestion of protein, carbohydrates, and fats; the latter portion consists of the islands of Langerhans, which produce insulin. Insulin is taken up by the bloodstream and is an important factor in the control of sugar metabolism in the body.

SYNONYM: *Pancreas* (NA).

PARATHYROID GLAND

The parathyroid gland is one of two such small paired endocrine glands, superior and inferior. They are usually situated in the connective tissue capsule on the posterior surface of the thyroid gland. They control the metabolism of calcium and phosphorus and secrete parathyroid hormone.

SYNONYM: *Glandula Parathyroidea* (NA).

PARAURETHRAL GLANDS

The paraurethral glands are relatively large glands situated just posterior and lateral to the urethral orifice.

SYNONYM: *Skene's Glands.*

PITUITARY GLAND

The pituitary gland is an endocrine gland situated in the sella turcica at the base of the brain. The gland is formed embryologically from two ectodermal rudiments—the dorsal diverticulum (Rathke's pouch) from the root of the buccal cavity and a ventral outgrowth from the base of the infundibulum of the diencephalon. The gland is composed of the anterior pituitary gland and the posterior pituitary gland.

SYNONYMS: *Hypophysis* (NA), *Glandula Pituitaria* (NA).

Anterior Pituitary

The anterior pituitary gland is the portion situated anteriorly in the sella turcica and comprises three regions: the pars infundibularis, pars intermedia, and pars distalis.

SYNONYMS: *Adenohypophysis* (NA), *Lobus Anterior* (NA).

PARS DISTALIS

The pars distalis is the portion of the anterior pituitary gland commonly known as the anterior lobe. The function of this portion depends on the hormonal factors passed to it from the hypothalamus through the portal vessels. The pars distalis secretes the gonadotropins, thyroid-stimulating hormone, and adrenocorticotropic hormone.

SYNONYM: *Pars Distalis* (NA).

PARS INTERMEDIA

The pars intermedia is a portion of the anterior pituitary gland that secretes melanocyte-stimulating hormone (MSH), which influences cutaneous pigmentation.

SYNONYM: *Pars Intermedia* (NA).

PARS INFUNDIBULARIS

The pars infundibularis is a portion of the anterior pituitary gland that is composed of a thin sheet of glandular and vascular tissue projecting along the infundibular stem.

SYNONYMS: *Pars Tuberalis, Pars Infundibularis* (NA).

Posterior Pituitary

The posterior pituitary gland is the portion that is situated posteriorly in the sella turcica and comprises three regions: median eminence of the tuber cinereum, relatively slender infundibular stem, and an enlarged infundibular process. The posterior pituitary plays a role in parturition, lactation, and control of water excretion by storing and liberating oxytocin and antidiuretic hormone.

SYNONYMS: *Neurohypophysis* (NA), *Lobus Posterior* (NA).

SEBACEOUS GLANDS, VULVAR

The vulvar sebaceous glands are composed of several saccular pouches surrounded by a connective tissue sheath in the dermis. The glands contain large polygonal nucleated cells. They open freely on the surfaces of the labia minora.

SUDORIFEROUS GLANDS, VULVAR

The vulvar sudoriferous glands are coiled glands that secrete fluid onto the surface of the vulva. There are two types: apocrine glands and eccrine glands.

SYNONYM: *Sweat Glands of Vulva.*

Apocrine Glands, Vulvar

The vulvar apocrine glands secrete an odorous fluid and are related to the hair follicles on the mons pubis, labia majora, and perineum. Their cells contribute part of their protoplasmic substance to secretion.

SYNONYM: *Large Coiled Sweat Glands of Vulva.*

Eccrine Glands, Vulvar

The vulvar eccrine glands consist of modified tubular glands that secrete a fluid on the surface of the vulva except on the mucocutaneous surfaces.

SYNONYM: *Small Coiled Sweat Glands of Vulva.*

THYROID GLAND

The thyroid gland is a ductless gland situated in front and to the sides of the upper part of the trachea. It has two lateral lobes joined by a narrow central portion, the isthmus. The blood supply comes from branches of the external carotid and subclavian arteries. The nerve supply is derived from the middle and inferior cervical ganglia of the sympathetic nervous system. The thyroid secretes the hormones thyroxin and triiodothyronine.

SYNONYM: *Glandula Thyroidea* (NA).

THYROID GLAND, ACCESSORY

The accessory thyroid gland is an isolated mass of thyroid tissue sometimes present in the side of the neck, just above the hyoid bone, or even as low as the aortic arch.

SYNONYM: *Glandula Thyroidea Accessoria* (NA).

URETHRAL GLANDS

The urethral glands are many small glands that open into the urethra. In the female, the largest of these glands are called the paraurethral glands.

SYNONYMS: *Morgagni's Gland, Littre's Gland, Glandulae Urethrales* (NA).

VAGINAL GLAND

The vaginal gland is one of the minute glands in the mucous membrane of the vagina. Vaginal glands are not true glands.

VESICAL GLAND

The vesical gland is one of several mucous follicles in the mucous membrane near the neck of the bladder. It is not a true gland.

SYNONYM: *Glandula Vesicalis.*

VESTIBULAR GLAND, MAJOR

The major vestibular gland is a racemose gland situated deep beneath the fascia of each labium major. The orifice of each gland is located at the middle of the lateral margin of the vaginal orifice. The main duct is lined by stratified transitional epithelium. The acini of the glands are lined by mucus-secreting epithelium.

SYNONYMS: *Bartholin's Gland, Duverney's Gland, Vulvovaginal Gland, Glandula Vestibularis Major* (NA).

VESTIBULAR GLAND, MINOR

The minor vestibular gland is one of the minute mucus-secreting glands on the surface of the vestibule.

SYNONYM: *Glandulae Vestibulares Minores* (NA).

Joints

JOINT

The joint is the place of union, usually more or less movable, between two or more bones.

SYNONYM: *Articulatio* (NA).

PUBIC SYMPHYSIS

The pubic symphysis is an articulation between the pubic bones. It is an amphiarthrodial joint formed between the two oval articular surfaces of the bones. The connective tissue supports of this articulation are the superior pubic and arcuate pubic ligaments and the interpubic fibrocartilaginous lamina.

SYNONYMS: *Symphysis Pubis, Pubic Joint, Articulation of the Pubic Bones, Symphysis Pubica* (NA).

SACROCOCCYGEAL FIBROCARTILAGE

The sacrococcygeal fibrocartilage is interposed between the contiguous surfaces of the sacrum and coccyx. It is thinner than the fibrocartilage between the bodies of the vertebrae, and its central part is firmer. It is somewhat thicker in front and behind than at the sides. Occasionally, the coccyx is freely movable on the sacrum, most notably during pregnancy. In such cases, a synovial membrane is present.

SACROCOCCYGEAL JOINT

The sacrococcygeal joint is an amphiarthrodial joint formed between the oval surface of the apex of the sacrum and the base of the coccyx. It is homologous with the joints between the bodies of the vertebrae and is connected by similar ligaments. These ligaments are the anterior sacrococcygeal, posterior sacrococcygeal, and lateral sacrococcygeal ligaments, and an interarticular ligament.

SYNONYMS: *Articulation of the Sacrum and Coccyx, Junctura Sacrococcygea* (NA).

SACROILIAC ARTICULATION

The sacroiliac articulation is an amphiarthrodial joint formed between the articular surfaces of the sacrum and the ilium. The articular surface of each bone is covered with a thin plate of cartilage, thicker on the sacrum than on the ilium. These cartilaginous plates are in close contact with each other and to a certain extent are united by irregular patches of softer fibrocartilage, and at their upper and posterior part by fine

39

interosseous fibers. In a considerable part of their extent, especially at advanced ages, they are separated by a space containing synovia-like fluid, and the joint presents the characteristics of diarthrosis. The ligaments of the joint are the anterior sacroiliac, posterior sacroiliac, and the interosseous.

SYNONYMS: *Sacroiliac Joint, Sacroiliac Synchondrosis, Articulatio Sacroiliaca* (NA).

Fossae

FOSSA
A fossa is a depression below the surface level of a part.
SYNONYM: *Fossa* (NA).

FOSSA OVALIS OF THIGH
The fossa ovalis of the thigh is an oval aperture in the fascia lata in the proximal part of the thigh, below the medial end of the inguinal ligament. The great saphenous vein passes through it just before it joins the femoral vein.
SYNONYMS: *Fossa Ovalis Femoris, Saphenous Opening, Hiatus Saphenus* (NA).

INGUINAL FOSSA, LATERAL
The lateral inguinal fossa is a depression in the peritoneal surface of the anterior abdominal wall, lateral to the ridge formed by the inferior epigastric artery. It corresponds to the position of the deep inguinal ring.
SYNONYM: *Fossa Inguinalis Lateralis* (NA).

INGUINAL FOSSA, MEDIAL
The medial inguinal fossa is a depression on the peritoneal surface of the anterior abdominal wall between the ridges formed by the inferior epigastric and the obliterated internal iliac arteries.
SYNONYM: *Fossa Inguinalis Medialis* (NA).

ISCHIORECTAL FOSSA
The ischiorectal fossa is somewhat prismatic, in the shape of a wedge, with its base at the perineum and its apex deep in the pelvis where the levator ani and obturator internus muscles come together.
SYNONYM: *Fossa Ischiorectalis* (NA).

NAVICULAR FOSSA OF VULVA
The navicular fossa of the vulva is a shallow depression between the hymen and frenulum of the labia minora.
SYNONYM: *Fossa Vestibuli Vaginae* (NA).

OVARIAN FOSSA
The ovarian fossa is a depression in the lateral wall of the pelvis occupied by the ovary. It is behind the broad ligament in the angle between the elevations produced by the diverging internal and external iliac arteries.
SYNONYM: *Claudius' Fossa.*

PARARECTAL FOSSA

The pararectal fossa is a depression on either side of the rectum formed by the reflection of the peritoneum to the posterior pelvic wall.

PARAVESICAL FOSSA

The paravesical fossa is a depression in the peritoneum on either side of the bladder.

SCARPA'S TRIANGLE

Scarpa's triangle is an anatomic area in the anterior aspect of the thigh bounded superiorly by the inguinal ligament, laterally by the sartorius muscle, and medially by the adductor longus muscle.

SYNONYMS: *Femoral Triangle, Trigonum Femorale* (NA).

SUPRAVESICAL FOSSA

The supravesical fossa is the depression on the peritoneal surface of the anterior abdominal wall between the median and medial umbilical folds.

SYNONYM: *Fossa Supravesicalis* (NA).

Ligaments

LIGAMENT

A ligament is a band or sheet of fibrous tissue connecting two or more bones, cartilages, or other structures, or serving as a support for fascia or muscles.

SYNONYM: *Ligamentum* (NA).

ANOCOCCYGEAL LIGAMENT

The anococcygeal ligament is a musculofibrous band passing from the anus to the coccyx.

SYNONYM: *Ligamentum Anococcygeum* (NA).

ARCUATE PUBIC LIGAMENT

The arcuate pubic ligament is a thick, triangular arch of ligamentous fibers connecting the two pubic bones below and forming the upper boundary of the pubic arch. Above, it is blended with the interpubic fibrocartilaginous lamina; laterally, it is attached to the inferior rami of the pubic bones; below, it is free and separated from the fascia of the urogenital diaphragm.

SYNONYMS: *Inferior Pubic Ligament, Subpubic Ligament, Ligamentum Arcuatum Pubis* (NA).

ARTERIAL LIGAMENT

The arterial ligament is a short, thick, strong fibromuscular cord that extends from the pulmonary artery to the arch of the aorta. It is the remains of the ductus arteriosus.

SYNONYM: *Ligamentum Arteriosum* (NA).

BROAD LIGAMENT

The broad ligament is one of two thin fibrous sheets, covered on both surfaces with peritoneum, that extends from each side of the uterus to the lateral wall of the pelvis. It is thicker at its inferior pelvic attachment than toward its free border.

SYNONYM: *Ligamentum Latum Uteri* (NA).

Mesometrium

The mesometrium is the portion of the broad ligament below the mesovarium.

SYNONYM: *Mesometrium* (NA).

43

Mesosalpinx
The mesosalpinx consists of the layers of the broad ligament above the mesovarium that enclose the fallopian tube.

SYNONYM: *Mesosalpinx* (NA).

Mesovarium
The mesovarium is a short peritoneal fold connecting the anterior border of the ovary with the posterior layer of the broad ligament.

SYNONYM: *Mesovarium* (NA).

CARDINAL LIGAMENT
The cardinal ligament is a fibrous sheet of subserous fascia imbedded in the adipose tissue on each side of the lower cervix uteri and vagina. The cardinal ligament extends across the pelvic floor as a deeper continuation of the broad ligament.

SYNONYMS: *Mackenrodt's Ligament, Ligamentum Transversalis Colli, Cervical Ligament of the Uterus.*

ILIOLUMBAR LIGAMENT
The iliolumbar ligament is attached above to the lower front part of the transverse process of the fifth lumbar vertebra. It radiates as it passes laterally and is attached by two main bands to the pelvis. The lower band runs to the base of the sacrum, blending with the anterior sacroiliac ligament. The upper band is attached to the crest of the ilium, immediately in front of the sacroiliac articulation, and is continuous above with the lumbodorsal fascia. In front, it is in relation with the psoas major muscle; behind, with the muscles occupying the vertebral groove; above, with the quadratus lumborum.

SYNONYM: *Ligamentum Iliolumbale* (NA).

INGUINAL LIGAMENT
The inguinal ligament is a fibrous band extending from the anterior superior iliac spine to the pubic tubercle.

SYNONYMS: *Poupart's Ligament, Ligamentum Inguinale* (NA).

LATERAL FALSE LIGAMENT
The lateral false ligament consists of peritoneal folds extending between the sides of the bladder and the lateral walls of the pelvic cavity.

MIDDLE UMBILICAL LIGAMENT
The middle umbilical ligament is a fibrous cord extending from the apex of the bladder to the umbilicus. It represents the remnants of the urachus.

SYNONYM: *Ligamentum Umbilicale Medianum* (NA).

OVARIAN LIGAMENT
The ovarian ligament is a cord containing some nonstriped muscular fibers. It lies within the broad ligament and extends from the lower pole of the ovary to the uterus below the attachment of the fallopian tube.

SYNONYM: *Ligamentum Ovarii Proprium* (NA).

POSTERIOR FALSE LIGAMENT

The posterior false ligament contains the obliterated internal iliac arteries, ureters, vessels, and nerves passing to the bladder.

SYNONYMS: *Uterovesical Ligament, Uterovesical Plica, Sacrogenital Fold.*

PUBOVESICAL LIGAMENTS

The pubovesical ligaments are a condensation of the connective tissue that extends from the lower part of the anterior wall of the bladder and upper urethra, through the space of Retzius, to the posterior surface of the pubic bones at the sides of the pubic symphysis.

SYNONYM: *Ligamentum Pubovesicale* (NA).

RECTOVESICAL LIGAMENTS

The rectovesical ligaments are condensations of subserous fascia underlying the posterior false ligaments. They secure the base of the bladder posteriorly to the sides of the rectum and the sacrum.

ROUND LIGAMENTS OF UTERUS

The round ligaments of the uterus are fibromuscular bands that extend from the superior lateral surface of the uterus downward, laterally, and forward through the inguinal canal to terminate in the labia majora.

SYNONYM: *Ligamentum Teres Uteri* (NA).

SACROCOCCYGEAL LIGAMENT, ANTERIOR

The anterior sacrococcygeal ligament consists of a few irregular fibers that descend from the anterior surface of the sacrum to the front of the coccyx, blending with the periosteum.

SYNONYM: *Ligamentum Sacrococcygeum Ventrale* (NA).

SACROCOCCYGEAL LIGAMENT, LATERAL

The lateral sacrococcygeal ligament exists on either side of and connects the transverse process of the coccyx to the lower lateral angle of the sacrum. It completes the foramen for the fifth sacral nerve.

SYNONYMS: *Intertransverse Ligament, Ligamentum Sacrococcygeum Laterale* (NA).

SACROCOCCYGEAL LIGAMENT, POSTERIOR

The posterior sacrococcygeal ligament is a flat band that arises from the margin of the lower orifice of the sacral canal and descends to be inserted into the posterior surface of the coccyx. This ligament completes the lower and back part of the sacral canal and is divisible into a short deep portion and a longer superficial part. It is in relation, behind, with the gluteus maximus muscle.

SACROILIAC LIGAMENTS, ANTERIOR

The anterior sacroiliac ligaments consist of numerous thin bands that connect the anterior surface of the lateral part of the sacrum to the margin of the auricular surface of the ilium and to the preauricular sulcus.

SYNONYM: *Ligamenta Sacroiliaca Ventralia* (NA).

SACROILIAC LIGAMENT, INTEROSSEOUS

The interosseous sacroiliac ligament lies deep to the posterior ligament and consists of a series of short, strong fibers connecting the tuberosities of the sacrum and the ilium.

SYNONYM: *Ligamenta Sacroiliaca Interossea* (NA).

SACROILIAC LIGAMENT, POSTERIOR

The posterior sacroiliac ligament is situated in a deep depression between the sacrum and ilium behind. It is strong and forms the chief bond of union between the bones. It consists of numerous fasciculi, which pass between the bones in various directions. The upper part (short posterior sacroiliac ligament) is nearly horizontal and passes from the first and second transverse tubercles on the back of the sacrum to the tuberosity of the ilium. The lower part (long posterior sacroiliac ligament) is oblique. It is attached by one extremity to the third transverse tubercle of the back of the sacrum and by the other to the posterior superior spine of the ilium.

SYNONYM: *Ligamenta Sacroiliaca Dorsalia* (NA).

SACROSPINOUS LIGAMENT

The sacrospinous ligament is thin and triangular. It is attached by its apex to the spine of the ischium, and medially by its broad base, to the lateral margins of the sacrum and coccyx.

SYNONYMS: *Anterior Sacrosciatic Ligament, Ligamentum Sacrospinale* (NA).

SACROTUBEROUS LIGAMENT

The sacrotuberous ligament is situated at the lower and dorsal part of the pelvis. It is flat and triangular, narrower in the middle than at the ends. It is attached by its broad base to the posterior inferior spine of the ilium, to the fourth and fifth transverse tubercles of the sacrum, and to the lower part of the lateral margin of the sacrum and the coccyx. Passing obliquely downward, forward, and laterad, it becomes narrow and thick. At its insertion into the inner margin of the tuberosity of the ischium, the sacrotuberous ligament increases in breadth and extends forward along the inner margin of the ramus as the falciform process, the free concave edge of which gives attachment to the obturator fascia. One surface is turned toward the perineum, the other toward the obturator internus muscle. The lower border of the ligament is directly continuous with the tendon of origin of the long head of the biceps femoris and is believed to be the proximal end of this tendon.

SYNONYMS: *Posterior Sacrosciatic Ligament, Ligamentum Sacrotuberale* (NA).

SUPERIOR PUBIC LIGAMENT
The superior pubic ligament connects the two pubic bones superiorly, extending laterally as far as the pubic tubercles.

SYNONYM: *Ligamentum Pubicum Superius* (NA).

SUSPENSORY LIGAMENTS OF BREAST
The suspensory ligaments of the breast consist of fibrous bands that secure the skin of the breast to the deep layer of the superficial fascia.

SYNONYMS: *Cooper's Suspensory Ligaments, Ligamenta Suspensoria Mammae* (NA).

SUSPENSORY LIGAMENT OF CLITORIS
The suspensory ligament of the clitoris is a fibrous band extending from the pubic symphysis to the clitoris.

SYNONYM: *Ligamentum Suspensorium Clitoridis* (NA).

SUSPENSORY LIGAMENT OF OVARY
The suspensory ligament of the ovary is a fold of peritoneum, attached to the tubal extremity of the ovary, that extends upward over the iliac vessels and contains the ovarian vessels.

SYNONYMS: *Infundibulopelvic Ligament, Ligamentum Suspensorium Ovarii* (NA).

TRANSVERSE LIGAMENT OF PELVIS
The transverse ligament of the pelvis consists of fibers crossing the perineum from one ischial tuberosity to the other.

SYNONYM: *Ligamentum Transversum Perinei* (NA).

UTEROSACRAL LIGAMENT
The uterosacral ligament is a prominent fibrous band of subserous fascia that takes a curved course along the lateral wall of the pelvis from the cervix uteri to the sacrum. It is a posterior continuation of the tissue that forms the cardinal ligament. It is attached to the deep fascia and periosteum of the sacrum and contains the rectouterine muscle. The ligaments on the two sides project out from the wall as crescentic shelves that narrow the diameter of the cavity in front of the lower rectum and mark it off as the rectouterine pouch.

VENOSUS LIGAMENT
The venosus ligament is the obliterated ductus venosus passing through the liver to the vena cava.

SYNONYMS: *Ligamentum Ductus Venosi, Ligament of Arantius, Ligamentum Venosum* (NA).

SECTION 1: ANATOMY

Muscles

ABDOMINAL MUSCLE, EXTERNAL OBLIQUE
The external oblique abdominal muscle is a muscle arising from the costal cartilages of the lower eight ribs and inserting into the crest of the ilium and the linea alba.

SYNONYM: *Musculus Obliquus Externus Abdominis* (NA).

ABDOMINAL MUSCLE, INTERNAL OBLIQUE
The internal oblique abdominal muscle is a muscle arising from the inguinal ligament, iliac fascia, iliac crest, and lumbar aponeurosis. It inserts into the inferior borders of the cartilages of the lower three or four ribs and the linea alba.

SYNONYM: *Musculus Obliquus Internus Abdominis* (NA).

ABDOMINAL MUSCLE, TRANSVERSE
The transverse abdominal muscle is a muscle arising from the lower six costal cartilages, lumbodorsal fascia, iliac crest, and inguinal ligament. It inserts into the linea alba and conjoined tendon.

SYNONYM: *Musculus Transversus Abdominis* (NA).

ANAL SPHINCTER, EXTERNAL
The external anal sphincter is a flat, elliptical bundle of muscle fibers surrounding the lower margin of the anus. It arises from the anococcygeal body, encircles the terminal portion of the anal canal, and inserts into the perineal body. It normally closes the inferior aperture of the anus.

SYNONYM: *Musculus Sphincter Ani Externus* (NA).

ANAL SPHINCTER, INTERNAL
The internal anal sphincter is a ring of muscle composed chiefly of involuntary muscle fibers. It is situated superior to the external sphincter, and is contiguous to but not a part of it. It is a sphincter like its homologue.

SYNONYM: *Musculus Sphincter Ani Internus* (NA).

BULBOSPONGIOSUS MUSCLE
The bulbospongiosus muscle is a paired muscle, one on each side of the vagina. Its function in the female is to constrict the lumen of the vagina near the introitus, and to constrict the bulbous urethra (in both

sexes). In the female, some fibers terminate in the corpora cavernosa of the clitoris.

SYNONYMS: *Constrictor Cunni, Sphincter Vaginae, Bulbocavernosus Muscle, Musculus Bulbospongiosus* (NA).

COCCYGEUS MUSCLE

The coccygeus muscle is a paired muscle lying between the levator ani muscle anteriorly and the piriformis muscle posteriorly. It assists in closing the posterior portion of the pelvic outlet and is considered a part of the pelvic floor. It supports the coccyx.

SYNONYM: *Musculus Coccygeus* (NA).

CREMASTER MUSCLE

The cremaster muscle is a muscle arising from the internal oblique abdominal muscle and the inguinal ligament. It inserts into the round ligament of the uterus.

SYNONYM: *Musculus Cremaster* (NA).

DETRUSOR URINAE MUSCLE

The detrusor urinae muscle is the external longitudinal layer of the muscular coat of the bladder.

DIAPHRAGM, PELVIC

The pelvic diaphragm is the main support of the pelvic viscera. The obturator internus and the piriformis muscles are not strictly components of the pelvic diaphragm. They are mentioned here because the fascia of the obturator internus contributes much to the fascia of the pelvis, and because the piriformis muscle, posterior to the coccygeus, completes the posterior closure of the inferior aperture (outlet) of the pelvis. Each of these muscles originates in the true pelvis but becomes inserted into the lower extremity, outside the pelvic cavity. The levator ani muscle on each side is covered, both on its superior surface (superior levator fascia) and its inferior surface (anal fascia), by a layer of dense fascia, collectively termed *pelvic fascia* or *levator fascia*. These fascial layers, at each side of the pelvis, fuse with each other and with the fascia covering the inner surface of each obturator internus muscle. The ridge created by this triple fusion of several fascial layers has an unmistakable appearance. It extends downward and dorsad on each side to the ischial spines. It is referred to as the *arcus tendineous of the levatores ani,* or the *white line of fused fascia.* Slightly below and medial to the white line, the superior levator fascia thickens to form a ridge, or base, of fascia, the *tela endopelvina of the visceral fascia,* that divides into four layers. One layer invests the bladder; the second lies loosely between the lower uterine segment, upper portion of the vagina, and the bladder. The third layer lies between the vagina and the rectum, and the fourth is situated posterior to the rectum.

SYNONYM: *Diaphragma Pelvis* (NA).

DIAPHRAGM, UROGENITAL

The urogenital diaphragm is composed of two flat layers of thin fascia in the anterior urogenital triangle of the perineum on each side of the midline. Between the two layers are enclosed the structures of the deep compartment. The superficial compartment lies between the layer of fascia that is the floor of the deep compartment and the dense layer of the deep superficial fascia known as *Colles' fascia*. Thus the floor of the superficial (inferior) compartment is Colles' fascia. Its roof is the inferior layer of the fascia of the urogenital diaphragm, which is likewise the floor of the deep (superior) compartment. The roof of the superior compartment is contiguous to the inferior fascia of the levator ani muscle.

SYNONYMS: *Triangular Ligament, Urogenital Trigone, Diaphragma Urogenitale* (NA).

GEMELLUS MUSCLE, SUPERIOR

The superior gemellus muscle arises from the outer surface of the spine of the ischium. It blends with the upper part of the tendon of the obturator internus and is inserted with it into the medial surface of the greater trochanter.

SYNONYM: *Musculus Gemellus Superior* (NA).

ISCHIOCAVERNOSUS MUSCLE

The ischiocavernosus muscle is the erector muscle of the clitoris; it occupies the lateral portion of the superficial compartment of the urogenital diaphragm. Arising from the tuberosity and ramus of the ischium, it inserts into the sides and inferior surface of the crus of the clitoris.

SYNONYMS: *Erector Clitoridis, Musculus Ischiocavernosus* (NA).

LEVATOR ANI MUSCLE

The levator ani muscle is the main support of the pelvic floor and pelvic viscera. Mainly, it consists of the iliococcygeus portion and the pubococcygeus portion. With its superior and inferior layers of fascia, it is called the pelvic diaphragm.

SYNONYM: *Musculus Levator Ani* (NA).

Iliococcygeus Muscle

The iliococcygeus muscle of the levator ani is the lateral portion of the levator ani muscle. It arises from the white line of the tendinous arch of the obturator internus fascia. It inserts into the perineal body, the anococcygeal body, and into the margin of the coccyx.

SYNONYM: *Musculus Iliococcygeus* (NA).

Pubococcygeus Muscle

The pubococcygeus muscle of the levator ani is the medial portion of the levator ani muscle. It originates from the pubis on either side of the vagina and proceeds posteriorly. Some fibers mingle with longitudinal fibers of the vaginal wall and with the bulbospongiosus fibers. Others decussate in the perineal body; the main portion mingles somewhat with the external sphincter but mainly with the anococcygeal body posterior to the sphincter.

SYNONYM: *Musculus Pubococcygeus* (NA).

PECTORALIS MAJOR MUSCLE

The pectoralis major muscle is a thick fan-shaped muscle situated at the upper and forepart of the chest.

SYNONYM: *Musculus Pectoralis Major* (NA).

PECTORALIS MINOR MUSCLE

The pectoralis minor muscle is a thin triangular muscle situated at the upper part of the thorax beneath the pectoralis major muscle.

SYNONYM: *Musculus Pectoralis Minor* (NA).

PERINEAL BODY

The perineal body is the wedge-shaped composite of all the soft tissues that together compose the septum separating the vagina from the anus. It constitutes only a part of the perineum.

SYNONYMS: *Obstetric Perineum, Central Perineal Body, Central Tendon of the Perineum, Median Raphe, Centrum Tendineum Perinei* (NA).

PIRIFORMIS MUSCLE

The piriformis muscle is a flat, pyramidal muscle, lying almost parallel with the posterior margin of the gluteus medius. It is situated partly within the pelvis against its posterior wall and partly at the back of the hip joint.

SYNONYM: *Musculus Piriformis* (NA).

PSOAS MAJOR MUSCLE

The psoas major muscle is a long, fusiform muscle. It arises from the bodies of the vertebrae and intervertebral disks from the 12th thoracic to the fifth lumbar vertebra, and from the transverse processes of the lumbar vertebrae. It inserts into the lesser trochanter of the femur.

SYNONYM: *Musculus Psoas Major* (NA).

PUBORECTAL MUSCLE

The puborectal muscle is composed of fibers of the pubococcygeus muscle that mingle with the external anal sphincter and the anus.

SYNONYM: *Musculus Puborectalis* (NA).

PUBOVESICAL MUSCLE

The pubovesical muscle consists of a few smooth muscle fibers, by which the base of the bladder is attached to the internal investing layer of deep fascia on the pubic bone.

SYNONYM: *Musculus Pubovesicalis* (NA).

PYRAMIDALIS MUSCLE

The pyramidalis muscle is a muscle arising from the pubis and superior pubic ligament and inserting into the linea alba.

SYNONYM: *Musculus Pyramidalis* (NA).

RECTOCOCCYGEUS MUSCLE
The rectococcygeus muscle is one of two bands of muscular tissue arising from the coccyx and blending with the posterior longitudinal muscle of the posterior anal wall.

SYNONYM: *Musculus Rectococcygeus* (NA).

RECTOUTERINE MUSCLE
The rectouterine muscle is a nonstriped muscle in the rectouterine fold.

SYNONYM: *Musculus Rectouterinus* (NA).

RECTOVESICAL MUSCLE
The rectovesical muscle is composed of nonstriped muscle fibers in the sacrogenital folds that run from the bladder fundus to the sides of the rectum. Usually, it is absent in the female.

SYNONYM: *Musculus Rectovesicalis* (NA).

RECTUS ABDOMINIS MUSCLE
The rectus abdominis muscle is a muscle that arises from the pubic crest and pubic symphysis. It inserts into the xiphoid process and fifth to seventh costal cartilages.

SYNONYM: *Musculus Rectus Abdominis* (NA).

TRANSVERSE PERINEAL MUSCLE, DEEP
The deep transverse perineal muscle is a paired muscle. It lies in the deep compartment of the anterior triangle and sends a few fibers to the vaginal wall. Mainly, like its more superficial homologue, it maintains the integrity of the perineal body.

SYNONYM: *Musculus Transversus Perinei Profundus* (NA).

TRANSVERSE PERINEAL MUSCLE, SUPERFICIAL
The superficial transverse perineal muscle is a narrow, paired muscle in the superficial (inferior) compartment of the anterior triangle. It supports the perineal body.

SYNONYM: *Musculus Transversus Perinei Superficialis* (NA).

URETHRAL SPHINCTER MUSCLE
The urethral sphincter muscle is a delicate muscle located in the deep compartment of the anterior triangle. It acts as a compressor, or sphincter, of the urethra.

SYNONYMS: *Sphincter Urethrae Membranaceae, Constrictor Urethrae, Musculus Sphincter Urethrae* (NA).

LINES

LINE
A line is a long narrow mark, strip, or streak, distinguished in anatomy from the adjacent tissues by color, texture, or elevation.
SYNONYM: *Linea* (NA).

ARCUATE LINE
The arcuate line is the semicircular line marking the lower edge of the posterior sheath of the rectus abdominis muscle.
SYNONYMS: *Line of Douglas, Linea Arcuata* (NA).

BLACK LINE
The black line is the pigmented white line of the abdomen in a pregnant woman.
SYNONYM: *Linea Nigra.*

DENTATE LINE
The dentate line is a sinuous line following the level of the anal valves and crossing the bases of the columns between them. It marks the junction of the zone of the anal canal lined with stratified squamous epithelium and the zone lined with columnar epithelium.
SYNONYM: *Pectinate Line.*

ILIOPECTINEAL LINE
The iliopectineal line is the ridge on the pubis and ilium marking the brim of the true pelvis.
SYNONYMS: *Linea Innominata, Linea Terminalis* (NA).

LINEA ALBICANS
The linea albicans is a stretch line or streak of atrophy in the skin, resulting from stretching due to pregnancy, ascites, or tumor.
SYNONYM: *White Line.*

MILK LINE
The milk line is the embryonic line composed of ridges of thickened epithelium extending from the axillary to the inguinal region, along which the breasts will form.

NÉLATON'S LINE
Nélaton's line is a line drawn from the anterosuperior part of the ilium to the tuberosity of the ischium.

RAPHE

A raphe is a line or seam situated at the meeting point of sheets of fascia or skin.

SYNONYM: *Raphe* (NA).

WHITE LINE OF ABDOMEN

The white line of the abdomen is the name given to the portion of the anterior abdominal aponeurosis or rectus sheath in the middle line. It represents the insertion of the external oblique, internal oblique, and transverse abdominal muscles by the fusion of their aponeuroses with those of the opposite side. The three aponeuroses are fused into a single tendinous band that extends from the xiphoid process to the pubic symphysis.

SYNONYM: *Linea Alba* (NA).

WHITE LINE OF OBTURATOR INTERNUS FASCIA

The white line of obturator internus fascia is a thickened band of the obturator fascia attached posteriorly to the spine of the ischium and anteriorly to the pubic bone at the anterior margin of the obturator membrane.

SYNONYM: *Arcus Tendineus Musculi Levatoris Ani* (NA).

Nerves

NERVE
A nerve is a cordlike structure through which stimuli are transmitted from the central nervous system to the periphery, or the reverse.
SYNONYM: *Nervus* (NA).

Afferent Nerve
An afferent nerve conveys impulses from the periphery to the central nervous system.

Efferent Nerve
An efferent nerve conveys impulses from the central nervous system to the periphery.

ANOCOCCYGEAL NERVES
The anococcygeal nerves are several small nerves arising from the lower portion of the pudendal plexus (coccygeal plexus), supplying the posterior portion of the levator ani muscle and skin over the coccyx.
SYNONYM: *Nervi Anococcygei* (NA).

CLITORAL NERVE
The clitoral nerve originates from the pudendal nerve and is distributed to the skin, crura, and corpus cavernosum of the clitoris.
SYNONYMS: *Cavernous Nerve of the Clitoris, Nervi Cavernosi Clitoridis* (NA).

COCCYGEAL NERVE
The coccygeal nerve is a small nerve, the lowest of the spinal nerves, entering into the formation of the pudendal plexus.
SYNONYM: *Nervus Coccygeus* (NA).

DORSAL NERVE OF CLITORIS
The dorsal nerve of the clitoris is the deep terminal branch of the pudendal nerve supplying especially the glans clitoris.
SYNONYM: *Nervus Dorsalis Clitoridis* (NA).

FEMORAL CUTANEOUS NERVE, LATERAL
The lateral femoral cutaneous nerve arises from the second and third lumbar nerves, passes forward beneath the iliac fascia to the anterior superior spine, and extends a short distance down the front of the thigh, supplying the skin of this region and of the outer side of the buttock.
SYNONYM: *Nervus Cutaneus Femoris Lateralis* (NA).

FEMORAL CUTANEOUS NERVE, POSTERIOR

The posterior femoral cutaneous nerve arises from the first three sacral nerves, accompanies the sciatic nerve to the lower border of the gluteus maximus muscle, and then supplies the skin of the posterior surface of the thigh and of the popliteal region. It gives off a perineal branch that passes to the labia majora.

SYNONYMS: *Small Sciatic Nerve, Nervus Cutaneus Femoris Posterior* (NA).

FEMORAL NERVE

The femoral nerve arises from the second, third, and fourth lumbar nerves in the substance of the psoas major muscle, and passing down, enters the thigh lateral to the femoral vessels, breaking up in Scarpa's triangle into several terminal branches. It supplies the muscles and skin of the thigh.

SYNONYMS: *Anterior Crural Nerve, Nervus Femoralis* (NA).

GENITOFEMORAL NERVE

The genitofemoral nerve arises by two roots from the first and second lumbar nerves, passes downward with the iliac vessels, and divides above the inguinal ligament into genital and femoral branches.

SYNONYMS: *Genitocrural Nerve, Nervus Genitofemoralis* (NA).

GLUTEAL NERVE, INFERIOR

The inferior gluteal nerve arises from the fifth lumbar and first and second sacral nerves and supplies the gluteus maximus muscle.

SYNONYM: *Nervus Gluteus Inferior* (NA).

GLUTEAL NERVE, SUPERIOR

The superior gluteal nerve arises from the fourth and fifth lumbar and first sacral nerves and supplies the gluteus medius and minimus muscles.

SYNONYM: *Nervus Gluteus Superior* (NA).

HYPOGASTRIC NERVE

The hypogastric nerve is one of two nerve trunks, right and left, that lead from the superior hypogastric plexus into the pelvis to join the inferior hypogastric plexuses.

SYNONYM: *Nervus Hypogastricus* (NA).

ILIOHYPOGASTRIC NERVE

The iliohypogastric nerve arises from the first lumbar nerve, passes through the psoas major muscle, and then forward above the crest of the ilium. It penetrates the posterior part of the transverse abdominal muscle and divides into a lateral and an anterior cutaneous branch. It supplies the abdominal muscles and the skin of the lower part of the anterior abdominal wall.

SYNONYM: *Nervus Iliohypogastricus* (NA).

ILIOINGUINAL NERVE
The ilioinguinal nerve arises from the first lumbar nerve and supplies the muscles of the abdominal wall and skin of the mons pubis and labia majora.
SYNONYM: *Nervus Ilioinguinalis* (NA).

LABIAL NERVES, ANTERIOR
The anterior labial nerves are branches of the ilioinguinal nerve. They pierce the internal oblique muscle, distributing filaments to it. The anterior labial nerves are distributed to the skin over the upper and medial parts of the thigh, the mons pubis, and the labia majora.
SYNONYM: *Nervi Labiales Anteriores* (NA).

LABIAL NERVES, MEDIAL AND LATERAL POSTERIOR
The medial and lateral posterior labial nerves are the superficial branches of the perineal nerve. They pierce the fascia of the urogenital diaphragm and are distributed to the skin of the labia majora.
SYNONYMS: *Superficial Branches of the Perineal Nerves, Nervi Labiales Posteriores* (NA).

LUMBAR NERVES
The lumbar nerves consist of five nerves on each side, emerging from the lumbar portion of the spinal cord. The first four nerves enter into the formation of the lumbar plexus, the fourth and fifth into that of the sacral plexus. The fourth lumbar nerve, being forked to enter into the formation of the two plexuses, is called the *nervus furcalis.*
SYNONYM: *Nervi Lumbales* (NA).

LUMBOSACRAL TRUNK
The lumbosacral trunk is a large nerve formed by the union of the fifth lumbar and first sacral nerves with a branch from the fourth lumbar nerve. These enter into the formation of the sacral plexus.
SYNONYM: *Truncus Lumbosacralis* (NA).

NERVE SUPPLY OF BLADDER
The nerve supply of the bladder consists of sympathetic fibers originating from the first and second lumbar segments of the spinal cord, and parasympathetic fibers that arise from the second, third, and possibly fourth sacral segments. Efferent sympathetic fibers pass by way of the presacral nerve, dividing and passing through the hypogastric ganglia to reach the bladder near the entrance of the ureters.

OBTURATOR NERVE
The obturator nerve arises from the second, third, and fourth lumbar nerves by three roots in the psoas major muscle, passes downward and forward below the brim of the pelvis, and enters the thigh through the obturator foramen. It supplies muscles and skin on the medial side of the thigh.
SYNONYM: *Nervus Obturatorius* (NA).

PERINEAL NERVE
The perineal nerve is the larger and more superficial of the two terminal branches of the pudendal nerve. It accompanies the perineal artery and divides at the urogenital diaphragm into the superficial and deep branches.

SYNONYM: *Nervi Perineales* (NA).

PERINEAL NERVE, DEEP BRANCH
The deep branch of the perineal nerve supplies the superficial transverse perineal, the deep transverse perineal, bulbospongiosus, ischiocavernosus, and the urethral sphincter muscles.

PHRENIC NERVE
The phrenic nerve is a motor nerve arising from the third, fourth, and fifth cervical segments of the cord. It innervates the diaphragm.

SYNONYM: *Nervus Phrenicus* (NA).

PUDENDAL NERVE
The pudendal nerve arises from the second, third, and fourth sacral nerves. It passes through the greater sciatic foramen and accompanies the internal pudendal vessels. Its branches are the inferior rectal nerve, the perineal nerve, and the dorsal nerve of the clitoris.

SYNONYMS: *Pudic Nerve, Nervus Pudendus* (NA).

RECTAL NERVE, INFERIOR
The inferior rectal nerve consists of several branches of the pudendal nerve that pass to the external anal sphincter and skin of the anal region.

SYNONYMS: *Inferior Hemorrhoidal Nerve, Nervi Rectales Inferiores* (NA).

SCIATIC NERVE
The sciatic nerve is the largest nerve in the body. It supplies the skin of the foot and most of the leg, the muscles of the back of the thigh, and all muscles of the leg and foot. The sciatic nerve contributes filaments to all the joints of the lower extremities.

SYNONYMS: *Great Sciatic Nerve, Nervus Ischiadicus* (NA).

SPLANCHNIC NERVE, GREATER
The greater splanchnic nerve arises from the fifth or sixth to the ninth or tenth thoracic ganglia and passes downward along the sides of the bodies of the vertebrae to join the celiac plexus.

SYNONYM: *Nervus Splanchnicus Major* (NA).

SPLANCHNIC NERVES, PELVIC
The pelvic splanchnic nerves are branches of the second, third, and fourth sacral nerves that join the inferior hypogastric plexus. They carry parasympathetic and sensory fibers.

SYNONYM: *Nervi Splanchnici Pelvini* (NA).

VAGINAL NERVES

The vaginal nerves arise from the lower part of the pudendal plexus, run along the vaginal arteries, and supply the vagina and erectile tissue of the clitoris and vestibular bulb.

SYNONYM: *Nervi Vaginales* (NA).

GANGLIA

GANGLION

A ganglion is any collection or mass of nerve cells that serves as a center of nervous influence.

SYNONYM: *Ganglion* (NA).

COCCYGEAL GANGLION

The coccygeal ganglion is an unpaired ganglion of the sympathetic trunk.

SYNONYM: *Ganglion Impar* (NA).

GREAT CERVICAL GANGLION

The great cervical ganglion is a triangular mass of ganglionic cells and nerve fibers lying behind and at the sides of the uterine cervix and upper part of the vagina.

SYNONYM: *Frankenhäuser's Ganglion.*

LUMBAR GANGLION

The lumbar ganglion consists of four or more ganglia on the inner border of the psoas major muscle on either side of the pelvis. They form, with the sacral and coccygeal ganglions and their connecting cords, the abdominopelvic sympathetic trunk.

SYNONYM: *Ganglia Lumbalia* (NA).

PARASYMPATHETIC GANGLION

The parasympathetic ganglion is composed of various small ganglia lying close to the organs of the thorax, abdomen, and pelvis.

PELVIC GANGLION

The pelvic ganglion is one of two ganglia on each side of the cervix uteri, connected with the sacral and hypogastric plexuses.

SYNONYMS: *Hypogastric Ganglion, Ganglia Pelvina* (NA).

RENAL GANGLION

The renal ganglion is a ganglion around the renal artery.

SYNONYM: *Ganglia Renalia* (NA).

SACRAL GANGLION

The sacral ganglion consists of three or four ganglia on either side of the pelvis constituting, with the coccygeal ganglion and the connecting cords, the pelvic portion of the sympathetic trunk.

SYNONYM: *Ganglia Sacralia* (NA).

SPLANCHNIC GANGLION
The splanchnic ganglion is occasionally found in the great splanchnic nerve.

SYNONYM: *Ganglion Splanchnicum* (NA).

PLEXUSES

PLEXUS
A plexus is a network or interjoining of nerves, of veins, or of lymphatic vessels.

ABDOMINAL AORTIC PLEXUS
The abdominal aortic plexus is formed by branches derived on either side from the celiac plexus and ganglia, and receives filaments from some of the lumbar splanchnic nerves. It is situated on the sides and front of the aorta, between the origins of the superior and inferior mesenteric arteries.

SYNONYMS: *Aortic Plexus, Plexus Aorticus Abdominalis* (NA).

CELIAC PLEXUS
The celiac plexus is the largest of the autonomic plexuses lying in front of the aorta at the level of origin of the celiac artery, behind the stomach. It is formed by the splanchnic and the vagus nerves and cords from the celiac and superior mesenteric ganglia. Through its connection with the other abdominal plexuses, it sends branches to all abdominal viscera.

SYNONYMS: *Solar Plexus, Plexus Celiacus* (NA).

COCCYGEAL PLEXUS
The coccygeal plexus is a small plexus formed by the fourth and fifth sacral and the coccygeal nerves, usually regarded as forming part of the pudendal plexus. It gives origin to the anococcygeal nerves.

SYNONYM: *Plexus Coccygeus* (NA).

HYPOGASTRIC PLEXUS, INFERIOR
The inferior hypogastric plexus is the autonomic plexus in the pelvis that is distributed to the pelvic viscera. It receives the hypogastric nerves and the pelvic splanchnic nerves.

SYNONYMS: *Pelvic Plexus, Plexus Pelvinus* (NA), *Plexus Hypogastricus Inferior* (NA).

HYPOGASTRIC PLEXUS, SUPERIOR
The superior hypogastric plexus is a continuation of the abdominal aortic plexus downward across the fifth lumbar vertebra into the pelvis, where it divides into two hypogastric nerves at the sides of the rectum. These join the inferior hypogastric plexus to supply the pelvic viscera.

SYNONYMS: *Nervus Presacralis* (NA), *Plexus Hypogastricus Superior* (NA).

LUMBOSACRAL PLEXUS

The lumbosacral plexus is formed by the union of the ventral primary divisions of the lumbar, sacral, and coccygeal nerves. It is usually divided into lumbar and sacral plexuses.

SYNONYM: *Plexus Lumbosacralis* (NA).

Lumbar Plexus

The lumbar plexus is formed by the first four lumbar nerves. It lies dorsal to the psoas major muscle.

SYNONYM: *Plexus Lumbalis* (NA).

Sacral Plexus

The sacral plexus is formed by the fourth and fifth lumbar and first, second, and third sacral nerves. It lies on the inner surface of the posterior wall of the pelvis. Its nerves supply the lower extremities.

SYNONYMS: *Sciatic Plexus, Plexus Sacralis* (NA).

MIDDLE RECTAL PLEXUS

The middle rectal plexus is the autonomic plexus along the rectum, derived from the inferior hypogastric plexus.

SYNONYMS: *Middle Hemorrhoidal Plexus, Plexus Rectales Medii* (NA).

OVARIAN PLEXUS

The ovarian plexus arises from the renal plexus. It runs along the ovarian arteries and supplies the ovaries, tubes, and fundus of the uterus.

SYNONYM: *Plexus Ovaricus* (NA).

PUDENDAL PLEXUS

The pudendal plexus is formed generally by the anterior branches of the second, third, and fourth sacral nerves, but it is subject to variation so that it may include branches of the first or fifth sacral nerves. It lies in the posterior hollow of the pelvis on the anterior surface of the piriformis muscle. From it are derived visceral branches, muscular branches, and the pudendal nerve. It is sometimes considered a part of the sacral plexus.

SUPERIOR RECTAL PLEXUS

The superior rectal plexus is derived from the inferior mesenteric plexus that accompanies the superior rectal artery.

SYNONYMS: *Superior Hemorrhoidal Plexus, Plexus Rectalis Superior* (NA).

URETERIC PLEXUS

The ureteric plexus is derived from the celiac plexus that accompanies the ureter.

SYNONYM: *Plexus Uretericus* (NA).

UTEROVAGINAL PLEXUS

The uterovaginal plexus lies on each side of the uterine cervix. It is derived from the inferior hypogastric plexus and the third and fourth sacral nerves.

SYNONYM: *Plexus Uterovaginalis* (NA).

VESICAL PLEXUS

The vesical plexus is an autonomic plexus on the bladder.

SYNONYM: *Plexus Vesicales* (NA).

Folds

FOLD
A fold is one of several anatomic structures in which there is a plication of the parts.
SYNONYM: *Plica* (NA).

ARBOR VITAE UTERI
The arbor vitae uteri are two longitudinal ridges in the mucous membrane of the endocervix. They are located on the anterior and posterior wall and numerous rugae or secondary folds branch off.
SYNONYM: *Plicae Palmatae* (NA).

INTERURETERIC FOLD
The interureteric fold is a fold of mucous membrane extending from the orifice of the ureter on either side to the median line of the bladder.
SYNONYMS: *Plica Ureterica, Plica Interureterica* (NA).

PLICA AMPULLARIS
The plica ampullaris is one of the folds of mucous membrane at the fimbriated end of the fallopian tube.

PLICA SIGMOIDEA
The plica sigmoidea is one of the transverse folds of mucous membrane in the cecum and colon.
SYNONYM: *Plicae Semilunares Coli* (NA).

PLICAE TUBARIAE
The plicae tubariae are numerous longitudinal folds in the mucous membrane of the fallopian tube.
SYNONYM: *Plicae Tubariae* (NA).

RECTOUTERINE FOLD
The rectouterine fold is a fold of peritoneum that extends from the rectum to the base of the broad ligament on either side, forming the lateral boundary of the rectouterine pouch.
SYNONYMS: *Douglas' Fold, Plica Rectouterina* (NA).

RECTOVAGINAL FOLD
The rectovaginal fold is a fold of peritoneum extending from the rectum to the vagina. It is the lower portion of the rectouterine fold.
SYNONYM: *Plica Rectovaginalis* (NA).

TRANSVERSE VESICAL FOLD
The transverse vesical fold is a fold of peritoneum appearing when the bladder is empty, but absent when the bladder is full.

SYNONYM: *Plica Vesicalis Transversa* (NA).

UMBILICAL FOLD, LATERAL
The lateral umbilical fold is the ridge on the peritoneal surface of the anterior abdominal wall formed by the inferior epigastric vessels.

SYNONYMS: *Epigastric Fold, Plica Umbilicalis Lateralis* (NA).

UMBILICAL FOLD, MEDIAL
The medial umbilical fold is a fold of peritoneum covering the obliterated umbilical artery on either side of the urachus on the anterior wall of the abdomen.

SYNONYMS: *Plica Hypogastrica, Plica Umbilicalis Medialis* (NA).

UMBILICAL FOLD, MIDDLE
The middle umbilical fold is a fold of peritoneum that covers the urachus or the remains of the allantois on the anterior wall of the abdomen.

SYNONYMS: *Plica Urachi, Plica Umbilicalis Mediana* (NA).

VALVES OF HOUSTON
The valves of Houston are three or four crescentic folds situated horizontally in the rectal mucous membrane. One fold is situated near the rectosigmoid junction on the right side; a second one projects from the left side at a slightly lower level; a third is directed backward from the anterior wall at the level of the fundus of the urinary bladder.

SYNONYMS: *Kohlrausch Valves, Transverse Folds of Rectum, Rectal Valves, Plicae Transversales Recti* (NA).

Pouches

PERINEAL POUCH, DEEP
The deep perineal pouch is the space between the superior and inferior fascial layers of the urogenital diaphragm.

SYNONYMS: *Deep Perineal Space, Spatium Perinei Profundum* (NA).

PERINEAL POUCH, SUPERIOR
The superior perineal pouch is the superficial compartment of the perineum. It is bounded above by the inferior fascia of the urogenital diaphragm and below by Colles' fascia.

SYNONYM: *Spatium Perinei Superficiale* (NA).

RECTOUTERINE POUCH
The rectouterine pouch is formed by the caudal portion of the parietal peritoneum. Its anterior boundary is the supravaginal cervix and posterior fornix of the vagina; its posterior boundary, the rectum; and its lateral boundary, the sacrogenital folds covering the uterosacral ligaments.

SYNONYMS: *Douglas' Cul-de-Sac, Douglas' Pouch, Rectogenital Pouch, Rectouterine Excavation, Excavatio Rectouterina* (NA).

RETROINGUINAL SPACE
The retroinguinal space is the triangular space between the fascia transversalis in the inguinal region and the peritoneum.

SYNONYMS: *Bogros' Space, Spatium Retroinguinale.*

RETROPERITONEAL SPACE
The retroperitoneal space is the area between the muscles of the posterior abdominal wall and the parietal peritoneum.

SYNONYM: *Spatium Retroperitoneale* (NA).

RETZIUS' SPACE
Retzius' space is the area of loose connective tissue between the bladder, the pubis, and anterior abdominal wall.

SYNONYMS: *Retropubic Space, Spatium Retropubicum* (NA).

VESICOUTERINE POUCH
The vesicouterine pouch is the depression in the peritoneum between the bladder and uterus.

SYNONYMS: *Uterovesical Pouch, Excavatio Vesicouterina* (NA).

Section 2: *Anatomy of Generative Organs*

Breast

BREAST

The breast is a modified sweat gland. Its size varies, but in most instances it extends from the second to the sixth rib and from the sternum to the anterior axillary line, with an axillary tail in the upper outer portion. The mammary tissue lies directly over the pectoralis major muscle and is separated from its outer fascia by a layer of adipose tissue. This layer is continuous with the fatty stroma of the gland itself. The breast is composed of the stroma and the parenchyma. The physiology of the breast is greatly affected by secretion of the anterior pituitary and by the secretions from the follicles and corpus luteum of the ovary. Follicle-stimulating hormone (FSH), acting on the ovary, stimulates follicular growth and estrogen output, which in turn stimulates the growth of mammary ducts and periductal stroma. After ovulation, luteinizing hormone (LH) stimulates the formation of the corpus luteum and output of progesterone, which then stimulates the growth of the mammary lobules. The lactogenic hormone of the anterior pituitary acts directly on the mammary gland to initiate lactation. Once initiated, lactation is stimulated and maintained by the act of suckling through the *milk-ejection reflex,* which is mediated by oxytocin. During lactation, follicular ripening and ovulation are suppressed. Conversely, large doses of estrogen tend to inhibit breast secretion.

SYNONYMS: *Mammary Gland, Mamma* (NA), *Glandula Mammaria* (NA).

ACINI OF BREAST

The acini of the breast are the secreting elements of the breast that produce milk after birth of the fetus. The terminal tubules and acini are more numerous in childbearing years, the greatest development occurring during pregnancy and lactation.

AREOLAR GLAND

The areolar gland is one of several cutaneous glands forming small, rounded projections from the surface of the areola of the breast.

SYNONYMS: *Montgomery's Gland, Glandulae Areolares* (NA).

BLOOD SUPPLY OF BREAST

The blood supply of the breast is furnished medially by the perforating branches of the internal thoracic arteries and veins, superiorly by the superior thoracic and arteries to the pectoralis major and pectoralis minor muscles, and laterally by the lateral thoracic artery, lateral thoracic vein, and branches of the interstitial arteries and veins.

COLOSTRUM

Colostrum is the watery secretion from the breast during the first few postpartum days. It is also secreted occasionally during pregnancy after the third to fourth gestational month. It changes to milk after stimulation of the breast by prolactin, generally following the fourth postpartum day. However, a copious flow of milk often may occur 24 to 48 hours postpartum, especially if the infant is allowed to nurse freely. Colostrum is made up of fat globules, a watery fluid, and the so-called *colostrum corpuscles*. Colostrum corpuscles are round, ovoid, or stellate cells that sometimes show ameboid movement and have one to three nuclei. They contain numerous fine fat globules and are believed to be changed gland epithelium, leukocytes, or mast cells that have gathered up fat globules. They remain four to six days. Colostrum contains very little, if any, casein, but nearly 15 per cent lactalbumin and lactoglobulin, with much fat.

HUMAN MILK

Human milk has a characteristic odor and sweet taste. Its specific gravity varies from 1.026 to 1.036. It is neutral or alkaline. On microscopic study, innumerable fine fat droplets and occasionally a glandular epithelial cell or leukocyte is observed. The composition of human milk varies from day to day and from hour to hour; generally 87.5 per cent water and 12.5 per cent solids, of which 6.2 per cent is milk sugar, 3.8 per cent fat, 2.3 per cent proteins (lactoglobulin, 1.3 per cent, and casein, 1 per cent), and 0.7 per cent salts.

SYNONYM: *Breast Milk.*

LACTIFEROUS SINUS

The lactiferous sinus is a dilation of the mammary duct just before it enters the nipple.

SYNONYM: *Sinus Lactiferi* (NA).

LYMPHATIC VESSELS OF BREAST

The lymphatic vessels of the breast are separated into two planes—the superficial or subareolar plexus of lymphatic vessels and the deep or fascial plexus. Both originate in the interlobular spaces and in the walls of the mammary ducts. The superficial plexus collects lymph from the central parts of the gland, the skin, areola, and nipple, and it drains laterally toward the axilla. The drainage passes to the central axillary lymph nodes. From there, the drainage is to the subclavian lymph nodes at the apex of the axilla, where the axillary and subclavian veins join. The deep fascial plexus extends through the pectoral muscles to Rotter's nodes, and then to the subclavian lymph nodes. This is known as *Groszman's pathway*. The rest of the fascial plexus, for the most part, extends medially along the internal thoracic artery via the internal mammary lymph nodes to the anterior mediastinal lymph nodes. Other paths of lymphatic drainage proceed from the lower and medial portion of the breast. One of these is the paramammary route of Gerota, through the lymphatic vessels of the abdomen to the liver or subdiaphragmatic lymph nodes. Another is a cross-mammary pathway, via superficial lymphatic vessels to the opposite breast and opposite axilla. From the lower medial portion of the gland some lymphatic vessels of the fascial group drain, passing beneath the sternum, to the anterior mediastinal lymph nodes situated in front of the aorta.

MAMMARY DUCTS

There are 15 to 20 mammary ducts. They dilate to form the ampullae just before reaching the surface of the skin and opening into the nipple. They extend radially from the nipple toward the chest wall. Secondary tubules arising from them end in the acinar structures of the breast.

SYNONYMS: *Milk Duct, Ductus Lactiferi* (NA).

NIPPLE

The nipple is an elevated structure that receives and contains the openings of the mammary ducts. The nipple, surrounded by the areola, is covered by modified mucous membrane containing the areolar glands.

SYNONYM: *Papilla Mammae* (NA).

PARENCHYMA OF BREAST

The parenchyma of the breast is the breast tissue composed of the mammary ducts, tubules, and acinar structures.

SYNONYM: *Corpus Mammae* (NA).

STROMA OF BREAST

The stroma of the breast is a mixture of fibrous and fatty tissue that determines the size and consistency of the breast when the woman is not lactating or pregnant. The enveloping fascia is continuous with the pectoral fascia and subdivides the breast into lobules sending strands to the overlying skin.

Fallopian Tubes

FALLOPIAN TUBES

The fallopian tubes are two muscular passages that transport ova from the ovaries to the uterus. They extend from the cornua of the uterus to the ovaries. Each tube is divided into four parts: interstitial, isthmic, ampullar, and infundibular. The walls of the tubes are composed of three layers: mucosa, muscular, and serosa.

SYNONYMS: *Oviduct, Tuba Uterina* (NA).

Ampullar Portion of Fallopian Tube

The ampullar portion of the fallopian tube is the trumpet-like, thin-walled portion between the isthmic and fimbriated parts of the tube.

SYNONYM: *Ampulla Tubae Uterinae* (NA).

Infundibular Portion of Fallopian Tube

The infundibular portion of the fallopian tube is the funnel-shaped distal portion. Its orifice is surrounded by fimbriae.

SYNONYM: *Infundibulum Tubae Uterinae* (NA).

Interstitial Portion of Fallopian Tube

The interstitial portion of the fallopian tube is the portion contained in the muscular wall of the uterine cornu. The uterine os of the tube is less than a millimeter in diameter.

SYNONYMS: *Intramural Portion of Fallopian Tube, Pars Uterina* (NA).

Isthmic Portion of Fallopian Tube

The isthmic portion of the fallopian tube is the narrow, cordlike portion between the interstitial and ampullar portions. It constitutes one-third of the extrauterine length of the tube.

SYNONYM: *Isthmus Tubae Uterinae* (NA).

ABDOMINAL OSTIUM

The abdominal ostium is the orifice of the infundibular portion of the fallopian tube.

SYNONYM: *Ostium Abdominale Tubae Uterinae* (NA).

CILIA OF FALLOPIAN TUBE

The cilia of the fallopian tube are hairlike processes of the cells of the tubal mucosa. They measure 7 to 8μ in length. Their function is to promote tubal transmigration of ova.

FIMBRIAE OF FALLOPIAN TUBE
The fimbriae of the fallopian tube are the finger-like projections of the infundibular portion of the fallopian tube.
SYNONYM: *Fimbriae Tubae* (NA).

FIMBRIA OVARICA
The fimbria ovarica is the longest fimbria of the infundibular portion of the fallopian tube.
SYNONYM: *Fimbria Ovarica* (NA).

LYMPHATIC VESSELS OF FALLOPIAN TUBE
The lymphatic vessels of the fallopian tube pass partly with the lymphatic vessels of the ovary and partly with those of the uterus.

MUCOSA OF FALLOPIAN TUBE
The mucosa of the fallopian tube is the lining epithelium of the tube containing ciliated, nonciliated, and intercalary cells. The epithelium undergoes cyclic changes similar to those in the endometrium.
SYNONYM: *Tubal Epithelium.*

MUSCULAR COAT OF FALLOPIAN TUBE
The muscular coat of the fallopian tube is composed of outer longitudinal and inner circular layers of muscle.

Circular Muscle Layer of Fallopian Tube
The circular muscle layer of the fallopian tube is the inner layer of muscle that encircles the tube. This layer becomes less distinct at the fimbriated extremity and is replaced by an interlacing network of muscular fibers.

Longitudinal Muscle Layer of Fallopian Tube
The longitudinal muscle layer of the fallopian tube is the layer of muscle fibers that parallels the tube and forms the outer wall. It becomes less distinct at the fimbriated extremity and is replaced by an interlacing network of muscle fibers.

PLICA AMPULLARIS
The plica ampullaris is one of the folds of mucous membrane at the fimbriated end of the fallopian tube.

PLICAE TUBARIAE
The plicae tubariae are numerous longitudinal folds in the mucous membrane of the fallopian tube.
SYNONYM: *Plicae Tubariae* (NA).

UTERINE OSTIUM
The uterine ostium is the uterine opening of the fallopian tube.
SYNONYM: *Ostium Uterinum Tubae* (NA).

SECTION 2: ANATOMY OF GENERATIVE ORGANS

Ovary

OVARIES

The ovaries are two ovoid structures situated on each side of the pelvis just below the distal end of the fallopian tubes. They measure about 3.5 cm in length, 2 cm in width, and about 1.5 cm in thickness. They each weigh about 4 to 8 gm, but may vary markedly in size, shape, and weight. The ovaries are suspended by the mesovarium, the suspensory ligaments of the ovary, and the ovarian ligaments. The two portions of the ovary are the outer cortex and the central portion or medulla. The surface of each ovary is covered by a superficial condensed layer of connective tissue containing a few involuntary muscle fibers. This covering is designated as the tunica albuginea of the ovary. The blood supply is derived from the ovarian arteries and ovarian branches of the uterine artery. The venous drainage is through the ovarian vein.

SYNONYM: *Ovarium* (NA).

ANTRUM OF OVARY

The antrum of the ovary is a cavity in the layer of follicle cells, and is filled with fluid known as the liquor folliculi.

CORONA RADIATA

The corona radiata is a layer of radially arranged granulosa cells that remains temporarily attached to the primary oocyte following its separation from the wall of the follicle. It is derived from part of the cumulus oophorus.

CORPUS ALBICANS

The corpus albicans is a retrogressed corpus luteum. It appears as a whitish, hyalinized, convoluted structure that slowly decreases in size.

SYNONYMS: *Corpus Candicans, Corpus Albicans* (NA).

CORPUS LUTEUM

The corpus luteum is the yellow endocrine body formed in the ovary at the site of a ruptured ovarian follicle. The life history of the corpus luteum begins immediately after ovulation. The stages of development are as follows: proliferation, vascularization, maturity, and retrogression.

Proliferation

Proliferation is the stage immediately following the rupture of the ovarian follicle. The granulosa layer shows evidence of beginning transformation into the large, polyhedral, often vacuolated cells

72

known as *lutein cells*. There is a zone of blood vessels known as the *perigranulosal vascular wreath* between the granulosa and theca layers. The color of the corpus luteum at this stage is a grayish yellow.

SYNONYMS: *Stage I of Corpus Luteum Development, Hyperemic Stage of Corpus Luteum Development.*

Vascularization

Vascularization is the phase characterized by the invasion of the lutein cells by blood vessels from the theca. These channels extend to the lumen, and hemorrhage is the normal feature of this phase. The theca interna has undergone regressive changes, its cells having shrunk through disappearance of the lipoid content.

SYNONYM: *Stage II of Corpus Luteum Development.*

Maturity

Maturity is the stage that parallels the progestational phase in the endometrium. Grossly, the corpus luteum appears yellow and reaches 10 to 20 mm in diameter. The theca cells often show luteinization, and the inner edge of the lutein zone is invaded by fibroblastic tissue.

SYNONYM: *Stage III of Corpus Luteum Development.*

Retrogression

Retrogression is the stage at which the corpus luteum has obtained its maximum development, probably as early as four to six days before the menstrual period. Regression of the corpus is marked by fatty degeneration, fibrosis, hyalinization of the lutein zone, and cicatricial tissue formation within the cavity. The end product is the corpus albicans.

CORTEX OF OVARY

The cortex of the ovary is the outer portion. It varies in thickness, depending on the patient's age. It has three layers: the germinal epithelium, the tunica albuginea, and the cortical stroma.

SYNONYM: *Zona Parenchymatosa.*

Cortical Stroma of Ovary

The cortical stroma of the ovary is composed of compactly placed spindle cells, connective tissue, follicular elements, and their derivatives.

Germinal Epithelium of Ovary

The germinal epithelium of the ovary is a single layer of cuboidal epithelium covering the cortex of the ovary. It is usually absent in the adult but often appears in chronic inflammation.

SYNONYM: *Germinal Epithelium of Waldeyer.*

Tunica Albuginea of Ovary

The tunica albuginea of the ovary is the layer of condensed connective tissue beneath the germinal epithelium of the external ovarian surface.

CUMULUS OOPHORUS
The cumulus oophorus is a mass of follicular or granulosa cells that surrounds the female germ cell.
SYNONYMS: *Cumulus Ovaricus, Cumulus Proligerus, Discus Proligerus, Cumulus Oophorus* (NA).

FOLLICLE
A follicle is a group of cells usually containing a fluid-filled cavity.

FOLLICULAR CELL
A follicular cell is one of the cells that line the ovarian follicle.
SYNONYM: *Follicular Epithelial Cell.*

FOLLICULAR STIGMA
The follicular stigma is the site on the surface of the ovary where the graafian follicle ruptures to permit extrusion of its contents.

GRAAFIAN FOLLICLE
The graafian follicle is an ovarian follicle possessing an antrum.
SYNONYMS: *Vesicular Follicle, Folliculus Oophorus Vesiculosus, Folliculi Ovarici Vesiculosi* (NA).

Anovular Graafian Follicle
An anovular graafian follicle is an ovarian follicle without an ovum.

Atretic Graafian Follicle
An atretic graafian follicle is an ovarian follicle that has failed to mature.

HILUM OF OVARY
The hilum of the ovary is the oblong groove or depression along the anterior margin at the insertion of the mesovarium. Blood vessels and nerves enter and leave through the hilum.
SYNONYM: *Hilus Ovarii* (NA).

LIQUOR FOLLICULI
The liquor folliculi is the fluid present in an ovarian follicle.

LOWER POLE OF OVARY
The lower pole of the ovary is the narrow pointed end that is directed inferiorly toward the uterus.
SYNONYMS: *Uterine Extremity, Extremitas Uterina* (NA).

LYMPHATIC VESSELS OF OVARY
The lymphatic vessels of the ovary ascend with the ovarian artery to the lateral and preaortic lymph nodes.

MEDULLA OF OVARY
The medulla of the ovary is the central portion of the ovary. It consists primarily of a connective-tissue matrix surrounding the major ovarian blood vessels and lymphatic vessels. It also contains the rete ovarii. The medulla is potentially androgenic in contrast to the cortex, which has an estrogenic role.
SYNONYM: *Zona Vasculosa.*

OOGONIUM
The oogonium is a primitive female germ cell containing a diploid number of chromosomes. It may reproduce itself by mitotic division, or may become a primary oocyte preparatory to undergoing meiotic division.

OVARIAN FOLLICLE
An ovarian follicle is a vascular body in the ovary that contains an ovum. It can either be a primordial follicle or a graafian follicle.

OVARIAN FOSSA
The ovarian fossa is a depression in the lateral wall of the pelvis occupied by the ovary. It is behind the broad ligament in the angle between the elevations produced by the diverging internal and external iliac arteries.
SYNONYM: *Claudius' Fossa.*

OVUM
Ovum is a general term referring to the female germ cell at any stage of development.
SYNONYM: *Ovum* (NA).

PAROOPHORON
The paroophoron consists of vestigial remains of the mesonephric tubules. The paroophoron is situated in the broad ligament between the parovarium and the uterus.
SYNONYM: *Paroophoron* (NA).

PAROVARIUM
The parovarium is the lateral portion of the vestigial remains of the mesonephric tubules. The parovarium lies in the mesosalpinx between the ovary and the fallopian tube.
SYNONYMS: *Organ of Rosenmüller, Epoophoron* (NA).

PERIVITELLINE SPACE
The perivitelline space is the space between the plasma membrane of the female germ cell and the zona pellucida.

PRIMORDIAL FOLLICLE
The primordial follicle is a young ovarian follicle before the formation of the antrum with its contained liquor folliculi.
SYNONYM: *Folliculi Ovarici Primarii* (NA).

RETE OVARII

Rete ovarii are the narrow slitlike tubules of the ovary that are lined by a flat epithelium and without surrounding muscle tissue.

THECA CELLS

Theca cells are cells that surround the granulosa cells and form the outer part of the wall of an ovarian follicle.

THECA FOLLICULI

The theca folliculi is the outer layer of connective tissue that covers a graafian follicle. It is divided into a poorly defined outer layer, the theca externa, and a sharply demarcated inner layer, the theca interna.

Theca Externa

The theca externa is the layer of theca cells that forms the outer part of the wall of an ovarian follicle.

Theca Interna

The theca interna is the layer of theca cells lying between the granulosa cells and the theca externa.

THECA-LUTEIN CELL

A theca-lutein cell is one of the cells of the corpus luteum derived from the theca interna.

UPPER POLE OF OVARY

The upper pole of the ovary is the rounded end of the ovary directed toward the fimbriated end of the fallopian tube.

SYNONYMS: *Tubal Extremity, Fimbrial Pole, Extremitas Tubaria* (NA).

ZONA PELLUCIDA

The zona pellucida is a clear, thick membrane that forms around the plasma membrane of the female germ cell and persists until the blastocyst is well developed.

SYNONYM: *Oolemma.*

Uterus

UTERUS

The uterus is a hollow, muscular, pear-shaped organ located in the pelvis between the bladder and rectum. The nulliparous uterus is approximately 5.5 to 8.0 cm in length, 3.5 to 5.0 cm in breadth at its upper portion, and about 2.0 to 2.5 cm in thickness. The portion of the uterus above the isthmus is called the corpus (body) and that below, the cervix. The wall of the uterus is composed of three coats: endometrium (mucosa), muscle, and serosa. The cavity is small in comparison to the thickness of its muscular wall. The cervical canal begins at the internal cervical os and ends at the external cervical os. The fallopian tubes enter the superior lateral borders of the corpus of the uterus. The portion of the corpus above the insertion of the tubes is designated as the fundus. The uterus is supported in the pelvic cavity by the broad, round, cardinal, and uterosacral ligaments along with the vesicouterine folds. The functions of the uterus are: menstruation; reception, retention, and nourishment of the fertilized ovum; and the expulsion of the products of conception by muscular contraction.

SYNONYM: *Uterus* (NA).

ANATOMIC INTERNAL OS

The anatomic internal os is the lower boundary of the corpus uteri and is recognized by constriction of the uterus at this point.

CERVIX

The cervix is the lower constricted segment of the uterus. It is approximately 4 cm in length. The vagina is attached obliquely around the center of the periphery of the cervix. This attachment divides the cervix into two parts: the supravaginal portion and infravaginal portion.

SYNONYM: *Cervix Uteri* (NA).

CORNU

The cornu is the portion of the corpus uteri that surrounds the insertion of the fallopian tube.

CORPUS UTERI

The corpus uteri is the portion of the uterus above the isthmus. It gradually narrows from the fundus to the isthmus. The anterior surface is flattened and is covered by peritoneum. The posterior surface is convex transversely, and is covered by peritoneum, which continues down to the cervix and vagina. The fundus is convex in all directions and covered by peritoneum. The sides of the corpus are not directly covered by peritoneum, but receive the attachments of the broad ligaments. The fallopian tube pierces the uterine wall at the cornu. The corpus uteri is composed of three layers: endometrium (mucosa), muscle, and serosa.

SYNONYMS: *Body of Uterus, Corpus Uteri* (NA).

ENDOMETRIUM

The endometrium is the mucous membrane that lines the uterine cavity. It is a specialized form of tissue characterized by a remarkable lability and a sensitivity to the ovarian steroids. The component parts of the endometrium are the glands, stroma, lymphoid follicles, and blood vessels. The endometrium is divided into the functional zone and basalis layer. It undergoes constant hormonally controlled changes during each menstrual cycle. These fundamental phases are: postmenstrual, proliferative, secretory, premenstrual, and menstrual.

SYNONYM: *Endometrium* (NA).

EXTERNAL LONGITUDINAL MUSCLE LAYER OF UTERUS

The external longitudinal muscle layer of the uterus is situated on the external surface of the anterior and posterior uterine walls. Contraction of this layer decreases the longitudinal diameter of the uterus.

FUNDUS OF UTERUS

The fundus is the portion of the corpus uteri above the insertion of the fallopian tubes.

SYNONYM: *Fundus Uteri* (NA).

INNER CIRCULAR MUSCLE LAYER OF UTERUS

The inner circular muscle layer of the uterus is situated on the inner aspect of the uterine wall. These fibers intermingle with the longitudinal and transverse fibers. Contraction of this layer decreases the transverse diameter of the uterus.

ISTHMUS OF UTERUS

The isthmus of the uterus is an area of constriction between the corpus uteri and cervix. At the junction of the corpus uteri and isthmus is the anatomic internal os. At the junction of the isthmus and cervix is the internal cervical os.

SYNONYMS: *Uterocervical Junction, Isthmus Uteri* (NA).

LYMPHATIC VESSELS OF UTERUS

The lymphatic vessels of the uterus consist of two sets, superficial and deep. The superficial vessels are situated beneath the peritoneum, and the deep vessels are situated in the substance of the organ. The lymphatic vessels of the cervix run in three directions: transversely to the external iliac lymph nodes, posterolaterally to the internal iliac lymph nodes, and dorsad to the common iliac lymph nodes. Most of the lymphatic vessels of the corpus and fundus of the uterus pass lateral in the broad ligaments, and continue up with the ovarian lymphatic vessels to the lateral and preaortic lymph nodes. A few lymphatic vessels run to the external iliac lymph nodes, and one or two to the superficial inguinal lymph nodes. In the nongravid uterus, the lymphatic vessels are very small, but during gestation they are greatly enlarged.

PARAMETRIUM

The parametrium is the connective tissue surrounding the uterus. It extends laterally from the fibrous subserous coat of the supracervical portion of the uterus to the layers of the broad ligament.

SYNONYM: *Parametrium* (NA).

RECTOUTERINE POUCH

The rectouterine pouch is formed by the caudal portion of the parietal peritoneum. Its anterior boundary is the supravaginal cervix and posterior fornix of the vagina; its posterior boundary, the rectum; and its lateral boundary, the sacrogenital folds covering the uterosacral ligaments.

SYNONYMS: *Douglas' Cul-de-Sac, Douglas' Pouch, Rectogenital Pouch, Rectouterine Excavation, Excavatio Rectouterina* (NA).

UTERINE AXIS

The uterine axis is an imaginary line passing lengthwise through the center of the uterus.

UTERINE SEROSA

The uterine serosa is derived from the peritoneum. It invests the fundus and the whole posterior surface of the uterus, but covers the anterior surface only as far as the junction of the corpus and the cervix. In the lower fourth of the posterior surface, the peritoneum, though covering the uterus, is not closely connected with it, being separated from it by a layer of loose cellular tissue and large veins.

SYNONYMS: *Serous Coat of Uterus, Perimetrium* (NA).

ENDOMETRIUM

ENDOMETRIUM

The endometrium is the mucous membrane that lines the uterine cavity. It is a specialized form of tissue, characterized by a remarkable lability and a sensitivity to the ovarian steroids. The component parts of the endometrium are the glands, stroma, lymphoid follicles, and blood vessels. The endometrium is divided into the functional zone and basalis layer. It undergoes constant hormonally controlled changes during each menstrual cycle. These fundamental phases are: postmenstrual, proliferative, secretory, premenstrual, and menstrual.

SYNONYM: *Endometrium* (NA).

BASALIS LAYER OF ENDOMETRIUM

The basalis layer of the endometrium is the deep layer. It is composed of young undifferentiated cells unresponsive to progesterone. This layer is responsive to estrogen in the premenstrual phase of the cycle and is not desquamated in toto at menstruation. The basalis layer is responsible for the growth and regeneration of the endometrium.

ENDOMETRIAL ARTERIES
The endometrial arteries consist of the endometrial coiled arteries and the endometrial basal arteries.

Endometrial Arteries, Basal
The endometrial basal arteries are branches of the radial arteries that supply the basalis layer of the endometrium. The basal arteries are not affected by hormonal influences. These arteries supply blood to the regenerating endometrium.

Endometrial Arteries, Coiled
The endometrial coiled arteries are essentially a continuation of the radial arteries. The coiled arteries supply the functional zone of the endometrium and are sensitive to the biphasic stimulation of the ovarian steroids. These arteries furnish the nutritional substances to the endometrial glands and stroma, and they exhibit a period of vasoconstriction creating ischemia in endometrial segments, tissue sloughing, and menstrual bleeding.
SYNONYM: *Endometrial Spiral Arterioles.*

ENDOMETRIAL GLANDS
The endometrial glands are the secretory structures of the endometrium. In the immediate postmenstrual phase, they are straight, narrow, and collapsed. In the proliferative phase, they begin to grow. The epithelial cells of the glands are of the low columnar type. There is no evidence of secretory activity. During the secretory phase, the glands are larger and longer. The epithelial cells of the glands are secretory. Vacuolization occurs beneath the nuclei of these cells, pushing the nuclei to the midportion of the cells. Later in the same phase, vacuoles disappear and nuclei recede to the basal membrane. In the premenstrual phase, the epithelial cells of the glands are of the low columnar type and possess frayed edges. The glands are wide, tortuous, and filled with secretory material. The glands metabolize glucose and store glycogen in increasing amounts. The maximum storage and metabolism of glycogen occurs from the 17th to the 19th day of the cycle. This is followed by regression.
SYNONYMS: *Uterine Glands, Glandulae Uterinae* (NA).

ENDOMETRIAL STROMA
The endometrial stroma is the supporting tissue of the endometrium. In the proliferative phase of the cycle, the stroma is rather dense and compact, but premenstrually there is increased edema and vascularity with actual hypertrophy of the cells. The cells become enlarged and polyhedral.
SYNONYM: *Uterine Stroma.*

ENDOMETRIAL SUBNUCLEAR VACUOLE
The endometrial subnuclear vacuole is a clear zone in the glandular epithelium containing various metabolic substances. The nucleus is ele-

vated to the upper portion of the epithelial cell. These vacuoles appear at the time of ovulation and in the early stages of progesterone activity.

ENDOMETRIAL VENULE

An endometrial venule is a venous channel of the endometrium. It drains the surface epithelium and capillary network of the tissue.

FUNCTIONAL ZONE OF ENDOMETRIUM

The functional zone of the endometrium is the superficial layer of the endometrium, consisting of the compact layer (stratum compactum) and the spongy layer (stratum spongiosum). The functional zone of the endometrium participates in the cyclic phenomena of menstruation.

LYMPHOID FOLLICLES

The lymphoid follicles are collections of round cells in the endometrial stroma. They resemble lymphoid tissue.

MYOMETRIAL ARCUATE ARTERIES

The myometrial arcuate arteries are branches of the uterine and ovarian arteries. They terminate in myometrial radial arteries.

MYOMETRIAL RADIAL ARTERIES

The myometrial radial arteries are a continuation of the myometrial arcuate arteries. They penetrate the endometrium and divide into the larger endometrial coiled arteries and the smaller endometrial basal arteries.

UTERINE FLUID

The uterine fluid is secreted by the endometrial glands during the secretory phase of the menstrual cycle. This fluid provides nutritive substances.

SYNONYM: *Endometrial Fluid.*

CERVIX

CERVIX

The cervix is the lower constricted segment of the uterus. It is approximately 4 cm in length. The vagina is attached obliquely around the center of the periphery of the cervix. This attachment divides the cervix into two parts: the infravaginal portion and the supravaginal portion.

SYNONYM: *Cervix Uteri* (NA).

Infravaginal Cervix

The infravaginal cervix is the portion below the attachment of the vagina.

SYNONYM: *Portio Vaginalis* (NA).

Supravaginal Cervix

The supravaginal cervix is the portion above the attachment of the vagina.

SYNONYMS: *Portioabdominalis, Portio Supravaginalis* (NA).

ANTERIOR LIP OF CERVIX
The anterior lip of the cervix is the area of the cervix anterior to the external os.
SYNONYM: *Labium Anterius* (NA).

ARBOR VITAE UTERI
The arbor vitae uteri are two longitudinal ridges in the mucous membrane of the endocervix. They are located on the anterior and posterior wall and numerous rugae or secondary folds branch off.
SYNONYM: *Plicae Palmatae* (NA).

CERVICAL CANAL
The cervical canal is a fusiform passage extending from the internal os to the external os of the cervix.
SYNONYM: *Canalis Cervicis Uteri* (NA).

CERVICAL GLAND
The cervical gland is a branched mucus-secreting gland of the cervical mucosa.
SYNONYM: *Glandula Cervicales Uteri* (NA).

CERVICAL LAMINA PROPRIA
The cervical lamina propria is the layer of connective tissue below the mucous membrane of the cervix.

CERVICAL MUCUS
Cervical mucus is a secretion of the endocervix during the menstrual cycle and pregnancy. Its composition is altered during the menstrual cycle by the action of estrogen and progesterone. It contains enzymes, mucus, leukocytes, cervical and vaginal cells, and other substances. During pregnancy, it serves as a plug, providing a mechanical and antibacterial barrier to the uterine cavity.
SYNONYMS: *Cervical Secretion, Cervical Plug, Mucous Plug.*

CERVICAL MUCUS ARBORIZATION
Cervical mucus arborization is the specific palm-leaf pattern created by the drying and resulting crystallization of cervical mucus due to electrolyte action on protein. It occurs in the proliferative phase of the menstrual cycle.
SYNONYM: *Ferning.*

CERVICAL OS, EXTERNAL
The external cervical os is the external opening of the cervical canal.
SYNONYM: *Ostium Uteri* (NA).

CERVICAL OS, INTERNAL
The internal cervical os is the internal opening of the cervical canal at the junction of the isthmus and the cervix.
SYNONYM: *Histologic Internal Os.*

CERVICAL STROMA
The cervical stroma is composed of connective tissue and muscle cells in the deeper portion of the cervix. This admixture increases near the internal os.

CIRCULAR MUSCLE LAYER OF CERVIX
The circular muscle layer of the cervix consists of muscle fibers scattered through dense tangled collagen.

ENDOCERVIX
The endocervix is the mucous membrane lining the cervical canal.
SYNONYM: *Cervical Mucous Membrane.*

FIBROMUSCULAR JUNCTION
The fibromuscular junction is the area between the muscular elements of the uterine wall and the fibrous tissue of the cervix. It has considerable functional significance in that it may produce a sphincter-like action, relaxing under estrogen influence and contracting under progesterone action.

GERMINAL CELL LAYER OF CERVIX
The germinal cell layer of the cervix is the layer of cells adjacent to the basement membrane of the cervix. These cells are seldom observed in vaginal smears.

ISTHMUS OF UTERUS
The isthmus of the uterus is an area of constriction between the corpus uteri and cervix. At the junction of the corpus uteri and isthmus is the anatomic internal os. At the junction of the isthmus and cervix is the internal cervical os.
SYNONYMS: *Uterocervical Junction, Isthmus Uteri* (NA).

POSTERIOR LIP OF CERVIX
The posterior lip of the cervix is the area of the cervix posterior to the external os.
SYNONYM: *Labium Posterius* (NA).

SPINNBARKEIT
Spinnbarkeit is a term used to denote cervical mucus of decreased viscosity. It is indicative of ovulation in some women.

SQUAMOCOLUMNAR JUNCTION
The squamocolumnar junction is the location on the endocervix where there is a transition from stratified squamous epithelium to columnar epithelium.

TRANSITIONAL LAYER OF CELLS OF CERVIX
The transitional layer of cells of the cervix is the layer of cells adjacent to the germinal layer of the cervical epithelium.

Vulva

VULVA
The vulva is the external genitalia of the female; it includes the mons pubis, labia majora, labia minora, clitoris, and the vestibule.
SYNONYMS: *Pudendum Muliebre, Pudendum Femininum* (NA).

ANTERIOR COMMISSURE
The anterior commissure is the junction of the labia majora above the clitoris.
SYNONYM: *Commissura Labiorum Anterior* (NA).

BULB OF VESTIBULE
The bulb of the vestibule consists of two elongated masses of erectile tissue located on either side of the vaginal orifice and joined in front by a narrow median band.
SYNONYM: *Bulbus Vestibuli* (NA).

CLITORIS
The clitoris is a small, cylindrical, erectile body, rarely exceeding 2 cm in length. It is situated at the most anterior portion of the vulva and projects between the branched extremities of the labia minora, which form the prepuce and frenulum. It consists of a glans, a corpus, and two crura. It is the homologue of the penis in the male, but does not possess a corpus spongiosum and is not perforated by the urethra.
SYNONYM: *Clitoris* (NA).

DERMIS OF VULVA
The dermis of the vulva consists of connective tissue with a varying amount of elastic fibers and numerous blood vessels, lymphatic vessels, and nerves. The connective tissue is arranged in two layers: a deep or reticular layer and a superficial or papillary layer.

Papillary Layer
The papillary layer of the vulvar dermis consists of numerous small, highly sensitive vascular eminences, the papillae, which rise perpendicularly from its surface.
SYNONYM: *Superficial Layer of Vulvar Dermis.*

Reticular Layer
The reticular layer of the vulvar dermis consists of fibroelastic connective tissue, composed chiefly of collagenous bundles. It also contains elastic fibers.
SYNONYM: *Deep Layer of Vulvar Dermis.*

84

END BULBS

End bulbs are oval or irregular spherical bodies in which the sensory nerve fibers terminate. They are located in the mucous membrane and sensitive regions of the vulva.

EPIDERMIS OF VULVA

The epidermis of the vulva is the superficial or outer layer of epithelial cells. It consists of stratified squamous epithelium that is arranged in five layers from within, outward, as follows: germinal cell layer, prickle cell layer, granular cell layer, clear cell layer, and horny cell layer.

Germinal Cell Layer

The germinal cell layer of the vulvar epidermis is a single layer of columnar cells that rests on the basement membrane. This layer constitutes the reproductive source from which all epidermoid cells are derived.

SYNONYM: *Basal Cell Layer.*

Prickle Cell Layer

The prickle cell layer of the vulvar epidermis is a layer of cells superimposed on the germinal cell layer. These cells form channels by which tissue fluids are circulated for cellular nutrition.

Granular Cell Layer

The granular cell layer of the vulvar epidermis is the layer of cells situated above the prickle cell layer. It consists of one or two rows of flattened cells that contain granules of eleidin.

Clear Cell Layer

The clear cell layer of the vulvar epidermis is the layer of the epidermis situated just above the granular cell layer. It consists of two or three layers of flat clear cells with atrophied nuclei.

Horny Cell Layer

The horny cell layer of the vulvar epidermis is the layer of cells that is superficial to the clear cell layer. It consists of several layers of flat epithelial cells.

ESCUTCHEON

The escutcheon is the pattern of hair growth covering the genitalia and lower abdomen. It is considered a secondary sexual characteristic.

FOURCHETTE

The fourchette is a thin fold of skin immediately behind the hymen. It is formed by the merging of the labia minora and the labia majora.

SYNONYM: *Commissura Labiorum Posterior* (NA).

INTROITUS

The introitus is the entrance to the vagina.

SYNONYMS: *Vaginal Orifice, Ostium Vaginae* (NA).

LABIA MAJORA

The labia majora are the longitudinal folds of fat that form the lateral boundaries of the vulva. The skin of the more prominent portion is pigmented. The major folds are rich in hair follicles and sebaceous and sudoriferous glands.

SYNONYM: *Labium Majus Pudendi* (NA).

LABIA MINORA

The labia minora are the longitudinal folds situated between the labia majora. The folds are composed of firm connective tissue with many large veins and some nonstriped muscle fibers resembling erectile tissue. Posteriorly, they join the labia majora to form the fourchette. Anteriorly, these folds separate, enclosing the clitoris and forming the frenulum posteriorly and the prepuce anteriorly.

SYNONYMS: *Nympha, Labium Minus Pudendi* (NA).

MEISSNER'S CORPUSCLES

Meissner's corpuscles are small, oval, sensitive structures present in the vulvar papillae.

SYNONYM: *Tactile Corpuscles.*

MONS PUBIS

The mons pubis is a cushion of fat covered by skin. It rests on the anterior surface of the pubic symphysis.

SYNONYMS: *Mons Veneris, Pubic Mound, Mons Pubis* (NA).

PACINIAN CORPUSCLES

Pacinian corpuscles are large oval bodies found in the deeper connective tissue of the labia majora and in the cavernous bodies of the clitoris.

PARAURETHRAL DUCTS

The paraurethral ducts are tiny tortuous canals that traverse just beneath the urethra for a distance of about 1.5 cm. The ducts are lined by one or two layers of transitional secretory epithelium. The paraurethral ducts open at the urethral orifice.

SYNONYMS: *Skene's Ducts, Schüller's Ducts, Ductus Paraurethrales* (NA).

PARAURETHRAL GLANDS

The paraurethral glands are relatively large glands situated just posterior and lateral to the urethral orifice.

SYNONYM: *Skene's Glands.*

SEBACEOUS GLANDS, VULVAR

The vulvar sebaceous glands are composed of several saccular pouches surrounded by a connective tissue sheath in the dermis. The glands contain large polygonal nucleated cells. They open freely on the surfaces of the labia minora.

SUDORIFEROUS GLANDS, VULVAR

The vulvar sudoriferous glands are coiled glands that secrete fluid onto the surface of the vulva. There are two types: apocrine glands and eccrine glands.

SYNONYM: *Sweat Glands of Vulva.*

Apocrine Glands, Vulvar

The vulvar apocrine glands secrete an odorous fluid and are related to the hair follicles on the mons pubis, labia majora, and perineum. Their cells contribute part of their protoplasmic substance to secretion.

SYNONYM: *Large Coiled Sweat Glands of Vulva.*

Eccrine Glands, Vulvar

The vulvar eccrine glands consist of modified tubular glands that secrete a fluid on the surface of the vulva except on the mucocutaneous surfaces.

SYNONYM: *Small Coiled Sweat Glands of Vulva.*

VESTIBULAR GLAND, MAJOR

The major vestibular gland is a racemose gland situated deep beneath the fascia of each labium major. The orifice of each gland is located at the middle of the lateral margin of the vaginal orifice. The main duct is lined by stratified transitional epithelium. The acini of the glands are lined by mucus-secreting epithelium.

SYNONYMS: *Bartholin's Gland, Duverney's Gland, Vulvovaginal Gland, Glandula Vestibularis Major* (NA).

VESTIBULAR GLAND, MINOR

The minor vestibular gland is one of the minute mucus-secreting glands on the surface of the vestibule.

SYNONYM: *Glandulae Vestibulares Minores* (NA).

VESTIBULE

The vestibule is the almond-shaped area enclosed by the labia minora. It extends from the clitoris to the fourchette and contains the urethral and vaginal orifices and openings of the ducts of the major vestibular gland and paraurethral glands.

SYNONYMS: *Vulvar Vestibule, Vestibulum Vaginae* (NA).

VULVAR SLIT

The vulvar slit is the opening or cleft between the labia majora.

SYNONYMS: *Pudendal Slit, Urogenital Cleft, Rima Vulvae, Rima Pudendi* (NA).

CLITORIS

CLITORIS

The clitoris is a small, cylindrical, erectile body, rarely exceeding 2 cm in length. It is situated at the most anterior portion of the vulva

and projects between the branched extremities of the labia minora, which form the prepuce and frenulum. It consists of a glans, a corpus, and two crura. It is the homologue of the penis in the male, but does not possess a corpus spongiosum and is not perforated by the urethra.
SYNONYM: *Clitoris* (NA).

Corpus of Clitoris
The corpus of the clitoris is the body of the clitoris. It contains two corpora cavernosa composed of erectile tissue and enclosed by a dense layer of fibrous membrane.
SYNONYM: *Corpus Clitoridis* (NA).

Crura of Clitoris
The crura of the clitoris are the continuations of the corpora cavernosa of the clitoris. The crura diverge from the body of the clitoris posteriorly and are attached to the pubic arch.
SYNONYM: *Crura Clitoridis* (NA).

Glans of Clitoris
The glans of the clitoris is the mass of erectile tissue capping the body of the clitoris.
SYNONYM: *Glans Clitoridis* (NA).

CORPUS CAVERNOSUM OF CLITORIS
The corpus cavernosum of the clitoris is one of the two parallel columns of erectile tissue forming the body of the clitoris.
SYNONYM: *Corpus Cavernosum Clitoridis* (NA).

FASCIA OF CLITORIS
The fascia of the clitoris is the firm fibrous sheath covering the crura of the clitoris.
SYNONYM: *Fascia Clitoridis* (NA).

FRENULUM OF CLITORIS
The frenulum of the clitoris is the fold of skin on the under surface of the clitoris.
SYNONYM: *Frenulum Clitoridis* (NA).

GENITAL CORPUSCLES
The genital corpuscles resemble end bulbs but are much larger. They are situated on the clitoris and anus.

PREPUCE OF CLITORIS
The prepuce of the clitoris is the external fold of the labia minora forming the cap over the glans of the clitoris.
SYNONYM: *Preputium Clitoridis* (NA).

SEPTUM OF CORPUS CAVERNOSUM
The septum of the corpus cavernosum is an incomplete fibrous comb-like wall between the corpora cavernosa.
SYNONYM: *Septum Corporum Cavernosorum* (NA).

HYMEN

HYMEN
    The hymen is a thin crescentic or annular mucous membrane that partially or completely occludes the external vaginal orifice.
    SYNONYM: *Hymen* (NA).

ANNULAR HYMEN
    An annular hymen is a hymen that has a circular opening.
    SYNONYM: *Hymen Annularis.*

BIFENESTRATE HYMEN
    A bifenestrate hymen is a hymen in which there are two openings separated by a wide band of tissue.
    SYNONYMS: *Hymen Bifenestratus, Hymen Biforis.*

CARUNCULAE MYRTIFORMES
    Carunculae myrtiformes are the numerous mucous membrane projections of the hymen after its rupture. They surround the vaginal orifice.
    SYNONYM: *Carunculae Hymenales* (NA).

CRESCENTIC HYMEN
    A crescentic hymen is a hymen with a long, half-moon appearance.
    SYNONYMS: *Hymen Crescentarius, Hymen Lunar.*

CRIBRIFORM HYMEN
    A cribriform hymen is a hymen with a number of small perforations.
    SYNONYM: *Hymen Cribriformis.*

DENTICULAR HYMEN
    A denticular hymen is a hymen with an opening that has serrated edges resembling teeth.
    SYNONYMS: *Denticulate Hymen, Hymen Denticulatus.*

IMPERFORATE HYMEN
    An imperforate hymen is a hymen without an opening. The vagina is completely occluded by a thin membrane of connective tissue.
    SYNONYM: *Hymen Imperforatus.*

INFANTILE HYMEN
    An infantile hymen is a thick resistant hymen with a small orifice.

INFUNDIBULIFORM HYMEN
    An infundibuliform hymen is a funnel-shaped hymen.
    SYNONYM: *Hymen Infundibuliformis.*

SCULPTATE HYMEN
    A sculptate hymen is a hymen with irregular and ragged edges.
    SYNONYM: *Hymen Sculptatus.*

SEMILUNAR HYMEN

A semilunar hymen is a hymen that has a crescent-shaped opening.
SYNONYM: *Hymen Semilunaris.*

SEPTATE HYMEN

A septate hymen is a hymen with two openings separated by a narrow band of tissue.
SYNONYM: *Hymen Septus.*

SUBSEPTATE HYMEN

A subseptate hymen is a hymen that is partially closed by a band of adventitious tissue.
SYNONYM: *Hymen Subseptus.*

VERTICAL HYMEN

A vertical hymen is a hymen in which the opening is perpendicular.
SYNONYM: *Hymen Verticalis.*

PERINEUM

PERINEUM

The perineum corresponds to the inferior aperture or outlet of the bony pelvis. The perineum includes all the soft parts, both muscle and fascia, that occupy that space.
SYNONYM: *Perineum* (NA).

ANAL SPHINCTER, EXTERNAL

The external anal sphincter is a flat, elliptical bundle of muscle fibers surrounding the lower margin of the anus. It arises from the anococcygeal body, encircles the terminal portion of the anal canal, and inserts into the perineal body. It normally closes the inferior aperture of the anus.
SYNONYM: *Musculus Sphincter Ani Externus* (NA).

ANAL SPHINCTER, INTERNAL

The internal anal sphincter is a ring of muscle composed chiefly of involuntary muscle fibers. It is situated superior to the external sphincter, and is contiguous to but not a part of it. It is a sphincter like its homologue.
SYNONYM: *Musculus Sphincter Ani Internus* (NA).

COLLES' FASCIA

Colles' fascia is a strong membrane in the urogenital region. It has a light yellow color owing to its content of elastic fibers, and it is smooth in texture. Ventrally, it is directly continuous with the deep layer of subcutaneous abdominal fascia (Scarpa's fascia) in the groove between the labium and thigh. Laterally, it is firmly adherent to the medial surface of the thigh along the ischiopubic ramus at the origin of the adductor muscles. Dorsally, it dips inward toward the ischiorectal fossa

around the posterior border of the superficial transverse perineal muscle
and becomes firmly attached to the deep fascia along the posterior border
of the deep transverse perineal muscle. It is attached also, with all the
other layers, to the perineal body. There is a distinct fascial cleft between
Colles' fascia and the external perineal fascia (deep fascia) over the
bulbocavernosus, ischiocavernosus, and superficial transverse perineal
muscles. This superficial perineal cleft is continuous with the cleft under
Scarpa's fascia on the anterior abdominal wall, but it is closed off laterally
and posteriorly by the attachments just described.

SYNONYM: *Fascia Perinei Superficialis* (NA).

CORPUS SPONGIOSUM OF FEMALE URETHRA

The corpus spongiosum of the female urethra is a thin layer of erectile
tissue surrounding the urethra, between the muscular coat and the
mucosa. It contains a plexus of veins and some fibers of smooth muscle.

DIAPHRAGM, PELVIC

The pelvic diaphragm is the main support of the pelvic viscera. The
obturator internus and the piriformis muscles are not strictly components
of the pelvic diaphragm. They are mentioned here because the fascia of
the obturator internus contributes much to the fascia of the pelvis, and
because the piriformis muscle, posterior to the coccygeus, completes the
posterior closure of the inferior aperture (outlet) of the pelvis. Each of
these muscles originates in the true pelvis but becomes inserted into the
lower extremity, outside the pelvic cavity. The levator ani muscle on
each side is covered, both on its superior surface (superior levator fascia)
and its inferior surface (anal fascia), by a layer of dense fascia, collectively termed *pelvic fascia* or *levator fascia*. These fascial layers, at each
side of the pelvis, fuse with each other and with the fascia covering the
inner surface of each obturator internus muscle. The ridge created by
this triple fusion of several fascial layers has an unmistakable appearance. It extends downward and dorsad on each side to the ischial
spines. It is referred to as the *arcus tendineus of the levatores ani,* or
the *white line of fused fascia.* Slightly below and medial to the white
line, the superior levator fascia thickens to form a ridge, or base, of
fascia, the *tela endopelvina of the visceral fascia,* that divides into four
layers. One layer invests the bladder; the second lies loosely between the
lower uterine segment, upper portion of the vagina, and the bladder.
The third layer lies between the vagina and rectum, and the fourth is
situated posterior to the rectum.

SYNONYM: *Diaphragma Pelvis* (NA).

DIAPHRAGM, UROGENITAL

The urogenital diaphragm is composed of two flat layers of thin fascia
in the anterior urogenital triangle of the perineum on each side of the
midline. Between the two layers are enclosed the structures of the
deep compartment. The superficial compartment lies between the layer
of fascia that is the floor of the deep compartment and the dense

layer of the deep superficial fascia known as *Colles' fascia.* Thus the floor of the superficial (inferior) compartment is Colles' fascia. Its roof is the inferior layer of the fascia of the urogenital diaphragm, which is likewise the floor of the deep (superior) compartment. The roof of the superior compartment is contiguous to the inferior fascia of the levator ani muscle.

SYNONYMS: *Triangular Ligament, Urogenital Trigone, Diaphragma Urogenitale* (NA).

Superficial Compartment of Urogenital Diaphragm

The superficial compartment of the urogenital diaphragm is composed of the ischiocavernosus, the bulbospongiosus, and the superficial transverse perineal muscles.

Deep Compartment of Urogenital Diaphragm

The deep compartment of the urogenital diaphragm is composed of the sphincter muscle of the membranous urethra and the deep transverse perineal muscle.

LYMPHATIC VESSELS OF PERINEUM AND EXTERNAL GENITALIA

The lymphatic vessels of the perineum and external genitalia follow the course of the external pudendal vessels; they end in the superficial inguinal and subinguinal lymph nodes. The lymphatic vessels of the clitoris terminate partly in the deep subinguinal lymph nodes and partly in the external iliac lymph nodes.

MUSCLE, BULBOSPONGIOSUS

The bulbospongiosus muscle is a paired muscle, one on each side of the vagina. Its function in the female is to constrict the lumen of the vagina near the introitus, and to constrict the bulbous urethra (in both sexes). In the female, some fibers terminate in the corpora cavernosa of the clitoris.

SYNONYMS: *Constrictor Cunni, Sphincter Vaginae, Bulbocavernosus Muscle, Musculus Bulbospongiosus* (NA).

MUSCLE, COCCYGEUS

The coccygeus muscle is a paired muscle lying between the levator ani muscle anteriorly and the piriformis muscle posteriorly. It assists in closing the posterior portion of the pelvic outlet and is considered a part of the pelvic floor. It supports the coccyx.

SYNONYM: *Musculus Coccygeus* (NA).

MUSCLE, ISCHIOCAVERNOSUS

The ischiocavernosus muscle is the erector muscle of the clitoris; it occupies the lateral portion of the superficial compartment of the urogenital diaphragm. Arising from the tuberosity and ramus of the ischium, it inserts into the sides and inferior surface of the crus of the clitoris.

SYNONYMS: *Erector Clitoridis, Musculus Ischiocavernosus* (NA).

MUSCLE, LEVATOR ANI

The levator ani muscle is the main support of the pelvic floor and pelvic viscera. Mainly, it consists of the iliococcygeus portion and the pubococcygeus portion. With its superior and inferior layers of fascia, it is called the pelvic diaphragm.

SYNONYM: *Musculus Levator Ani* (NA).

Iliococcygeus Muscle

The iliococcygeus muscle of the levator ani is the lateral portion of the levator ani muscle. It arises from the white line of the tendinous arch of the obturator internus fascia. It inserts into the perineal body, the anococcygeal body, and into the margin of the coccyx.

SYNONYM: *Musculus Iliococcygeus* (NA).

Pubococcygeus Muscle

The pubococcygeus muscle of the levator ani is the medial portion of the levator ani muscle. It originates from the pubis on either side of the vagina and proceeds posteriorly. Some fibers mingle with longitudinal fibers of the vaginal wall and with the bulbospongiosus fibers. Others decussate in the perineal body; the main portion mingles somewhat with the external sphincter but mainly with the anococcygeal body posterior to the sphincter.

SYNONYM: *Musculus Pubococcygeus* (NA).

MUSCLE, PUBORECTAL

The puborectal muscle is composed of fibers of the pubococcygeal muscle that mingle with the external anal sphincter and the anus.

SYNONYM: *Musculus Puborectalis* (NA).

MUSCLE, PUBOVESICAL

The pubovesical muscle consists of a few smooth muscle fibers, by which the base of the bladder is attached to the internal investing layer of deep fascia on the pubic bone.

SYNONYM: *Musculus Pubovesicalis* (NA).

MUSCLE, RECTOCOCCYGEUS

The rectococcygeus muscle is one of two bands of muscular tissue arising from the coccyx and blending with the posterior longitudinal muscle of the posterior anal wall.

SYNONYM: *Musculus Rectococcygeus* (NA).

MUSCLE, RECTOUTERINE

The rectouterine muscle is a nonstriped muscle in the rectouterine fold.

SYNONYM: *Musculus Rectouterinus* (NA).

MUSCLE, RECTOVESICAL

The rectovesical muscle is composed of nonstriped muscle fibers in the sacrogenital folds that run from the bladder fundus to the sides of the rectum. Usually, it is absent in the female.

SYNONYM: *Musculus Rectovesicalis* (NA).

MUSCLE, TRANSVERSE PERINEAL, DEEP
The deep transverse perineal muscle is a paired muscle. It lies in the deep compartment of the anterior triangle and sends a few fibers to the vaginal wall. Mainly, like its more superficial homologue, it maintains the integrity of the perineal body.

SYNONYM: *Musculus Transversus Perinei Profundus* (NA).

MUSCLE, TRANSVERSE PERINEAL, SUPERFICIAL
The superficial transverse perineal muscle is a narrow, paired muscle in the superficial (inferior) compartment of the anterior triangle. It supports the perineal body.

SYNONYM: *Musculus Transversus Perinei Superficialis* (NA).

MUSCLE, URETHRAL SPHINCTER
The urethral sphincter muscle is a delicate muscle located in the deep compartment of the anterior triangle. It acts as a compressor, or sphincter, of the urethra.

SYNONYMS: *Sphincter Urethrae Membranaceae, Constrictor Urethrae, Musculus Sphincter Urethrae* (NA).

PERINEAL BODY
The perineal body is the wedge-shaped composite of all the soft tissues that together compose the septum separating the vagina from the anus. It constitutes only a part of the perineum.

SYNONYMS: *Obstetric Perineum, Central Perineal Body, Central Tendon of the Perineum, Median Raphe, Centrum Tendineum Perinei* (NA).

WHITE LINE OF OBTURATOR INTERNUS FASCIA
The white line of obturator internus fascia is a thickened band of the obturator fascia attached posteriorly to the spine of the ischium and anteriorly to the pubic bone at the anterior margin of the obturator membrane.

SYNONYM: *Arcus Tendineus Musculi Levatoris Ani* (NA).

VAGINA

VAGINA
The vagina is a musculomembranous canal extending from the vestibule to the cervix of the uterus. The vagina generally measures 6 to 7.5 cm along its anterior wall and 9 cm along the posterior wall. The vaginal wall has three layers: internal mucous membrane, middle muscular layer, and external connective tissue layer.

SYNONYM: *Vagina* (NA).

COLUMNS OF VAGINA
The columns of the vagina are two longitudinal ridges in the vaginal mucosa, one anterior and one posterior.

SYNONYMS: *Columna Vaginalis, Vaginal Longitudinal Ridge, Columnae Rugarum* (NA).

CONNECTIVE TISSUE LAYER OF VAGINA
The connective tissue layer of the vagina is a layer of tissue that surrounds the vagina and contains a large plexus of blood vessels and occasional small lymphoid nodules.

GERMINAL LAYER OF CELLS OF VAGINA
The germinal layer of cells of the vagina forms the basal layer of epithelial cells of the vaginal mucosa. Germinal cells are rarely found on vaginal smears.

INNER BASAL LAYER OF CELLS OF VAGINA
The inner basal layer of cells of the vagina is composed of small round cells of the vaginal mucosa. They have deeply staining cyanophilic cytoplasm.

INTROITUS
The introitus is the entrance to the vagina.
SYNONYMS: *Vaginal Orifice, Ostium Vaginae* (NA).

LYMPHATIC VESSELS OF VAGINA
The lymphatic vessels of the vagina are carried in three directions: those of the upper part of the vagina to the external iliac lymph nodes, those of the middle part to the internal iliac lymph nodes, and those of the lower part to the common iliac lymph nodes. Small nodes are situated along the course of the vessels from the middle and lower parts. Some lymphatic vessels from the lower part of the vagina join those of the vulva and pass to the superficial inguinal lymph nodes. The lymphatic vessels of the vagina anastomose with those of the cervix, vulva, and rectum, but not with those of the bladder.

PARACOLPIUM
The paracolpium comprises the tissues alongside the vagina.

RUGAE
The rugae are numerous transverse folds of the vaginal mucosa.
SYNONYMS: *Vaginal Folds, Rugae Vaginales* (NA).

UTEROVAGINAL CANAL
The uterovaginal canal is the canal formed by fusion of the paramesonephric ducts.
SYNONYM: *Leuckart's Canal.*

VAGINAL CARINA
The vaginal carina is the lower part of the anterior vaginal column accentuated by the subadjacent urethra.
SYNONYMS: *Urethral Ridge, Carina Vaginae, Carina Urethralis Vaginae* (NA).

VAGINAL FORNIX

The vaginal fornix is an arch or pocket at the upper end of the vagina. SYNONYMS: *Vaginal Vault, Vaginal Apex, Fornix Vaginae* (NA).

Vaginal Fornix, Anterior

The anterior vaginal fornix is the space at the upper end of the vagina, anterior to the cervix of the uterus and posterior to the bladder.

Vaginal Fornix, Lateral

The lateral vaginal fornix is the space at the upper end of the vagina, on either side of the cervix of the uterus.

Vaginal Fornix, Posterior

The posterior vaginal fornix is the space at the upper end of the vagina, behind the cervix of the uterus, in front of the rectum, and below the rectouterine pouch.

VAGINAL GLAND

A vaginal gland is one of the minute glands in the mucous membrane of the vagina. Vaginal glands are not true glands.

VAGINAL MUCOUS MEMBRANE

The vaginal mucous membrane is the lining membrane of the vagina. It is composed of layers of stratified squamous epithelium that are responsive to ovarian steroids. The mucous membrane has two longitudinal folds that extend laterally to form rugae. It is composed of three layers of cells beginning at the basement membrane: germinal, transitional or basal, and superficial.

VAGINAL MUSCULAR LAYERS

The vaginal muscular layers are composed of an external longitudinal and an inner circular muscle layer. At the lower end of the vagina is a band of striped muscle fibers.

Circular Muscle Layer of Vagina

The circular muscle layer of the vagina is the inner layer of muscle surrounding the vagina.

Longitudinal Muscle Layer of Vagina

The longitudinal muscle layer of the vagina is the outer layer of muscle that runs parallel with the vaginal lumen.

VAGINAL WALL, ANTERIOR

The anterior vaginal wall is situated posterior to the bladder and urethra. SYNONYM: *Paries Anterior* (NA).

VAGINAL WALL, POSTERIOR

The posterior vaginal wall is situated anterior to the rectum and anus. SYNONYM: *Paries Posterior* (NA).

Bladder

BLADDER

The bladder is a distensible musculomembranous organ that serves as a receptacle for urine. It is located dorsal to the pubic symphysis and ventral to the uterus. It is covered by loose connective tissue except at the trigone and base, where the areolar layer is thicker and stronger. The detrusor urinae muscle comprises all the bladder musculature except the trigone. The bladder is lined with transitional epithelium upon a loose lamina propria except at the trigone. The arterial supply is derived from the inferior and pudendal arteries. Veins drain into the vesico-vaginal and pubic plexuses. The lymphatic vessels drain into the internal iliac and inguinal lymph nodes in association with lymphatic vessels about the neck of the bladder.

SYNONYM: *Vesica Urinaria* (NA).

Apex of Bladder

The apex of the bladder is the junction of the superior and infero-lateral surfaces of the bladder. It is continuous with the middle umbilical ligament.

SYNONYMS: *Vertex of Bladder, Apex Vesicae* (NA).

Body of Bladder

The body of the bladder is the part of the bladder between the apex and the fundus.

SYNONYM: *Corpus Vesicae* (NA).

Fundus of Bladder

The fundus of the bladder is the base or posterior portion of the bladder.

SYNONYM: *Fundus Vesicae* (NA).

BLADDER MUCOSA

The bladder mucosa is composed of transitional epithelium on a loose base, except at the trigone.

BLADDER SPHINCTER

The bladder sphincter is a thickening of the middle muscular layer of the bladder around the urethral opening.

INTERURETERIC FOLD

The interureteric fold is a fold of mucous membrane extending from the orifice of the ureter on either side to the median line of the bladder.

SYNONYMS: *Plica Ureterica, Plica Interureterica* (NA).

LIGAMENT, LATERAL FALSE
The lateral false ligament consists of peritoneal folds extending between the sides of the bladder and the lateral walls of the pelvic cavity.

LIGAMENT, MIDDLE UMBILICAL
The middle umbilical ligament is a fibrous cord extending from the apex of the bladder to the umbilicus. It represents the remnants of the urachus.

SYNONYM: *Ligamentum Umbilicale Medianum* (NA).

LIGAMENT, POSTERIOR FALSE
The posterior false ligament contains the obliterated internal iliac arteries, ureters, vessels, and nerves passing to the bladder.

SYNONYMS: *Uterovesical Ligament, Uterovesical Plica, Sacrogenital Fold.*

LIGAMENTS, PUBOVESICAL
The pubovesical ligaments are a condensation of the connective tissue that extends from the lower part of the anterior wall of the bladder and upper urethra, through the space of Retzius, to the posterior surface of the pubic bones at the sides of the pubic symphysis.

SYNONYM: *Ligamentum Pubovesicale* (NA).

LIGAMENTS, RECTOVESICAL
The rectovesical ligaments are condensations of the subserous fascia underlying the posterior false ligaments. They secure the base of the bladder posteriorly to the sides of the rectum and the sacrum.

LYMPHATIC VESSELS OF BLADDER
The lymphatic vessels of the bladder originate in two plexuses—intramuscular and extramuscular—for it is generally acknowledged that the mucous membrane is devoid of lymphatic vessels. The efferent vessels are arranged in two groups, one from the anterior and another from the posterior surface of the bladder. The vessels from the anterior surface pass to the external iliac lymph nodes. The vessels from the posterior surface pass to the internal, external, and common iliac lymph nodes; those draining the upper part of this surface traverse the lateral vesical lymph nodes.

LYMPHATIC VESSELS OF URETER
The lymphatic vessels of the ureter run in different directions. Those from its upper portion end partly in the efferent lymphatic vessels of the kidney and partly in the lateral aortic lymph nodes. The lymphatic vessels from the portion immediately above the brim of the lesser pelvis are drained into the common iliac lymph nodes; the vessels from the intrapelvic portion of the tube either join the efferents from the bladder or end in the internal iliac lymph nodes.

TORUS URETERICUS
The torus uretericus is a smooth ridge in the bladder wall stretching between the ureteral orifices. It forms the base of the trigone.

TRANSVERSE VESICAL FOLD
The transverse vesical fold is a fold of peritoneum appearing when the bladder is empty, but absent when the bladder is full.
SYNONYM: *Plica Vesicalis Transversa* (NA).

TRIGONE
The trigone is the triangular area of the bladder between the ureteral orifices and the internal urethral opening.
SYNONYM: *Trigonum Vesicae* (NA).

URACHUS
The urachus is the allantoic duct that opens into the apex of the bladder. It involutes to form a cord. Occasionally, the urachus remains patent and forms a tube opening at the umbilicus. Anomalies of the urachus consist of various forms of patent urachus, including urachal fistulas and cysts.
SYNONYM: *Urachus* (NA).

URETER
The ureter is one of the two tubes that convey urine from the kidneys to the urinary bladder. The ureter forms, as it lies in relation to the wall of the pelvis, the posterior boundary of a shallow depression named the *ovarian fossa*, in which the ovary is situated. It then runs mediad and forward on the lateral aspect of the cervix and upper part of the vagina to reach the fundus of the bladder. In this part of its course, it is accompanied for about 2.5 cm by the uterine artery, which then crosses over the ureter and ascends between the two layers of the broad ligament. The ureter is situated about 2 cm from the side of the cervix of the uterus.
SYNONYM: *Ureter* (NA).

VESICAL GLAND
The vesical gland is one of several mucous follicles in the mucous membrane near the neck of the bladder. It is not a true gland.
SYNONYM: *Glandula Vesicalis*.

URETHRA

URETHRA
The urethra is a tubular structure 3 to 5.5 cm in length and 7 to 10 mm in diameter. It extends from the urethral opening of the bladder to the urinary meatus and lies close to the anterior vaginal wall. It is composed of inner longitudinal and outer circular muscular layers and mucous membrane lining. The urethra is divided into three portions: membranous, pelvic, and vaginal.
SYNONYMS: *Urethra Muliebris, Urethra Feminina* (NA).

Membranous Portion of Urethra

The membranous portion of the urethra is that section of the urethra between the layers of the urogenital diaphragm.

Pelvic Portion of Urethra

The pelvic portion of the urethra is that section of the urethra between the bladder and the urogenital diaphragm.

Vaginal Portion of Urethra

The vaginal portion of the urethra is that section of the urethra between the urogenital diaphragm and the urethral orifice.

CORPUS SPONGIOSUM OF FEMALE URETHRA

The corpus spongiosum of the female urethra is a thin layer of erectile tissue surrounding the urethra, between the muscular coat and the mucosa. It contains a plexus of veins and some fibers of smooth muscle.

LYMPHATIC VESSELS OF URETHRA

The lymphatic vessels of the urethra pass to the internal iliac lymph nodes.

MUCOUS MEMBRANE LINING OF URETHRA

The mucous membrane lining of the urethra is composed for the most part of transitional epithelium except near the external orifice. Stratified squamous epithelium of the vaginal mucosa extends into the canal for a short distance. The mucosa of the urethra contains branched tubular glands.

MUSCULAR LAYER OF URETHRA

The muscular layer of the urethra is composed of an inner and an outer longitudinal muscle layer and a circular muscle layer.

PARAURETHRAL DUCTS

The paraurethral ducts are tiny tortuous canals that traverse just beneath the urethra for a distance of about 1.5 cm. The ducts are lined by one or two layers of transitional secretory epithelium. The paraurethral ducts open at the urethral orifice.

SYNONYMS: *Skene's Ducts, Schüller's Ducts, Ductus Paraurethrales* (NA).

PARAURETHRAL GLANDS

The paraurethral glands are relatively large glands situated just posterior and lateral to the urethral orifice.

SYNONYM: *Skene's Glands.*

URETHRAL CREST

The urethral crest is a longitudinal fold of the posterior urethral wall.

SYNONYM: *Crista Urethralis* (NA).

URETHRAL GLANDS

The urethral glands are many small glands that open into the urethra. In the female, the largest of these glands are called the paraurethral glands.

SYNONYMS: *Morgagni's Gland, Littre's Gland, Glandulae Urethrales (NA).*

URETHRAL ORIFICE

The urethral orifice is the outlet of the urethra. The orifice is situated posterior to the frenulum of the clitoris and anterior to the vaginal orifice.

SYNONYMS: *Urethral Meatus, Ostium Urethrae Externum (NA).*

URETHRAL SPHINCTER MUSCLE

The urethral sphincter muscle is a delicate muscle located in the deep compartment of the anterior triangle. It acts as a compressor, or sphincter, of the urethra.

SYNONYMS: *Sphincter Urethrae Membranaceae, Constrictor Urethrae, Musculus Sphincter Urethrae (NA).*

Rectum

RECTUM

The rectum is the portion of the large bowel that begins where the pelvic mesocolon ends. It is composed of two parts. The first part is 10 to 12 cm long and extends forward following the curve of the sacrum and coccyx. The second portion (anal canal) begins on the pelvic floor and curves downward and backward to the anus. The anal canal is from 2.5 to 3.5 cm in length and passes through the pelvic floor. The lower end is entirely surrounded by the two sphincter muscles. The rectum has a well-defined longitudinal muscle layer that is better developed anteriorly and posteriorly than laterally. Structures of importance are the valves of Houston, anal columns, crypts, and papillae. The blood supply is from the superior and middle rectal arteries. The inferior rectal branch of the internal pudendal artery provides the blood below the anorectal line. The innervation is sympathetic above the dentate line; below the anoderm area, it is part of the central nervous system.

SYNONYM: *Rectum* (NA).

ANAL SPHINCTER, INTERNAL

The internal anal sphincter is a ring of muscle composed chiefly of involuntary muscle fibers. It is situated superior to the external sphincter, and is contiguous to but not a part of it. It is a sphincter like its homologue.

SYNONYM: *Musculus Sphincter Ani Internus* (NA).

LEVATOR ANI MUSCLE

The levator ani muscle is the main support of the pelvic floor and pelvic viscera. Mainly, it consists of the iliococcygeus portion and the pubococcygeus portion. With its superior and inferior layers of fascia, it is called the pelvic diaphragm.

SYNONYM: *Musculus Levator Ani* (NA).

Iliococcygeus Muscle

The iliococcygeus muscle of the levator ani is the lateral portion of the levator ani muscle. It arises from the white line of the tendinous arch of the obturator internus fascia. It inserts into the perineal body, the anococcygeal body, and into the margin of the coccyx.

SYNONYM: *Musculus Iliococcygeus* (NA).

Pubococcygeus Muscle

The pubococcygeus muscle of the levator ani is the medial portion of the levator ani muscle. It originates from the pubis on either side of the vagina and proceeds posteriorly. Some fibers mingle with longitudinal fibers of the vaginal wall and with the bulbospongiosus fibers. Others decussate in the perineal body; the main portion mingles somewhat with the external sphincter but mainly with the anococcygeal body posterior to the sphincter.

SYNONYM: *Musculus Pubococcygeus* (NA).

LONGITUDINAL MUSCLE LAYER OF RECTUM

The longitudinal muscle layer of the rectum consists of muscle fibers that are parallel to the rectum. They are better developed anteriorly and posteriorly than laterally.

LYMPHATIC VESSELS OF RECTUM

The lymphatic vessels of the rectum traverse the pararectal glands and pass to those in the sigmoid mesocolon; the efferents of the latter terminate in the preaortic lymph nodes around the origin of the inferior mesenteric artery.

PUBORECTAL MUSCLE

The puborectal muscle is composed of fibers of the pubococcygeal muscle that mingle with the external anal sphincter and the anus.

SYNONYM: *Musculus Puborectalis* (NA).

RECTOCOCCYGEUS MUSCLE

The rectococcygeus muscle is one of two bands of muscular tissue arising from the coccyx and blending with the posterior longitudinal muscle of the posterior anal wall.

SYNONYM: *Musculus Rectococcygeus* (NA).

RECTOUTERINE MUSCLE

The rectouterine muscle is a nonstriped muscle in the rectouterine fold.

SYNONYM: *Musculus Rectouterinus* (NA).

RECTOVESICAL MUSCLE

The rectovesical muscle is composed of nonstriped muscle fibers in the sacrogenital folds that run from the bladder fundus to the sides of the rectum. Usually, it is absent in the female.

SYNONYM: *Musculus Rectovesicalis* (NA).

VALVES OF HOUSTON

The valves of Houston are three or four crescentic folds situated horizontally in the rectal mucous membrane. One fold is situated near the beginning of the rectum on the right side; a second one projects from the left side at a slightly lower level; a third is directed backward from the anterior wall at the level of the fundus of the urinary bladder.

SYNONYMS: *Kohlrausch Valves, Transverse Folds of Rectum, Rectal Valves, Plicae Transversales Recti* (NA).

ANUS

ANUS

The anus is the external opening of the intestinal tract. Sphincters surround the terminal portion of the anal canal. The internal anal sphincter is a thickening of the circular muscle fibers of the rectum. The voluntary muscles of the rectum and anus are the external anal sphincter, levator ani, and rectococcygeal muscles. The nerve supply is from the fourth sacral nerve and small branch of the internal pudendal nerve.

SYNONYM: *Anus* (NA).

ANAL COLUMNS

The anal columns are situated in the anal canal and consist of a series of longitudinal folds of mucous membrane containing some smooth muscle fibers. The folds become more prominent downward and just above the anus. The columns are united by an archlike fold of mucous membrane.

SYNONYMS: *Anal Columns of Morgagni, Rectal Columns of Morgagni, Columnae Anales* (NA).

ANAL CRYPTS

Anal crypts are small fossae behind the anal valves.

ANAL PAPILLAE

The anal papillae are small papillary fibrous structures on the anal surface of the rectal folds.

ANAL SINUSES

The anal sinuses are furrows in the lumen of the anal canal that separate the anal columns from one another. They end in the anal valves.

SYNONYMS: *Rectal Sinuses, Sinus Anales* (NA).

ANAL SPHINCTER, EXTERNAL

The external anal sphincter is a flat, elliptical bundle of muscle fibers surrounding the lower margin of the anus. It arises from the anococcygeal body, encircles the terminal portion of the anal canal, and inserts into the perineal body. It normally closes the inferior aperture of the anus.

SYNONYM: *Musculus Sphincter Ani Externus* (NA).

ANAL VALVES

The anal valves are folds of the mucous membrane of the anal columns.

SYNONYM: *Valvulae Anales* (NA).

CIRCUMANAL GLAND

The circumanal gland is one of the large apocrine sweat glands surrounding the anus.

SYNONYM: *Glandula Circumanalis* (NA).

GENITAL CORPUSCLES

The genital corpuscles resemble end bulbs but are much larger. They are situated on the clitoris and anus.

Section 3: *Diseases and Conditions of Generative Organs*

SECTION 3: DISEASES AND CONDITIONS OF GENERATIVE ORGANS

Breast

ABSCESS, BREAST

A breast abscess is a late, usually suppurative, sequel to acute mastitis.

ABSCESS, SUBMAMMARY

A submammary abscess is a form of mastitis in which the infection passes directly through the gland to the areolar tissue.

SYNONYMS: *Submammary Mastitis, Retromammary Mastitis.*

ADENOSIS, SCLEROSING, MAMMARY

Mammary sclerosing adenosis is characterized by multiple, firm, tender nodules in the breast, small cysts, increased fibrous tissue, and mastodynia. Microscopically, spilling of the epithelial cells into the stroma can be observed.

AGALACTIA

Agalactia is the absence of lactation.

AMASTIA

Amastia is the absence of breasts.

COMEDOMASTITIS

Comedomastitis is a condition, generally in elderly women, in which it feels as if there were a mass of worms beneath the areola. Toothpaste-like debris can be expressed from the retracted nipple. It results from inspissation of desquamated debris. Comedomastitis is sometimes difficult to distinguish from comedocarcinoma.

SYNONYMS: *Ductule Ectasia, Mammary Duct Ectasia.*

DYSPLASIA, MAMMARY

Mammary dysplasia is abnormal tissue development, primarily a reflection of ovarian hormonal imbalance.

ENGORGEMENT, BREAST

Breast engorgement is a temporary inflammatory condition caused by increased blood flow preceding the formation of milk. It is characterized by fullness, redness, and hardness of the breast.

SYNONYMS: *Caked Breast, Stagnation Mastitis.*

FATTY NECROSIS, MAMMARY

Mammary fatty necrosis is a peculiar and unusual breast tumor occasionally encountered in fat, pendulous breasts following injury. A history of physical violence to the breasts, however, is elicited in less than half the women with this condition. Mammary fatty necrosis may be associated with a suppurative disease of the breast, with carcinoma, with ischemia produced by pressure, and with breast biopsy procedures. Symptoms may be present for months or years. A hard, somewhat fixed lump in the absence of discoloration of the skin easily may be clinically misinterpreted as a malignant tumor. In the early stages, the lesion appears as a well-defined, firm, solid, homogeneous, lardaceous substance. As necrosis progresses, it may change to a light yellow, orange, brown, or brownish red color, depending on the presence or absence of hemorrhage. Cyst formation, hemorrhage, calcification, stellate scarring, and fixation are almost constant in the old lesion. Histologic architecture of acute inflammation in the adipose tissue may be more striking than fat necrosis. Polymorphonuclear cells, plasma cells, lymphocytes, and monocytes are constant. The monocytes may be of epithelioid or foam type, but they generally form foreign-body giant cells. Early stages of the disease present opaque fat cells (fat saponification), and later there is found true necrosis, with cholesterol crystals (sharp, angular clefts) and calcifications present.

GALACTORRHEA

Galactorrhea is the constant leakage of milk from the breast.

HYPERTROPHY, MAMMARY

Mammary hypertrophy is enlargement of the breast. It may be bilateral or unilateral. The breast becomes enormous because of increased fibrous stroma and hypertrophied ducts. This condition is irreversible and can be treated only by plastic surgery. The most dramatic form of mammary hypertrophy is *gigantomastia of pregnancy.*

SYNONYMS: *Macromastia, Macromazia, Mastauxe.*

HYPERTROPHY, PRECOCIOUS MAMMARY

Precocious mammary hypertrophy is symmetrical, bilateral enlargement of the breasts. It is usually associated with endocrine disturbances.

HYPOMASTIA

Hypomastia is underdevelopment of the female breast. It may be associated with hypogonadism.

MAMMILLITIS

Mammillitis is inflammation of the nipple.

SYNONYMS: *Thelitis, Mammary Papillitis.*

MASTADENITIS

Mastadenitis is inflammation of the mammary gland.

MASTATROPHY

Mastatrophy is atrophy of the breast.

MASTITIS, ACUTE

Acute mastitis is acute inflammation of the breast usually associated with a cracked or fissured nipple and occurring in the period of lactation.

MASTITIS, GARGANTUAN

Gargantuan mastitis is chronic inflammation of the breast with great enlargement of the gland.

MASTITIS, GLANDULAR

Glandular mastitis is an inflammatory disease of the breast that involves the lactiferous tubules.

SYNONYMS: *Galactophoritis, Parenchymatous Mastitis.*

MASTITIS, INTERSTITIAL

Interstitial mastitis is an inflammatory disease of the breast in which bacteria gain access to the connective tissue through a crack or deep fissure. The infection occurs in the fat around the lobes or lobules.

SYNONYMS: *Phlegmonous Mastitis, Lymphangitis Mastitis.*

MASTITIS, PERIDUCTAL

Periductal mastitis is inflammation of tissues about the ducts of the mammary gland. It is caused by escape into the stroma of the secretion that results from abnormal hormonal stimulation of the gland.

MASTITIS, PLASMA CELL

Plasma cell mastitis is an inflammatory condition of the breast, usually affecting multiparas approaching menopause. Stasis and inspissation are present making this a chemical rather than a bacterial inflammation. Induration of the mass is questionable. The microscopic appearance is similar to that in tuberculosis. However, polymorphonuclear leukocytes and plasma cells are present. No caseation or bacilli can be observed. The lesion is very radiosensitive.

MASTITIS, PUERPERAL

Puerperal mastitis is an inflammation of the breast that occurs in the puerperium.

MASTITIS, SUPPURATIVE

Suppurative mastitis is inflammation of the breast due to infection with pyogenic bacteria.

MASTITIS, TUBERCULOUS

Tuberculous mastitis occurs infrequently, usually in a patient with an acute focus of tuberculosis elsewhere. It is characterized by painless induration and nodularity in the breast. The clinical course may be protracted; if so, multiple sinuses eventually form. There is involvement of the axillary lymph nodes. Biopsy is better than culture to establish the diagnosis. Grossly, caseation may be observed; microscopically, typical tubercles are seen.

MASTODYNIA

Mastodynia is breast pain. In the young, it is associated with areas of fibrosis and small cyst formation. In menopausal and obese women, it is due to pendulous breasts.

SYNONYMS: *Mastalgia, Mammary Neuralgia, Mazodynia, Mammalgia.*

MASTOPATHY, CYSTIC

Cystic mastopathy is a morbid condition of the mammary gland with the formation of cysts.

MASTOPTOSIS

Mastoptosis is ptosis or sagging of the breast.

MASTORRHAGIA

Mastorrhagia is hemorrhage from a breast.

MASTOSYRINX

Mastosyrinx is a fistula of the breast.

POLYGALACTIA

Polygalactia is the excessive flow of milk from the breast.

POLYMASTIA

Polymastia is a condition in which accessory breasts and nipples are present in various locations of the body.

SYNONYM: *Supernumerary Breasts.*

POLYTHELIA

Polythelia is the presence of accessory nipples along the milk line.

STEWART-TREVES SYNDROME

The Stewart-Treves syndrome is characterized by the late development of an angiosarcoma in an edematous upper extremity after radical breast surgery. The condition occurs in women between 44 and 68 years of age with no history of delayed healing, postoperative infection, or thrombosis. Postmastectomy edema usually appears in the arm on the operated side within a year and gradually spreads to involve the hand and fingers. Other manifestations include minor atrophy of the skin, hyperkeratoses, spontaneous telangiectasia, and febrile bouts with true erysipelas or erysipeloid changes. After an interval varying from 6 to 24 years, there appears a single, purplish red, subdermal, slightly raised, macular or polypoid lesion in the skin of the arm or antecubital area. Later, additional lesions develop on the forearm, hand, and thorax with all stages of ulceration, discharge, and healing. The lesions do not resemble the cutaneous nodules of recurrent mammary cancer and are distinct from the early mammary lesion. It is suggested that the syndrome is probably due to a systemic carcinogenic factor. Differential diagnosis should exclude metastatic carcinoma and Kaposi's sarcoma.

SYNONYM: *Postmastectomy Lymphangiosarcoma Syndrome.*

Fallopian Tubes and Ovaries

HYDROSALPINX
Hydrosalpinx is an accumulation of serous fluid in the fallopian tube, often resulting from a pyosalpinx. The tube is enlarged with thin walls, and the fimbriated end is inverted and obliterated.

OOPHORITIS
Oophoritis is an inflammation of the ovary, generally associated with pelvic inflammatory disease.
SYNONYM: *Ovaritis.*

OVARIUM BIPARTITUM
Ovarium bipartitum is an ovary separated into two parts.

OVARIUM DISJUNCTUM
Ovarium disjunctum is an ovary more or less completely divided into two parts.

OVARIUM GYRATUM
Ovarium gyratum is an ovary showing curved or irregular grooves or furrows.

OVARIUM LOBATUM
Ovarium lobatum is an ovary divided by furrows into two or more parts or lobes.

OVARY, ACCESSORY
An accessory ovary is ovarian tissue situated near the normally placed ovary. It may be connected to the normal ovary and seems to have developed from it.

OVARY, SUPERNUMERARY
A supernumerary ovary is an extra ovary entirely separate from the other ovaries.

POLYCYSTIC OVARIAN DISEASE
Polycystic ovarian disease is an entity associated with polycystic ovaries and clinical symptoms and signs such as oligomenorrhea, anovulation, infertility, and hirsutism. Grossly, the ovaries are enlarged and oyster gray, with a firm, smooth cortex indicating no evidence of ovula-

111

tion or corpus luteum formation. The tunica albuginea is thickened, tough, and fibrous. Many trapped follicles in all stages of development are present underneath the tunica albuginea. Microscopically, multiple cysts are present in the cortex without corpus luteum formation. Marked hyperplasia of the theca interna of the atretic follicles is frequent. Urinary 17-ketosteroids and plasma testosterone levels are usually normal or slightly elevated. Gonadotropin levels vary. The condition is associated with a defect in ovarian steroidogenesis favoring the production of androgenic steroids at the expense of the estrogens. The underlying cause is not known. A relative enzyme deficiency in the ovary has been postulated. In the differential diagnosis, it is important to rule out other conditions that may be associated with bilateral cystic ovaries and hirsutism, including adrenogenital syndrome, Cushing's syndrome, and pituitary or hypothalamic lesions.

SYNONYMS: *Stein-Leventhal Syndrome, Stein's Syndrome, Bilateral Polycystic Ovarian Syndrome, Sclerocystic Disease of the Ovaries.*

PYOSALPINX
Pyosalpinx is a suppurative inflammation of the fallopian tube. It may be a sequel to gonorrhea or postpartum infection. It is a result of blockage of the tubal lumen at the fimbriated and isthmic ends or obstruction of various segments of the tube. The tube is distended owing to pus accumulation. Generally, the tube adheres to the surrounding structures. The lumen is filled with purulent material; the mucous membrane is edematous and flattened. Microscopically, the stroma is invaded by small round and plasma cells. There may be bizarre patterns of cells representing adenomatous changes owing to the fusion of plicae and the entrapping of epithelium.

SALPINGITIS
Salpingitis is an inflammation of the fallopian tube. It may be acute, subacute, or chronic.

Salpingitis, Acute
Acute salpingitis is an infection of the fallopian tube that may be gonorrheal or pyogenic.

Salpingitis, Subacute
Subacute salpingitis is a stage of infection intermediate between acute and chronic salpingitis.

Salpingitis, Chronic
Chronic salpingitis is a stage of infection of the fallopian tube following the subacute stage. This type may be manifested in four forms: pyosalpinx, hydrosalpinx, chronic interstitial salpingitis, or salpingitis isthmica nodosa.

SALPINGITIS, CHRONIC INTERSTITIAL

Chronic interstitial salpingitis is a form of chronic salpingitis characterized by enlargement of the tube due to increased thickening of the wall. The ostium is closed and the fimbriae adhere to the surrounding structures. Microscopically, there is extensive infiltration of all layers of the tube, especially the mucosa, with round and plasma cells. The epithelium may be intact but generally there are areas of denudation. The epithelium is actually proliferative or pseudostratified. There is an increase in the number of indifferent cells and mitosis does not take place.

SALPINGITIS, FOREIGN BODY

Foreign body salpingitis is an inflammatory reaction created by introduction of foreign material such as suture material or Lipiodol into the fallopian tubes. This reaction is characterized microscopically by the formation of giant cells in the tissue.

SALPINGITIS, GONORRHEAL

Gonorrheal salpingitis is a form of acute salpingitis that is a sequel to acute gonorrheal infection of the lower genital tract. The mucous membrane is the primary focus of the pathologic changes. It becomes reddened and swollen and gives forth a purulent exudate. Microscopically, the chief features are infiltration with polymorphonuclear leukocytes, hyperemia, and edema. In severe cases, the epithelium shows degeneration.

SALPINGITIS, GRANULOMATOUS

Granulomatous salpingitis is a proliferation of the tubal mucosa. It may be caused by syphilis.

SALPINGITIS, GRANULOMATOUS, SPECIFIC

Specific granulomatous salpingitis is a marked proliferation of the tubal mucosa caused generally by the *Mycobacterium tuberculosis*. This salpingitis resembles carcinoma.

SALPINGITIS ISTHMICA NODOSA

Salpingitis isthmica nodosa is a condition of the fallopian tube characterized by one or more nodular thickenings of the tunica muscularis of the isthmus of the tube. In some cases, evidence of inflammation is present; in others, the condition is found without inflammation. Salpingitis isthmica nodosa is characterized grossly by the presence of beadlike swellings, especially in the isthmic portion of the tube. It is generally bilateral and produces few if any clinical symptoms. It is an important cause of sterility. Microscopically, numerous, discrete glandlike spaces are scattered through the myosalpinx, with thickening of the surrounding muscle.

SYNONYM: *Adenosalpingitis.*

SALPINGITIS, PYOGENIC

Pyogenic salpingitis is a form of acute salpingitis. It generally occurs in conjunction with puerperal infection. Microscopically, the mucosa is normal or only slightly infiltrated with great thickening of the muscularis as a result of edema and leukocytic infiltration. Usually some degree of acute fibrinous peritonitis of the tubal serosa is observed.

SALPINGOCELE

Salpingocele is hernial protrusion of the fallopian tube.

SALPINGOLITHIASIS

Salpingolithiasis is the presence of calcareous deposits in the wall of the fallopian tube.

SALPINGOOOPHORITIS

Salpingooophoritis is an inflammation of a fallopian tube and ovary.

SALPINGOOOPHOROCELE

Salpingooophorocele is a hernia containing a fallopian tube and ovary.

SALPINGOOOPHOROPERITONITIS

Salpingooophoroperitonitis is an inflammation of the fallopian tube, ovary, and peritoneum by *Neisseria gonorrhoeae*.

SECTION 3: DISEASES AND CONDITIONS OF GENERATIVE ORGANS

Uterus, Endometrium, and Cervix

AMETRIA

Ametria is congenital absence of the uterus.

ANAPLASIA, ENDOMETRIAL

Endometrial anaplasia is a form of hyperplasia of the endometrium characterized by proliferation of the glands with marked intraluminal tufting and budding, unusual mitotic activity, and obliteration of the stroma. It may be a precursor of adenocarcinoma of the endometrium.

SYNONYM: *Pseudomalignant Endometrium.*

APLASIA, UTERINE

Uterine aplasia is imperfect development or congenital absence of the uterus.

SYNONYM: *Uterine Agenesis.*

ASHERMANN SYNDROME

Ashermann syndrome is a condition of intrauterine adhesions and infection generally created by frequent and vigorous curettage. The endometrial cavity is practically obliterated and amenorrhea is a persistent sign.

SYNONYM: *Traumatic Intrauterine Synechiae.*

CERVICITIS

Cervicitis is inflammation of the cervix; it may be acute or chronic.

SYNONYM: *Trachelitis.*

Cervicitis, Acute

Acute cervicitis is an infection of the endocervix caused by a variety of organisms. Clinically, the cervix is reddened and congested, with edema and swelling of the endocervical mucosa. These anatomic changes result in a profuse purulent vaginal discharge. Microscopically, the vessels are congested and infiltration of the subepithelial and perigranular tissues with polymorphonuclear leukocytes can be observed.

SYNONYM: *Acute Endocervicitis.*

Cervicitis, Chronic

Chronic cervicitis is a chronic infection of the endocervix caused by a variety of organisms. The cervix may appear normal, or in most cases, there is a chronic inflammatory process of the entire endocervix. These reactions are the common cause of leukorrhea. Microscopically, chronic cervicitis is characterized by extensive sub-epithelial infiltration, with many round cells and plasma cells.

SYNONYM: *Chronic Endocervicitis.*

CONDYLOMA ACUMINATUM, CERVICAL

Cervical condyloma acuminatum is a venereal wart or a growth on the cervix producing an irritating vaginal discharge. It consists of a fibrous overgrowth that is covered by thickened epithelium. It also may occur on the perineum, vulva, and vagina.

ENDOMETRITIS

Endometritis is an inflammation of the endometrium. The classifications—acute and chronic—are broad divisions of the more specific types of endometritis.

Endometritis, Acute

Acute endometritis is acute inflammation of the endometrium, usually due to bacterial infection of the tissue.

Endometritis, Chronic

Chronic endometritis is a chronic infection of the endometrium. This condition may be associated with retained products of conception, submucous fibroids, intrauterine devices, or prolonged infection associated with chronic salpingitis. The upper functional layer of the endometrium may be primarily involved, but infection may extend into the myometrium. Microscopically, the tissue demonstrates round and plasma cell infiltration, new blood vessels, granulation tissue, and distortion of the endometrial glands.

Endometritis, Gonorrheal

Gonorrheal endometritis is an infection of the endometrium caused by *Neisseria gonorrhoeae*. It generally results from infection of the lower genital tract. The organism makes its way to the fallopian tube by way of the endometrium.

Endometritis, Postabortal

Postabortal endometritis is inflammation of the endometrium following spontaneous or induced abortion. Uterine bleeding, fever, and an enlarged tender uterus are some of the clinical signs of this disease. Microscopically, chorionic villi and decidual cells, together with other findings of acute and chronic inflammation, are diagnostic of this condition.

Endometritis, Puerperal

Puerperal endometritis is infection of the endometrium in association with puerperal infection. The endometrium is swollen, hyperemic, and edematous. In the severe type, bacterial toxin causes destructive effects on the endometrium, with necrosis and ulceration. Thrombosis of the uterine vessels may result in thrombophlebitis of the uterine and pelvic vessels. Septic emboli may pass to other structures, causing distant abscess and bloodstream infection.

Endometritis, Senile

Senile endometritis is an infection superimposed on postmenopausal endometrial atrophy. The endometrium is thin. Patches of squamous epithelium replace the normal columnar epithelium, and occasionally the entire endometrial surface is covered by stratified epithelium.

Endometritis, Syncytial

Syncytial endometritis is an accentuation of the morphologic features of the placental site. The endometrium and myometrium are infiltrated by trophoblastic cells with varying degrees of inflammation. The lesion is usually benign.

Endometritis, Tuberçulous

Tuberculous endometritis is an infection of the endometrium caused by *Mycobacterium tuberculosis*. The fallopian tube is usually involved first. The microscopic findings are those of chronic inflammation; tubercles or clusters of tubercles are present with the characteristic epithelioid and giant cells. Ulceration and granulomatous changes, and caseation may be found. Few full-term pregnancies occur after this disease.

ENDOMETRIUM, UNRIPE

Unripe endometrium is a condition of the endometrium in which the functional layer remains in the proliferative phase.

EROSION, CERVICAL

Cervical erosion is a condition caused by chemical irritation or an inflammatory process and characterized by ulceration of the everted columnar epithelium of the endocervix and the squamous epithelium of the vaginal portion of the cervix.

EVERSION, CERVICAL

Cervical eversion is external evidence of a chronic inflammatory process of the cervical canal. It is characterized by the rolling out or pouting of the swollen and congested cervical mucosa.

GRAVID UTERUS, INCARCERATED

An incarcerated gravid uterus is a uterus that is confined in the hollow of the sacrum by adhesions or by its size. The uterus is generally retroverted.

HEMATOMETRA

Hematometra is a collection or retention of blood in the uterine cavity.
SYNONYM: *Hemometra.*

HYDROMETROCOLPOS

Hydrometrocolpos is an accumulation of watery fluid in the uterus and vagina.

HYPERPLASIA, ENDOMETRIAL

Endometrial hyperplasia is a condition in which there is an abnormal growth response in the endometrium due to a relatively excessive, unopposed estrogenic stimulus. The degree of response depends not only on the amount and duration of estrogenic stimulus but also on the degree of receptivity of the individual endometrium. Endometrial hyperplasia is related to failure of ovulation.

Hyperplasia, Adenomatous Endometrial

Adenomatous endometrial hyperplasia is an extreme degree of proliferation of the glandular epithelium. Glands increase in number so that there is only a small amount of stroma between them. Cellular patterns in the glands change from one layer of cuboidal or columnar cells to an irregular pallisading in localized areas within the glands. The epithelial cells are hyperchromatic, some mitotic activity is evident, giant cells are absent, the basement membrane is completely intact, and stroma is not invaded.

Hyperplasia, Cystic Endometrial

Cystic endometrial hyperplasia is a type of proliferative hyperplasia characterized by cystically dilated but active glands lined by a single layer of columnar epithelium or by pseudostratified epithelium. The stroma is composed of cells with very scanty cytoplasm, but the striking feature is the presence of large, thin-walled stromal sinusoids. It is from these that the bleeding occurs in endometrial hyperplasia. Grossly, the hyperplastic endometrium is soft, pale pink to yellow, and irregularly thickened, forming prominent polypoid areas.

Hyperplasia, Postmenopausal Endometrial

Postmenopausal endometrial hyperplasia is characterized by variations in the cellular activity of the endothelium. It is caused by estrogen stimulation, generally from extragenital sources. Various forms of hyperplasia may be present.

Hyperplasia, Proliferative Endometrial

Proliferative endometrial hyperplasia is a condition in which the endometrium remains in the proliferative phase owing to failure of ovulation. It is associated with functional uterine bleeding of an endocrine imbalance type.

Hyperplasia, Secretory Endometrial

Secretory endometrial hyperplasia is a variation in the histologic patterns of the endometrium with an increase in both epithelial and stromal elements. Surface and glandular epithelial cells are tall with heavily stained nuclei. There may be areas of marked necrotic change with round cell infiltration and vessel thrombosis. Patches of active hyperplasia and polypoid formation in various combinations may be observed in different parts of the same endometrium. There may be stratification or pseudostratification of the nuclei in the glandular epithelium.

HYPERTROPHY, MYOMETRIAL
Myometrial hypertrophy is uterine muscle hypertrophy causing symmetrical enlargement of the uterus.
SYNONYM: *Fibrosis Uteri* (obsolete).

HYSTERALGIA
Hysteralgia is pain in the uterus.
SYNONYMS: *Hysterodynia, Metralgia, Metrodynia, Uteralgia, Uterodynia.*

HYSTERATRESIA
Hysteratresia is congenital absence or pathologic closure of the uterus.

HYSTEROSPASM
Hysterospasm is spasm of the uterus.

LYMPHOGRANULOMA VENEREUM, CERVICAL
Cervical lymphogranuloma venereum is caused by a virus-like organism of the psittacosis-lymphogranuloma group. It is characterized by transient ulceration of the cervix and lymphadenopathy. The Frei test together with the clinical picture enables one to establish the diagnosis.

METAPLASIA, SQUAMOUS, ENDOMETRIAL
Endometrial squamous metaplasia is the replacement of endometrial columnar epithelium by squamous epithelium. This is an uncommon phenomenon and generally occurs in elderly patients. It may result in squamous cell carcinoma.
SYNONYM: *Ichthyosis Uteri.*

METROCELE
A metrocele is a hernia of the uterus.
SYNONYM: *Hysterocele.*

METROLYMPHANGITIS
Metrolymphangitis is an inflammation of the uterine lymphatic vessels.

METROPERITONITIS
Metroperitonitis is inflammation of the peritoneum about the uterus.

METRORRHAGIA
Metrorrhagia is irregular, acyclic uterine bleeding.

METROSALPINGITIS
Metrosalpingitis is inflammation of the uterus and one or both of the fallopian tubes.

METROSTAXIS
Metrostaxis is a small but persistent hemorrhage from the uterus.

MYOMETRITIS

Myometritis is an inflammatory condition of the myometrium that generally follows endometrial infection. It may be acute or chronic.

Myometritis, Acute

Acute myometritis is a severe form of infection of the myometrium resulting from a puerperal streptococcal infection. There is marked edema, muscle hypertrophy, and leukocytic infiltration.

Myometritis, Chronic

Chronic myometritis is a prolonged infection of the myometrium characterized by infiltration of plasma cells and edema between the muscle bundles. Grossly, the uterus is enlarged and boggy with resultant bleeding, discharge, and pain.

PYOMETRA

Pyometra is a condition in which the endometrial cavity becomes filled with pus. This results from an inflammatory process of the endometrium with a concomitant stenosis of the cervix. The uterus is distended and thin-walled. There may be no special symptoms. Pyometra may occur with cervical or uterine carcinoma, or following benign conditions, cervical amputation, or radiation therapy.

SYPHILIS, CERVICAL

Cervical syphilis is an indurated ulceration of the cervix. It is generally a primary lesion and is diagnosed by the presence of spirochetes on a dark-field microscopic examination.

SYNONYM: *Chancre of Cervix.*

TUBERCULOSIS, CERVICAL

Cervical tuberculosis is either an ulcerative or hyperplastic lesion of the cervix that may simulate carcinoma. It is generally a secondary manifestation of genital tuberculosis, almost always resulting from involvement of the fallopian tubes. Microscopically, the lesion is characterized by chronic inflammatory processes with infiltration of giant cells and epithelioid cells.

UTERINE BLEEDING, FUNCTIONAL

Functional uterine bleeding is abnormal bleeding unassociated with tumor, inflammation, or pregnancy. It is characterized by complete irregularity of the menstrual cycle and prolonged menses, frequently alternating with periods of amenorrhea. Functional uterine bleeding is usually associated with ovarian dysfunction and anovulation.

SYNONYM: *Dysfunctional Uterine Bleeding.*

UTERINE POSITIONS

Anteflexion, Uterine

Uterine anteflexion is a position of the uterus in which the corpus is tilted forward creating an angulation between the corpus and cervix.

Anteversion, Uterine
Uterine anteversion is a position in which the entire uterus is tilted forward without angulation between the corpus and cervix.

Dextroversion, Uterine
Uterine dextroversion is deviation of the uterus from its normal position to the right side.

Displacement, Uterine
Uterine displacement is a change from a normal to an abnormal uterine position.
SYNONYMS: *Metrectopia, Uterine Malposition.*

Lateroflexion, Uterine
Uterine lateroflexion is deviation of the corpus uteri from its normal position to one side, creating an angulation between the corpus and the cervix.

Lateroversion, Uterine
Uterine lateroversion is a deviation of the uterus to one side without angulation between the corpus and cervix.

Retrocession, Uterine
Uterine retrocession is a posterior location of the uterus so that it occupies a position much closer to the sacrum than normal.
SYNONYM: *Uterine Retroposition.*

Retroflexion, Uterine
Uterine retroflexion is a backward deviation of the corpus uteri from its normal position.

Retroversion, Uterine
Uterine retroversion is the position in which the entire uterus is tilted backward without angulation between the corpus and cervix.

UTERUS ACOLLIS
Uterus acollis is a uterus without a cervix.

UTERUS, ANOMALOUS
An anomalous uterus is a malformed uterus resulting from abnormal development or fusion of one or both of the paramesonephric ducts.

UTERUS, ARCUATE
An arcuate uterus is a malformed uterus characterized by a depression in the fundus.
SYNONYM: *Saddle-Shaped Uterus.*

UTERUS BICAMERATUS VETULARUM
Uterus bicameratus vetularum is a condition in which fluid accumulates in and distends the cervix and corpus uteri, the two cervical ora being sealed by adhesions.

UTERUS, BICORNUATE
A bicornuate uterus is a uterus that is divided into two compartments owing to an arrest in development.
SYNONYMS: *Uterus Bifidus, Uterus Bicornis.*

UTERUS BIFORIS
Uterus biforis is a uterus with a normal corpus and a septate cervix.
SYNONYMS: *Uterus Subseptus, Double-mouthed Uterus.*

UTERUS, CAPPED
A capped uterus is a uterus with tonic muscular contraction of the fundus.

UTERUS, COCHLEATE
A cochleate uterus is an acutely flexed adult uterus with a small globular body and a conical cervix.

UTERUS, CORDATE
A cordate uterus is a heart-shaped uterus.
SYNONYM: *Uterus Cordiformis.*

UTERUS DIDELPHYS
Uterus didelphys is two distinct uteri, side by side, with a double vagina. It results from failure of fusion of the paramesonephric ducts.
SYNONYM: *Uterus Duplex.*

UTERUS DUPLEX BICORNIS BICOLLIS
Uterus duplex bicornis bicollis is a complete double uterus with a normal vagina.

UTERUS, FETAL
A fetal uterus is an abnormally formed uterus in which the length of the cervix exceeds the size of the corpus.

UTERUS INCUDIFORMIS
Uterus incudiformis is a bicornuate uterus in which the fundus is broad and flat.
SYNONYMS: *Uterus Planifundalis, Uterus Triangularis.*

UTERUS, INFANTILE
An infantile uterus is a small uterus of normal shape but with arrested development.
SYNONYM: *Pubescent Uterus.*

UTERUS PARVICOLLIS
Uterus parvicollis is a uterus with a normal corpus but a disproportionately small cervix, particularly the portio vaginalis.

UTERUS, PROLAPSED

A prolapsed uterus is a uterus that has descended into the vagina. This results from relaxation and atony of the muscular and fascial structures of the pelvic floor, usually after childbirth or advanced age. There are three types: first-degree, second-degree, and third-degree.

SYNONYMS: *Prolapsus Uteri, Procidentia Descensus Uteri, Metroptosis, Metrocolpocele, Metroptosia, Hysteroptosia, Hysteroptosis.*

First-Degree Uterine Prolapse

First-degree uterine prolapse is a descent of the uterus in which the cervix is within the vaginal orifice.

SYNONYM: *Vault Prolapse.*

Second-Degree Uterine Prolapse

Second-degree uterine prolapse is a descent of the uterus in which the cervix partially or totally appears outside of the vaginal orifice.

Third-Degree Uterine Prolapse

Third-degree uterine prolapse is a complete descent of the entire uterus beyond the vaginal orifice.

UTERUS, PROLAPSED, CONGENITAL

A congenital prolapsed uterus is a uterus that has descended into the vagina in a nulliparous woman. This is assumed to be the result of congenital weakness of the pelvic structures.

UTERUS, SEPTATE

A septate uterus is a uterus that is divided into two cavities by an anteroposterior septum.

SYNONYMS: *Uterus Septus, Uterus Bipartitus, Uterus Bilocularis, Bipartite Uterus.*

UTERUS UNICORNIS

Uterus unicornis is a uterus in which only one lateral half is present. The other is underdeveloped or absent. It is due to the absence of one paramesonephric duct.

SECTION 3: DISEASES AND CONDITIONS OF GENERATIVE ORGANS

Vulva and Vagina

ABSCESS, BARTHOLIN'S GLAND
A Bartholin's gland abscess is an abscess formation within a major vestibular gland or its ductal system. It is a common sequel to bartholinitis, or may result from infection of the contents of a Bartholin duct cyst, or obstruction of a major vestibular duct. It is clinically characterized by redness, swelling, fluctuation, and pain.

SYNONYMS: *Vulvovaginal Gland Abscess, Major Vestibular Gland Abscess.*

ABSCESS, SKENE'S DUCT
A Skene's duct abscess is an inflammatory process with the accumulation of purulent material within the paraurethral duct consequent to occlusion of the duct and infection.

SYNONYM: *Paraurethral Duct Abscess.*

ACANTHOSIS NIGRICANS, BENIGN
Benign acanthosis nigricans is a dermatosis grossly similar to malignant acanthosis nigricans, but unlike the latter, it is not associated with a malignant tumor. It may be present at birth but more often it arises later in childhood or at puberty.

ACANTHOSIS NIGRICANS, MALIGNANT
Malignant acanthosis nigricans is a rare dermatosis characterized by hyperpigmentation and roughness of the skin of the vulva and surrounding regions. It is usually associated with an internal adenocarcinoma.

SYNONYM: *Keratosis Nigricans.*

ACTINOMYCOSIS
Actinomycosis is a chronic infectious disease caused by *Actinomyces israelii.* It is characterized by the formation of granulomatous lesions that break down and form abscesses discharging through numerous sinuses. There may be secondary involvement of the female pelvis.

ADENITIS, BARTHOLIN'S
Bartholin's adenitis is inflammation and infection of a major vestibular gland. It is frequently due to gonorrheal infection, although other bacterial organisms may be responsible. The gland becomes turgid, swollen, and painful, and a purulent exudate may be expressed from the duct.

SYNONYM: *Bartholinitis.*

ATRESIA, VAGINAL
Vaginal atresia is the absence or closure of the vagina.

BALANITIS
Balanitis is inflammation of the glans of the clitoris.

BALANOCHLAMYDITIS
Balanochlamyditis is an inflammatory condition of the glans and prepuce of the clitoris.

BEHÇET'S DISEASE
Behçet's disease is a chronic relapsing granulomatous disease of the vulva characterized by painful aphthous ulcers simultaneously occurring on the oral mucosa. No specific organism is isolated.

CANDIDIASIS, GENITAL
Genital candidiasis is an acute or subacute infection of the skin or mucous membranes of the vulva or vagina by a yeastlike fungus such as *Candida albicans.* It is relatively common and is characterized by pruritus, reddening of the mucous membrane, discharge, and often has scattered or confluent white thrush patches.
   SYNONYMS: *Moniliasis, Monilial Vaginitis, Candidal Vaginitis, Vaginal Thrush, Yeast Vulvovaginitis.*

CARBUNCLE, VULVAR
A vulvar carbuncle is a pyoderma of the vulvar skin in which several adjoining hair follicles become infected, suppurate, intercommunicate with each other, and have multiple openings onto the skin surface.

CELLULITIS, VULVAR
Vulvar cellulitis is inflammation of cellular tissue, especially of the loose subcutaneous tissue of the vulva. It is most often seen following episiotomy and other surgical procedures. It is characterized by swelling, tenderness, and erythema about the episiotomy or surgical site.

CHANCROID
Chancroid is a venereal infection usually characterized by multiple, painful, well-defined ulcers with an erythematous halo. It is caused by *Hemophilus ducreyi.*
   SYNONYMS: *Soft Chancre, Ulcus Molle.*

CLITORIDAUXE
Clitoridauxe is an enlargement of the clitoris.

CLITORIDITIS
Clitoriditis is inflammation of the clitoris.

CLITORISM
Clitorism is the prolonged and usually painful erection of the clitoris. It is the analogue of priapism.

COCCIDIOIDOMYCOSIS, VULVAR

Vulvar coccidioidomycosis is a very rare, deep mycotic infection of the vulva. It is characterized by the appearance of erythema nodosum-like nodules, papules, pustules, verrucose growths, and fungating ulcers. It is caused by *Coccidioides immitis*.

COLPALGIA

Colpalgia is pain in the vagina.

COLPATRESIA

Colpatresia is occlusion or imperforation of the vagina.

COLPECTASIA

Colpectasia is distention or stretching of the vagina.

COLPODYNIA

Colpodynia is neuralgic pain in the vagina.
SYNONYM: *Vaginodynia*.

COLPOSTENOSIS

Colpostenosis is a narrowing of the lumen of the vagina.
SYNONYM: *Vaginal Stenosis*.

COLPOXEROSIS

Colpoxerosis is an abnormal dryness of the mucous membrane of the vagina.

DERMATITIS, MEDICATION

Medication dermatitis is an eruption of the skin or mucous membrane following oral or parenteral administration of a drug to which the patient is allergic.
SYNONYMS: *Dermatitis Medicamentosa, Drug Eruption*.

DERMATITIS, VULVAR SEBORRHEIC

Vulvar seborrheic dermatitis is a dermatosis characterized by pruritus and by the presence on the vulva of one or more erythematous spots covered with greasy, yellow scales. It is usually associated with similar lesions of the scalp and face.

ECTHYMA, VULVAR

Vulvar ecthyma is a pustular infection of the skin of the vulva similar to impetigo, although it involves the full thickness of the epidermis and the superficial layers of the corium. Most of the cases are caused by a streptococcus.

EDEMA, VULVAR

Vulvar edema is swelling of the vulva due to the accumulation of subcutaneous fluid. It may be produced by prolonged pressure, infections, general metabolic disease, nephritis, ascites, cardiac failure, lymphatic obstruction, often by preeclampsia, and by trauma. It also may be produced by the pressure caused by prolonged apposition of the thighs in multiple sclerosis.

ELEPHANTIASIS, VULVAR

Vulvar elephantiasis is enlargement of the external genitalia due to hypertrophy and thickening of the skin and subcutaneous tissues or lymphedema. It is generally a sequel to filariasis or lymphogranuloma venereum.

ERYSIPELAS, VULVAR

Vulvar erysipelas is a rapidly spreading, acute infection of the skin of the vulva caused by invasion of the superficial lymphatic vessels by a beta hemolytic streptococcus. It is usually the result of bacterial inoculation incident to trauma. It is an exceedingly rare condition.

ERYTHEMA MULTIFORME

Erythema multiforme is an acute or subacute inflammatory eruption of the vulvar skin or vaginal mucous membrane, consisting of erythematous macules or papules, wheals, vesicles, and sometimes bullae. Although the cause generally remains obscure, drug sensitivity is common.
SYNONYMS: *Herpes Iris, Erythema Multiforme Bullosum.*

ERYTHRASMA

Erythrasma is a superficial skin infection characterized by small, cir- cumscribed, reddish brown, scaly macules that may coalesce to form plaques on the inner sides of the thigh and adjacent genitalia. The lesions fluoresce under Wood's light. It is caused by *Corynebacterium minutissimum.*

ESTHIOMENE

Esthiomene is chronic ulceration and elephantiasis of the labia and clitoris due to lymphogranuloma venereum.

FISSURE, VULVAR

A vulvar fissure is a split in the mucous membrane or skin of the vulva, usually in natural folds.

FISTULA, RECTOVAGINAL

A rectovaginal fistula is an abnormal passage between the rectum and the vagina. It is usually caused by obstetric injuries, incomplete healing of an episiotomy, rectocele repair, radium therapy, or uterine cancer.

FISTULA, SIGMOIDOVAGINAL

A sigmoidovaginal fistula is an abnormal passage between the sigmoid colon and the vagina. It occurs as a complication of hysterectomy, pelvic abscess, carcinoma, or diverticulitis.

FISTULA, URETEROVAGINAL

A ureterovaginal fistula is an abnormal passage between a ureter and the vagina. It is usually a delayed complication following total abdominal, vaginal, or radical hysterectomy. It may be congenital.

FISTULA, VESICOVAGINAL

A vesicovaginal fistula is an opening or communication between the bladder and vagina. A vesicovaginal fistula is caused by obstetric injuries, pelvic operations, roentgen-ray or radium therapy, and inflammation and malignant neoplasms of the urinary bladder, cervix, and vagina. The communication usually involves the posterior wall of the bladder and upper anterior wall of the vagina.

FOLLICULITIS, VULVAR

Vulvar folliculitis is a persistent infection of the pilosebaceous ducts and hair follicles usually by a staphylococcus. There are two types: superficial, in which the infection is limited to the upper part of a pilosebaceous duct; and deep, in which the infection has involved the entire hair follicle and the sebaceous glands.

FURUNCLE, VULVAR

A vulvar furuncle is a local pyogenic infection involving tissues beyond the hair follicles. It is similar to folliculitis but involves the perifollicular tissues.

FURUNCULOSIS, VULVAR

Vulvar furunculosis is the continuous or intermittent appearance of furuncles over a period of months or years.

GONORRHEA

Gonorrhea is an infection of the genitalia caused by *Neisseria gonorrhoeae*. To begin with, the infection is limited to structures below the internal cervical os.

GRANULOMA INGUINALE

Granuloma inguinale is one of the venereal diseases of the vulva and surrounding tissues caused by the bacterium *Donovania granulomatis*. It is characterized by an extensive, destructive, ulcerating, granulomatous lesion of the vulva, perianal tissues, and inguinal region. Microscopically, it is characterized by the presence of the specific Donovan encapsulated bacilli within histiocytes or tissue spaces.

SYNONYMS: *Granuloma Venereum, Granuloma Pudendi, Donovanosis, Venereal Granuloma.*

HEMATOCOLPOMETRA

Hematocolpometra is an accumulation of blood in the uterus and vagina resulting from an imperforate hymen or other lower vaginal obstruction.

HEMATOCOLPOS

Hematocolpos is an accumulation of menstrual blood in the vagina resulting from an imperforate hymen or other obstruction.

SYNONYM: *Retained Menstruation.*

HEMOPHILUS VAGINALIS VAGINITIS

Hemophilus vaginalis vaginitis is a vaginal infection caused by the bacterial parasite *Hemophilus vaginalis.* It is characterized by a malodorous, gray, homogeneous discharge. Irritative symptoms are minimal if present. It is thought that most of the vaginitides previously diagnosed "nonspecific" were attributable to this disease.

HERPES GENITALIS

Herpes genitalis is an acute herpetic inflammatory disease of the genitalia caused by the herpes simplex virus type 2. The chief symptoms are hyperesthesia, burning, itching, burning pain on urination, and frequently, exquisite tenderness. Multiple small vesicles that rapidly rupture and become superficial ulcers are characteristic.

SYNONYMS: *Herpes Progenitalis, Herpes Simplex of Vulva.*

HERPES ZOSTER

Herpes zoster is a rare disease of the vulva grossly similar to herpes genitalis. It is caused by a virus believed to be identical in some respects to the varicella virus. It is manifested by vesiculoulcerative eruptions, is unilateral, and follows paths of nerves. There is marked erythema of the skin around the vesicle.

SYNONYM: *Vulvar Shingles.*

HIDRADENITIS SUPPURATIVA, VULVAR

Vulvar hidradenitis suppurativa is a resistant, purulent infection of the apocrine glands often associated with abscesses, sinus tract formation, and scarring. Such infection may occur at any site where apocrine glands are present.

HOTTENTOT APRON

A Hottentot apron is excessive elongation of the labia minora seen in Hottentot women or associated with masturbation.

SYNONYM: *Velamen Vulvae.*

HYDROCOLPOS

Hydrocolpos is an accumulation of mucus or other nonsanguinous fluid within the vagina. The condition is caused by an imperforate hymen and other lower vaginal obstructions.

HYPERTROPHY, CLITORAL

Clitoral hypertrophy is enlargement of the clitoris due to stimulation by excessive amounts of androgen. Causes are congenital adrenal hyperplasia, masculinizing ovarian and adrenal tumors, and exogenous androgens.

HYPOPLASIA, CLITORAL

Clitoral hypoplasia is underdevelopment of the clitoris generally associated with endocrine disturbances.

HYPOPLASIA, VULVAR

Vulvar hypoplasia is failure of the normal development of the vulva, associated with endocrine disturbances.

IMPETIGO HERPETIFORMIS

Impetigo herpetiformis is a pyoderma of the vulva and other areas, complicating pregnancy. The eruptions are small, closely aggregated pustules that develop on an inflammatory base. There are severe symptoms and the condition may end in death.

INTERTRIGO

Intertrigo is a chronic dermatitis induced by friction between moist, opposed surfaces of the skin, particularly of the genitocrural folds and upper inner thighs. The inguinal folds and the intergluteal regions also may be affected. The clinical features are variable and may include erythema, maturation, lichenification, verrucose changes, and increased pigmentation.

KRAUROSIS VULVAE

Kraurosis vulvae is a term used in past years to denote the atrophic stage in leukoplakia. Kraurosis does not denote a specific disease entity. The term, if used at all, probably should denote only the contractive stages of lichen sclerosis et atrophicus.

LEUKODERMA, VULVAR

Vulvar leukoderma is an asymptomatic condition characterized by the appearance of depigmented areas of skin about the vulva. It is sometimes associated with similar lesions on other portions of the body. Except for a loss of pigment, the skin is normal. Vulvar leukoderma has been distinguished from vitiligo by some, in that leukoderma is acquired hypopigmentation occurring after inflammation, whereas vitiligo is congenital hypopigmentation and is often associated with similar lesions elsewhere.

LEUKOPLAKIA, VULVAR

Vulvar leukoplakia was thought for many years to be a specific premalignant condition of the vulva. More recently, the term has been acceptable only as a descriptive one to denote a visible white patch or plaque. Many conditions of the vulva are associated with such lesions.

LEUKORRHEA

Leukorrhea is a common gynecologic disorder characterized by an abnormal, nonbloody discharge from the genital tract.

LEUKORRHEA, PREMENARCHAL

Premenarchal leukorrhea is a physiologic type of leukorrhea that develops with the increased production of unopposed estrogen in the months or years immediately before menarche.

LICHEN PLANUS ERYTHEMATOSUS, VULVAR

Vulvar lichen planus erythematosus is a rare variety of lichen planus in which the papules are soft, red, vascular, and sensitive. The lesions are discrete on the vulva and are sometimes seen close to the urethral orifice.

LICHEN PLANUS VERRUCOSUS, VULVAR

Vulvar lichen planus verrucosus is a form of lichen planus in which the papules coalesce to form a wartlike patch near the vagina.

LICHEN PLANUS, VULVOVAGINAL

Vulvovaginal lichen planus is an inflammatory disease of the skin of the vulva and mucous membrane of the vagina. It is clinically characterized by smooth, flat, violaceous papules. On the vulva it may appear as a white, or leukoplakic, plaque.

LICHEN SCLEROSIS ET ATROPHICUS, VULVAR

Vulvar lichen sclerosis et atrophicus is a dystrophy of the vulvar skin and usually several characteristics are present: white plaques, thinning of the skin with a parchment or crinkled appearance, edema of foreskin and phimosis of the clitoris, atrophy of the labia minora, telangiectases, and fissures. It is occasionally associated with marked contracture of the vulvar tissues (kraurosis). Microscopically, it is identified by hyperkeratosis, thinning of the epithelium, a subepithelial zone of collagen, and chronic inflammatory infiltration beneath the collagen.

LUPUS VULGARIS, VULVAR

Vulvar lupus vulgaris is a form of cutaneous tuberculosis with the characteristic nodular lesions. It is generally found in other parts of the body but may be present on the buttocks, thighs, and genitalia.

LYMPHOGRANULOMA VENEREUM

Lymphogranuloma venereum is a venereal infection caused by a virus of the psittacosis-lymphogranuloma group. It is characterized by a transient genital ulcer, inguinal adenopathy, perirectal node involvement, and occasionally, rectal strictures. Genital elephantiasis may be a consequence of this disease.

SYNONYMS: *Lymphopathia Venereum, Lymphogranuloma Inguinale, Climatic Bubo, Poradenitis, Nicolas-Favre Disease, Fourth Venereal Disease.*

MELANOSIS, VULVAR

Vulvar melanosis is an abnormal dark brown pigmentation of the vulva due to the deposition of abnormal amounts of melanin in the skin.

MOLLUSCUM CONTAGIOSUM

Molluscum contagiosum is a viral infection that causes a proliferative process of the skin resembling a localized neoplasm. The lesions are usually multiple, the size of the growth varying from a pinhead to 1 cm in diameter. The typical lesion is a dome-shaped wavy papule. Numerous molluscum bodies consisting of viral particles are seen within the epithelial cells of the lesion.

NEURODERMATITIS, VULVAR

Vulvar neurodermatitis is a chronic superficial inflammation of the skin of the vulva. It is characterized by thickened, dry, desquamating, well-demarcated, excoriated plaques, of oval, irregular, or angular shape, associated with severe pruritis.

SYNONYMS: *Circumscribed Neurodermatitis, Lichen Simplex Chronicus.*

PARAVAGINITIS

Paravaginitis is inflammation of the tissues alongside of the vagina.
SYNONYM: *Paracolpitis.*

PEDICULOSIS PUBIS

Pediculosis pubis is an infestation of the hair-bearing area of the vulva by *Phthirus pubis,* the crab louse. The organism or its eggs can be visibly detected as they attach to the hair roots.

PRURITUS VULVAE

Pruritus vulvae is itching of the external genital organs of the female.

PSEUDOACANTHOSIS NIGRICANS

Pseudoacanthosis nigricans is a type of acanthosis nigricans that develops primarily in darkly pigmented, obese persons. The cutaneous changes resemble those of acanthosis nigricans. They usually disappear when the weight returns to normal and irritation factors are eliminated. It is not associated with a malignant tumor.

PSORIASIS, VULVAR

Vulvar psoriasis is a chronic, occasionally acute, relapsing, papulosquamous dermatosis affecting the skin of the vulva. The lesions consist of sharply demarcated erythematous papules or plaques covered with overlapping, shiny, or slightly opalescent scales.

SCABIES VULVAE

Scabies vulvae is a transmissible parasitic skin infection, characterized by superficial burrows, intense pruritus, and secondary inflammatory changes. It is caused by the itch mite.

SKENITIS

Skenitis is inflammation and infection of the paraurethral glands, characterized by swelling and soreness around the urethra. It may be the result of a gonococcal infection.

SYNONYM: *Paraurethral Gland Infection.*

SYPHILIS

Syphilis is a continuous infectious process caused by *Treponema pallidum*. It is initiated at the time of sexual contact and passes through well-known clinical stages: primary, secondary, latent, and tertiary (late). The lesions of syphilis are classified as primary (chancre), secondary (condylomata lata), and tertiary (gummata).

Chancre

Chancre is the primary lesion of syphilis. It may occur on the vulva. It often begins as a dull, red, hard, insensitive papule or area of infiltration that generally breaks down into an ulcer. Instead of the classic punched-out ulcer with rolled edges, many chancres of the vulva, vagina, and cervix are superficial ulcers without induration.

SYNONYM: *Hard Chancre.*

Condylomata Lata

Condylomata lata are secondary lesions of syphilis characterized by flat-topped papules that occur in groups. These eruptions are often ulcerated and are covered by a necrotic layer of epithelium that secretes a seropurulent fluid. The eruptions are found on the vulva, around the anus, and wherever contiguous skin folds produce heat and moisture.

SYNONYM: *Flat Condyloma.*

Gumma

The gumma is the usual lesion of tertiary syphilis. It appears as a nodule that enlarges, and because of necrosis of the overlying skin, ulcerates and sloughs.

TINEA CRURIS

Tinea cruris is a well-delineated superficial fungal infection extending from the crural fold over the adjacent upper inner thigh. Both sides may be affected but ordinarily the eruption is asymmetrical. Tinea cruris is caused by a variety of ringworms and may be confused with contact or seborrheic dermatitis, psoriasis, erythrasma, or candidiasis.

SYNONYMS: *Trichophytosis Vulvae, Eczema Marginatum, Tinea Vulvae, Ringworm of Vulva.*

TORULOPSIS GLABRATA VULVOVAGINITIS

Torulopsis glabrata vulvovaginitis is an uncommon, mild infection of the vulva and vagina by the fungus *Torulopsis glabrata*. The most common clinical feature is an increase in vaginal discharge. The color is white or slate; the consistency is less curdy than normal, and thrush patches do not form. Discharge, mild itching, and a mild burning sensation are the manifestations most often mentioned by the patient.

TRICHOMONIASIS

Trichomoniasis is a protozoan infection of the vagina, Skene's ducts, and lower urinary tract. The causative agent is *Trichomonas vaginalis*.

According to the severity of the infection, trichomoniasis may be classified as acute, asymptomatic, or chronic.

Trichomoniasis, Acute

Acute trichomoniasis is characterized by an abnormal vaginal discharge, gross tissue reactions of the vagina, vulva, or both, and generally irritative symptoms, particularly pruritis. Edema and erythema are the common gross abnormalities of the vulva, and the vagina usually exhibits one or more of the following signs: erythema, swollen papillae, petechiae, or ecchymoses.

Trichomoniasis, Asymptomatic

Asymptomatic trichomoniasis is the carrier stage of trichomoniasis. The patients usually have no clinical, bacteriologic, or histologic signs of the disease. Most patients with asymptomatic trichomoniasis give a history of past clinical disease, and almost all later experience exacerbations.

Trichomoniasis, Chronic

Chronic trichomoniasis is the most common variety of trichomoniasis. The vaginal secretions manifest abnormal volume, odor, consistency, pH, and pathogenic bacteria. Varying degrees of inflammatory infiltration may be observed in histologic sections of the vagina.

TUBERCULOSIS, VULVAR

Vulvar tuberculosis is an infection of the vulvar tissues by *Mycobacterium tuberculosis*. Grossly, it appears in three general types: tuberculous ulcers, lupus vulgaris, and scrofuloderma. Diagnosis may be confirmed by the microscopic finding of tubercles containing *Mycobacterium tuberculosis* in the tissue obtained by biopsy, by isolating the bacterium from scrapings, and by spiral cultures.

ULCER

An ulcer is a depressed lesion of the skin or a mucous membrane caused by disintegration of all superficial epithelial layers: thus the lesion reaches the dermis or submucosal tissues. It is often attended by suppuration. A wound with superficial loss of tissue from trauma is not primarily an ulcer, but may turn into one if healing stops or infection occurs.

Chronic Ulcer of Vagina

A chronic ulcer of the vagina is a persistent disintegration of the vaginal mucosa. The lesion may result from pressure of a foreign body or may result from a chronic infection.

Simple Acute Ulcer of Vulva

A simple acute ulcer of the vulva appears as a shallow, rounded or oval lesion of the vulva or lower vagina. The ulcers may be single or multiple and are readily amenable to simple antiseptic treatment.
SYNONYMS: *Ulcus Vulvae Acutum, Lipschütz Ulcer.*

VAGINISMUS

Vaginismus is a painful spasm of the vagina preventing satisfactory coitus or pelvic examination.

SYNONYMS: *Colpospasm, Vulvismus.*

VAGINITIS

Vaginitis, strictly interpreted, means inflammation of the mucous membrane of the vagina. Some parasitic infectious agents such as *Hemophilus vaginalis* live on vaginal serous secretions and desquamated debris to produce leukorrhea and malodor without causing morphologic changes in the tissues. But a broad interpretation of the term "vaginitis" permits the diseases resulting from these parasitic agents to be included under the classification.

VAGINITIS, ADHESIVE

Adhesive vaginitis is inflammation of the vagina with areas of exfoliation and ulceration of mucous membrane that subsequently adhere, causing varying degrees of obliteration of the lumen of the vagina.

VAGINITIS, AMEBIC

Amebic vaginitis is infection of the vulva, vagina, and cervix by *Entamoeba histolytica*. Ulcerations are apparent on the upper vagina and cervix although the vulva is rarely affected.

VAGINITIS, ATROPHIC

Atrophic vaginitis is a relatively frequent inflammation of the vaginal mucosa in postmenopausal women when estrogen levels fall below physiologic levels. The vaginal infection generally produces burning, itching, soreness, and in some patients, vaginal bleeding. The epithelium is thin, and may be ulcerated and subject to minimal bleeding.

SYNONYM: *Senile Vaginitis.*

VAGINITIS, DESQUAMATIVE INFLAMMATORY

Desquamative inflammatory vaginitis appears to be a specific entity of unknown etiology that displays some of the clinical and microscopic features of atrophic vaginitis, yet it develops in women with normal estrogen levels. It is characterized mainly by reddened superficial ulcerations that respond slowly to treatment; recrudescence is the rule.

VAGINITIS EMPHYSEMATOSA

Vaginitis emphysematosa is an unusual condition of the vagina characterized by multiple, discrete, gas-filled, cystoid cavities of the vaginal and cervical mucosa. The blebs are distended with a gas of unknown composition but with a known carbon dioxide content. It occurs more commonly in association with pregnancy, trichomoniasis, and *Hemophilus vaginalis* vaginitis.

SYNONYMS: *Emphysematous Vaginitis, Emphysematous Colpitis, Colpohyperplasia Cystica.*

VAGINITIS, POSTIRRADIATION

Postirradiation vaginitis results from physical trauma to the vagina produced by radium applicators and packs, from the irradiation per se of the vagina, and from irradiation castration.

VAGINOCELE

Vaginocele is a hernia protruding into the vagina.
SYNONYM: *Colpocele.*

VULVITIS

Vulvitis is inflammation of the vulva.
SYNONYM: *Edeitis.*

VULVITIS, DIABETIC

Diabetic vulvitis is a special variety of chronic vulvar dermatitis that develops only in diabetics and is probably related to chronic and recurrent candidiasis. It is characterized by chronic pruritus, irritation, burning, dysuria, and dyspareunia, all of which tend to persist in varying degrees after treatment for the diabetes and candidiasis.

VULVITIS, ECZEMATOID

Eczematoid vulvitis is an acute or chronic inflammatory reaction of the female external genital structures. It is characterized by multiform lesions, moist or dry, and accompanied by itching, burning, and various paresthesias. It may be an allergic reaction. It is often seen in patients who have been overtreated with topical agents used for a specific vaginitis.

VULVOVAGINITIS

Vulvovaginitis is inflammation of the vulva and vagina.

VULVOVAGINITIS, BACTERIAL

Bacterial vulvovaginitis is inflammation of the vulva and vagina by nonvenereal bacteria such as *Hemophilus vaginalis, Proteus, Pseudomonas, Streptococcus,* and *Staphylococcus.*

VULVOVAGINITIS, CONTACT

Contact vulvovaginitis is a cutaneous eruption on the vulva or mucous membrane of the vagina due to external irritants. It may be edematous, erythematous, or vesicular. Chemical irritants are frequent causes.

SECTION 3: DISEASES AND CONDITIONS OF GENERATIVE ORGANS

Bladder and Urethra

ABSCESS, SUBURETHRAL
A suburethral abscess is an abscess formation beneath the urethra in association with infection and occlusion of the paraurethral glands and ducts.

ACYSTIA
Acystia is the congenital absence of the urinary bladder.

AMYLOIDOSIS
Amyloidosis is marked amyloid infiltration of the bladder wall. Grossly, the lesions are elevated, flat, yellowish or pinkish brown, with smooth or roughened hyperemic surfaces. Some are ulcerated and hemorrhagic. Microscopically, an almost acellular homogeneous material is seen that has an affinity for amyloid stains. The membrana propria is replaced by amyloid substances.

BLADDER, ATONIC
An atonic bladder is a bladder characterized by failure of muscle contraction due to disturbance of innervation.

BLADDER, AUTONOMIC
An autonomic bladder is a bladder characterized by periodic reflex micturition free from voluntary control.

BLADDER, CORD
Cord bladder is a neurogenic dysfunction of the bladder resulting from paresis of the bladder. It is marked by weakness of the detrusor muscle with weakness of the sphincters and the general presence of residual urine.

BLADDER, EXSTROPHY OF
Exstrophy of the bladder is an anomaly in which the anterior wall of the bladder and the overlying anterior abdominal wall are absent so that the inner surface of the posterior wall is everted. This protrudes in the region of the lower anterior wall of the abdomen. It occurs about once in 50,000 births and seven times more frequently in the male. Only a few patients have survived well into adult life.

BLADDER, FASCICULATE

A fasciculate bladder is a bladder with hypertrophied walls, the muscular bundles standing out like interlacing cords beneath the vesical mucosa.

BLADDER, IRRITABLE

An irritable bladder is a bladder abnormally sensitive to the presence of small amounts of urine, producing a constant desire to urinate.

SYNONYM: *Cysterethism.*

BLADDER, NEUROGENIC

A neurogenic bladder is a malfunctioning bladder caused by damaged innervation.

CALCULI, VESICAL

Vesical calculi are stones of the bladder. Calculi developing in the urinary bladder may be of inflammatory or noninflammatory origin. Among the most common causes are imperfect emptying of the bladder due to obstruction or paralysis, infection, foreign bodies, an inadequate amount of vitamin A, or faulty metabolism of calcium, uric acid, cystine, or xanthine. Vesical calculi may be single or multiple, and variable in size. Complications of vesical stones are obstruction, bladder hypertrophy, hydronephrosis, or pyelonephritis.

SYNONYM: *Cystoliths.*

COLPOCYSTOCELE

A colpocystocele is a herniation of the bladder into the vagina.

CYST, URETHRAL

A urethral cyst generally arises from an inflammatory occlusion of the urethral glands. It usually results in a swelling between the urethra and vagina.

CYSTALGIA

Cystalgia is pain in the bladder.

SYNONYM: *Cystodynia.*

CYSTATROPHIA

Cystatrophia is atrophy of the bladder.

CYSTAUXE

Cystauxe is enlargement of the bladder. It may be due to stricture of the urethra, obstruction of the vesical neck, or neurogenic dysfunction. If obstruction is of long duration, the dilatation may be accompanied by compensatory hypertrophy.

CYSTISTAXIS

Cystistaxis is an oozing of blood from the mucous membrane of the bladder due to inflammation, tumors, calculi, blood dyscrasias, parasites, foreign bodies, or trauma.

CYSTITIS
Cystitis is an acute or chronic inflammation of the urinary bladder. It is rarely a primary condition and is usually secondary to an infection of the kidney or urethra. The direct agents causing cystitis are: bacteria, chemical irritants, mechanical irritants, parasites, and fungi.

CYSTITIS, ABACTERIAL
Abacterial cystitis is usually associated with Reiter's disease, in which there may also be bilateral conjunctivitis and polyarticular arthritis. The urine contains many polymorphonuclear neutrophils and no bacteria. Bacterial cultures of urine are repeatedly negative. The mucosa is edematous, somewhat hyperemic, and may contain superficial ulcers.

CYSTITIS, ACUTE
Acute cystitis may be catarrhal, fibrinopurulent, purulent, diphtheritic, ulcerative, hemorrhagic, or gangrenous. In mild inflammation, the mucosa is hyperemic, edematous, and infiltrated with lymphocytes and a few polymorphonuclear neutrophils. In moderate and severe forms, there is marked hyperemia of the tunica propria. This is followed by multiple hemorrhages in the tunica propria, and superficial ulceration of the mucosa may develop. As the inflammation progresses the bladder wall becomes more thickened and infiltrated with neutrophilic leukocytes. At times there is a diffuse purulent cystitis or there may be small intramural abscesses. When necrosis supervenes, the picture is that of a hemorrhagic gangrenous cystitis. The surface becomes shaggy owing to adherent fibrin, mucopurulent exudate, and projecting necrotic tissue.

CYSTITIS, ACUTE HEMORRHAGIC
Acute hemorrhagic cystitis is an acute bladder inflammation of such intensity that bleeding from the mucosa results.

CYSTITIS, BULLOUS
Bullous cystitis is an inflammatory condition with marked mucosal and submucosal edema manifested by large bullae that at times may simulate polyps. It occurs in a variety of inflammatory conditions, but it is most commonly seen in uremia and early irradiation cystitis. It may be local or may involve the entire bladder. The bladder wall is thick and edematous, and the mucosa is thrown into folds and polypoid masses.

CYSTITIS, CHRONIC
Chronic cystitis is a chronic inflammation of one or all of the layers of the bladder. It may follow one or repeated attacks of acute cystitis. The capacity of the bladder is decreased owing to fibrosis, thickening of the wall, and decreased elasticity. The mucosa is rather dull and frequently roughened and contains focal areas of dilated blood vessels. The gross and microscopic changes of chronic cystitis with its acute exacerbations vary markedly and depend on: individual variability of tissue reaction, intensity of the infection, and the causative agent.

CYSTITIS COLLI
Cystitis colli is an inflammation of the vesical neck.

CYSTITIS, CYSTIC
Cystic cystitis consists of single or multiple cysts projecting above the mucosal surface of the bladder. These lesions are usually associated with chronic cystitis. Microscopic studies reveal epithelial sprouts arising from the mucosa and extending into the tunica propria. The proximal part of the epithelial downgrowth thins out to form an epithelial stalk. The stalk eventually becomes severed, resulting in free transitional epithelial bodies known as *epithelial nests*. The central cells are transformed into mucus-secreting cuboidal or columnar epithelial cells that at first rest on transitional cells. Ultimately, the underlying transitional cells disappear and a glandular or cystic structure is formed, lined by cuboidal or columnar cells. Some sprouts become cystic without being detached from the mucosa. Some cysts remain microscopic in dimension; others enlarge, push upward, and project above the surface. The contents may be watery or thick and viscid.

CYSTITIS, EMPHYSEMATOUS
Emphysematous cystitis is a rather rare condition in which the mucosa is studded with gas-filled vesicles. It occurs most frequently in diabetic patients. It may be due either to bacterial fermentation of glucose present in the mucosa and submucosa or to enzymatic action of these tissues when bacteria are absent. In nondiabetic cases, the formation of vesicles is due to clostridial gas-forming bacilli. Grossly, the mucosa may show various gradations of hyperemia, with prominent silvery bubbles ranging from 1 to 10 mm in diameter. Microscopically, most of the vesicles are situated beneath the mucosa, and their walls are composed of compressed fibrous tissue.

CYSTITIS, ENCRUSTED
Encrusted cystitis is an alkaline-encrusted cystitis that may become a stubborn chronic infection. Most cases occur in women after parturition. The inflamed bladder is invaded by urea-splitting bacteria, causing production of ammonia and consequently the precipitation of urinary salts. The crystals settle on any injured portion of the bladder, forming whitish or grayish white, granular, flat or slightly elevated patches (crusts).

CYSTITIS, EXFOLIATIVE
Exfoliative cystitis is an inflammation of the bladder with sloughing of the mucosa.

CYSTITIS, FOLLICULAR
Follicular cystitis is characterized by aggregations of numerous tiny, grayish or yellowish, elevated nodules, some of which are surrounded by a reddish zone. Microscopically, there are numerous discrete collections of lymphocytes in the submucosa. Well-defined follicles of larger lympho-

cytes with pale nuclei are in the center of the collections. The trigone is the most frequent seat of this rare disease.

CYSTITIS, GANGRENOUS

Gangrenous cystitis occurs in severe infections, trauma, extravesical pressure (pregnancy, tumors, etc.), x-ray and radium reactions, circulatory obstruction of adjacent arteries, and injection of chemicals. This serious infection occurs more frequently in women. It may involve either the mucosa alone or all layers of the bladder. The mucous surface appears rough, shaggy, dirty, and grayish with purplish and black areas. The mucosa may be cast off in fragments or in one piece.

CYSTITIS, GLANDULAR

Glandular cystitis is a lesion usually located in the trigone. It frequently occurs in exstrophied bladders. The tunica propria contains simple glands or glandlike spaces lined with cuboidal or columnar epithelial cells. The glandular structures may open on the mucosal surface. The most frequent type of gland is lined with tall columnar mucus-secreting epithelial cells. They originate either from cloacal rests or metaplastic changes of the bladder mucosa in a manner similar to that in the genesis of cystic cystitis.

CYSTITIS, INTERSTITIAL

Interstitial cystitis is a lesion of unknown cause occurring almost exclusively in women. It is often associated with endocervicitis, lymphatic obstruction, and bladder spasm in women under nervous tension. The lesion, single or multiple, usually begins in the dome or anterior wall of the bladder. Grossly, the involved area appears thick, has an uneven, usually smooth surface with a faint ulcerated or excoriated area. Microscopically, the surface epithelium is flattened, thin, or denuded in the ulcer-bearing area. In the early stages, the submucous connective tissue is edematous and infiltrated with lymphocytes. Later an increased amount of fibrous tissue develops in the tunica propria and the intermuscular stroma. As the lesion spreads, there is increased fibrosis, with cicatricial contraction so that the capacity of the bladder becomes diminished. In advanced fibrosis, the bladder may shrink to a capacity of only 2 or 3 ounces of urine.

SYNONYMS: *Hunner's Ulcer, Localized Submucous Fibrosis.*

CYSTITIS, IRRADIATION

Irradiation cystitis is produced by exposure to roentgen ray or radium. In the early stage, a bullous cystitis may involve the posterior wall. Later, small granulomatous red excrescences appear. Indolent ulcers with marginal telangiectasia may develop months or years after irradiation. Microscopically, there is telangiectasia of the veins and lymphatic vessels, hyaline fibrosis, and thickening of the arteries. The mucosa is usually atrophic or may undergo squamous cell metaplasia. Complications are ureteral strictures and vesicorectal and vesicovaginal fistulas.

CYSTITIS, PHLEGMONOUS

Phlegmonous cystitis is rare and is comparable to phlegmonous gastritis. The purulent exudate may be local and circumscribed, and become an intramural abscess, or the entire wall may be diffusely infiltrated with polymorphonuclear leukocytes.

CYSTITIS, TUBERCULOUS

Tuberculous cystitis may be associated with general miliary tuberculosis. Most cases of tuberculous cystitis are due to implantation of tubercle bacilli from the upper urinary tract. Early lesions appear as miliary tubercles around the orifices of the ureters. The tubercles break down to form minute ulcers that coalesce, forming large irregular ulcers. Widespread ulceration with concomitant fibrosis causes contraction of the bladder.

CYSTOCELE

A cystocele is a hernia of the bladder through the inguinal or femoral rings. Congenital or acquired weakenings of the abdominal wall, increased intraabdominal pressure (gravid uterus), overdistention of the bladder, and trauma are some of the most important factors influencing the development of bladder herniation.

CYSTOENTEROCELE

A cystoenterocele is a hernial protrusion of portions of the bladder and of the intestine.

CYSTOEPIPLOCELE

Cystoepiplocele is a hernial protrusion of a portion of the bladder and of the omentum.

CYSTOLITHIASIS

Cystolithiasis is the presence of calculi or stones in the urinary bladder.

CYSTOPARALYSIS

Cystoparalysis is paralysis of the bladder.
SYNONYM: *Cystoplegia.*

CYSTOPTOSIS

Cystoptosis is prolapse of the mucous membrane of the bladder into the urethra.

CYSTOPYELITIS

Cystopyelitis is an inflammation of both the bladder and the kidney pelvis.

CYSTOPYELONEPHRITIS

Cystopyelonephritis is an inflammation of the bladder, pelvis of the kidney, and the kidney substance.

CYSTORRHAGIA
Cystorrhagia is hemorrhage from the bladder due to tumors, inflammation, calculi, blood dyscrasias, parasites, foreign bodies, or trauma.

CYSTORRHEA
Cystorrhea is a mucous discharge from the bladder.

CYSTOSPASM
Cystospasm is a spasmodic contraction of the bladder producing pain.

CYSTOURETERITIS
Cystoureteritis is inflammation of the bladder and one or both ureters.

CYSTOURETHRITIS
Cystourethritis is inflammation of the bladder and the urethra.

CYSTOURETHROCELE
Cystourethrocele is relaxation or prolapse of the urinary bladder and urethra.

DIVERTICULUM, URETHRAL
A urethral diverticulum is a sac, filled with urine or a purulent substance, that generally extends from the posterior wall of the urethra into the urethrovaginal septum.

DIVERTICULUM, VESICAL
A vesical diverticulum is an outpouching of the bladder wall. It may be single or multiple, congenital or acquired, and of the true or false type. A true diverticulum is usually a congenital outpouching in which the wall contains all the layers of the bladder. A false diverticulum is usually acquired and is formed by herniation of the inner lining through a defect of the outer lining. Infection may lead to vesical diverticulitis, ulceration, and lithiasis.

DYSFUNCTION, NEUROGENIC BLADDER
Neurogenic bladder dysfunction is caused by diseases of the nervous system that in turn cause paralysis, atony, or hypertonicity of the urinary bladder. The lesions may be central or peripheral.

Central Lesions
Central lesions that cause bladder dysfunction are traumatic and neoplastic diseases of the brain and spinal cord, and inflammatory and noninflammatory degenerative diseases such as neurosyphilis (tabes dorsalis, paresis, and rarely, gumma), multiple sclerosis, poliomyelitis, transverse myelitis, ataxic paraplegia, spina bifida, and rarely, thrombosis and infarction. The mucosa is pale and smooth and shows threadlike trabeculation.

Peripheral Nerve Lesions

Peripheral nerve lesions causing neurogenic bladder dysfunction are found in spina bifida occulta, peripheral neuritis, infectious neuronitis, and in some infectious diseases with high fevers such as scarlet fever and diphtheria.

DYSURIA

Dysuria is painful urination.

ENDOMETRIOSIS, VESICAL

Vesical endometriosis is the presence of endometrial tissue in the urinary bladder. The lesions appear as reddish, bluish, or bluish black elevations in which small cysts may be recognized. Their usual size is 1 to 2 cm in diameter, but they may appear as tumors of several centimeters in diameter. The mucosa around and sometimes over the lesion is congested, edematous, and folded. During menstruation, the lesions are larger, more congested, bluish, and cystic. Active bleeding may occur. Microscopically, isolated endometrial glands surrounded by an endometrial stroma are seen. The structures lie in the tunica propria and muscularis.

EPICYSTITIS

Epicystitis is inflammation of the structures above the bladder.

FISTULA, UMBILICOURACHOCYSTIC

An umbilicourachocystic fistula is a condition that develops as a result of nondescent of the bladder. Frequently, a granuloma may form in the umbilicus.

FISTULA, URACHOUMBILICAL

An urachoumbilical fistula may be congenital or acquired. The congenital type communicates with the umbilicus and not with the bladder. The acquired urachoumbilical fistula results from increased intravesical pressure, usually at the junction of the bladder and urachus. Urine escapes between the transversalis fascia and peritoneum and may perforate the floor of the umbilicus.

FISTULA, VESICOENTERIC

A vesicoenteric fistula is a communication between the bladder and rectum, sigmoid, jejunum, ileum, or appendix. It occurs in both sexes but is more common in the male. These fistulas may result from trauma, inflammatory or neoplastic diseases, roentgen and radium rays, or erosion of a vesical calculus.

FISTULA, VESICOUTERINE

A vesicouterine fistula is a communication between the bladder and uterus. It may occur after cesarean section, neoplastic diseases, or radiation therapy.

FISTULA, VESICOVAGINAL

A vesicovaginal fistula is an opening or communication between the bladder and vagina caused by obstetric injuries, pelvic operations, roentgen or radium therapy, or inflammation and malignant neoplasm of the urinary bladder, cervix, or vagina. The size of the opening may vary from pinpoint to several centimeters. The communication usually involves the posterior wall of the bladder and upper anterior wall of the vagina. The walls are discolored and undergo marked inflammatory changes; in radium cases, there is considerable sloughing.

HYPERTROPHY OF BLADDER

Hypertrophy of the bladder is thickening of the wall of the urinary bladder. It may be concentric or eccentric.

Concentric Hypertrophy of Bladder

Concentric hypertrophy of the bladder is usually due to irritation as in inflammation, calculi, and foreign bodies. The bladder maintains its normal capacity.

Eccentric Hypertrophy of Bladder

Eccentric hypertrophy of the bladder is predominantly due to obstruction to the outflow of urine. The thickening of the wall is due to hypertrophy of the interlacing bands of smooth muscle and an increase of connective tissue. Externally the bladder appears wrinkled; internally there is prominent crisscrossing of hypertrophied muscle bundles, often described as trabeculation of the bladder. Between the muscle bundles there are small pockets or cellules.

LEUKOPLAKIA, VESICAL

Vesical leukoplakia is a disease producing a smooth, dead-white, sharply demarcated patch representing an area of epidermoid transformation of the transitional cells of the bladder mucosa. The patch may be single, multiple, or may in very rare cases involve the entire mucosa. It is definitely associated with chronic cystitis of long duration. Microscopic sections reveal two types of lesions. In one type, there is a thickened layer of well-differentiated, stratified, squamous epithelial cells. In the second type, the layer of squamous epithelial cells shows activity or proliferation of the basal portion. The nuclei may be elongated and hyperchromatic, frequently showing mitotic figures. Such lesions have been considered precancerous, thus supporting the popular belief that they give rise to malignant neoplasms. A few cases of squamous cell carcinoma associated with leukoplakia have been reported.

MALAKOPLAKIA, VESICAL

Vesical malakoplakia is an uncommon granulomatous inflammation occurring predominantly in women past 30 years of age who have had frequent bouts of cystitis. The lesions are multiple, discrete or confluent, soft, grayish yellow or yellowish brown, well-defined, slightly raised plaques or nodules, frequently having depressed centers, and often surrounded by a zone of hyperemia. They vary from 1 mm to more than 5 cm in diameter. Microscopically, the lesions are granulomatous. In addition to the usual inflammatory cellular elements, there are many large and medium-size, rounded and polyhedral cells having abundant granular and vacuolated cytoplasm and well-defined cell membranes. The most characteristic feature of malakoplakia is the presence of calcospherites which, if uniform in size and not laminated, have the appearance of yeastlike fungi. They reveal high calcium content with von Kossa stain. Hemosiderin may be demonstrated in them using the Gomori iron reaction.

MYCOSES, VESICAL

Vesical mycoses are rare infections of the urinary bladder. They are usually secondary to an invasion by actinomyces from adjacent visceral involvement or implantation from renal actinomycosis. Grossly, the lesions may resemble tuberculosis, and actinomyces may be demonstrated microscopically in the granulation tissue. Monilial cystitis has been reported with general candidiasis. In females, monilia may invade the bladder by way of the urethra in cases of monilial vaginitis. Grossly, the mucosa contains soft, pearl-white, slightly elevated patches. These patches are quite firmly adherent to the mucosa, which bleeds when they are removed. Many yeastlike spores and occasional filaments are present in scrapings from the patches. Other yeasts and molds may become secondary invaders and produce lesions in the bladder.

PARACYSTITIS

Paracystitis is an inflammation of the connective tissue and other structures lying near the urinary bladder.

PERICYSTITIS

Pericystitis is an inflammation of the tissues surrounding the urinary bladder.

PROCTOCYSTOCELE

A proctocystocele is herniation of the bladder into the rectum.

PROLAPSE, URETHRAL

A urethral prolapse is a prolapse of the urethral mucosa. Absence of pediculation, hyperesthesia, and infiltration distinguishes this lesion from a caruncle or malignancy. This condition may occur in infancy and can be corrected surgically.

SYNONYM: *Urethrocele.*

PROLAPSE, VESICAL

A vesical prolapse is an inversion and herniation of the upper part of the bladder through the urethra. It is caused by relaxation of supporting ligaments and sphincters, an aftermath of difficult labor, with an increase in intraabdominal pressure. Gangrene may develop rapidly because of pressure on the blood vessels. A vesical prolapse occurs only in the female.

REFLUX, VESICOURETERAL
Vesicoureteral reflux is the backward flow of urine from the bladder into a ureter.

STENOSIS, BLADDER NECK
Bladder neck stenosis is an obstruction to the flow of urine. It may be congenital or acquired. In congenital stenosis, a diaphragm composed of muscle and fibrous tissue obstructs the proximal end of the urethra. The acquired type occurs almost exclusively in males as a result of scarring and narrowing of the bladder neck and prostatic urethra. Microscopically, the congenital diaphragm is composed of normal muscle and fibrous tissue devoid of inflammation, whereas the acquired type contains very few muscle fibers, much fibrous tissue, and inflammatory cellular infiltration.
SYNONYM: *Marion's Disease.*

URETHRALGIA
Urethralgia is pain in the urethra.
SYNONYM: *Urethrodynia.*

URETHRATRESIA
Urethratresia is occlusion or atresia of the urethra.

URETHREMORRHAGIA
Urethremorrhagia is bleeding from the urethra.
SYNONYM: *Urethrorrhagia.*

URETHREMPHRAXIS
Urethremphraxis is obstruction of the free flow of urine through to the urethra.

URETHRISM
Urethrism is irritability or spasmodic stricture of the urethra.
SYNONYM: *Urethrismus.*

URETHRITIS
Urethritis is inflammation of the urethra.

URETHRITIS VENEREA
Urethritis venerea is gonorrhea of the urethra.

URETHROCYSTITIS
Urethrocystitis is inflammation of the urethra and bladder.

URETHROLITHIASIS
Urethrolithiasis is a condition in which calculi are found in the urethra. They are either dislodged bladder calculi, or when primary, they originate in a urethral diverticulum.

URETHROPHYMA

Urethrophyma is any circumscribed swelling of the urethra.

URETHRORRHEA

Urethrorrhea is an abnormal discharge of mucus or purulent material from the urethra.

SYNONYM: *Blennorrhea.*

URETHROSPASM

Urethrospasm is a spasmodic contraction of the muscular fibers surrounding the urethra.

Rectum and Anus

FISSURE, ANAL

An anal fissure is a slitlike ulcer at and proximal to the anal verge, and characterized by intermittent pain.

FISTULA, ANORECTAL

An anorectal fistula is a pathologic tract between the anorectum and some adjacent viscus or skin surface.

HEMORRHOID

A hemorrhoid is a varicose dilatation involving one or more branches of the hemorrhoidal plexus of veins.

External Hemorrhoid

An external hemorrhoid is a varicose dilatation of one or more branches of the middle and inferior rectal veins beneath the skin of the anal canal and anal verge.

Internal Hemorrhoid

An internal hemorrhoid is a varicose dilatation of one or more branches of the superior rectal veins beneath the mucous membrane of the rectum and proximal to the dentate line.

PAPILLITIS, ANAL

Anal papillitis is inflammation and hypertrophy of an anal papilla with protrusion into the anal canal.

POLYP, ANAL

An anal polyp is an outgrowth from the mucous membrane of the anus.

PROCTAGRA

Proctagra is a pain in the anus.

PROCTATRESIA

Proctatresia is imperforation of the anus.
SYNONYM: *Imperforate Anus.*

PROCTECTASIA

Proctectasia is dilatation of the anus or rectum.

PROCTENCLEISIS
Proctencleisis is a stricture of the anus or rectum.
SYNONYMS: *Proctostenosis, Rectostenosis.*

PROCTITIS
Proctitis is an inflammation of the mucous membrane and deeper layers of the rectum.
SYNONYM: *Rectitis.*

PROCTODYNIA
Proctodynia is pain in the rectum.
SYNONYM: *Proctalgia.*

PROCTOMENIA
Proctomenia is vicarious menstruation involving the rectum.

PROCTOPARALYSIS
Proctoparalysis is paralysis of the anus, resulting in fecal incontinence.

PROCTOPHOBIA
Proctophobia is a fear of rectal disease.

PROCTOPOLYPUS
Proctopolypus is a polyp of the rectum.

PROCTOSTASIS
Proctostasis is constipation due to anesthesia of the rectum to the stimulus of defecation.

PRURITUS ANI
Pruritus ani is more or less intense itching at the anus and is unassociated with other lesions except those caused by intertrigo and scratching.

RECTOCELE
A rectocele is a herniation of the rectum into the vagina, usually resulting from trauma to the levator ani muscles and supporting fascia.
SYNONYM: *Proctocele.*

RECTOCYSTOCELE
A rectocystocele is a herniation of the bladder into the rectum.

RECTUM, PROLAPSED
A prolapsed rectum is the abnormal descent of all layers of the rectum with or without protrusion through the anal canal.
SYNONYMS: *Proctoptosis, Proctoptoma.*

SPHINCTER, ANAL, INCOMPETENT
An incompetent anal sphincter is an anal sphincter that cannot control bowel contents, resulting in fecal incontinence.

Section 4: *Benign and Malignant Neoplasms*

SECTION 4: BENIGN AND MALIGNANT NEOPLASMS

Staging of Tumors

The Committee on Terminology of The American College of Obstetricians and Gynecologists has studied intensively the various classifications of malignant diseases of the generative organs. The Committee has further discussed these classifications on many occasions with cancer committees of national and international organizations. The Committee recommends the use of the classification of gynecologic malignancies which was published by the International Federation of Gynecology and Obstetrics in 1971. The Committee has made some editorial additions to a few of the definitions as originally worded in the International Federation of Gynecology and Obstetrics' classification. The classification of malignant disease of the fallopian tube is proposed by The American College of Obstetricians and Gynecologists' Committee on Terminology.

GENERAL RULES FOR STAGING MALIGNANCY
OF THE GENERATIVE ORGANS

1. The staging of every malignancy of the generative organs should be determined before definitive therapy, and the malignancy should be classified accordingly.

2. Examinations that can be performed in all hospitals by all physicians and surgeons should be used to determine the stage of the malignancy.

3. The procedures should consist of a clinical examination including pelvic and rectal examinations with palpation and inspection, and examinations such as cytologic examination, histologic examination, biopsy, fractional curettage, colposcopy, hysteroscopy, roentgen examination of the lungs and skeleton, and intravenous urography. Pertinent diagnostic procedures and examinations under anesthesia should be performed.

4. The neoplasm must be confirmed histologically.

5. The staging should not be changed after definitive therapy, interim response to treatment, or postmortem findings.

6. When staging is in doubt, the lesser stage of the disease should be assigned.

7. Statistics relating to efficacy of therapy should be reported separately for noninvasive carcinoma (Stage 0, carcinoma in situ) and for invasive malignancy.

153

ANAPLASIA

Anaplasia is failure of cellular maturation with loss of structural differentiation and polarity, the presence of nuclear hyperchromatism, and increased numbers of mitotic figures.

SQUAMOUS METAPLASIA

Squamous metaplasia is benign focal or diffuse replacement of columnar epithelium by cells resembling squamous cells.

OBSOLETE TERMS:

Atypia, atypical epithelial hyperplasia, atypical metaplasia, atypism, basal cell hyperplasia, koilocytotic atypia, reserve cell hyperplasia.

STAGING OF CARCINOMA OF FALLOPIAN TUBE

Stage 0
The carcinoma is confined to the epithelium of the fallopian tubes.

Stage I
The carcinoma is confined to the fallopian tubes.

STAGE I_a
The carcinoma is confined to one fallopian tube with no ascites.

STAGE I_b
The carcinoma is confined to both fallopian tubes with no ascites.

STAGE I_c
The carcinoma is confined to one or both fallopian tubes. Ascites is present with malignant cells in the fluid.

Stage II
The carcinoma extends to other intraperitoneal organs or tissues within the true pelvis.

STAGE II_a
The carcinoma extends only to the uterus, or ovaries, or both.

STAGE II_b
The carcinoma extends to the uterus or ovaries and to other intraperitoneal organs or tissues within the true pelvis.

Stage III
The carcinoma extends to the uterus or ovaries and to other intraperitoneal organs and tissues beyond the true pelvis (for example, omentum, the small intestine, or mesentery).

Stage IV
The carcinoma metastasizes to organs or tissues outside the peritoneal cavity.

STAGING OF CARCINOMA OF OVARY

Staging of carcinoma of the ovary should be based on clinical examination and observation at laparotomy. Germ cell tumors, hormone-produc-

ing neoplasms, and metastatic carcinomas should be excluded from therapeutic statistical reporting on ovarian epithelial tumors.

Stage I
The carcinoma is confined to the ovaries.

STAGE I$_a$

The carcinoma is confined to one ovary without ascites.
(i) Capsule ruptured; (ii) capsule not ruptured.

STAGE I$_b$

The carcinoma is confined to both ovaries without ascites.
(i) Capsule ruptured; (ii) capsule not ruptured.

STAGE I$_c$

The carcinoma is confined to one or both ovaries with ascites
and the presence of malignant cells in the fluid. (i) Capsule
ruptured; (ii) capsule not ruptured.

Stage II
The carcinoma involves one or both ovaries with pelvic extension.

STAGE II$_a$

The carcinoma extends and/or metastasizes to the uterus
and/or fallopian tubes only.

STAGE II$_b$

The carcinoma extends to other pelvic tissues.

Stage III
The carcinoma involves one or both ovaries with widespread intraperitoneal metastasis to the abdomen (the omentum, the small intestine, and its mesentery).

Stage IV
The carcinoma involves one or both ovaries with distant metastasis
outside the peritoneal cavity.

Special Category
a. Unexplored cases in which extraperitoneal tumors thought to
be of ovarian origin have developed.

b. Patients in whom exploratory surgery has shown widespread
intraperitoneal carcinoma believed to be of ovarian origin.

STAGING OF CARCINOMA OF CORPUS UTERI*
Carcinoma of the corpus uteri should be so classified when the primary
site of growth is located in the corpus. Mixed mesenchymal tumors and
the so-called carcinoma sarcoma should be excluded.

Stage 0
The carcinoma is confined to the endometrium (carcinoma in situ).

---

* On occasion, it may be difficult to decide whether the cancer originates in the
endocervix or in the corpus and endocervix. If a clear differentiation of origin is
not possible from the findings at fractional curettage, then those cancers that are
adenocarcinomas should be classified as carcinoma of the corpus, and those that
are squamous carcinomas as carcinoma of the cervix.

Stage I
The carcinoma is confined to the corpus of the uterus.

STAGE I$_a$
The carcinoma is present in a uterus measuring up to 8 cm in length from the external os to the upper limit of the uterine cavity.

STAGE I$_b$
The carcinoma is present in a uterus measuring more than 8 cm in length from the external os to the upper limit of the uterine cavity.

The carcinoma should be subdivided according to the histologic structures in the tissues:

G1 = Highly differentiated adenomatous carcinoma.

G2 = Differentiated adenomatous carcinoma with partly solid areas.

G3 = Predominantly solid or entirely undifferentiated carcinoma.

Stage II
The carcinoma involves the corpus and the cervix, but does not extend beyond the uterus.

Stage III
The carcinoma extends beyond the uterus, but is confined within the true pelvis.

Stage IV
The carcinoma extends outside the true pelvis, or obviously involves the mucosa of the bladder or rectum. A bullous edema as such does not permit allotment of a case to Stage IV.

STAGING OF CARCINOMA OF CERVIX

Stage 0
The carcinoma is confined to the epithelium (carcinoma in situ). Cases of Stage 0 should not be included in any statistical classification.

Stage I
The carcinoma is strictly confined to the cervix.

STAGE I$_{a-1}$
A tumor with a tongue of minimal invasion to a depth of less than 1 mm into the adjacent stroma in continuity with surface epithelium or lining epithelium.

STAGE I$_{a-2}$
A tumor with free (discontinuous) invasion greater than 1 mm.

STAGE I$_b$
All other cases of Stage I.

Stage II
The carcinoma extends beyond the cervix, infiltrating the endometrium, the upper two-thirds of the vagina, or the parametrium, but not to the pelvic wall.

STAGE II$_a$
The carcinoma infiltrates the upper two-thirds of the vagina or the endometrium.

STAGE II$_b$
The carcinoma infiltrates the parametrium.

Stage III
The carcinoma extends onto the pelvic wall or the distal one-third of the vagina.

STAGE III$_a$
The carcinoma involves the distal one-third of the vagina.

STAGE III$_b$
The carcinoma extends onto the pelvic wall.

Stage IV
The carcinoma extends beyond the true pelvis or infiltrates the mucosa of the bladder or of the rectum.

STAGE IV$_a$
The carcinoma infiltrates the mucosa of the contiguous organs (bladder or rectum).

STAGE IV$_b$
The carcinoma extends to distant organs.

STAGING OF CARCINOMA OF VULVA
Carcinoma of the vulva should be so classified when the primary site of growth is on the vulva. A tumor present on the vulva as secondary growth from extragenital sites should be excluded from registration (for example, malignant melanoma).

CATEGORIES OF CARCINOMA OF THE VULVA*

T—Tumor or Primary Lesion and Its Extent
T1
The carcinoma is strictly confined to the vulva and is 2 cm or less in its largest diameter.

---

* Categories of carcinoma of the vulva employing the tumor-node-metastasis classification as proposed by the International Union Against Cancer.

T2

The carcinoma is confined to the vulva and is more than 2 cm in its largest diameter.

T3

The carcinoma is of any size with adjacent spread to the urethra and/or vagina and/or to the anus.

T4

The tumor is of any size and infiltrates the bladder mucosa or rectal mucosa including the upper half of the urethral mucosa, or is fixed to the pelvic bones.

N—Lymph Nodes of the Region and Their Condition

N0

There are no palpable lymph nodes.

N1

The lymph nodes palpable in either groin are discrete, mobile, of normal size, and not clinically suggestive of neoplasm.

N2

The lymph nodes palpable in either or both groins are enlarged, firm, and mobile, and are clinically suggestive of neoplasm.

N3

The lymph nodes palpable in either or both groins are fixed, confluent, or ulcerated.

M—Distant Metastases

M0

There is no clinical evidence of metastases.

$M1_a$

There are palpable deep pelvic lymph nodes.

$M1_b$

There is clinical evidence of metastases beyond the pelvis.

STAGING OF CARCINOMA OF VAGINA

Carcinoma of the vagina should be so classified when the primary site of growth is in the vagina. Tumors occurring in the vagina as secondary growth from either genital or extragenital sites should be excluded from the registration. A growth that has extended to the portio of the cervix and reached the area of the external os should be classified as carcinoma of the uterine cervix. A growth that has extended to the vulva should be classified as a carcinoma of the vulva. A growth located in the urethra should be classified as carcinoma of the urethra.

Stage 0

The carcinoma is limited to the epithelium of the vagina (carcinoma in situ).

Stage I

The carcinoma is limited to the vaginal wall.

STAGE I$_a$

The carcinoma is confined to the vaginal wall and is 2 cm or less in its greatest diameter.

STAGE I$_b$

The carcinoma is more than 2 cm in its greatest diameter but involves less than the entire vaginal wall in the longitudinal axis.

STAGE I$_c$

The carcinoma involves the entire vaginal wall in the longitudinal axis.

Stage II

The carcinoma infiltrates the paravaginal tissue but does not reach the pelvic wall.

Stage III

The carcinoma extends to and is fixed to the pelvic wall.

Stage IV

The carcinoma extends beyond the true pelvis or involves the mucosa of the bladder or of the rectum.

STAGE IV$_a$

The carcinoma extends to or involves the mucosa of the bladder or of the rectum.

STAGE IV$_b$

The carcinoma extends outside the true pelvis—for example, metastasizes to the inguinal lymph nodes, lymph nodes above the pelvic brim, or to distant sites.

Classification of Tumors

CLASSIFICATION OF TUMORS OF FALLOPIAN TUBE

Benign Tumors

EPITHELIAL ORIGIN
Endometriosis
Polyp*
Papilloma*
Dysgerminoma

ENDOTHELIAL OR MESOTHELIAL ORIGIN
Adenomatoid tumor
Hemangioma
Inclusion cyst*
Lymphangioma

MESODERMAL ORIGIN
Chondroma*
Lipoma
Leiomyoma (fibromyoma)
Osteoma*

TERATOID ORIGIN
Benign cystic teratoma (dermoid cyst)
Struma salpingis

MISCELLANEOUS
Granulosa cell tumor
Hilus cell hyperplasia*
Sertoli-Leydig tumor*
Xanthoma*
Mesonephroma

Malignant Tumors

Primary carcinoma
Secondary carcinoma
Choriocarcinoma
Sarcoma

---

* Tumors that have been reported but not pathologically confirmed.

CLASSIFICATION OF TUMORS OF OVARY

PHYSIOLOGIC OVARIAN CYSTS
  Follicular cyst
  Corpus luteum cyst
  Theca-lutein cyst
  Corpus albicans cyst

EPITHELIAL ORIGIN
  Serous cystoma
    Benign serous cystadenoma
    Serous cystadenoma with proliferative activity of the epithelial
      cells and nuclear abnormalities but with no infiltrative destruc-
      tive growth (low malignant potential)
    Serous cystadenocarcinoma
  Mucinous cystoma
    Benign mucinous cystadenoma
    Mucinous cystadenoma with proliferating activity of the epithelial
      cells and nuclear abnormalities but with no infiltrative destruc-
      tive growth (low malignant potential)
    Mucinous cystadenocarcinoma

ENDOMETRIAL TUMORS (similar to adenocarcinoma of endometrium)
  Benign endometrial cyst
  Endometrial tumors with proliferating activity of the epithelial cells
    and nuclear abnormalities but with no infiltrative destructive
    growth (low malignant potential)
  Endometrial adenocarcinoma

MESONEPHRIC TUMORS
  Benign mesonephric tumors
  Mesonephric tumors with proliferating activity of the epithelial cells
    and nuclear abnormalities but with no infiltrative destructive
    growth (low malignant potential)
  Mesonephric cystadenocarcinoma

UNCLASSIFIED CARCINOMA (tumors that cannot be assigned to one of
  the groups)

MESODERMAL
  Fibroma
  Fibrosarcoma
  Rhabdomyosarcoma
  Lymphoma

GONADAL STROMAL TUMORS
  Granulosa-theca cell tumors
    Granulosa cell tumor
    Thecoma
    Luteoma
  Arrhenoblastoma
  Gynandroblastoma

GERM CELL TUMORS
  Dysgerminoma
  Primary ovarian choriocarcinoma
  Endometrial sinus tumor
  Benign cystic teratoma (dermoid)
    Struma ovarii
  Malignant teratoma
  Gonadoblastoma
  Teratocarcinoma

CONGENITAL REST TUMORS
  Adrenal rest tumor
  Mesometanephric rest tumor
  Brenner tumor
  Hilar cell tumor

PRIMARY SOLID CARCINOMA
  Carcinoma
  Adenocarcinoma

SECONDARY MALIGNANT NEOPLASM (Metastatic)
  Krukenberg tumor

CLASSIFICATION OF TUMORS OF CORPUS UTERI

Benign

ENDOMETRIUM
  Endometrial polyp

MYOMETRIUM
  Leiomyoma
  Benign metastasizing leiomyoma
  Hemangiopericytoma
  Lipoma

Malignant

ENDOMETRIUM
  Carcinoma in situ
  Invasive carcinoma
    Adenoacanthoma
  Pedunculated adenomyoma
  Malignant mixed müllerian tumor
    Endometrial carcinosarcoma

MYOMETRIUM
  Leiomyosarcoma
  Malignant mixed müllerian tumor
    Rhabdomyosarcoma*
    Endometrial stromal sarcoma

---

* Rare tumor of the uterus

CLASSIFICATION OF TUMORS OF CERVIX

QUESTIONABLE NEOPLASTIC NATURE
  Polyp
  Papilloma
      Cockscomb polyp
      Condyloma acuminatum
      True cervical papilloma

EPITHELIAL ORIGIN
  Squamous cell carcinoma in situ
  Squamous cell carcinoma
  Adenocarcinoma
      Adenoacanthoma
      Mesometanephroma

MESODERMAL ORIGIN
  Leiomyoma
  Leiomyosarcoma*

MIXED MÜLLERIAN ORIGIN
  Botryoid tumor

RARE TUMORS
  Lymphoma
  Hemangioma
  Hemangioendothelioma
  Ganglioneuroma
  Malignant melanoma

CLASSIFICATION OF TUMORS OF VULVA

Benign Tumors

EPITHELIAL ORIGIN
  Condyloma acuminatum
  Papilloma
  Acrochordon
  Seborrheic keratosis
  Endometriosis
  Pigmented nevus
  Sebaceous adenoma
  Basal cell epithelioma
  Inclusion cyst
  Epidermal cyst
  Pilonidal cyst
  Sebaceous cyst
  Hidradenoma
  Syringoma

---

* Rare tumor of the cervix

MESODERMAL ORIGIN
  Fibroma
  Lipoma
  Neurofibroma
  Leiomyoma
  Granular cell myoblastoma
  Hemangioma
    Strawberry hemangioma
    Cavernous hemangioma
    Senile hemangioma
    Angiokeratoma
    Pyogenic granuloma
  Lymphangioma
    Lymphangioma simplex
    Lymphangioma cavernosum
    Lymphangioma circumscriptum
  Bartholin Duct Cyst

EMBRYONIC ORIGIN
  Embryonic cyst

Malignant Tumors

EPITHELIAL ORIGIN
  Carcinoma in situ
    Bowen's disease
    Erythroplasia of Queyrat
    Extramammary Paget's disease
    Amelanotic melanoma
  Papillary carcinoma in situ
  Melanoma
  Invasive carcinoma
    Basal cell carcinoma
    Squamous cell carcinoma
  Hidradenocarcinoma
  Bartholin gland carcinoma

MESODERMAL ORIGIN
  Sarcoma
    Rhabdomyosarcoma
    Liposarcoma
    Lymphosarcoma
    Fibrosarcoma
  Bartholin gland sarcoma

CLASSIFICATION OF TUMORS OF VAGINA

EPITHELIAL ORIGIN
  Papilloma
  Polyp

Cysts
    Inclusion cyst
    Gartner duct cyst
Adenosis
Primary carcinoma

MESODERMAL ORIGIN
    Leiomyoma
    Sarcoma
    Melanoma
    Fibroma*
    Myoblastic myoma*
    Neurofibroma*
    Fibroleiomyoma*
    Neuroepithelioma*

MIXED MÜLLERIAN ORIGIN
    Sarcoma botryoides

TERATOID ORIGIN
    Benign cystic teratoma

MISCELLANEOUS
    Endometriosis

METASTATIC
    Metastatic carcinoma

---

* Rare tumors of the vagina

SECTION 4: BENIGN AND MALIGNANT NEOPLASMS

Tumors

BREAST

ACUTE INFLAMMATORY CARCINOMA OF BREAST

Acute inflammatory carcinoma of the breast is a condition occurring in the obese pendulous breasts of young women, especially during lactation. It very closely resembles acute inflammation of the breast. It is generally associated with outstanding signs and symptoms of inflammation—both local and general. It is sudden in onset, showing a rapidly developing discoloration and induration of the breast. An intense reddish purple hue develops that may extend onto the chest wall or to the opposite breast. The skin is hot and dry and frequently shows a diffuse scaling. It has a particularly indurated feel. The crusted nipple is generally retracted, being barely visible. On gross examination, a very thick edematous skin and breast stroma are readily identified. In rare instances, a large, centrally situated, poorly defined mass can be identified; this generally has the characteristics of an infiltrating adenocarcinoma. Histologic characteristics are not specific, but infiltration of the subepidermal lymphatic vessels and lymph nodes is the identifying feature. Similar minute clusters of neoplastic cells infiltrate throughout the breast substance.

SYNONYMS: *Erysipeloid Carcinoma, Carcinomatous Mastitis.*

ADENOCARCINOMA OF BREAST

Adenocarcinoma of the breast is characterized by an extremely hard, fixed, infiltrating nodule with a slightly concave cut surface marked by grayish and yellowish streaking. Its early infiltration produces fixation, dimpling of the skin, retraction of the nipple, and axillary metastasis. The histologic character is that of a very prominent central hyalinized fibrosis associated with minute, angular, cleftlike spaces containing few closely packed epithelial cells. These may form minute columns or threadlike groups. When the cells are found in larger groups or broad columns, the tumor is known as *carcinoma simplex*. The cells are moderate in size and are generally deeply stained; the distinction between cytoplasm and nuclei is frequently obscure. Periductal and perivascular infiltration is most common.

ADENOMA OF BREAST

Adenoma of the breast differs from the other tumors in its remarkable epithelial proliferation of mature, irregular, closely packed glands outlined by tall, partly secreting epithelium.

166

CARCINOMA OF BREAST

Carcinoma of the breast may affect either breast, accessory breast tissue, or the male gland. Most cancers are discovered shortly before, during, or just after the menopause. The cause of mammary cancer is not completely known. Malignant tumors arise most frequently in the upper outer quadrant of the breast. There are two important gross types of breast carcinoma: (1) The classic example is that of a single, hard, poorly movable, nonelastic, easily cut nodule. Sections have a dry, gritty, opaque surface marked by radiating, translucent lines of connective tissue accompanied by small yellowish or opaque grayish dots and streaks. The central portion of the tumor is slightly concave, and the margins extend into the stroma, between which the fat lobules may protrude above the level of the tumor. Therefore, the border may be scalloped. The concave surface, the chalky streaks, the pouting fat tissue, and the blending of the tumor with the stroma in a radiating fashion are the paramount characteristics. The tissue appears extremely turgid and is not elastic or flexible. The infiltration of the connective tissue produces a contraction of the dermal papillae and of Cooper's ligaments, thereby developing the orange-peel appearance of the skin. Periductal invasion causes retraction of the nipple. Intimate fixation to breast stroma and sometimes to the underlying fascia makes the tumor limited in movement. (2) The other gross type is that of an opaque, white or pink, soft, highly cellular tissue that uniformly bulges above the cut surface and has an encephaloid character. This is particularly likely to be accompanied by cyst formation and hemorrhage. More than 90 per cent of malignant mammary tumors arise from the epithelium of the duct system, either the large or the small channels.

CARCINOMA OF MAMMARY DUCT

Carcinoma of the mammary duct is quite similar to comedocarcinoma, but it ordinarily lacks the central necrosis of the tumor cell disks. It is commonly associated with pain or discharge from the nipple and involvement of axillary nodes. The gross appearance is similar to that of comedocarcinoma, but small tumor-cell masses may be expressed rather than ribbons of pasty material. The microscopic picture is that of a profuse growth of the duct epithelium forming large clear cells with large nuclei, prominent nucleoli, and frequent mitoses. Minute papilloid projections and accessory acinar formation are more prominent than in comedocarcinoma. Pleomorphism is noteworthy.

CARCINOSARCOMA OF BREAST

Carcinosarcoma of the breast is an infiltrating epithelial malignant tumor in which histologic characteristics of a sarcoma are mimicked.

COMEDOCARCINOMA OF BREAST

Comedocarcinoma of the breast is characterized by plugs of pasty material expressed from the surface of the tumor. It averages 5 cm in diameter, is rather soft, and in only 15 per cent of the cases has involved axillary lymph nodes. A central location of the tumor is associated with cloudy nipple discharge in approximately one-third of the cases. Skin ulceration and retraction of the nipple are very late findings. It occurs particularly in women after the menopause and is more frequently associated with chronic cystic mastitis than with other carcinomas. It arises from the small or intermediate ducts. In its growth, the ducts of a given portion of the breast become filled with plugs of tumor cells. The tumor is usually somewhat circumscribed, quite firm and grayish. It has an infiltrating gross appearance, but it is not as hard as the scirrhous carcinoma. The tumor areas present grayish dots, from which ribbon-like plugs of yellowish gray pasty material or solid tumor plugs are extruded on pressure. Microscopic characteristics are those of many cores of highly cellular epithelial tissue, generally containing a central granular amorphous eosinophilic necrosis. Occasionally, there is liquefaction of some of the cells in the epithelial layer, resembling accessory acinar formation. The cells are generally small and dark, and they have dense nuclei. Cells nearer the center may be larger and less intensely stained. Hyperchromatism, mitoses, and loss of polarity are quite prominent.

CYSTIC DISEASE OF BREAST
Cystic disease of the breast presents as a round, smooth, tense, movable mass averaging 3 to 4 cm in diameter that can be transilluminated and may be fluctuant. The area is closer to the center of the breast than in adenosis. Sections show an exaggerated pattern of adenosis. Cysts are variable, multiple, and large, and they protrude into the stromal fat. They are somewhat translucent, causing the light brownish contents to appear bluish through the cyst wall. The shotty areas are also larger, harder, and more yellowish. Microscopically, the irregular lobules are small, the acini are few, and the ductules are dilated and filled with amorphous granular material. Epithelial involution is the most important diagnostic characteristic, to which there are two exceptions: the occasionally persistent focus of hyperplasia or papilloma formation, and the hyperplasia of apocrine-like glands. The glands are variable and large. The lining acidophilic epithelium is very tall and commonly presents plump papillary projections. Nuclei are nearly basilar in position and are round and stain lightly. Knobby free margins of the tall cells are characteristic. Lymphocytic or mononuclear infiltrations around ducts, smaller cysts, and in the lobules are both prominent and constant.
    SYNONYMS: *Blue Dome Cyst of the Breast, Fibrocystic Disease.*

DYSPLASIA OF BREAST
Dysplasia of the breast is essentially an abnormal interplay of parenchyma and stroma, developed and expressed by failure of reciprocal proliferation and involution—that is, anatomic consequences of abnormal physiology. The paramount change centers about the breast lobule of sexual maturity. The condition, therefore, is not very active in postmenopausal life, nor is it a disease of the male breast. It is, moreover, neither inflammatory nor neoplastic, and the irrevocable term of chronic

cystic mastitis is not generic. Anatomic changes in this condition are reflections of ovarian hormonal imbalance (corpus luteum deficiency with relative or absolute hyperestrinism) acting on the susceptible breast over a long period. Basically, the condition is a lumpiness and cysts of the mammary gland. It is found in women, chiefly in the last decade of reproductive life, but although developing in this period, the disorder may not have prominent symptoms or be recognized until after the menopause. It is commonly bilateral and associated with premenstrual pain. The upper outer quadrant of the breast is chiefly involved. The hormonal irregularity is also evident in sterility or irregular menstruation. Failure of pregnancy and lactation or disturbances attending these physiologic processes predispose to mammary dysplasia, whereas normal pregnancy and lactation are the best therapies. In many cases, the disorder apparently subsides spontaneously. On the basis of histologic interplay (in the lobule) between epithelium, myoepithelium, lobular connective tissue, stromal connective tissue, and inflammatory cells, mammary dysplasia may be multiform. Pronounced mixtures of these tissues occur frequently in a single lesion.

Adenosis of Breast

Adenosis of the breast has a characteristic gross appearance. The breast is rather small and fibrous. It has an easily palpable, exaggerated parenchyma with sharp peripheral boundaries. The nodularity to palpation, which is quite characteristic, is mostly peripheral. The gland cuts with difficulty. Involved areas resemble mazoplasia, but have three differences: (1) minute pinhead to pea-size clear cysts; (2) small, rubbery-hard, finely granular, speckled, shotlike areas containing yellowish, grumose plugs closely associated with the cysts; and (3) irregular clustering of enlarged tan-pink lobules forming a discrete area of increased consistency. Microscopically, diffuse fibrosis with loss of distinction between intralobular and periductal connective tissue and the general stroma is characteristic. Many ductules are dilated and contain clear or cloudy fluid. The epithelium is usually hyperplastic and lines the proliferating ductules with several layers of cells.

Mazoplasia

Mazoplasia is grossly characterized by involvement of the mammary gland by a periodic swelling and diffuse granularity of the affected area. Cutting is somewhat difficult, and sections so made present a white, poorly demarcated, dense, irregular, stiff, tough substance marked by minute pinkish dots of the parenchyma. Microscopically, the essential change is a moderate thickening and increase of the lobular stroma and its fusion with the general connective tissue. The ducts are dilated, and the lobules are variable in size and irregular in outline. The epithelium may be nearly normal or multilayered, secretory or vacuolated, flat or desquamating.

SYNONYMS: *Fibrous Mastopathy, Mammary Hyperplasia, Lobular Hyperplasia.*

FIBROADENOMA OF BREAST

Fibroadenoma of the breast is a slowly growing, estrogen-induced, benign tumor in females, most often before the age of 30. It begins as mammary dysplasia with an overgrowth of young myxomatous intralobular connective tissue and variable epithelial proliferations. Menopause usually results in cessation of the growth of the tumor; pregnancy and lactation cause it to grow readily. The tumor is usually solitary but occasionally multiple, bilateral, or recurring. The skin overlying the tumor and the axillary lymph nodes shows no change. The tumor is movable, solid, rubbery, and smooth or lobulated. Its average size is about 3.5 cm. It does not transilluminate. The gross appearance is distinctly different from that of any other mammary tumor. A sharp distinct edge outlines the decidedly elevated, flat, or slightly convex cut (or sectioned) surface. Firmer lesions are grayish white; softer ones are pink. The surface made by section may present a fine granularity or a delicately fissured geographic pattern.

GALACTOCELE

A galactocele develops in young females during lactation. The contents are truly milky or inspissated. It develops presumably because of duct obstruction. The cyst wall may show areas of necrosis, round cell infiltration, and condensation of the adjacent stroma. It is rare.

SYNONYM: *Milk Cyst.*

INTRACANALICULAR FIBROADENOMA OF BREAST

Intracanalicular fibroadenoma of the breast is characterized by active and proliferating connective tissue. Large polypoid masses growing into the parenchymal channels, thereby becoming covered by epithelium, produce a mosaic of distorted myxomatous disks. The epithelium is intimately connected to these projections and is continuous with that of the duct. It is atrophic at points of physical contact, and heaped up or multilayered in dilated segments of the elongated tortuous ductules. Huge formations of this type, 10 cm or greater in diameter, are known as *giant intracanalicular myxoma* and *cystosarcoma phyllodes.*

LIPOMA OF BREAST

Lipoma of the breast is a common tumor. The mass is discrete and soft, and it may resemble a cystic lesion. It is not tender. These tumors are well encapsulated. The cyst surface is a uniform, shiny yellow. Lobulations may be present. Microscopically, typical fat cells establish the diagnosis.

LOBULAR CARCINOMA OF BREAST

Lobular carcinoma of the breast is a carcinoma in which an unusual pattern of cancer centers in one or more of the lobules without forming a distinct tumor mass. It appears to begin in the lobular duct and to extend into the acini, if such have developed. The diagnosis is made microscopically, because grossly in the noninfiltrating lesion there is only a suggestion of increased density, as well as prominent lobules in a small area of the breast tissue.

MEDULLARY CARCINOMA OF BREAST

Medullary carcinoma of the breast is characterized by a deeply situated, midzonal, circumscribed, movable mass. The skin may be stretched over the bulging mass, but it does not show dimpling and is generally free from ulceration. The gross lesion appears as a soft, partially cystic or hemorrhagic, bulky, somewhat opaque, white tumor. It is generally spherical and is usually larger than 5 cm in diameter. The microscopic picture is that of a highly cellular tumor composed of large, oval or polygonal cells with slightly basophilic cytoplasm and vesicular nuclei with prominent nucleoli. Minute foci of keratin may be present. Various round or oval masses and thick papilloid stalks of epithelial cells are common. Usually a generous lymphocyte infiltration accompanies the epithelial cells—an important histologic characteristic.

SYNONYMS: *Cancer Cyst, Neomammary Cancer.*

MUCINOUS CARCINOMA OF BREAST

Mucinous carcinoma of the breast is not a common lesion. It grows rather slowly and is associated with late metastasis and lack of nipple retraction. Grossly, the tumor is fairly well demarcated but not encapsulated. It produces a spherical, moderately firm mass, with a translucent, moist, gelatinous, or slimy surface marked by a delicately interlacing pattern of more solid, opaque tissue. It is very slippery, and small particles of mucoid material can easily be removed from the tumor by scraping. The typical microscopic picture is that of a multilocular cyst-like formation. The spaces contain a light grayish, blue-staining, amorphous material. Between such cystic spaces, the breast stroma and parenchyma may be infiltrated by columns and nests of deeply staining epithelial cells. These have round, solid nuclei, eccentrically placed. The cytoplasm contains a single vacuole. Signet-ring forms are produced by large amounts of intracellular mucoid substance.

SYNONYMS: *Colloid Carcinoma, Gelatinous Carcinoma.*

PAGET'S DISEASE OF BREAST

Paget's disease of the breast is a chronic eczematoid thelitis associated with a central duct carcinoma. It has a course of long duration that begins with symptoms of burning, itching, or soreness of the nipple, followed by physical findings of hyperemia and enlargement. This change extends to the areola and is accompanied by fissuring, weeping or oozing, crust formation, and eventually ulceration and destruction of the nipple. Occasionally, the nipple changes are preceded by a definable lump in the breast. Gross examination of the tissue beneath the nipple area shows dilated, thick ducts containing grumose, pasty material. The nipple and cutaneous manifestations of the disease are characterized by the presence of very large, pale, vacuolated cells (Paget cells) in the rete pegs of the epithelium. These may show large hyperchromatic nuclei and mitoses. The epidermis therefore, has a moth-eaten histologic appearance.

PAPILLARY ADENOCARCINOMA OF BREAST

Papillary adenocarcinoma of the breast is a centrally located tumor that grows slowly and frequently is 5 cm or more in diameter. It is commonly associated with discharge from the nipple and the presence of a large, soft, bulky nodule. With central hemorrhage or cyst formation, it may be fluctuant. In the late stages, it loses its movable characteristics and ulcerates through the skin. Axillary node involvement is quite late and not prominent. The microscopic architecture is papillary in type, showing a communicating dendritic pattern. The cells are variable, in some instances forming large sheets and in other instances forming single cell layers. Lymphoid cells about the borders are not unusual. Histologic invasion is evident at the attachment of the papillary mass and is characterized by cells of moderate hyperchromatism, lack of polarity, and frequent mitoses. Invasion is the best evidence of malignancy.

PAPILLOMA OF BREAST

Papilloma of the breast may be intraductal or intracystic, and it occurs predominantly in parous women at or shortly before the menopause. The papilloma appears as a firm, granular, raspberry-like nodule, filling a duct or forming a small nipple-like projection on the wall of a cyst beneath the areola. A cloudy sanguineous fluid fills the cyst or duct and accounts for the spontaneous or induced bleeding from the nipple in more than half the cases. Papillomas are commonly multiple. The microscopic structure usually shows a delicately branching villous pattern of narrow vascularized connective-tissue stalks covered by a single or multilayered, uniform cuboidal epithelium. Lesions with broad fibrous stalks have minimal epithelium. Conversely, pronounced cellular proliferations produce epithelial bridging and cribriform designs without significant stroma. Papillomas of the breast are benign lesions whose potential for development of malignancy has been both affirmed and denied.

PERICANALICULAR FIBROADENOMA OF BREAST

Pericanalicular fibroadenoma of the breast has a dense stroma. Both epithelium and stroma in proliferation make up the tumor. The ductules and lobules are hyperplastic and distorted by connective-tissue growth. More typical are sweeping, encircling bands of dense connective tissue about the ductules and glands.

SARCOMA OF BREAST

Sarcoma of the breast is generally preceded by a slowly growing fibroadenoma. The sudden enlargement of a pre-existent tumor, without physical characteristics of a carcinoma and in the absence of axillary lymph node involvement, is a significant clinical finding. It is a large lesion, 5 cm or more in diameter, and firmer than a carcinoma of similar size. Grossly, the tumor is fairly well circumscribed, fleshy, and occasionally cystic; it presents various interlacing reticular patterns. Whorls of connective tissue with variable pleomorphism, mitoses, and loose myxomatous connective tissue are the usual histologic features. However, at times the myxomatous stroma is inconspicuous, and a compact, highly cellular, pleomorphic, fibrosarcomatous proliferation is present.

SCLEROSING ADENOMATOSIS OF BREAST

Sclerosing adenomatosis of the breast is characterized by separation and disorganization of the lobules by advanced intralobular fibrosis accompanied by epithelial proliferation resembling glandular growth and invasion. Such a lobule presents a filigree pattern and is frequently associated with myoepithelial hyperplasia. Although the lesion is benign, its histologic appearance may easily be misinterpreted as cancer.

SYNONYM: *Fibrosing Adenoma.*

FALLOPIAN TUBES

ADENOMATOID TUMOR OF FALLOPIAN TUBE

An adenomatoid tumor of the fallopian tube is a small circumscribed tumor confined to the muscular wall and composed of small glandlike spaces lined by cells of mesothelial, endothelial, or even epithelial appearance. Grossly, these tumors are less than 3 cm in diameter, usually occur immediately beneath the serosa, and are well circumscribed, but rarely, if ever, encapsulated. On section they are homogeneous and white to pinkish gray. Microscopically, the cells vary from flattened endothelium-like elements to a cuboidal or low columnar type, enclosing gland or vessel-like spaces of varying size and shape. Sometimes the cells may be in solid cords. The cells may be vacuolated, containing mucinoid material. The stroma is fibromuscular, and it appears to be an integral part of the tumor. These tumors have all been found incidentally, so that there is no clinical syndrome. The lesion is generally benign.

BENIGN CYSTIC TERATOMA OF FALLOPIAN TUBE

Benign cystic teratoma of the fallopian tube is rare, probably originating from a germ cell that lodged in the tubal primordium rather than completing its migration to the gonad. This tumor appears as a swelling on the tube; it varies from 1 to 17 cm. It is generally unilateral and cystic, arising intraluminally by a pedicle. Microscopically, the neoplasm contains skin and its derivatives, muscle, bone, and endodermal derivatives.

SYNONYM: *Dermoid Cyst of Fallopian Tube.*

Struma Salpingis

Struma salpingis is a rare tumor, usually part of a dermoid cyst, that contains tissue resembling adult thyroid tissue and may contain psammoma bodies.

CHORIOCARCINOMA OF FALLOPIAN TUBE

Choriocarcinoma of the fallopian tube is a malignant neoplasm that may arise primarily from ectopic pregnancy or secondarily from a choriocarcinoma of the uterus or ovary. Microscopically, the appearance of primary tubal choriocarcinoma differs in no way from that arising in the endometrium. Although cases in which villi are present have been reported, for the most part the villus pattern is absent, and sheets of bizarre, proliferating syncytial and cytotrophoblastic cells invade and destroy the surrounding musculature. Direct invasion or metastases from the fundal lesion show the same characteristic changes.

SYNONYM: *Tubal Chorioepithelioma.*

DYSGERMINOMA OF FALLOPIAN TUBE

Dysgerminoma of the fallopian tube is a rare neoplasm that has arisen from accessory ovarian tissue within the mesosalpinx or the wall of the tube, or from a misplaced primordial germ cell.

ENDOMETRIOSIS OF FALLOPIAN TUBE

Endometriosis of the fallopian tube is the presence of endometrial tissue on the serosal surface or within the lumen of the fallopian tube. The cause of endometriosis of the surface of the tube is probably similar to that in the ovary, whereas in the tubal lumen endometriosis probably arises by differentiation of potential endometrial stroma or possibly by heteroplasia of the tubal mucosa. The appearance of the endometriotic serosal surface of the tube is typical. It consists of scattered, irregular, red to black nodules 0.1 to 0.3 cm in diameter, with a variable amount of scarring. When endometriosis occurs within the tube, it presents as hemorrhagic, pouting mucosa on sectioning. Typical endometrial glands and stroma, with varying amounts of old and fresh hemorrhage, occur on the serosal surface of the tube and may replace both the tubal epithelium and stroma within the lumen. The presence of definite endometrial stroma in these locations is illustrated by the focal pseudo-decidual reaction, which usually occurs in both sites during normal pregnancy, although there is no evidence of true endometriosis. These pseudodecidual cells are large, with refractile borders and relatively small nuclei. They should be distinguished from metastatic tumor.

GRANULOSA CELL TUMOR OF FALLOPIAN TUBE

A granulosa cell tumor of the fallopian tube is a neoplasm that has arisen from misplaced ovarian tissue. It may contain lutein cells, as well as granulosa cells.

HEMANGIOMA OF FALLOPIAN TUBE

Hemangioma of the fallopian tube is a rare tumor arising from the vascular endothelium and resembling hemangiomas in other areas of the body. This tumor must not be confused with a group of congested veins.

LEIOMYOMA OF FALLOPIAN TUBE

Leiomyoma of the fallopian tube is a rare smooth muscle tumor. Grossly, the clinical picture may simulate salpingitis isthmica nodosa, adenomyosis, or adenomatoid tumors. The tumor may vary in size, is generally single, and may be submucous, interstitial, or subserosal. It may undergo the following degenerative changes: cystic change, edema, hyalinization, and calcification. Microscopically, it is well demarcated from surrounding tissue and has the same whorled pattern of muscle cells as leiomyomas elsewhere.

LIPOMA OF FALLOPIAN TUBE

Lipoma of the fallopian tube is a rare lesion, asymptomatic and generally discovered in the course of pelvic surgery for other conditions. Most cases occur in the distal portion of the tube. Although all layers of the tube have been involved, it seems most logical that the fatty tissues of the serosal region would be the primary site of origin.

LYMPHANGIOMA OF FALLOPIAN TUBE

Lymphangioma of the fallopian tube is a small tumor that may be confused with an adenomatoid tumor. The distinction is difficult unless good cuboidal glandlike tissue is present to indicate an adenomatoid tumor.

MESONEPHROMA OF FALLOPIAN TUBE

Mesonephroma of the fallopian tube is a very rare neoplasm that arises from mesonephric elements persisting in the broad ligament. It may be confused with an adenomatoid tumor.

PRIMARY CARCINOMA OF FALLOPIAN TUBE

Primary carcinoma of the fallopian tube is rare. The common pelvic diseases frequently mask carcinoma of the tube clinically. Salpingitis is usually present in the tube in which the malignant tumor occurs, but it is not a constant finding in the other tube. The clinical picture of primary tubal carcinoma is not pathognomonic, but the most common symptom is vaginal discharge. This may be watery, bloodstained, or leukorrheic. Occasionally, the discharge may be even very profuse; however, the syndrome *hydrops tubae profluens*, which is the relief of pain and disappearance of a mass accompanied by profuse vaginal discharge, is neither pathognomonic nor a constant finding in tubal carcinoma, but is more likely to occur with hydrosalpinx. Pain is another common symptom, and a history of menstrual irregularities is usual. The tumor may be purple, soft and doughy, or moderately to extremely firm, depending on the degree of fibrous tissue deposition. On section, the tumor is granular, gray to yellow, and friable to cheesy. It is usually situated in the distal third of the tube and may fungate through the fimbriated end if it remains open. The ostium of the tube tends to become occluded or adherent to the homolateral ovary; this averts spillage of cells until the tumor is quite large.

SARCOMA OF FALLOPIAN TUBE

Sarcoma of the fallopian tube is a very rare malignant neoplasm. Premenopausally, the symptoms are generally menorrhagia, metrorrhagia, or both, associated with a serosanguineous or semipurulent vaginal discharge. Postmenopausally, there may be a dischrage that is usually blood-stained and occasionally profuse and watery. Pain, probably the most constant and conspicuous symptom, may be either distinctly pelvic or diffusely abdominal. Gastrointestinal symptoms may accompany the pain. Other symptoms are abdominal distention or enlargement, malaise, loss of weight, and emaciation. Grossly, the tumor may be bilateral. It is soft and papillary, and adheres to surrounding structures. Microscopically, the cells are similar to sarcoma elsewhere in the body.

SECONDARY CARCINOMA OF FALLOPIAN TUBE

Secondary carcinoma of the fallopian tube is a neoplasm that has developed from other sources, usually the ovary or uterine corpus. Grossly, these metastatic tumors may be bilateral or unilateral, without predilection for either side. The size of metastases varies widely. Chronic salpingitis is present in about one-third of the cases. Microscopically, secondary carcinoma resembles the primary tumor. The lymphatic vessels and lymph nodes of the tunica muscularis and of the mesosalpinx are usually involved. The lymphatic vessels and lymph nodes of the endosalpinx and the endosalpinx itself are more rarely involved. The prognosis is the same as that in primary carcinoma.

SYNONYM: *Metastatic Carcinoma of Fallopian Tube.*

OVARIES

ADENOCARCINOMA OF OVARY

Adenocarcinoma of the ovary is a primary solid ovarian carcinoma in which the cellular elements are quite similar to the glandular pattern of adenocarcinoma of the endometrium. The glandular cells may be arranged in clumps and buried in layers of actively functioning epithelial cells. These tumors do not produce hormones. The prognosis is poor.

ADRENAL REST TUMOR OF OVARY

An adrenal rest tumor of the ovary is a rare, usually benign tumor that grossly and histologically resembles the cortical tissue of the adrenal gland. Grossly, the tumor is unilateral, encapsulated, and lobulated owing to fibrous septa arising from the capsule. It is located near the hilum of the ovary rather than in the cortex. Microscopically, it shows nests or cords of uniform, vividly eosinophilic, polyhedral, sharply defined cells having prominent irregular nuclei. The resemblance of these tumors to adrenal cortex can be striking. The tumor is generally not malignant, and oophorectomy relieves the symptoms.

SYNONYMS: *Adrenocorticoid Tumor, Adrenal Adenoma, Hypernephroid Tumor, Virilizing Lipoid Cell Tumor, Masculinizing Luteoma.*

ARRHENOBLASTOMA

Arrhenoblastoma is a potentially maligant, predominantly unilateral, mesenchymal tumor of the ovary that resembles varying aspects of the embryonic testis. It causes clinical defeminization and virilization usually in proportion to the amount, maturity, and function of the male-hormone-producng interstitial stroma. This tumor occurs chiefly in young, previously normal women of childbearing age. The gross appearance of an arrhenoblastoma is not pathognomonic. They vary from microscopic size to 28 cm, averaging from 12 to 14 cm. Most are unilateral, the right ovary being slightly favored, and occasionally there are multiple foci in one ovary. The external surface of the tumor is usually smooth, moist, glistening, and blue to yellow. The smaller tumors are usually firm, because of the mesenchymal or fibrous nature of the tumor; if larger, they may be soft because of necrosis, hemorrhage, or cyst formation. The appearance of the cut surface is variable. Small tumors tend to be solid, fibrous, white to gray, with a yellow cast if there is fat within the tumor tissue. Large tumors have significant areas of necrosis and hemorrhage. Solid tumors show a tendency to lobulation. Cysts, small or large, single or multiple, are smooth or ragged, but they do not have papillary projections. The fluid is clear or blood-tinged and may be somewhat mucinous.

BENIGN CYSTIC TERATOMA OF OVARY

Benign cystic teratoma of the ovary is a neoplasm that arises from primordial germ cells by parthenogenetic development at any point along the line of migration of the germ cell. It is composed of any combination of well-differentiated ectodermal, mesodermal, and entodermal elements. Grossly, it is round, smooth, and generally unilocular. Its contents may be a tangled mass of hair with thick greasy fluid, or mucinous thick material if the cyst is lined with brain tissue. Various other structures may be represented in the tumor, such as bone or cartilage. In some instances malignant changes may occur. It is the most common ovarian tumor associated with pregnancy. The prognosis is generally good after surgical removal.

SYNONYM: *Dermoid Cyst.*

Struma Ovarii

Struma ovarii is a cystic teratoma of the ovary composed mostly or even entirely of thyroid tissues. Microscopically, thyroid follicles in various stages of activity are found, generally containing abundant colloid material. Secondary malignant changes in these tumors may occur. Clinically, the signs and symptoms of hyperthyroidism may exist, together with symptoms of pelvic tumor. Ascites may also occur.

SYNONYM: *Teratoma Strumoides Thyroideale Ovarii.*

BRENNER TUMOR

The Brenner tumor is an ovarian fibroepithelial tumor composed of nests of transitional type (pseudosquamous) epithelium infiltrating a dense fibrous stroma that does not produce hormones. Grossly, the neoplasm varies from microscopic size to tumors of considerable weight and size. This neoplasm may be solid or cystic with a smooth serosal surface, but it may also be irregularly lobulated. It is firm, and the cut surface is gray-white with whorled areas. Microscopically, there is abundant fibrillary connective tissue and typical epithelial nests composed of compact polyhedral squamous (transitional) cells. The nuclei are oval with distinct nucleoli. The epithelial nests may become cystic, the epithelial cells changing to a cuboidal or low columnar type. Glycogen and mucus are present in the epithelial cells. Clinically, the patient may experience only an enlargement of the abdomen due to the growing tumor. Mucinous cystomas are found in one-third of the patients. Simple excision is curative.

CARCINOMA ARISING FROM DERMOID CYST
Carcinoma arising from a dermoid cyst is a rare malignant solid squamous cell tumor of the ovary. It arises from an ulcerated area of the lining of a benign cystic teratoma. Microscopically, it is composed of epidermoid cells with nests of differentiated spindle type cells with epithelial pearl formation.

CARCINOMA OF OVARY
Carcinoma of the ovary is a type of primary solid tumor. It is characterized by the absence of an adenomatous pattern. Various terms may be used to describe it—for example, papillary, medullary, alveolar, and scirrhous. Microscopically, a solid pattern may coexist with a predominantly cystic one. The prognosis is poor.

CARCINOSARCOMA OF OVARY
Carcinosarcoma of the ovary is a very rare ovarian neoplasm that recapitulates the various potentials of müllerian epithelium and mesenchyme.

CORPUS LUTEUM CYST
A corpus luteum cyst arises from a *corpus luteum hematoma*. The hematoma develops if bleeding into the center of the corpus luteum is excessive during its early stages of development. Although the blood is subsequently reabsorbed and replaced by serous fluid, the cyst remains. It varies from 3 to 10 cm in diameter, but the average cyst seldom is more than 3 to 4 cm. The thin wall is bright yellow when the cyst is first formed, but with regression it becomes gray or white and increasingly transparent. The serous fluid in the cyst may be clear, brownish, or colorless. Microscopically, the wall contains typical polygonal luteinized cells, but with age these may largely disappear and be replaced by connective tissue. A variant of the corpus luteum cyst is the *corpus albicans cyst*.

CYSTADENOFIBROMA OF OVARY
Cystadenofibroma of the ovary is a benign fibroepithelial neoplasm whose epithelial component is derived from germinal epithelium and

connective tissue from either the cortical stroma, the tunica albuginea, or both. The neoplasm may be solid or cystic, large or small, benign or malignant. The cyst may contain clear or straw-colored fluid. Papillary excrescenses may be present on the inner or outer surface. The cysts are lined with cuboidal or columnar epithelium that is often ciliated. There are three types, which are related to the three types of cystomas, ie, serous, mucinous, and endometrioid. The cytoplasm is eosinophilic and usually homogeneous. Papillae, when present, are composed of dense fibrous tissue.

DYSGERMINOMA

Dysgerminoma is an uncommon type of solid ovarian neoplasm that arises from primordial germ cells before their differentiation into definitive sex cells. Grossly, the size may vary, some being a few centimeters in diameter and others massive. The tumor is covered with a smooth, dense capsule and is soft or doughy. Microscopically, the tumor is composed of large, rounded polyhedral cells arranged in nests. There may be rather extensive lymphocytic infiltration, and giant cells may be found in the substance of the tumor. The tumor appears most often before puberty or during adolescence, and it is the most common ovarian cancer associated with pregnancy. There are inconsistencies in its clinical manifestation.

ENDODERMAL SINUS TUMOR OF OVARY

An endodermal sinus tumor of the ovary is considered by some to recapitulate stages in the phylogenetic development of extraembryonic structures such as the allantois and yolk sac. These tumors have sometimes been described as embryonal carcinoma of the ovary, but these latter tumors very often contain a variety of germ cell tumor patterns. Grossly, the tumors vary from several to 25 cm or more in diameter, but usually they are about 15 cm. Usually the surface is smooth, but there may be extension of the tumor. The cut surface is soft, friable, and variable in color. It may be cystic with necrotic foci. Microscopically, the characteristic feature is a glomeruloid unit, with a central, thin-walled vessel surrounded by loose connective tissue with a covering of cuboidal or columnar cells that seem to project into a cavity lined by endothelial cells. Otherwise the tumor is composed of loose mesenchymal tissue of stellate cells that tend to form a system of communicating cavities and channels.

SYNONYM: *Schiller's Mesonephroma Ovarii.*

ENDOMETRIAL CYSTADENOCARCINOMA OF OVARY

Endometrial cystadenocarcinoma of the ovary is derived from an endometrial cystoma, the benign form of this tumor. The usually unilateral tumor may show direct transitional evidence of being derived from benign endometriosis and may, on occasion, show the typical pattern of adenoacanthoma.

ENDOMETRIAL CYSTOMA OF OVARY

An endometrial cystoma of the ovary originates in areas of ovarian endometriosis and may be multilocular. The cysts are frequently bilateral and rarely exceed 10 cm in diameter. Typically, the cyst wall is fairly thick with a gray-white appearance that conceals the tarry brown-black color of its contents. If the wall is thinner, and in smaller cysts, the accumulated old blood will give the tumor a bluish tinge. The cyst wall is often somewhat irregular and characteristically has areas of typical endometrial glands and stroma with evidences of old and recent hemorrhage. In some cases, pressures within the cyst are sufficient to cause atrophy of the characteristic lining, resulting in a scarred connective tissue capsule with no distinguishable histologic features. Malignant transformation, though possible, occurs very rarely.

SYNONYM: *Chocolate Cyst of Ovary.*

FIBROMA OF OVARY

A fibroma of the ovary is a benign neoplasm composed of fibroblasts and variable amounts of collagen. These tumors arise from the ovarian cortex, the connective tissue of the capsule, or around blood vessels. Grossly, the neoplasm is dense, hard, homogeneous, and fibrous, with occasional cystic and edematous areas. Calcification of these tumors may result. Microscopically, the cellular content is similar to that of the stromal cells of the ovarian cortex. The cells are thin, spindle-shaped, and arranged in bundles. Clinically, the patient experiences a slow, gradual increase in the size of the abdomen owing to the growing tumor. This may occasionally be accompanied by ascites and hydrothorax. Excision is generally curative. It appears in association with Meigs' syndrome.

FIBROSARCOMA OF OVARY

Fibrosarcoma of the ovary is a rare malignant connective tissue neoplasm that generally occurs in elderly patients. Grossly, the neoplasm is generally unilateral, round, nodular, or lobulated. The cut surface is firm and gray-white. There may be necrosis in the center of the tumor. Microscopically, the cellular pattern varies from that of a cellular fibroma to that of a pleomorphic sarcoma. Clinically, symptoms of a pelvic tumor, swelling of the abdomen, urinary disturbances, and occasionally uterine bleeding are present. Surgical removal may be curative for the low-grade malignant tumor. Radiotherapy is of uncertain value, but it probably is not effective.

FOLLICULAR CYST

A follicular cyst is an ovarian follicle that has become filled with an excessive amount of liquor folliculi. It is nonmalignant and results when ovulation does not occur on schedule, or when the follicle is located deep in the substance of the ovary so that spontaneous rupture of the follicle cannot occur. Grossly, the follicle is small but may reach a considerable size, producing clinical symptoms of pain and irregular menstrual bleeding. Follicular cysts may be single or multiple. Microscopically, the wall may be composed of either granulosa or theca interna cells, with or without luteinization, or theca externa cells, with or without hyalinization. Not infrequently, hemorrhage into the cyst cavity takes place producing a *follicular hematoma.*

GERMINAL INCLUSION CYST OF OVARY

A germinal inclusion cyst of the ovary is formed by the invagination and isolation of small segments of the germinal epithelium from the ovarian surface. They occur predominantly in older patients, and because they seldom exceed 1 cm in diameter, they are usually discovered when the ovary is examined after removal for some other reason. Grossly, they appear as small single cystic spaces immediately beneath the surface of the ovary. They contain clear serous fluid and are lined by a single layer of cuboidal or low columnar epithelium. They have no known malignant potential.

GONADOBLASTOMA

Gonadoblastoma is most conveniently placed with the germ cell tumors, although it recapitulates the whole embryonic gonad in that it contains germ cells, Sertoli-granulosa cells, and Leydig-theca cells. Patients with these tumors have primary amenorrhea and lack sexual development. Features may be eunochoidal, Turner's syndrome may be present, and the patients are masculinized. Patients have a male sex chromatin pattern, 46/XY, or sex chromosome mosaicism, XO/XY. Grossly, the tumor is similar to a dysgerminoma. Often there is disseminated calcification. Microscopically, the tumor contains germ cells, which may be in nests with lymphoid stroma with an outer rim of Sertoli-granulosa cells or may surround spaces containing eosinophilic material. The stroma may be cellular or may contain large polyhedral cells of the Leydig-theca type.

GRANULOSA-THECA CELL TUMORS OF OVARY

The granulosa-theca cell tumors of the ovary are functioning tumors that produce feminizing hormones. They are composed of various elements of the wall of the graafian follicle that differ in proportional relationship and stages of activity, maturity, and regression. Microscopically, there are widely varying patterns of growth. At least six types have been described—macrofolliculoid, microfolliculoid, cylindromatous, sarcomatous, pseudoadenomatous, and tubular. They all are composed of uniform deeply staining cells with a large nucleus and rather scant cytoplasm. These cells tend to be arranged in rosettes or clusters very much like primordial follicles. Occasionally, a more specific two-layered follicle, the *Call-Exner body,* may be demonstrated. These functioning tumors are designated as granulosa cell tumors, thecomas, or luteomas.

SYNONYMS: *Feminizing Solid Ovarian Tumors, Feminizing Mesenchymomas.*

Granulosa Cell Tumor

A granulosa cell tumor is a functional ovarian tumor that produces feminizing hormones. Grossly, these tumors vary from only a few millimeters in diameter to tumors filling a large part of the abdominal cavity and weighing more than 30 pounds. They usually are of moderate size. When small, they are apt to be solid, but the larger tumors often have one or many cystic cavities. The intervening solid tissue is friable or granular, and grayish and sometimes yellowish. Microscopically, the diagnosis of granulosa cell tumor is based on the granulosal character of the constituent cells and on the growth characteristics of these cells, which are quite like those of normal granulosa. For example, tiny cystic areas of liquefaction, corresponding to the *Call-Exner bodies* so characteristic of the granulosa tend to form. The epithelial elements may dominate the picture in diffuse varieties of the tumor with only a small amount of trabeculating connective tissue, often hyalinized. In such cases, the epithelial cells tend to be arranged in rosette-like or horseshoe-shaped clusters, resembling the primitive follicles.

Thecoma

A thecoma is a functional ovarian tumor that produces feminizing endocrine substances. It is solid due to increased connective tissue of cortical stromal origin. Grossly, the tumor is fibrous with occasional small cystic areas and is yellow with pale scarred areas interspersed. Microscopically, it is composed of spindle-shaped cells, predominantly theca cells with bands of collagen. The cells stain deep yellow for fat indicating the presence of ovarian steroids. This tumor generally develops during the postmenopausal period. The neoplasm produces irregularities in the menstrual cycle, breast enlargement, and occasionally increased libido. It is basically benign, although adenocarcinoma of the endometrium may be associated with it.

Luteoma

A luteoma is a very rare variant of the granulosa-theca cell ovarian neoplasm that probably represents a luteinized granulosa cell tumor. It is solid with a smooth capsule. The cut surface is orange-yellow, buttery in consistency, with some cystic degeneration and hemorrhage. Microscopically, the cells resemble miniature cells of the corpus luteum. There are areas of cuboidal and polygonal cells that stain deep yellow for fat. There is a variable endocrine function of this neoplasm. It may produce virilizing or mild feminizing effects (progesterone). It may be malignant. It may be associated with pregnancy—the *luteoma of pregnancy*—although this is not a true tumor but hyperplasia in that it regresses after pregnancy.

SYNONYM: *Luteinized Granulosa-Theca Cell Tumor.*

GYNANDROBLASTOMA

Gyandroblastoma is a rare ovarian neoplasm that produces simultaneous androgenic and estrogenic manifestations. Grossly, it may vary from

1 cm to 20 cm. On the cut surface, small, solid, yellow areas may be noted. These tumors are generally nonmalignant but may exhibit malignant changes. Clinically, the patients show varying degrees of hirsutism and uterine bleeding associated with hyperplasia of the endometrium.

HILAR CELL TUMOR

A hilar cell tumor is a rare benign neoplasm located in the hilum of the ovary. Grossly, it may be homogeneous and fleshy, or soft and friable. Microscopically, the cellular elements appear like those of the Leydig cells in the testis. Their nuclear and cytoplasmic detail and lipid content are similar. Both contain lipochrome pigment and crystalloids, indistinguishable microchemically from the albuminoid crystalloids of Reinke in the interstitial cells of the testis. The cells may be elongated, oval, or polygonal. The cytoplasm is eosinophilic. Clinically, this tumor is sometimes associated with masculinization and other endocrine changes, with increased ketosteroid excretion in some cases. Excision is generally curative.

KRUKENBERG TUMOR

The Krukenberg tumor is a bilateral metastatic ovarian neoplasm whose primary location is the gastrointestinal tract, usually the stomach. The ovarian symptoms and signs usually precede those of the gastrointestinal tract. Grossly, this neoplasm is a smooth, nonirritating, irregular, nodular, solid mass with cystic degeneration. The cut surface may be myxomatous, with areas of necrosis and hemorrhage. Microscopically, the neoplasm generally consists of large round or polyhedral cells or clear cells having mucinous cytoplasm that crowds the nucleus to one side of the cell, the signet-ring cells. Clinically, symptoms are those of a malignant tumor of the ovary. The prognosis is poor, and treatment is mostly palliative.

LYMPHOMA OF OVARY

Lymphoma of the ovary is usually bilateral, grossly nodular, and brainlike, varying from gray to reddish gray. The various types are lymphocytic lymphoma, lymphoblastoma, reticulum cell lymphoma, and giant follicular lymphoma.

MALIGNANT TERATOMA OF OVARY

A malignant teratoma of the ovary is a rather uncommon malignant ovarian neoplasm whose origin is a primitive unfertilized ovum. This tumor is composed of undifferentiated and differentiated malignant derivations of ectoderm, mesoderm, and entoderm. Grossly, a malignant teratoma is usually unilateral. It may maintain the shape of the ovary, or present as a pedunculated, rounded, ovoid, or nodular mass. Adhesions are common, but may present a variety of colors: gray, yellow, red, blue, or brown. It is usually soft, but may be firm, spongy, or cystic. Cysts may contain either slimy colloid or fatty material. Frequently, there are hemorrhagic foci within solid tissue and within the cysts. Microscopically, the picture is extremely varied. Well-differentiated cellular areas and completely undifferentiated parts may be seen. Prognosis is poor regardless of treatment.

MESOMETANEPHRIC REST TUMOR OF OVARY

The mesometanephric rest tumor of the ovary is an uncommon malignant ovarian neoplasm that morphologically resembles the tubules, glomeruli, or both, of the metanephros or mesonephros. Grossly, the neoplasm is smooth and semisolid with cystic areas. It may adhere to its surrounding structures. The microscopic features are the presence of glomeruloid structures covered with flattened or cuboidal epithelium. Other cells resembling primitive kidney tubules may be present. The prognosis is poor, regardless of therapy.

SYNONYMS: *Mesonephroma, Adenocarcinoma of Schiller (ovarian).*

MUCINOUS CYSTADENOCARCINOMA

Mucinous cystadenocarcinoma is a malignant cystic or semisolid tumor. Rarely, one is solid. This tumor may develop from a mucinous cystadenoma, or it may be malignant at the onset. The cysts are lined with tall columnar epithelial cells; in others, the epithelium consists of many layers of cells that have lost normal structure entirely. In the more undifferentiated tumors, one may see sheets and nests of tumor cells that have very little resemblance to the parent structure.

SYNONYM: *Pseudomucinous Cystadenocarcinoma.*

MUCINOUS CYSTADENOMA

Mucinous cystadenoma is a benign, unilocular or multilocular, cystic ovarian neoplasm derived generally from germinal epithelium. It may be a one-way teratoma simulating the gastrointestinal tract. The tumor may range from 1 to 50 cm in diameter. Grossly, the tumor has a more or less lobulated appearance with a smooth exterior and a pale color. It generally does not adhere to the surrounding structures. The contents are usually clear and straw-colored unless hemorrhage has occurred, and they may vary from viscid to gelatinous. Microscopically, the epithelial lining is composed of tall columnar cells resembling mucosa of the uterine cervix or intestinal tract. Goblet cells that secrete mucin are located between the columnar cells.

SYNONYM: *Pseudomucinous Cystadenoma.*

PRIMARY OVARIAN CHORIOCARCINOMA

Primary ovarian choriocarcinoma is a very rare malignant ovarian neoplasm that has its origin in the primordial germ cell and is composed of syncytiotrophoblastic and cytotrophoblastic elements. Grossly, the tumor may be smooth, or coarse and nodular, covered by a thin capsule. Microscopically, the tumor has the typically interlacing plexiform pattern of syncytiotrophoblast surrounding or covering cytotrophoblastic cells. There may be blood-filled spaces similar to the intervillous spaces of an early placenta. Clinically, the signs and symptoms are those of an enlarging abdominal tumor, occasionally accompanied by acute abdominal pain if hemorrhage or rupture of the tumor has occurred. Prognosis is extremely poor, regardless of therapy.

RHABDOMYOSARCOMA OF OVARY

Rhabdomyosarcoma of the ovary is a rare malignant ovarian neoplasm that may occur in any decade of life. Grossly, the neoplasm is generally large, solid or cystic, and is gray-white to red. Microscopically, straplike cells with cross-striations are always identified. Clinically, the patient complains of enlargement of the abdomen, uterine bleeding, and pressure. Prognosis is extremely poor.

SEROUS CYST OF OVARY

A serous cyst of the ovary is thin-walled and unilateral. The cyst has no papillary projections and contains clear or yellowish fluid. It does not adhere to the surrounding structures. Grossly, it is a unilocular cyst with a smooth, shining internal surface. Microscopically, the wall is lined with low cuboidal epithelium without anaplasia.

SYNONYM: *Simple Cystoma.*

SEROUS CYSTADENOCARCINOMA

Serous cystadenocarcinoma is a malignant cystic or semicystic ovarian neoplasm. It usually occurs bilaterally. The external surface is generally covered with papillary excrescences. These growths may also occur within each individual loculus. Microscopically, the papillary patterns are predominantly epithelial overgrowths with some differentiated and undifferentiated papillary serous cystadenocarcinoma cells. Psammoma bodies may be present. The tumor generally adheres to surrounding structures and produces ascites.

SEROUS CYSTADENOMA

Serous cystadenoma is a unilocular, parvilocular, or multilocular cystic ovarian neoplasm derived from germinal epithelium. It is often bilateral, papillary, and may be malignant or benign. The fluid content of the cyst is thin, watery, and serous, containing a serum protein. The cysts may vary greatly in size, some partially filling the abdominal cavity. Microscopically, the epithelial lining varies from the simple cuboidal type of germinal epithelium to epithelium resembling various segments of the fallopian tube. The stroma of the serous cystoma varies from an edematous to a densely fibrous type, the latter presumably derived from the tunica albuginea. The stroma also may be predominantly cortical in type. These neoplasms may also possess *psammoma bodies,* which are concentrically laminated calcareous structures within the intercellular stroma adjacent to the epithelium.

TERATOCARCINOMA OF OVARY

Teratocarcinoma of the ovary is an undifferentiated carcinoma usually with large irregular cells unlike those of müllerian carcinomas or any other recognizable type of carcinoma from any other part of the body. The origin is similar to that of a malignant teratoma, but there is an overgrowth or exclusive growth of epithelial elements. Grossly, this tumor is similar to malignant teratoma or to dysgerminoma. Prognosis is poor, regardless of the treatment.

THECA-LUTEIN CYST

A theca-lutein cyst is a follicular cyst of the ovary associated with hydatidiform mole and choriocarcinoma. The cyst is generally multiple and bilateral. It is produced by chorionic gonadotropin secreted by the trophoblastic tissue. Grossly, it is bluish and multilocular. Microscopically, the cyst shows marked luteinization of the theca interna zone.

UTERUS AND ENDOMETRIUM

ADENOACANTHOMA OF UTERUS

Adenoacanthoma of the uterus is an adenocarcinoma with areas that are undergoing metaplasia to squamous epithelium. The microscopic appearance is that of a mixed adenocarcinoma and squamous cell carcinoma.

BENIGN METASTASIZING LEIOMYOMA OF UTERUS

Benign metastasizing leiomyoma of the uterus is a very rare condition in which a leiomyoma, appearing benign histologically, extends locally via lymphatic vessels or blood vessels and may even produce distant metastases.

CARCINOMA IN SITU OF ENDOMETRIUM

Carcinoma in situ of the endometrium has no definite gross appearance, the endometrium showing the features of the hyperplasia in which it is arising. Microscopically, there are groups of pale glands back to back, obliterating the intervening stroma. Although carcinoma in situ is found in association with or precedes invasive carcinoma and is morphologically similar to this cancer, it is not identical. It is to be distinguished from typical microscopic adenocarcinoma, which is confined to the endometrium without evidence of myometrial invasion.

ENDOMETRIAL STROMAL SARCOMA

Endometrial stromal sarcoma is a pale, polypoid, fleshy tumor usually arising from the uterine fundus. Occasionally, there may be diffuse myometrial invasion without a polypoid tumor. Usually the tumor is fairly sharply demarcated from more normal endometrium. Microscopically, it is composed of cells that are fusiform on longitudinal section and round on cross-section. Cytoplasm may be scanty, the cells resembling those of the endometrial stroma in the proliferative phase, or more abundant, so that the constituent cells resemble decidua. There may be giant cells. The prognosis is poor, although somewhat better in the sarcomas that seem to arise in a leiomyoma.

HEMANGIOPERICYTOMA OF UTERUS

Hemangiopericytoma is a rare tumor of the uterus. It is composed of nonneoplastic capillary endothelium surrounded by collars of neoplastic capillary pericytes of Zimmermann. Hemangiopericytoma is grossly similar to the leiomyoma, but it is usually less discrete, softer, and more yellow, and it is often mistaken for leiomyosarcoma. Microscopically, there are capillaries, often collapsed and surrounded by a sheath of reticulum that separates them from the collars of fusiform pericytes containing uniform round or oval nuclei but few mitoses. No malignant variant has been reported in the uterus.

SYNONYM: *Endolymphatic Stromal Myosis.*

INVASIVE CARCINOMA OF ENDOMETRIUM

Invasive carcinoma of the endometrium is usually glandular, but sometimes is associated with squamous elements. The peak incidence is in the sixth decade. There is an increased incidence of diabetes mellitus, obesity, breast carcinoma, thyroid disease, and estrogenically hyperactive ovarian lesions in association with endometrial carcinoma. It often develops as the result of long-continued, noncyclic stimulation of the endometrium by estrogen (and possibly progesterone), usually of ovarian origin. Endometrial carcinoma does not arise from normal endometrium, but it may arise from abnormal foci within otherwise normal endometrium. Grossly, there are two types of carcinomas of the endometrium: diffuse and discrete. The diffuse variety may be confined to the endometrium but spread widely through it. It may be polypoid, pale, firm, friable, and lacking the glistening mucosal surface of cystic hyperplasia. There may be surface ulceration, or the surface may be hemorrhagic, or shiny as a result of mucus production. The discrete form may occur anywhere in the uterus—most frequently in the posterior wall—and may be papillary, polypoid, or slightly raised from the surrounding endometrium. Discrete tumors are sometimes localized to the endometrium, but they usually have invaded the myometrium. Endometrial carcinoma may be well, moderately well, or poorly differentiated. In the better differentiated varieties, glands may vary in size, often having subsidiary gland lumina actually within their walls. Endometrial carcinoma is slow to invade the myometrium, but occasionally may penetrate the wall and extend to adjacent intestine or to the broad ligament. The most common distant metastases are to the lungs and liver. The prognosis is related to the extent of the tumor and is better if the tumor is well differentiated.

LEIOMYOMA UTERI

Leiomyoma uteri is a well-circumscribed but nonencapsulated benign uterine tumor, composed mainly of muscle but with a variable fibrous connective tissue element. Grossly, leiomyomas may occur anywhere within the uterus, being subserosal (sometimes pedunculated), intramural, or submucosal. Usually they are multiple, but they may be single. Leiomyomas are well demarcated from the surrounding muscle, which they may flatten to form a false capsule, but they have no true capsule. Microscopically, the leiomyoma is composed of groups and bundles of smooth muscle fibers in a twisted, whorled pattern.

LEIOMYOSARCOMA OF UTERUS

Leiomyosarcoma of the uterus usually arises in the central part of a leiomyoma, but it may arise at the edge and cause early loss of the sharp line of demarcation. Grossly, the tumor may vary from a single nodule to diffuse myometrial involvement. It may extend through the serosal surface to adhere to adjacent structures, or it may project as a polypoid structure into the endometrial cavity. On section, the tumor is of equally varied appearance. It may be indistinguishable from a leiomyoma, although usually some feature suggests a difference, such as focal loss of the whorled pattern, variation in color, or focal bulging above the level of the cut surface. The diffuse type of leiomyosarcoma is homogeneous, varying from yellow to pink to gray, and it is often hemorrhagic, necrotic, or pultaceous. Microscopically, leiomyosarcomas are generally similar to sarcomas; the constituent cells are spindle, round, and giant forms. Usually these are combined in varying proportions, and division of tumors into cell types is impossible. The single most important feature appears to be the number of mitoses.

LIPOMA OF UTERUS

Lipoma is a rare tumor of the uterus, composed of adult adipose tissue, often with collagenous and muscular tissue, well demarcated from the surrounding myometrium. Grossly and microscopically, these tumors are similar to lipomas elsewhere.

MALIGNANT MIXED MÜLLERIAN TUMORS OF VAGINA, CERVIX, AND UTERUS

Malignant mixed müllerian tumors are a group of neoplasms arising in the mucosal stroma of the vagina, cervix, and uterus from birth to old age. They exhibit variable combinations of sarcomatous and carcinomatous elements conditioned by the embryonic potentialities of the urogenital mesenchyme and the müllerian epithelium derived therefrom. They usually are designated: as sarcoma botryoides in the infant or child and are confined mainly to the vagina; as botryoid tumors of the cervix in women within the reproductive period; and as mixed mesodermal tumors or carcinosarcomas in postmenopausal women, in whom these tumors are largely confined to the endometrium but may arise in the cervix.

Sarcoma Botryoides

Sarcoma botryoides is intimately related to, if not identical with, the polypoid rhabdomyosarcoma of the bladder, most of which occur in the young. Other forms are probably histogenetically related to and may histologically simulate Wilms' tumor. Sarcoma botryoides is a soft, bulky, polypoid, and coarsely lobulated tumor. It varies from pink to red to purple-gray, may be single or multiple, and may be small or large, often filling the vagina and presenting at the vulva. The cut surface varies from moderately firm, pale, fibrous stroma to translucent, myxomatous tissue showing variable amounts of hemorrhage.

Botryoid Tumor

A botryoid tumor occurring in the cervix or uterus may be diffuse or polypoid. The polypoid appearance of the tumor seems to depend on the presence of a distensible cavity within which it can grow, for the polypoid appearance is not present in the metastases or in local pelvic recurrence.

Endometrial Carcinosarcoma

Endometrial carcinosarcoma is a histologic variant of malignant mixed müllerian tumors. It occurs in menopausal and postmenopausal patients, is polypoid, pedunculated or sessile, single or multiple, and often sharply demarcated from the myometrium. The tumor varies from 2 to 3 cm when multiple and up to 6 cm in its greatest diameter when single. Its external surface is coarsely lobulated, smooth or ulcerated, soft to firm, occasionally friable, and varies from red to yellow-gray. The cut surface may be smooth, bulging, homogeneous, or variable, depending on the proportion of epithelial elements. Necrosis and hemorrhage are usually present.

PEDUNCULATED ADENOMYOMA OF UTERUS

Pedunculated adenomyoma of the uterus is characterized by a mixture of normal endometrium and fragments of uterine muscle containing endometrial type glands without any surrounding endometrial stroma. Glands are usually irregular, and squamous elements are common. The lesions may persist after curettage and show myometrial invasion. Pedunculated adenomyomas usually occur in young patients, often in those with infertility problems.

POLYP OF ENDOMETRIUM

A polyp of the endometrium may be single or multiple and varies from a few millimeters to several centimeters in diameter. It usually arises from the middle or basal third of the endometrium and may or may not be covered by functioning endometrium.

CERVIX

ADENOACANTHOMA OF CERVIX

Adenoacanthoma of the cervix is a variant of adenocarcinoma containing histologically benign squamous elements, which apparently develop by a process of metaplasia. Adenoacanthoma must be distinguished from the simultaneous occurrence of a squamous cell carcinoma and an adenocarcinoma in the same cervix.

ADENOCARCINOMA OF CERVIX

Adenocarcinoma of the cervix is an epithelial neoplasm arising from the endocervical mucosa or its glands, and may be situated anywhere between the internal and external os. There are no specific gross features distinguishing adenocarcinoma from squamous cell carcinoma. However, in the early lesions, location in the endocervix may suggest the glandular nature of the tumor. Usually the tumor appears to have arisen in the endocervix, but obviously may have arisen from glands on the portio vaginalis or may appear to have arisen diffusely through the cervix. The tumors are most commonly papillary (40 per cent), or ulcerative (34 per cent), but they may also be nodular or polypoid. The type arising in the endocervical canal and growing into the cervical stroma may be free from symptoms until the tumor erodes onto the portio vaginalis. The diffuse variety may result in marked enlargement and extreme friability of the cervix. Microscopically, the pattern is extremely varied. The well-differentiated adenocarcinomas may be of the cervical gland type, gyriform type, or papillary type, or show an endometrioid pattern or tubal-type pattern. When not very well differentiated, these tumors may be very difficult to diagnose. The moderately poorly differentiated type may have a goblet cell pattern or be of the signet-ring type. The undifferentiated tumors do not have a significant pattern.

DYSPLASIA OF CERVICAL EPITHELIUM

Dysplasia of the cervical epithelium is failure of cellular maturation of all except the superficial layers of the cervical epithelium. There are varying degrees of dysplasia.

GANGLIONEUROMA OF CERVIX

Ganglioneuroma of the cervix is extremely rare. One case has been reported in which there was a tiny polypoid cervical lesion composed largely of Schwann cells with some ganglion cells.

HEMANGIOENDOTHELIOMA OF CERVIX

Hemangioendothelioma of the cervix is extremely rare. Cervical hemangioendotheliomas constitute 0.1 per cent of malignant cervical tumors and are radiosensitive.

HEMANGIOMA OF CERVIX

Hemangioma of the cervix is a rare tumor that presents as a wine-colored lesion of the cervix, fading on pressure. Microscopically, there are dilated venous spaces, chiefly beneath the portio vaginalis.

LEIOMYOMA OF CERVIX

Leiomyoma of the cervix is rare, smooth, relatively avascular, and benign, composed of groups and bundles of smooth muscle fibers arranged in twists and whorls in an interlacing pattern. The gross and microscopic appearance of these tumors is similar to those occurring in the corpus uteri.

LYMPHOMA OF CERVIX

Lymphoma of the cervix is extremely rare. It probably is a direct result of the lack of lymphoid tissue in this area. Presumably it arises from the occasional germinal lymphoid follicles found in the cervix. Leukemic infiltration of the cervix may occur and result in vaginal bleeding as the presenting symptom of the disease.

MALIGNANT MELANOMA OF CERVIX

Malignant melanoma of the cervix is an extremely rare primary cervical tumor. The gross appearance is characteristic of the usual melanoma. The prognosis is poor.

MALIGNANT MIXED MÜLLERIAN TUMORS OF VAGINA, CERVIX, AND UTERUS

Malignant mixed müllerian tumors are a group of neoplasms arising in the mucosal stroma of the vagina, cervix, and uterus from birth to old age. They exhibit variable combinations of sarcomatous and carcinomatous elements conditioned by the embryonic potentialities of the urogenital mesenchyme and the müllerian epithelium derived therefrom. They are usually designated: as sarcoma botryoides in the infant or child and are confined mainly to the vagina; as botryoid tumors of the cervix in women within the reproductive period; and as mixed mesodermal tumors or carcinosarcomas in postmenopausal women, in whom these tumors are largely confined to the endometrium but may arise in the cervix.

Sarcoma Botryoides

Sarcoma botryoides is intimately related to, if not identical with, the polypoid rhabdomyosarcoma of the bladder, most of which occur in the young. Other forms are probably histogenetically related to and may histologically simulate Wilms' tumor. Sarcoma botryoides is a soft, bulky, polypoid, and coarsely lobulated tumor. It varies from pink to red to purple-gray, may be single or multiple, and may be small or large, often filling the vagina and presenting at the vulva. The cut surface varies from moderately firm, pale fibrous stroma to translucent, myxomatous tissue showing variable amounts of hemorrhage.

Botryoid Tumor

A botryoid tumor occurring in the cervix or uterus may be diffuse or polypoid. The polypoid appearance of the tumor seems to depend on the presence of a distensible cavity within which it can grow, for the polypoid appearance is not present in the metastases or in local pelvic recurrence.

Endometrial Carcinosarcoma

Endometrial carcinosarcoma is a histologic variant of malignant mixed müllerian tumors. It occurs in menopausal and postmenopausal patients, is polypoid, pedunculated or sessile, single or multiple, and often sharply demarcated from the myometrium. The tumor varies from 2 to 3 cm when multiple and up to 6 cm in its greatest diameter when single. Its external surface is coarsely lobulated, smooth or ulcerated, soft to firm, occasionally friable, and varies from red to yellow-gray. The cut surface may be smooth, bulging, homogeneous, or variable, depending on the proportion of epithelial elements. Necrosis and hemorrhage are usually present.

MESOMETANEPHROMA OF CERVIX

Mesometanephroma is an adenocarcinoma of the cervix that arises from the mesonephric (wolffian) duct remnants. The tumor may involve the anterolateral or posterolateral aspect of the cervix or include the entire structure. Microscopically, it may vary from a well-differentiated tubular carcinoma to a typical clear cell carcinoma of the hypernephroid or Grawitz type.

SYNONYM: *Adenocarcinoma of Schiller (cervical).*

MICROINVASIVE CARCINOMA OF CERVIX

Microinvasive carcinoma of the cervix is failure of cellular maturation of all layers of cervical epithelium with penetration of the basement membrane to a depth of less than 1 mm.

PAPILLOMA OF CERVIX

Papilloma of the cervix is an epithelial tumor in which the cells cover finger-like processes or ridges of stroma. Usually these are composed of stratified squamous epithelium with varying degrees of keratinization, covering connective-tissue stalks. The various types of neoplasm in the papilloma group are the cockscomb polyp, condyloma acuminatum, and the true papilloma.

Cockscomb Polyp

A cockscomb polyp is a papilloma of the cervix associated with pregnancy but of unknown cause. This warty, firm, usually single lesion of variable size grows rapidly during pregnancy but regresses spontaneously during the postpartum period. It usually disappears by the time uterine involution is complete.

Condyloma Acuminatum

Condyloma acuminatum is a venereal wart or a growth on the cervix, producing an irritating vaginal discharge. It consists of a fibrous overgrowth that is covered by thickened epithelium. It also may occur on the perineum, vulva, and vagina.

True Cervical Papilloma

A true cervical papilloma is usually single, small (0.2 to 0.7 cm), and is attached at or near the squamocolumnar junction by a broad base. It is potentially malignant, and it is often difficult to determine whether early cancer is present. Microscopically, there is connective-tissue stalk covered by squamous epithelium thrown into papillary folds.

POLYP OF CERVIX

A polyp of the cervix is a pedunculated growth from the mucous surface of the cervix. Polyps may arise from the portio vaginalis, the squamocolumnar junction, or the lower endocervix (usually the latter), and they often represent the overgrowth of one of the cervical folds (arbor vitae uteri). Polyps may be single or multiple and may be associated with chronic cervicitis, although this does not seem to be causative. Polyps are found most commonly in parous women in the fifth decade.

They vary from microscopic to 2 cm or more and are soft but sometimes shotty (due to nabothian cysts), pink to red, and sometimes ulcerated. Microscopically, there is a loose vascular connective tissue, the surface being covered by endocervical epithelium and with occasional cervical glands. The stroma is usually very inflamed. Cervical polyps have a low potential of malignancy.

SQUAMOUS CELL CARCINOMA IN SITU OF CERVIX

Squamous cell carcinoma in situ of the cervix is failure of cellular maturation of all layers of cervical epithelium, without penetration of the basement membrane. Grossly, there are no characteristic features of carcinoma in situ. Squamous cell carcinoma in situ usually arises on the endocervical side of the squamocolumnar junction and may extend upward into the endocervix, out to the portio vaginalis, or in both directions. The cervix is frequently distorted by eversion, erosion, or laceration, because this lesion usually occurs in women who have borne at least one child. In the nulliparous woman, carcinoma in situ is usually at the margin of a congenital erosion. Erosion is the most common associated finding, although the portio vaginalis may be covered with smooth, intact epithelium and appear completely normal. The cervix may bleed easily when touched with a cotton swab. Microscopically, the usually accepted histologic criteria of carcinoma in situ are those of morphologic malignancy in any squamous epithelium. These criteria include loss of stratification, loss of polarity, and cellular pleomorphism with increased and often abnormal mitotic activity throughout the epithelium rather than only in the basal one-third. Exception to the general rule of loss of stratification is the uncommon, well-differentiated squamous cell carcinoma in situ arising in or associated with abnormalities of keratinization, such as hyperkeratosis and parakeratosis.

SQUAMOUS CELL CARCINOMA OF CERVIX

Squamous cell carcinoma of the cervix is a malignant neoplasm that usually develops in the region of the squamocolumnar junction involving and penetrating the basement membrane into the stroma. The gross appearance varies. The apparently benign cervix may harbor a tumor that has extended into the endocervix and out into the cervical connective tissue, but without ulcerating through the epithelium of the portio vaginalis. This is often clinically unsuspected. The smallest lesion visible on the portio vaginalis is a firm granular area near the external os that bleeds with minimal trauma. There are three classic types: the excavating type, which results in an irregular, hard ulcer with sloughing base; the cauliflower type, which may vary considerably in size and has a coarsely nodular or papillary appearance, often with surface ulceration; and the flat, infiltrating type (most common), which may grow out on the cervix without ulcerating the cervical mucosa and may extend the length of the vagina without ulcerating the vaginal mucosa. It is hard and tough, when cut it shows a gritty consistency, and ulceration appears late. Microscopically, these tumors are nonkeratinizing and belong to the moderately well-differentiated squamous cell carcinomas.

VULVA

ACROCHORDON OF VULVA

Acrochordon of the vulva is a polypoid fibroepithelial lesion often arising on the vulva and adjacent medial aspect of the thigh, or perianally. The cause of acrochordon is unknown; it does not become malignant. The lesion is a soft, flesh-colored, gray-tan, wrinkled, polypoid structure devoid of hair. It may be pedicled or sessile and varies from several millimeters to 1 cm. The acrochordon is covered by gentle folds of mature, slightly hyperkeratotic epithelium. The stalk and substance of the tumor are composed of loose fibrous tissue containing scattered capillaries. Occasionally, a mild chronic inflammatory reaction is apparent within the stroma.

BARTHOLIN DUCT CYST

A Bartholin duct cyst arises in the duct system of the major vestibular glands. Most cysts involve only the main duct and thus are unilocular, although occasionally one or more loculi lie deep to the main cyst. Multilocular cysts result from occlusion of deeply situated minor ducts or acini of the ductal system, in addition to occlusion of the main duct. In an infected cyst, the contents become purulent, thus constituting a *Bartholin abscess.* All except the smallest cysts cause the entrance to the vestibule to be crescent-shaped. Most Bartholin duct cysts are visible, unilateral, nontender, tense, palpable masses situated in the posterior part of the labia majora, opposite the posterior fourchette. As a rule, they are 1 to 4 cm in diameter; a few become as large as 8 to 10 cm. Most cysts are round or ovoid, although a few have a bizarre configuration with finger-like projections. A cyst that has arisen from the main duct of a major vestibular gland is lined with transitional or squamous epithelium, whereas if it originated in an acinus, the lining consists of cuboidal epithelium. Within the cyst wall, the typical acini of the major vestibular glands are frequently present.

BARTHOLIN GLAND CARCINOMA

Bartholin gland carcinoma is a rare vulvar lesion. In its early stage, it is usually a hard, painless nodule deep in the labial fat and may be confused with an inflammatory process. It becomes attached to surrounding tissue, although skin involvement is late, and it tends to extend deeply into fat, muscle, and the pubic bones. The tumor may undergo necrosis, resulting in a fluctuant mass. The cut surface of the early lesion is firm and pale; the late lesion is loculated, containing stringy mucus separated by a delicate fibrous connective tissue.

BARTHOLIN GLAND SARCOMA

Bartholin gland sarcoma is extremely rare.

BASAL CELL EPITHELIOMA OF VULVA

Basal cell epithelioma of the vulva is a nevoid tumor (hamartoma) derived from immature, incompletely differentiated pluripotential cells.

Pruritus, burning, and chronic ulceration are its chief manifestations. As a rule, bleeding and a discharge are associated with large lesions. Occasionally, the presence of a mass is the patient's only complaint. The labia majora are the most common site. Typically, the vulvar tumors are slightly raised, slow-growing nodules with central ulcerations and pearly, rolled borders. They may or may not be pigmented. The base of the ulcers may be covered with a small amount of necrotic debris or small crusts. If untreated, the tumors may erode deeply into the under-lying tissues and into the bone of the pubic symphysis. In time, the ulcers may become infected, leading to secondary inguinal adenopathy. The tumor is composed of nests of closely packed, uniform oval or fusiform cells. The clusters of cells appear as single or multiple growths arising from the basal layer of the epidermis or from a hair shaft or glandular apparatus. Many are rimmed by a single layer of cells ar-ranged in a radial pattern. The nuclei of the cells are deeply basophilic and are surrounded by a small rim of cytoplasm. The cells resemble the basal cells of the epidermis, although they do not have intercellular bridges. Mitotic figures are often present.

CARCINOMA IN SITU OF VULVA

Carcinoma in situ of the vulva is a term used to include several clinicopathologic entities, namely, amelanotic melanoma, Bowen's dis-ease, erythroplasia of Queyrat, and extramammary Paget's disease.

Bowen's Disease

Bowen's disease is an epithelial lesion that may occur anywhere on the skin of middle-aged or elderly patients of either sex, without any predilection for the vulva. The lesions may be papular or plaquelike, slightly raised above the surface, and reddish brown. Early lesions are discrete, but later they coalesce to form large areas with a crusted or dull red, moist surface. Microscopically, the epithelium is markedly thickened with irregularity in size and shape of cells and numerous mitoses. Invasive carcinoma may occasionally develop from this lesion, but the disease is not sufficiently common to determine the prognosis statistically.

Erythroplasia of Queyrat

Erythroplasia of Queyrat is a rare lesion of the vulva that appears grossly as a red velvety patch of mucous membrane. It may be a variant of Bowen's disease.

Extramammary Paget's Disease

Extramammary Paget's disease is a rare dermatosis, limited to the skin of the axilla and the anogenital region of either sex. Clin-ically and pathologically, it resembles Paget's disease of the breast. The lesion is extremely rare but more commonly found on the labia majora. Grossly, the lesion is red, moist, and sharply demarcated, sometimes with superficial crust formation. The nearby vulva may be swollen and edematous. A firm underlying cancer of variable

size may be palpable. Microscopically, there are typical large, clear
Paget cells in the epidermis, within or just above the malpighian
layer. These cells may coalesce, resulting in loss of the more superficial layers of the squamous epithelium. The underlying carcinoma,
when found, is an adenocarcinoma of apocrine sweat gland origin.

Amelanotic Melanoma

Amelanotic melanoma is an intraepidermal form of melanoma
that simulates Paget's disease. The lesion is confined to the epidermis.
Groups of pale spherical to ovoid cells are present within the
epidermis, usually where it joins the underlying dermis.

CONDYLOMA ACUMINATUM OF VULVA

Condyloma acuminatum of the vulva is a projecting warty growth
on the external genitals or at the anus consisting of fibrous overgrowths
covered by thickened epithelium. The growths are usually associated
with discharges of chronic venereal disease.

SYNONYMS: *Pointed Wart, Venereal Wart, Verrucum Acuminata, Acumi-
nate Condyloma, Genital Wart.*

EMBRYONIC CYST OF VULVA

Embryonic cyst of the vulva is usually solitary, superficial, and thin-
walled. Most of these cysts are located in the hymen, vestibule, labia
minora, and periclitoral tissues. They are usually less than 2 cm in
diameter, although a few reach 10 cm. When they reach this large size,
they tend to be pedunculated. The smaller ones frequently resemble
clear nabothian cysts; others are yellow and soft. The contents are
mucinous.

ENDOMETRIOSIS OF VULVA

Endometriosis of the vulva is not a true neoplasm, but may simulate
one grossly and microscopically. It may arise in two ways, either by
metaplasia of the pelvic peritoneum accompanying the round ligament or
by implantation of viable endometrium following a surgical procedure.
The lesion may reach 1 to 2 cm and, grossly and microscopically, is
similar to endometriosis seen elsewhere.

EPIDERMAL CYST OF VULVA

An epidermal cyst of the vulva is the most common variety of cyst
found there. Epidermal cysts are epithelial cysts lined by squamous
epithelium and are known not to be caused by buried fragments of skin.
Most of these cysts arise from pilosebaceous ducts that have become
occluded. These ducts are lined with stratified squamous epithelium.
As a result of the obstruction, lesions similar to those caused by trau-
matically buried fragments of skin develop. Epidermal cysts of the
vulva arise chiefly in the labia majora, particularly the anterior half. As
a rule, they are multiple, grow slowly, and are round, nontender, and
deep-seated. Most are less than 5 mm in diameter; the largest lesions
seldom exceed 2 cm. The skin over the smaller lesions is thickened,

whereas over the larger cysts it is frequently loose and thin. The contents are usually inspissated and of a caseous or gritty consistency. The lining of the cysts consists of all layers of skin but is usually somewhat thin. The surface cells of the lining epithelium are keratinized, and the cysts usually contain laminated keratinized debris.

FIBROMA OF VULVA

Fibroma of the vulva is usually a firm, pedunculated mass and less often a small, firm, subcutaneous nodule. Fibroma of the vulva arises by a proliferation of fibroblasts and often undergoes myxomatous degeneration. On cross-section, the tumor exhibits a dense, gray-white, fibrous stroma. Microscopically, parallel and intertwining bundles of fibrous tissue may be observed. No mitotic figures are present.

GRANULAR CELL MYOBLASTOMA OF VULVA

Granular cell myoblastoma of the vulva is a benign, usually solitary, slow-growing, discrete nodule that tends to infiltrate the adjacent tissues. Granular cell myoblastomas rarely attain a large size, varying in diameter from 1 to 4 cm. They may lie deep within the tissue, though they are more often superficial and elevated, and occasionally the overlying skin is depigmented. Rarely, the tumor is pedunculated and resembles a papilloma. At times, the epidermis may ulcerate, leading to an erroneous diagnosis of carcinoma. Grossly, the tumor is often mistaken for a fibroma or epidermal cyst or other benign vulvar neoplasm. The tumor is firm, poorly encapsulated, and on section has a glistening surface that is gray-white to pale yellow. Microscopically, there are irregularly arranged bundles of large, pink-staining, round and polyhedral cells, with indistinct cell borders, the bundles being separated by bands of collagen fibers. The cytoplasm of the cells contains numerous eosinophilic granules 0.1 to 3.0μ in diameter. The nuclei vary from small to large and are dark-staining, centrally placed structures containing one or two nucleoli. The margins of the tumor are irregular, with bands of tumor cells extending into the contiguous tissues. The squamous epithelium overlying the tumor may be normal or atrophic, or it may exhibit a hyperplastic response that produces a pseudoepitheliomatous hyperplasia. This response may be pronounced, with rete pegs extending down into the tumor mass, thus presenting the appearance of squamous cell carcinoma. The granular cell myoblastoma is almost invariably benign, although locally infiltrative.

HEMANGIOMA OF VULVA

Hemangioma of the vulva is, in reality, a malformation of blood vessel origin rather than a true neoplasm. There are five different types: the angiokeratoma, cavernous hemangioma, pyogenic granuloma, senile hemangioma, and strawberry hemangioma.

Angiokeratoma

Angiokeratoma may be single or multiple. Angiokeratomas are usually dark red in color, although they may be bright red, brown, blue, or black. They may be slightly lobulated, irregular, or papular and may have a verrucose surface. In diameter, they may vary from 0.2 to 2.0 cm, though most are quite small. The lesions occasionally are confused with melanomas, vulvar warts, or nevi. The upper dermis contains enormously dilated capillaries, usually within the papillae, and the epidermis exhibits hyperkeratosis, parakeratosis, papillomatosis, and irregular elongation of the rete pegs. In areas, the dilated capillaries high in the papillae may be surrounded by a downward proliferation of the epidermis. Thrombosis, with organization and recanalization of the blood clot, is often a feature.

Cavernous Hemangioma

Cavernous hemangioma frequently appears during the first few months of life and increases in size until the child reaches the age of about 18 months. Thereafter it may remain static, or it may begin to regress and eventually almost disappear. Cavernous hemangiomas frequently are deep purple and are multilobular. In size and shape they vary widely, covering only a few square millimeters to several centimeters of the skin surface. The tumor masses may extend up into the vagina and bulge from beneath the vaginal mucosa into the vaginal canal. They are round or flat, lobulated or nodular, and extend deep into the subcutaneous tissue. In undergoing spontaneous involution, they may become fibrous. Microscopically, this tumor exhibits large, irregular blood spaces lined by a single layer of endothelial cells. The walls of the blood vessels are thickened by an overgrowth of adventitial cells. The dilated vessels may progressively ramify in the subcutaneous fat and into the underlying fascia and intermuscular septa.

Pyogenic Granuloma of Vulva

Pyogenic granuloma is a form of capillary hemangioma that may, on rare occasions, appear on the vulva. The tumor, usually single, may be sessile or pedunculated, and dull red to red-brown. It may grow rapidly, attaining a diameter of 0.5 to 2.0 cm and thereafter remain stationary. The surface may be smooth, although it is frequently covered with a crust. The nodule bleeds easily on traumatization. Microscopic study reveals a circumscribed, raised lesion covered by a thinned-out epidermis. The stroma contains numerous newly formed capillaries in varying degrees of dilation, surrounded by a loose, edematous stroma. The early lesions may not exhibit any inflammatory reaction, whereas the older lesions often are inflammatory and perhaps ulcerated, resulting from erosion of the thinned epidermis.

SYNONYM: *Granuloma Pyogenicum.*

Senile Hemangioma

Senile hemangioma is a tumor composed of soft, bright red to dark blue, compressible papules, usually no more than 2 to 3 cm in diameter. Microscopically, the tumor reveals the presence of numerous dilated capillaries lined by flattened endothelial cells. The capillaries are located in the superficial corium near the epidermis, frequently encroaching on the lining epithelium. The collagen around the vessels may exhibit some homogenization.

Strawberry Hemangioma

Strawberry hemangioma is an elevated, bright red to dark red soft tumor, varying in diameter from a few millimeters to several centimeters. The lesion is usually observed shortly after birth and after an initial growth period frequently undergoes spontaneous involution over several years. Microscopically, the tumor reveals dilation of the normal capillaries in the upper dermis, and the presence of newly formed vessels. In the early stages of growth, considerable capillary proliferation is present, with large, prominent endothelial cells. In older lesions, the endothelial cells flatten out, and the lumina of the capillaries widen. Later, fibrosis replaces the vessels and leads to gradual shrinkage of the tumor.

SYNONYM: *Nevus Vasculosus.*

HIDRADENOCARCINOMA OF VULVA

Hidradenocarcinoma of the vulva is an extremely rare malignant variant of hidradenoma. Very rarely, hidradenocarcinoma may be part of extramammary Paget's disease with involvement of the overlying skin.

HIDRADENOMA OF VULVA

Hidradenoma of the vulva is a rare and essentially asymptomatic small tumor arising from the apocrine sweat glands. The hidradenoma appears chiefly on the labia majora as a sharply circumscribed, elevated nodule, only occasionally larger than 1 cm. Such cysts are freely movable, and their consistency varies from hard to soft. Occasionally, pressure necrosis of the overlying skin causes umbilication. Red, granular, papillomatous tissue may protrude through the opening. Hidradenomas consist largely of irregular acini and tubules, usually separated by fine connective-tissue septa. Generally, the papillary projections are covered by a single layer of epithelial cells. These cells are usually tall columnar or cuboidal. They have a pale eosinophilic cytoplasm and a vesicular nucleus located near the base of the cell. Because of the pronounced glandular proliferation, the tumor may be mistaken for an adenocarcinoma. The distinction from carcinoma is based on the lack of cellular pleomorphism and marked multilayering of cells in the hidradenoma. Also, unlike carcinoma, invasion of the adjacent tissues is lacking.

SYNONYMS: *Hidradenoma Papilliferum, Hidradenoma Tubulare, Apocrine Adenoma.*

INCLUSION CYST OF VULVA

An inclusion cyst of the vulva is usually situated on the perineum, in the site of a previous operation. Viable stratified squamous epithelium, if buried beneath either skin or mucosa, may proliferate, secrete, and desquamate, forming the inclusion cyst.

INVASIVE CARCINOMA OF VULVA

Invasive carcinoma of the vulva is the most common malignant disease of the vulva, and may be either of the basal cell or squamous cell types.

Basal Cell Carcinoma of Vulva

Basal cell carcinoma of the vulva usually occurs on the labia majora. Two types have been described, a superficial plaque that may persist unchanged for some time, and the rodent ulcer, which begins as a small plaque and later ulcerates. Recently, a microscopic variant—*adenocystic basal cell carcinoma*—has been described. The superficial plaque occurs on the labia majora and has a rough brown or reddish, scaly, crusted surface, fairly well-demarcated. The lesion persists, sometimes for years, without changing its appearance. A rodent ulcer appears first as a small nodule, growing laterally and superficially, and ulcerating rather late. The ulcer has an irregular outline and is flat. The edge is slightly everted, irregular, fairly sharply defined, and has a beaded appearance. The base is smooth, red, shiny, and slightly friable. Extension is slow, lateral, and superficial. It is curable by excision.

Squamous Cell Carcinoma of Vulva

Squamous cell carcinoma of the vulva usually occurs on the labia majora. The tumor may be finely papillary, but usually has a granular, ulcerated surface. Usually there is adjacent induration due to an accompanying infection. Squamous cell carcinomas of the vulva are usually well differentiated, producing prickle-like cells and often with definite pearl formation. These may arise from unicentric or multicentric foci. Squamous cell carcinoma of the vulva metastasizes most usually via the lymphatic vessels but occasionally via the bloodstream. The "kiss" metastasis sometimes observed on the opposite labium is due to lymphatic extension. Vulvar carcinoma spreads first to the superficial inguinal and femoral lymph nodes, then to Cloquet's node, and finally to the medial group of the external iliac lymph nodes and nodes about the bifurcation of the aorta.

LEIOMYOMA OF VULVA

Leiomyoma of the vulva is a rare tumor of the vulva. Leiomyomas usually arise from the smooth muscle of the erectile tissue in the vulva, although they may also arise from the round ligament of the uterus. In the latter case, they are located in the anterior portion of the vulva. Leiomyomas appear as solitary, firm masses varying from less than 1 cm to more than 10 cm. The tumor may progressively enlarge until symptoms of pressure and ulceration appear. Frequently, the only symptom is recognition of the tumor mass by the patient. Microscopically, there are bundles of smooth muscle intertwining with fibrous tissue and producing a whorled pattern. The smooth muscle element usually predominates.

LIPOMA OF VULVA

Lipoma of the vulva is a soft, either sessile or pedunculated mass. Microscopically, it is composed of mature fat cells and usually has no well-defined connective-tissue capsule. Interspersed between individual and clusters of fat cells are varying amounts of connective tissue. A tumor containing abundant fibrous tissue is more correctly referred to as a *fibrolipoma*. Lipomas vary in size, the largest reported being 17 cm in diameter.

LYMPHANGIOMA OF VULVA

Lymphangioma of the vulva is a tumor of the lymphatic vessels and is analogous to tumors of the blood vessels. There are several types of lymphangiomas: lymphangioma cavernosum, lymphangioma circumscriptum, and lymphangioma simplex.

Lymphangioma Cavernosum

Lymphangioma cavernosum is a soft, compressible tumor that may produce diffuse enlargement of the affected side of the vulva and extend down over the perineum and even up into the vagina. The overlying skin is relatively normal. Microscopically, there are large, cystic spaces filled with lymph and lined with a single layer of endothelial cells present in the dermis and subcutaneous tissue and occasionally extending into the muscle. The connective tissue surrounding the lymphatic channels is hypertrophied.

Lymphangioma Circumscriptum

Lymphangioma circumscriptum is a form of lymphangioma in which there are local groups of small, thin-walled vesicles.

Lymphangioma Simplex

Lymphangioma simplex is a soft, compressible, gray-pink nodule. It may be solitary, or there may be multiple lesions. Swelling is usually diffuse. At times, a few straw-colored vesicles are apparent on the surface of the mass. The dermis contains lymph vessels of various sizes, in which lymph may or may not be present. The vessels have thin walls lined by endothelium.

MELANOMA OF VULVA

Melanoma of the vulva is a malignant tumor of the vulva. The histologic structure of melanomas is very diverse; the cells may be spherical, polyhedral, fusiform, or pleomorphic, and may be arranged in an epithelial, perivascular, or diffuse pattern. The entire tumor may or may not be pigmented, or variations in pigmentation may occur within the same tumor. Moreover, a single tumor may show all these histologic variants. The spread of melanoma of the vulva is unpredictable. There may or may not be extensive local growth prior to metastasis, either through the lymphatic vessels to local or distant lymph nodes or through the bloodstream to a variable number of other sites.

NEUROFIBROMA OF VULVA

Neurofibroma of the vulva arises from the neural sheath. The solitary neurofibroma is often referred to as a *neuronevus*. The tumors appear as small, fleshy, frequently flabby, pink-tan, polypoid masses. Seldom do they reach a large size. Neurofibromas are well circumscribed, though not encapsulated. They are composed of loose, wavy fibrils of pale blue-staining cells that tend to form whorls. Typically, the nuclei of the cells exhibit a palisaded arrangement.

PAPILLARY CARCINOMA IN SITU OF VULVA

Papillary carcinoma in situ of the vulva is a lesion quite distinct clinically from Bowen's disease, although occasionally there may be some overlapping in the histologic pattern. Basically the lesion is papillary, but it may vary from a granular area, through a papillary lesion grossly similar to and often misdiagnosed as condyloma acuminatum, to a large plaque with a rough papillary surface. In general, the lesion grows slowly in a lateral direction, invading the underlying stroma relatively late, if at all. Histologically, loss of polarity of cells and mitotic activity are prominent.

PAPILLOMA OF VULVA

Papilloma of the vulva is an uncommon, usually single, potentially malignant tumor occurring anywhere on the vulva during adult life. It is usually small, although it may attain a diameter of several centimeters. The outer surface has a wrinkled appearance, and small finger-like projections may develop on the surface. Repeated trauma and irritation may lead to ulceration. Microscopically, it is composed of papillary processes of squamous epithelium with a scanty central connective-tissue core. It should be distinguished from the usually multiple condylomata acuminata.

PIGMENTED NEVI OF VULVA

Pigmented nevi of the vulva may be divided into five clinical types: flat nevi, usually junctional; slightly elevated nevi, usually compound; papillomatous nevi, which may be compound, though most are intra-dermal; dome-shaped nevi, usually intradermal; and pedunculated nevi, which are intradermal. The pigmented nevi vary from a light tan to a dark brown to black. They may vary in diameter from 1 mm to 2 cm. Histologically, nevi are classified into three main groups: junctional, intradermal, and compound. The junctional nevus is characterized by an active formation of cells in the basal layer of the epidermis. These cells form more or less circumscribed nests. The nests may appear to be "dropping off" the epidermis, yet remain in contact with it. Although this type of nevus is the one most likely to become malignant, the danger of its transformation is slight if the nests of cells are well circumscribed. The compound nevus exhibits junctional activity, yet nests of nevus cells are present within the dermis. This tumor may also have malignant potential. The cells in the intradermal nevus are located within the dermis. Careful sectioning of the tissue, however, will generally reveal some foci of junctional activity, even though none have been suspected from routine sections. The nevus cell is oval or cuboidal. Its membrane is quite distinct, and the cytoplasm appears homogeneous. The cytoplasm of scattered cells may contain dark brown melanin. The nuclei, which may be round or oval, are large, vesicular, and pale. The nevus cells lying deep in the dermis may be fusiform and embedded in fibrous tissue. In addition, the dermis may contain multinucleated nevus cells.

PILONIDAL CYST OF VULVA

A pilonidal cyst of the vulva represents a foreign-body reaction to hair that has become buried beneath the skin surface, causing infection, granuloma, and sinus tracts. The superficial portion of the sinus tract is lined with squamous epithelium with or without hair follicles, hair shafts, and sebaceous glands. At a deeper level, the tract may be lined with granulation tissue. The tract eventually opens into an abscess filled with purulent exudate and hairs. The granulation tissues exhibit an acute inflammatory reaction throughout, as evidenced by the presence of large numbers of polymorphonuclear leukocytes, lymphocytes, and plasma cells. The contents usually include hair shafts, pus cells, epithelial cells, and necrotic debris. A surrounding cellulitis may be present.

SARCOMA OF VULVA

Sarcoma of the vulva is rare. The tumors may vary considerably in size, 1 to 15 cm, and may be diffuse or discrete. Initially they lie beneath the skin and then extend and ulcerate through the surface. Usually they are homogeneous and fleshy, but may be soft or firm, and white, yellow, or red. The rate of growth of an individual tumor may vary, remaining stationary for some time and then growing rapidly. Microscopically, it is usually some type of fibrosarcoma, but occasionally may be a lipo-sarcoma, lymphosarcoma, or rhabdomyosarcoma.

SEBACEOUS ADENOMA OF VULVA

Sebaceous adenoma of the vulva is a solitary, smooth, firm, elevated, round, or oval nodule, usually less than 1 cm in diameter. At times, it may be pedunculated. It may closely resemble a hidradenoma, epidermal inclusion cyst, sebaceous cyst, or a small cyst of embryonic origin. Microscopically, there are lobules of varying size and shape consisting of two types of cells. One type is identical with the cells found at the periphery of normal sebaceous glands; the other type is a mature sebaceous cell that has developed from the generative cells. The relative number of each type of cell in each lobule varies considerably, with transitional cells from the generative to the mature sebaceous type often being present. The tumor is sharply demarcated from the adjacent tissue and is usually surrounded by a connective-tissue capsule.

SEBACEOUS CYST OF VULVA

A sebaceous cyst of the vulva is clinically indistinguishable from an epidermal cyst. These cysts are rare. Most result from the accumulation of sebaceous secretions incident to obstruction of sebaceous gland ducts. Grossly, sebaceous cysts are usually spherical, nontender, and firm. The contents are cheesy or sebaceous. The cysts are often multiple, and are more likely to appear on the inner and anterior aspects of the labia majora, particularly about the clitoris. These cysts are lined with stratified epithelial cells without intercellular bridges and without keratinization. The epithelium exhibits no rete malpighii, as may epidermal cysts. The cysts are filled with an amorphous sebaceous material.

SEBORRHEIC KERATOSIS OF VULVA

Seborrheic keratosis of the vulva is a form of papilloma that appears as a solitary tumor or in association with similar growths elsewhere. Seborrheic keratoses are sharply circumscribed, slightly raised, verrucose lesions, usually papular but sometimes macular. They vary in diameter from minute to several centimeters, and they may appear singly or in clusters. They may be flesh-colored or black, though most are dark brown and appear greasy. The tumor consists of solid sheets or masses of epithelial cells surrounding connective tissue. The horny layer tends to invaginate the lesion, and cystic inclusions of horny material are observed in some areas. Infrequently, thin tracts of double rows of basal cells extend down from the epidermis, branching and interweaving to give the tumor an adenoid appearance.

SYRINGOMA OF VULVA

Syringoma of the vulva is a rather unusual lesion, frequently mistaken for Fox-Fordyce disease. The lesion develops at puberty or later in life, most often around the eyelids and less often on the chest, abdomen, and vulva. Syringoma is characterized by multiple or occasionally single, small, firm papules or cystic structures beneath the skin of the labia majora. Within the dermis are many small, cystic ducts, usually lined by two layers of epithelial cells. The cells tend to be flat, and the inner layer of cells frequently has a clear, vacuolated appearance. Solid strands of epithelial cells may also be seen within the dermis.

VAGINA

ADENOSIS OF VAGINA

Adenosis of the vagina is a rare condition characterized by the presence of definite mucous glands beneath the superficial squamous epithelium of the vaginal wall. The glands may be diffuse or circumscribed. They may be asymptomatic while the surface epithelium is intact, or discharging and bleeding when destroyed. These glands develop from müllerian tissue remaining after replacement of original vaginal mucosa by urogenital sinus epithelium. They should be distinguished from mesonephric remnants lying deep in the lateral vaginal wall.

BENIGN CYSTIC TERATOMA OF VAGINA

A benign cystic teratoma of the vagina occurs rarely and probably arises from a misplaced primordial germ cell that failed to reach its destination during its migration from the yolk-sac endoderm. Grossly and microscopically, it is similar to benign cystic teratoma arising in the ovary.

SYNONYM: *Dermoid Cyst of Vagina.*

CYSTS OF VAGINA

Cysts of the vagina are of two main types. Those arising from remnants of the mesonephros are lined by a cuboidal epithelium, although the cells may become flattened by the cyst contents. Cysts arising after surgery are of the epidermal inclusion type and are lined by squamous epithelium that is flattened and thinned out to a variable degree. Endometriosis may present as a hemorrhagic cyst. Occasionally, the epithelial lining may suggest paramesonephric origin. Vaginitis emphysematosa must be considered when cysts are multiple.

Gartner Duct Cyst

A Gartner duct cyst arises from the vestigial remains of the mesonephric canals, which as the so-called Gartner ducts course along the outer anterior aspect of the vaginal canal. The resulting cysts may be small, or they may become so large that they bulge from the vaginal outlet. They are always located on the anterolateral aspect of the canal. Microscopically, they are lined with a varying type of epithelium, cuboidal or columnar, ciliated or nonciliated, and sometimes stratified.

Inclusion Cyst of Vagina

An inclusion cyst of the vagina arises from inclusion beneath the surface of tags of mucosa resulting from perineal lacerations or from imperfect denudation in the course of perineal surgery. Such bits of mucosa become encysted, although the cysts are always small, rarely exceeding a few centimeters in diameter. They are not infrequently multiple. They are lined by a stratified squamous epithelium, and the content is usually cheesy. The cysts occur at the lower end of the vagina, usually on the posterior surface.

ENDOMETRIOSIS OF VAGINA

Endometriosis of the vagina is not a true neoplasm but it may simulate one. Usually associated with endometriosis elsewhere in the pelvis, it may arise spontaneously or after pelvic surgery. It may occur either in the mucosa or in the muscle of the vagina, in the latter case usually having extended from the pelvic peritoneum to the posterior fornix. A variable overgrowth of the muscle may occur, resulting in adenomyosis or an adenomyoma. Endometriosis in the vagina may undergo cyclic change and, extremely rarely, may give rise to an adenocarcinoma of endometrial type.

LEIOMYOMA OF VAGINA

A leiomyoma of the vagina is a rare benign tumor of connective tissue origin. It occurs usually in the fifth decade, but may occur in the pregnant patient. Grossly and microscopically, it is similar to these tumors found elsewhere in the female genital tract. It varies from 1.5 to 4.5 cm and is usually discrete and easily shelled out, but it may be diffuse.

MALIGNANT MIXED MÜLLERIAN TUMORS OF VAGINA, CERVIX, AND UTERUS

Malignant mixed müllerian tumors are a group of neoplasms arising in the mucosal stroma of the vagina, cervix, and uterus from birth to old age. They exhibit variable combinations of sarcomatous and carcinomatous elements conditioned by the embryonic potentialities of the urogenital mesenchyme and the müllerian epithelium derived therefrom. They are usually designated: as sarcoma botryoides in the infant or child and are confined mainly to the vagina; as botryoid tumors of the cervix in women within the reproductive period; and as mixed mesodermal tumors or carcinosarcomas in postmenopausal women, in whom these tumors are largely confined to the endometrium but may arise in the cervix.

Sarcoma Botryoides

Sarcoma botryoides is intimately related to, if not identical with, the polypoid rhabdomyosarcoma of the bladder, most of which occur in the young. Other forms are probably histogenetically related to and may histologically simulate Wilms' tumor. Sarcoma botryoides is a soft, bulky, polypoid, and coarsely lobulated tumor. It varies from pink to red to purple-gray, may be single or multiple, and may be small or large, often filling the vagina and presenting at the vulva. The cut surface varies from moderately firm, pale fibrous stroma to translucent myxomatous tissue showing variable amounts of hemorrhage.

Botryoid Tumor

A botryoid tumor occurring in the cervix or uterus may be diffuse or polypoid. The polypoid appearance of the tumor seems to depend on the presence of a distensible cavity within which it can grow, for the polypoid appearance is not present in the metastases or local pelvic recurrence.

Endometrial Carcinosarcoma

Endometrial carcinosarcoma is a histologic variant of malignant mixed müllerian tumors. It occurs in menopausal and postmenopausal patients, is polypoid, pedunculated or sessile, single or multiple, and often sharply demarcated from the myometrium. The tumor varies from 2 to 3 cm when multiple and up to 6 cm in its greatest diameter when single. Its external surface is coarsely lobulated, smooth or ulcerated, soft to firm, and occasionally friable, and it varies from red to yellow-gray. The cut surface may be smooth, bulging, homogeneous, or variable, depending on the proportion of epithelial elements. Necrosis and hemorrhage are usually present.

MELANOMA OF VAGINA

Melanoma of the vagina is among the rarest of vaginal tumors. The tumors range from 2 to 4 cm in diameter, and occur anywhere in the vagina. They may be nodular, plaquelike, or even papillary. Secondary ulceration is common. Because melanomas disseminate widely by way of the lymphatic vessels and the bloodstream, and because the tumor is radioresistant, the prognosis is poor.

METASTATIC CARCINOMA OF VAGINA

Metastatic carcinoma of the vagina is more common than primary carcinoma of the vagina. Secondary involvement of the vagina may be by (1) direct extension from the cervix, vulva, bladder, urethra, or rectum; (2) lymphatic permeation or embolization from the endometrium, cervix, bladder, or rectum; (3) vascular embolization from uterine carcinoma, renal hypernephroma, ovarian neoplasms, or choriocarcinoma; and (4) by direct implantation from the endometrium or cervix. Rarely, the vagina may have secondary blood-borne metastases from malignant neoplasms other than those mentioned. The most common secondary carcinoma of the vagina is from the cervix. The prognosis is poor, even with treatment of both the primary and the metastatic lesion.

SYNONYM: *Secondary Carcinoma of Vagina.*

PAPILLOMA OF VAGINA

Papilloma of the vagina is an uncommon single or multiple tumor that may simulate or give rise to carcinoma. It has the usual appearance, both grossly and microscopically, of a papilloma arising from squamous epithelium. It should be distinguished from condyloma acuminatum, which is usually multiple and of viral origin.

POLYP OF VAGINA

A polyp of the vagina is an uncommon vaginal tumor derived from the mucosal stroma and covered by vaginal epithelium. It sometimes contains glandlike structures. It does not appear to have any malignant potential.

PRIMARY CARCINOMA OF VAGINA

Primary carcinoma of the vagina is uncommon. Symptoms in order of frequency are vaginal discharge; dysuria; vaginal mass; pruritus; pelvic, abdominal, or coital pain; swelling of the legs; weakness; and loss of weight. Most vaginal carcinomas are of the squamous cell type. The remainder are adenocarcinomas that arise from endometriosis, adenomyosis, and mesonephric tubular and ductal remnants, or perhaps from adenosis of the vagina. Those rare adenocarcinomas arising from endometriosis resemble endometrial carcinoma. Those from mesonephric tubular and ductal elements resemble mesonephromas, with glandlike spaces lined by flattened cells or large cells with clear cytoplasm.

SARCOMA OF VAGINA

Sarcoma of the vagina is a rare malignant tumor. Sarcomas vary in size from 2 to 15 cm and may be located anywhere in the vaginal wall. They may be soft or firm, pale gray to pink, homogeneous, and well vascularized, with varying degrees of necrosis and hemorrhage. They may arise from the stroma of the mucosa or the vaginal wall itself. The microscopic pattern is varied. It has been reported specifically as that of myosarcoma, fibrosarcoma, myxosarcoma, and angiosarcoma. Prognosis is poor.

Section 5: *Selected Gynecologic Topics*

Gynecologic Operations

INCISIONS

COLPOHYSTEROTOMY
Colpohysterotomy is an incision into the uterus through the vagina.
SYNONYM: *Vaginal Hysterotomy.*

COLPOTOMY
Colpotomy is an incision made in the posterior fornix of the vagina into the rectouterine pouch to visualize pelvic structures, perform surgical procedures on tubes or ovaries, or to drain pelvic abscesses.
SYNONYMS: *Posterior Colpotomy, Culdotomy.*

COLPOURETEROTOMY
Colpoureterotomy is an incision into the ureter through the vagina.

CYSTOSTOMY
Cystostomy is the creation of a temporary or permanent opening into the bladder for drainage. It may be transvaginal (vaginal cystostomy) or suprapubic.

CYSTOTOMY
Cystotomy is an incision into the bladder. It may be done transvaginally or transabdominally.

HYMENOTOMY
Hymenotomy is division of an imperforate hymen.

HYSTEROTOMY
Hysterotomy is an incision into the uterus extending into the uterine cavity. It may be performed vaginally (*colpohysterotomy, vaginal hysterotomy*) or transabdominally.
SYNONYM: *Uterotomy.*

LAPAROTOMY
Laparotomy is a surgical incision into the abdominal cavity.

OOPHOROTOMY
Oophorotomy is an incision into an ovarian cyst.
SYNONYM: *Ovariotomy.*

PFANNENSTIEL INCISION
The Pfannenstiel incision is a low, transverse abdominal incision, dividing skin, subcutaneous tissue, and fascia transversely, and separating the rectus muscles in the midline vertically.

SALPINGOSTOMY
Salpingostomy is the creation of an opening in the fallopian tube to permit removal of tubal contents (tubal pregnancy, hydrosalpinx, etc.), leaving the defect open.

SALPINGOTOMY
Salpingotomy is an incision into a fallopian tube.

SCHUCHARDT INCISION
The Schuchardt incision is a mediolateral episiotomy dividing the levator muscle for exposure in vaginal surgery.

EXCISION OPERATIONS

BARTHOLIN'S CYSTECTOMY
Bartholin's cystectomy is the excision of a cyst of a major vestibular gland.

BIOPSY (CERVICAL, ENDOMETRIAL, OVARIAN, VULVAR, etc.)
A biopsy is the removal of a portion of tissue for pathologic examination.

CERVICECTOMY
Cervicectomy is surgical extirpation of the uterine cervix.
SYNONYMS: *Cervical Amputation, Trachelectomy.*

CLITORIDECTOMY
Clitoridectomy is the surgical excision of the clitoris.
SYNONYM: *Clitoral Amputation.*

CONIZATION (OF CERVIX)
Conization of the cervix is the removal of a cone of tissue around the external os, the apex of the cone extending up the endocervical canal.

CYSTECTOMY (TOTAL OR PARTIAL)
Total cystectomy is excision of the bladder. *Partial cystectomy* is resection of a portion of the bladder.

FEMALE CIRCUMCISION
Female circumcision is the surgical excision of the prepuce and frenulum of the clitoris.

GROIN DISSECTION
Groin dissection is the removal of inguinal lymph nodes (*superficial groin dissection*) or inguinal, iliac, hypogastric, femoral, and obturator lymph nodes (*radical groin dissection*). It may be carried out as a unilateral or bilateral procedure.

HYMENECTOMY
Hymenectomy is excision of the hymen.

HYSTERECTOMY
Hysterectomy is the surgical removal of the uterus. It may be performed either abdominally or vaginally and is classified as radical, subtotal, or total.

HYSTERECTOMY, ABDOMINAL
Abdominal hysterectomy is the removal of the uterus through an incision in the abdominal wall.

Subtotal Hysterectomy
Subtotal hysterectomy is the removal of the uterus at or above the level of the internal os.

SYNONYMS: *Supracervical Hysterectomy, Supravaginal Hysterectomy.*

Total Hysterectomy
Total hysterectomy is the removal of the corpus and cervix uteri.

HYSTERECTOMY, CESAREAN
Cesarean hysterectomy is an operation in which the fetus is removed through an incision in the abdomen and the uterus followed by either incomplete or complete hysterectomy.

SYNONYM: *Porro's Operation.*

HYSTERECTOMY, RADICAL
Radical hysterectomy is the total removal of the uterus, upper vagina, and parametrium for cancer.

Modified Radical Hysterectomy
Modified radical hysterectomy is an extended hysterectomy in which the ureters are exposed and retracted laterally without dissection from the ureteral bed. The paracervical tissue is removed more widely than usual, but medial to the ureters. A portion of the upper vagina is removed.

SYNONYM: *TeLinde Modification.*

Radical Wertheim Hysterectomy
The radical Wertheim hysterectomy requires mobilization of the ureters, with removal of the peritoneum of the rectouterine pouch, uterosacral ligaments, upper vagina, and paracervical and paravaginal tissues from their outer attachments near the pelvic wall.

Radical Hysterectomy and Pelvic Lymphadenectomy
Radical hysterectomy and pelvic lymphadenectomy includes, in addition to the Wertheim operation, bilateral removal of iliac, hypogastric, obturator lymph nodes, and paraaortic lymph nodes. The ureter may be replaced intraperitoneally (*Novak modification*),

resutured to the obliterated hypogastric (*Green modification*), or left attached by a thin web to the obliterated hypogastric (*Morris modification*). The *Brunschwig modification* includes removal of the hypogastric vessels.

SYNONYM: *Meigs' Operation.*

HYSTERECTOMY, VAGINAL

A vaginal hysterectomy is the removal of the uterus through the vagina.

Morcellation Operation

The morcellation operation is a vaginal hysterectomy in which the uterus is split into lateral halves, each of which is brought down in succession and removed.

Schauta-Amreich Operation

The Schauta-Amreich operation is an extended vaginal hysterectomy and bilateral adnexectomy, including the upper vagina and the maximum amount of paracervical tissue.

HYSTEROSALPINGOOOPHORECTOMY

Hysterosalpingooophorectomy is the surgical removal of the uterus, fallopian tubes, and the ovaries.

LITHOTOMY

Lithotomy is removal of a stone from the urinary bladder.

SYNONYM: *Lithectomy.*

MYOMECTOMY, ABDOMINAL

Abdominal myomectomy is the removal of a myoma from the uterus through an abdominal incision.

MYOMECTOMY, VAGINAL

Vaginal myomectomy is the removal of a myoma from the uterus through the vagina.

SYNONYM: *Colpomyomectomy.*

NEURECTOMY, PRESACRAL

A presacral neurectomy is excision of the presacral plexus for relief of severe dysmenorrhea.

SYNONYMS: *Presacral Sympathectomy, Cotte's Operation.*

OOPHORECTOMY

Oophorectomy is the surgical removal of an ovary. The operation may be unilateral or bilateral.

OOPHOROCYSTECTOMY

Oophorocystectomy is the excision of an ovarian cyst.

PELVIC EXENTERATION

Pelvic exenteration is the complete surgical removal of the pelvic viscera, including the rectum and/or bladder, and pelvic lymphadenectomy.

SYNONYMS: *Pelvic Evisceration, Brunschwig Procedure.*

Anterior Pelvic Exenteration

Anterior pelvic exenteration is complete surgical removal of the pelvic viscera anterior to the rectum, including pelvic lymphadenectomy, with urinary diversion.

Posterior Pelvic Exenteration

Posterior pelvic exenteration is complete removal of the pelvic viscera posterior to the bladder and urethra, including pelvic lymphadenectomy and sigmoid colostomy.

Total Pelvic Exenteration

Total pelvic exenteration is the complete removal of the pelvic viscera with ureterointestinal anastomoses and colostomy.

SYNONYM: *Brunschwig's Operation.*

PELVIC LYMPHADENECTOMY

Pelvic lymphadenectomy is the removal of the lymph nodes overlying the iliac vessels (iliac, hypogastric, and obturator lymph nodes). The operation may be carried out extraperitoneally (*Nathonson procedure*), or transperitoneally (*Taussig procedure*).

SALPINGECTOMY

Salpingectomy is the surgical removal of a fallopian tube. It may be complete or partial, unilateral or bilateral.

SALPINGOOOPHORECTOMY

Salpingooophorectomy is the surgical removal of an ovary and its fallopian tube. It may be unilateral or bilateral.

STURMDORF OPERATION

The Sturmdorf operation is conical excision of the endocervix with preservation of sufficient cervical mucosa to cover the exposed area of excision.

VAGINECTOMY

Vaginectomy is the excision of the vagina. It may be either partial or total.

SYNONYM: *Colpectomy.*

VULVECTOMY

Vulvectomy is excision of the vulva. It may be complete or partial (hemivulvectomy).

Radical Vulvectomy

A radical vulvectomy is the wide removal for cancer of all structures of the vulva, together with adjacent skin, a portion of the mons, and subcutaneous fat down to the deep fascia and muscles. It is usually accompanied by regional lymph node dissection through single or separate incisions.

Stanley Way Procedure

The Stanley Way procedure is a radical vulvectomy for cancer with bilateral, en bloc removal of pelvic and inguinal lymph nodes, with overlying skin, and vulva. The operation requires division of Poupart's ligament and is performed through a butterfly-shaped incision that precludes complete wound closure about the vulva.

Simple Vulvectomy

Simple vulvectomy, performed for benign disease, is the superficial removal of vulvar structures, including skin, mucous membrane, and superficial fat and connective tissue.

WEDGE RESECTION, OVARIAN

Ovarian wedge resection is surgical removal of a longitudinal wedge of ovarian cortex and stroma extending to the hilum.

PLASTIC OPERATIONS, REPAIRS, AND SUSPENSIONS

COLPOCYSTOPLASTY

Colpocystoplasty is a surgical plastic procedure to repair the vesicovaginal wall.

COLPOHYSTEROPEXY

Colpohysteropexy is a fixation of the uterus performed through the vagina.

SYNONYM: *Vaginal Hysteropexy.*

COLPOPEXY

Colpopexy is suspension of a relaxed and prolapsed vagina. It may be suspended by fixation to the abdominal wall, by attachment to the sacrum, by fascial strips, or by use of the round ligaments.

SYNONYMS: *Vaginopexy, Vaginal Suspension.*

COLPOPLASTY

Colpoplasty is any plastic operation involving the vagina.

COLPOPOIESIS

Colpopoiesis is the construction of an artificial vagina.

McIndoe Operation

The McIndoe operation is the construction of a vagina by use of a split-thickness graft over a vaginal stent or mold.

Williams Operation

The Williams operation entails construction of a vagina by incising each of the labia majora vertically to the perineum and suturing the edges together across a midline stent to give a labial tube for coitus.

COLPORRHAPHY

Colporrhaphy is the repair of a laceration or relaxation of the vagina.

Anterior Colporrhaphy

Anterior colporrhaphy is the repair of a cystocele or relaxation of the anterior wall of the vagina.

SYNONYM: *Cystocele Repair.*

Posterior Colporrhaphy

Posterior colporrhaphy is the repair of a rectocele or relaxation of the posterior wall of the vagina.

SYNONYM: *Rectocele Repair.*

CULDOPLASTY

Culdoplasty is a plastic procedure to repair relaxation of the posterior fornix of the vagina.

McCall Culdoplasty

The McCall culdoplasty entails suspension of the posterior fornix of the vagina and repair of enterocele by attaching the vaginal apex to transverse sutures placed across the rectouterine pouch.

CYSTOPEXY

Cystopexy is a surgical suspension of the urinary bladder to the pubic symphysis or to the abdominal wall.

GRACILIS MUSCLE TRANSPLANT OPERATION

The gracilis muscle transplant operation is a plastic procedure for the cure of vaginal fistulas using the gracilis muscle to close the defect.

SYNONYM: *Ingleman-Sundberg Operation.*

HYSTEROPEXY

Hysteropexy is the operative fixation of an abnormally positioned uterus. The operation may be performed by various methods—for example, shortening of the round ligaments, fixation to the abdominal wall, or plication of the uterosacral ligaments.

SYNONYMS: *Uterofixation, Uteropexy.*

Frommel's Operation

Frommel's operation is shortening of the uterosacral ligaments by the abdominal route, for retrodeviation.

Ventrofixation of Uterus

Ventrofixation of the uterus is suspension of the uterus by suturing the uterine fundus to the abdominal wall.

MANCHESTER-FOTHERGILL OPERATION

The Manchester-Fothergill operation is used to correct uterine prolapse. It entails elevation of the uterus by approximating the cardinal ligaments anterior to the cervix, cervical amputation, and an anterior colporrhaphy.

SYNONYM: *Fothergill-Donald Operation.*

METROPLASTY

Metroplasty is any plastic operation on the uterus.

SYNONYM: *Hysteroplasty.*

Strassmann Metroplasty

The Strassmann metroplasty is a technique for repair of a bicornuate uterus using a transverse incision. In the *Jones modification*, a V incision is used.

PERINEORRHAPHY

Perineorrhaphy is the surgical repair of a rectocele or perineal laceration.

SYNONYMS: *Posterior Repair, Colpoperineorrhaphy.*

SALPINGOPEXY

Salpingopexy is the operative fixation of a fallopian tube.

SALPINGOPLASTY

Salpingoplasty is the surgical plastic repair of a fallopian tube.

SYNONYM: *Tuboplasty.*

Cornual Reimplantation

Cornual reimplantation involves resection of a portion of a cornu of the uterus and obstructed interstitial portion of the tube, with reimplantation of the tube into the cornu.

Fimbrioplasty

Fimbrioplasty is the freeing up of the fimbria of a tube when obstruction is present.

Rock-Mulligan Hood Procedure

The Rock-Mulligan procedure entails placing small, plastic, umbrella-shaped hoods over the distal end of the fallopian tube after opening a clubbed tube and turning back a cuff.

TRACHELORRHAPHY

Trachelorrhaphy is the repair and suturing of a lacerated cervix.

SYNONYM: *Emmet's Operation.*

UTERINE SUSPENSION OPERATIONS

Uterine suspension is the correction of uterine retroversion or prolapse by use of the round ligaments.

Baldy-Webster Suspension

The Baldy-Webster suspension operation is anterior fixation of the uterine fundus by drawing a fold of each round ligament behind the uterus, through an opening in the broad ligament, and suturing these ligaments to the posterior wall of the uterine corpus.

Coffey Suspension (Meigs' Modification)

Meigs' modification of the Coffey suspension operation draws the uterine fundus forward by suturing a loop of each round ligament to the anterior wall of the uterus, the loops coming together in the midline.

Gilliam Suspension

The Gilliam suspension operation is correction of a retroverted uterus by drawing a loop of each round ligament through the abdominal wall and fixing the loops to the abdominal fascia.

SYNONYMS: *Doléris Suspension, Simpson Suspension, Crossen Suspension.*

Olshausen Suspension

The Olshausen suspension operation suspends the uterus by suturing the midportion of the round ligament to the anterior rectus sheath.

OPERATIONS FOR STRESS INCONTINENCE

KELLY PLICATION

The Kelly plication is a plication of the bladder neck and urethra for stress incontinence. It is usually accompanied by anterior colporrhaphy.

SYNONYM: *Kelly-Stoeckel Operation.*

LEVATOR MUSCLE SLING

The levator muscle sling is an anterior colporrhaphy supplemented by a sling formed by freeing up the levator muscles and approximating them beneath the bladder neck.

SYNONYMS: *Ingleman-Sundberg Procedure, Pubococcygeoplasty.*

MARSHALL-MARCHETTI-KRANTZ RETROPUBIC SUSPENSION

The Marshall-Marchetti-Krantz retropubic suspension is an operation for stress incontinence performed through the space of Retzius. Interrupted sutures are used to attach the periurethral tissue to the posterior surface of the pubic symphysis.

PEREYRA PERIURETHRAL SUSPENSION

The Pereyra periurethral suspension operation is a combined vaginal and suprapubic operation for stress incontinence. Through a small suprapubic incision, a special needle in a steel sheath is passed into the vaginal dissection through the tissue on both sides of the urethra. A double-needle arrangement enables a loop of suture material to pick up the periurethral fascia and lift it upward when sutured to the fascia of the anterior abdominal wall.

SUPRAPUBIC SLING OPERATION

The suprapubic sling operation, used to correct stress incontinence, is usually combined with anterior colporrhaphy, in which fascial strips from the anterior abdominal wall are detached at one end and passed beneath the urethra through the space of Retzius.

SYNONYMS: *Millin-Read Sling, Goebell-Stoeckel-Frangenheim Operation, Aldridge-Studdiford Operation.*

MISCELLANEOUS OPERATIONS

ASPIRATION, OVARIAN

Ovarian aspiration is the removal of fluids from an ovarian cyst by means of a hollow needle or trocar connected to a suction syringe.

BRICKER ILEAL CONDUIT

The Bricker ileal conduit is a urinary diversion procedure using a segment of terminal ileum into which the ureters have been implanted.

CAUTERIZATION, CERVICAL

Cervical cauterization is the induction of cellular necrosis in a portion of the cervix by means of physical or chemical agents.

COLPOCLEISIS

Colpocleisis is the surgical closure of the vaginal canal.

Partial Colpocleisis

Partial colpocleisis is an operation in which the vaginal canal is partially obliterated by suturing together areas of the anterior and posterior wall, denuded of vaginal mucosa, leaving a bilateral and posterior tunnel of intact vaginal mucosa to permit external egress of cervical and uterine secretions.

SYNONYM: *Le Fort's Operation.*

CRYOSURGERY

Cryosurgery is the use of freezing by means of special probes cooled with liquid nitrogen, Freon gas, or carbon dioxide.

CULDOCENTESIS

Culdocentesis is aspiration of fluid from the rectouterine pouch by puncture of the posterior fornix.

CULDOSCOPY

Culdoscopy is visual examination of the female pelvic viscera through the posterior vaginal fornix by means of an endoscope.

DILATATION AND CURETTAGE

Dilatation and curettage is dilation of the cervix followed by removal of the endometrium by means of a curet.

SYNONYM: *Recamier's Operation.*

ABBREVIATION: D & C.

Fractional Dilatation and Curettage

Fractional dilatation and curettage is removal of the mucous membrane of the endocervix by means of a curet followed by dilation of the cervix and removal of the endometrium with polyp forceps and also by means of a curet. The specimens are kept separate for laboratory examination.

Suction Curettage

Suction curettage is removal of uterine contents (pregnancy prior to 12 weeks, mole, incomplete abortion) by a hollow curet attached to a strong vacuum pump.

SYNONYM: *Vacuum Aspiration.*

ESTES OPERATION

Estes operation is implantation of an ovary into a uterine cornu to permit ovulation to occur directly into the endometrial cavity.

FULGURATION, CERVICAL

Cervical fulguration is the destruction of cervical tissue by electric current.

HYSTEROLYSIS

Hysterolysis is release of adhesions between the uterus and surrounding parts.

HYSTEROSALPINGOSTOMY

Hysterosalpingostomy is the operation of forming an anastomosis between the uterus and the distal portion of the fallopian tube after the excision of a strictured or obstructed portion of the tube.

LAPAROSCOPY

Laparoscopy is visual examination of the pelvis by means of an endoscope through the abdominal wall.

SYNONYM: *Peritoneoscopy.*

LASH'S OPERATION

Lash's operation is an operation for an incompetent cervix. A wedge of the internal cervical os is removed and the gaping internal os is sutured into a tighter canal structure.

MARSUPIALIZATION

Marsupialization is an operation used to cure a cyst by opening the tumor, evacuating the contents, and suturing the edges of the cyst to the edges of the external incision. This wound is kept open while the interior of the cyst suppurates and closes by granulation.

PARACENTESIS

Paracentesis is the withdrawal of ascitic fluid through the abdominal wall by needle, trochar, or catheter.

PARACERVICAL UTERINE DENERVATION

Paracervical uterine denervation is an operation in which the uterosacral ligaments are severed from the uterus at the cervicouterine junction for relief of severe dysmenorrhea.

SYNONYM: *Doyle's Operation.*

SALPINGOLYSIS

Salpingolysis is an operation to free the fallopian tube from surrounding and restricting adhesions.

SHIRODKAR'S OPERATION

Shirodkar's operation is a purse-string suturing of an incompetent cervical os.

TUBAL LIGATION, BILATERAL

Bilateral tubal ligation is a method of sterilization in which both fallopian tubes are occluded by applying constricting ligatures.

Irving Operation

The Irving operation is a method of sterilization in which the fallopian tube is ligated and divided. The proximal end is buried in the uterine musculature; the distal end is buried in the leaves of the broad ligament.

Madlener Operation

The Madlener operation is a method of sterilization in which the middle portion of the fallopian tube is crushed and ligated with nonabsorbable suture material.

Pomeroy Operation

The Pomeroy operation is a method of sterilization in which the fallopian tube is ligated with absorbable material at the middle portion, followed by resection of the intervening tubal loop.

URETERONEOCYSTOSTOMY

Ureteroneocystostomy is the reimplantation of the ureter into the bladder.

Roentgenology

AMNIOGRAPHY

Amniography is the injection of radiopaque media into the amniotic fluid to outline the fetus, the placenta, and the uterus in a roentgenogram.

BERMAN CLASSIFICATION OF PELVES

The Berman classification of pelves is a functional working classification based on pelvic size and shape related to the outcome of labor. The pelvis is evaluated in both its anteroposterior and transverse aspects. Each pelvic level is studied individually. The size is determined from the roentgen measurements and the shape from the pelvic architecture.

Pelvic Variations
   Ample or adequate pelves
   Contracted pelves
      Inlet contraction
      Midpelvic contraction
      Outlet contraction
      Upper pelvic contraction
      Lower pelvic contraction
      Complete pelvic contraction

Pelvic Deformities
   Congenital abnormality
   Musculoskeletal disease
   Pelvic trauma

CEPHALOPELVIMETRY

Cephalopelvimetry is the roentgenographic measurement of the dimensions of maternal pelvis and fetal head.

CHAIN CYSTOGRAM

A chain cystogram is a roentgenogram of the bladder to identify the course of the urethra and bladder neck using a beaded chain.

FETOGRAPHY

Fetography is roentgenography of the fetus in utero.

HALO SIGN

The halo sign is a roentgen finding seen both in the living and dead fetus. If the fetus is alive, it is always severely affected by hydrops fetalis. The halo sign is caused by edema that elevates the subcutaneous fat layer from the underlying bones of the fetal skull.

HYSTEROGRAPHY
Hysterography is a roentgenographic visualization of the uterus after instillation of a radiopaque medium into the uterine cavity.

HYSTEROSALPINGOGRAPHY
Hysterosalpingography is roentgenography of the uterus and fallopian tubes after injection of radiopaque material.

  SYNONYMS: *Uterosalpingography, Uterotubography, Hysterotubography, Metrotubography, Metrosalpingography.*

MAMMOGRAPHY
Mammography is roentgenography of the breasts, usually to detect cancer or fibrocystic disease.

PLACENTOGRAPHY
Placentography is roentgenography of the placenta after the injection of a radiopaque substance.

PLACENTOGRAPHY, INDIRECT
Indirect placentography is roentgenographic determination of the presence of placenta previa by estimating the distance between the presenting part of the fetus and the bladder, which has been filled with a radiopaque substance.

PNEUMOCYSTOGRAPHY
Pneumocystography is roentgenography of the bladder following injection of air.

PSEUDOHYDROCEPHALY
Pseudohydrocephaly is the distortion of a roentgenogram of a fetal skull that occurs when the fetal skull is exceedingly close to the x-ray tube and far from the film. It gives a false appearance of hydrocephalus.

PYELOGRAPHY
Pyelography is roentgenography of the ureter and pelvis of the kidney.
  SYNONYMS: *Pelviureterography, Ureteropyelography.*

RAD
A rad is a measure of the dose of radioisotopes. One rad corresponds to the absorption of 100 ergs of energy per gm and is roughly equivalent to a roentgen.

RADIOGRAPHY
Radiography is the making of a record or photograph by means of radioactivity.

RADIOISOTOPE
A radioisotope is a radioactive isotope produced artificially by a nuclear reactor. Such radioactive substances may be used as tracers.

RAYS, ALPHA

Alpha rays are streams of high-speed helium nuclei that have been ejected from radioactive substances.

RAYS, BETA

Beta rays are streams of electrons ejected from radioactive substances with velocities that may be as high as 0.98 of the velocity of light.

RAYS, GAMMA

Gamma rays are electromagnetic radiations consisting of high-energy photons and resulting from a nuclear reaction.

RAYS, ROENTGEN

Roentgen rays are electromagnetic vibrations of short wavelengths (from 5 Å down) or corresponding quanta (wave mechanics) that are produced when electrons moving at high velocity impinge on various substances, especially the heavy metals. Roentgen rays are able to penetrate most substances to some extent, some much more readily than others, and to affect a photographic plate. These qualities make it possible to use them in taking roentgenograms of various parts of the body thus revealing the presence and position of fractures, foreign bodies, or radiopaque substances that have been purposely introduced. They can also cause certain substances to fluoresce; this makes fluoroscopy possible by which the size, shape, and movement of various organs such as the heart, stomach, and intestines can be observed. By reason of the high energy of their quanta, they strongly ionize tissue through which they pass by means of the photoelectrons, both primary and secondary, which they liberate. Because of this physiologic effect, they are used in the treatment of various pathologic conditions.

SYNONYM: *X rays.*

ROBERT'S SIGN

Robert's sign is the presence of gas in the fetal circulation, which is demonstrated on a roentgenogram of the fetus in utero. It is rather pathognomonic of fetal death and also suggestive of spinal and skull deformities.

ROENTGEN

A roentgen is the international unit of x- or gamma-radiation. It is the quantity of x- or gamma-radiation such that the associated corpuscular emission per 0.001293 gm of air produces in air ions carrying 1 electrostatic unit of electrical charge of either sign.

ROENTGENOGRAPHY

Roentgenography is photography by means of roentgen rays.

SALPINGOGRAPHY

Salpingography is the roentgenographic demonstration of the fallopian tubes after injection of a solution of a radiopaque compound.

SPALDING-HORNER SIGN

The Spalding-Horner sign is an overlapping of the bones of the fetal skull together with decided curvature or angulation of the spine and the general crowding of the fetal skeleton which is demonstrated on a roentgenogram of the fetus in utero. The findings are almost pathognomonic of fetal death. These signs are best elicited with the patient in the erect position.

STEREOSCOPIC PELVIMETRY

Stereoscopic pelvimetry is roentgenographic measurement of the pelvic diameters by means of two films taken under the same conditions but with the x-ray tube shifted a standard predetermined distance, and subsequent correction of the distortion.

THERMOGRAPHY

Thermography is a method of measuring skin temperature by using films of cholesteric liquid crystals that are placed on the skin in a sensor film. These crystals reflect white light in a variety of iridescent colors related to ambient temperature. This method may be used to detect subcutaneous tumors and the location of the placenta.

THOMS CLASSIFICATION

The Thoms classification is based on the pelvic index, using the relationship of the anteroposterior and transverse inlet diameters without considering the lower pelvic architecture. The four basic types are brachypellic, mesatipellic, dolichopellic, and platypellic.

XERORADIOGRAPHY

Xeroradiography is a dry, totally photoelectric process for recording x-ray images, using metal plates coated with a semiconductor such as selenium.

X-RAY PELVIMETRY

X-ray pelvimetry is a method of estimating the size and shape of the pelvis by roentgenographic examination. It also gives a relative estimation of the size of the fetus and its presenting part.

SECTION 5: SELECTED GYNECOLOGIC TOPICS

Hormones and Steroids

HORMONE

A hormone is a specific chemical substance synthesized and secreted by endocrine glands. Hormones are released into the blood or body fluids to effect a response in target organs.

STEROID

A steroid is a hydrocarbon with a chemical structure consisting of a hydrogenated cyclopentanophenanthrene nucleus that may have an aliphatic or a cyclic side chain. All steroids possess oxygen groups on the nucleus, and the side chains may have an oxygen group(s). Steroids comprise a wide range of naturally occurring compounds including cholesterol, adrenocortical steroids, progesterone, androgens, estrogens, bile acids, cardiac aglycones, saponins, toad poisons, and the insect hormone ecdysone. The steroid molecule has three six-membered rings, A, B, and C, and one five-membered ring, D. The steroid hormones may be grouped as follows:

C_{21} compounds, with a methyl group at C-10 and C-13 and a two carbon side chain at C-17. The adrenocortical hormones and progesterone are examples.

C_{19} compounds, with methyl groups at C-10 and C-13. These include androgens, such as testosterone, and its metabolites.

C_{18} compounds, with an aromatic A ring and no methyl group at C-10: the estrogens.

ADRENAL CORTICOSTEROIDS

The adrenal corticosteroids are C_{21} steroid hormones synthesized by the adrenal gland; they affect the maintenance of homeostasis. They may be grouped as primarily mineralo- or glucocorticosteroids, depending on whether their effect is mainly on mineral (sodium retention and potassium excretion) or on carbohydrate metabolism. However, the difference is quantitative, not qualitative. Some general structure-function correlation can be made. The 11-oxycorticosteroids, which have an oxygen atom at C-11, particularly cortisol, cortisone, and corticosterone, have a more marked effect on carbohydrate metabolism than do the 11-deoxycorticosteroids, which have no oxygen atom at C-11. The 11-deoxycorticosteroids, especially deoxycorticosterone, have a greater effect on salt and water. Aldosterone is the exception, having a C-11 oxygen atom and being the steroid with the greatest mineralocorticoid effect. Corticosteroids enhance gluconeogenesis. They are catabolic—

that is, they inhibit protein synthesis. They mobilize fat. In addition, corticoids have an anti-inflammatory activity.

SYNONYM: *Adrenocorticoids.*

ADRENOCORTICOTROPIC HORMONE

Adrenocorticotropic hormone is a polypeptide hormone elaborated by the basophil cells of the human anterior pituitary. It controls the growth of the adrenal gland and stimulates it to secrete corticosteroids and some of the androgens and estrogens. Secretion of this hormone is controlled by a releasing factor from the hypothalamus. Cortisol depresses ACTH secretion so that an inverse relationship exists between the concentrations of ACTH and cortisol. A polypeptide with activity similar to natural ACTH and having 23 amino acids has been synthesized.

SYNONYMS: *Adrenocorticotrophin, Corticotrophin, Corticotropin, Adrenocorticotrophic Hormone.*

ABBREVIATION: ACTH.

ALDOSTERONE

Aldosterone is the major mineralocorticoid elaborated by the adrenal cortex; it is formed in the zona glomerulosa. Aldosterone is unique among the corticosteroids in that it has an aldehyde group on C-18; in solution it exists as a hemiacetal. It principally affects the kidney tubules and controls the excretion and reabsorption of sodium and potassium. It causes sodium retention and potassium excretion. The release of aldosterone is not directly influenced by ACTH, but it is controlled by the renin-angiotensin system.

SYNONYM: *Electrocortin.*

CHEMICAL NAME: 4-Pregnen-11β,21-diol-3,18,20-trione.

ANDROGEN

Androgens are compounds that cause the development and maintenance of function of male secondary sex structures. In both sexes, androgen increases the growth rate and contributes to the development of muscle mass, sexual hair, and seborrhea. Androgens are also potent anabolic agents. Naturally occurring androgens are C_{19} steroids and are produced by adrenal gland, testis, and ovary. They include testosterone, dihydrotestosterone, 5α-androstan-3α, 17β-diol, androstenedione, dehydroepiandrosterone, and androsterone.

SYNONYM: *Male Hormone.*

ANDROSTENEDIONE

Androstenedione is a C_{19} steroid produced by ovary, testis, and adrenal cortex. It is an androgen about one-fifth as potent as testosterone; it is uncertain whether this androgenic activity is due to a partial conversion to testosterone itself. Androstenedione and testosterone are interconvertible.

CHEMICAL NAME: 4-Androstene-3,17-dione.

ANDROSTERONE

Androsterone is an androgenic C_{19} steroid having a ketone group at C-17; it is about one-tenth as potent as testosterone. Androsterone is a metabolite of testosterone and of some adrenocorticoids. It is one of the major components of the so-called neutral 17-ketosteroids.

CHEMICAL NAME: 5α-Androstan-3α-ol-17-one.

CATECHOLAMINES

Catecholamines are dihydroxylated phenolic compounds. They are formed by hydroxylation and decarboxylation of the essential amino acid, phenylalanine. They include epinephrine, norepinephine, and dopamine.

CHOLESTEROL

Cholesterol is a C_{27} steroid having a branched side chain of eight carbon atoms at C-17. It can be completely synthesized in the body from acetate. It is an important intermediary in the biogenesis of steroid hormones and affects arteriosclerosis associated with thyroid deficiency and diabetes.

CHORIONIC GONADOTROPIN, HUMAN

Human chorionic gonadotropin is a glycoprotein produced by the Langhans cells of the chorionic villi of the placenta. It functions as a luteotropin in man, maintaining the corpus luteum and causing it to secrete progesterone and estrogen. It stimulates the male secondary sex structures by causing secretion of testicular steroids. Its ability to cause ovulation in several laboratory animals has been the basis of pregnancy tests.

SYNONYMS: *Human Chorionic Gonadotrophin, Chorionic Gonado-trophin.*

ABBREVIATION: HCG.

CORTICOID

Corticoid is a term applied to C_{21} steroid hormones of the adrenal cortex that affect carbohydrate metabolism and sodium balance. It is also applied to other natural or synthetic compounds having similar activity. Among the synthetic compounds having very high glucocorticoid activity are 1-dehydrocortisol (prednisolone), 1-dehydrocortisone (prednisone), and 9α-fluoro-16α-methyl prednisolone (dexamethasone).

CORTICOSTERONE

Corticosterone is a C_{21} steroid hormone produced by the fasciculata and reticularis zones of the adrenal cortex. It possesses some mineralo-corticoid activity, being third after aldosterone and deoxycorticosterone. It enhances gluconeogenesis and is catabolic.

SYNONYMS: *Compound B* (Kendall), *Compound H* (Reichstein).

CHEMICAL NAME: 4-Pregnen-11β,21-diol-3,20-dione.

CORTISOL

Cortisol is a C_{21} steroid hormone produced by the fasciculata and reticularis zones of the adrenal cortex. It is the major glucocorticoid in man. Its primary metabolic effect is to enhance gluconeogenesis. It enhances water diuresis. Cushing's Syndrome is the clinical picture produced by cortisol excess.

SYNONYMS: *Hydrocortisone, Compound F* (Kendall).

CHEMICAL NAME: 4-Pregnen-11β,17α,21-triol-3,20-dione.

CORTISONE

Cortisone is a C_{21} steroid hormone produced by the fasciculata and reticularis zones of the adrenal cortex. After cortisol, it is the most important glucocorticoid in man. Cortisone production predominates over cortisol in the first few days of life. Cortisone was the first naturally occurring glucocorticoid synthesized and produced commercially.

SYNONYMS: *Compound E* (Kendall), *Compound Fa* (Reichstein), *17-Hydroxy-11-dehydrocorticosterone.*

CHEMICAL NAME: 4-Pregnen-17α,21-diol,3,11,20-trione.

DEHYDROEPIANDROSTERONE

Dehydroepiandrosterone (DHEA) is a C_{19} steroid having a ketone group at C-17. It is formed in the fasciculata and reticularis zones of the adrenal cortex and in the ovary and testis. It is a weak androgen. DHEA is a precursor in the biosynthesis of other androgens and of estrogens. In pregnancy, dehydroepiandrosterone and its sulfate are important precursors for estrogen formation by the placenta.

SYNONYM: *Androstenolone.*

ABBREVIATION: DHEA.

CHEMICAL NAME: 5-Androsten-3β-ol-17-one.

DEOXYCORTICOSTERONE

Deoxycorticosterone is a C_{21} steroid hormone lacking an oxygen at C-11. It is biosynthesized in the fasciculata and reticularis zones of the adrenal cortex. It is the second most potent mineralocorticoid and is an intermediate in the synthesis of corticosterone and aldosterone. It has very little effect on carbohydrate metabolism. The hypertensive form of the adrenogenital syndrome due to 11β-hydroxylase deficiency may be associated with high levels of this corticoid.

SYNONYMS: *Desoxycorticosterone, Desoxycortone, Cortexone.*

ABBREVIATION: DOC.

CHEMICAL NAME: 4-Pregnen-21-ol-3,20-dione.

DIHYDROTESTOSTERONE

Dihydrotestosterone is a C_{19} androgenic steroid that is as potent (or more) than testosterone. It is formed from testosterone in the accessory organs of reproduction. It is present in the plasma of men and women, but whether it is a primary secretory product or is formed by extra gonadal interconversion is not known.

CHEMICAL NAME: 5α-Androstan-17β-ol-3-one.

EPINEPHRINE

Epinephrine is a catecholamine (a dihydroxylated phenolic compound) and is the principal hormone of the adrenal medulla. Many of its actions resemble those obtained by stimulation of the sympathetic nerves. It stimulates the heart and causes constriction or dilation of the blood vessels, bronchiolar relaxation, and relaxation of intestinal smooth muscle.

SYNONYMS: *Chromaffin Hormone, Sympathetic Hormone, Adrenaline.*

CHEMICAL NAME: L-1-(3,4-Dihydroxyphenyl)-2-methylaminoethanol.

ESTRADIOL-17β

Estradiol-17β is a C_{18} steroid hormone formed by the ovary, adrenal cortex, testis, and placenta. It is the principal estrogen in man.

SYNONYM: *Follicular Hormone.*

CHEMICAL NAME: 1,3,5(10)-Estratrien-3,17β-diol.

ESTRIOL

Estriol is a C_{18} steroid estrogen and is a metabolite of estradiol, estrone, and dehydroepiandrosterone. It is formed from estradiol and estrone in the liver, uterus, and placenta. In man, it is much less potent than estradiol and estrone.

CHEMICAL NAME: 1,3,5(10)-Estratrien-3,16α,17β-triol.

ESTROGENS

Estrogens are compounds that stimulate growth of and maintain the function of the female secondary sexual structures. In the human, naturally occurring estrogens are C_{18} steroids with a phenolic A ring. They are secreted by ovarian follicles, corpus luteum, adrenal cortex, testis, and placenta. The principal estrogens in man are: estradiol-17β, the most active; estrone, an oxidized form of estradiol; and estriol, the form that is further hydroxylated and probably the main metabolite of the other estrogens. Estrogens, with progesterone, stimulate the growth of the endometrium and play a major role in maintaining pregnancy and growth of mammary tissue. Several nonsteroidal synthetic compounds such as diethylstilbestrol, benzestrol, dienestrol, and hexestrol are potent estrogens.

SYNONYM: *Female Hormone.*

ESTRONE

Estrone is a C_{18} steroid hormone with a ketone group at C-17. It is the second most active estrogen in man. Estrone and estradiol are interconvertible.

CHEMICAL NAME: 1,3,5(10)-Estratrien-3-ol-17-one.

FOLLICLE-STIMULATING HORMONE

Follicle-stimulating hormone (FSH) is a glycoprotein synthesized by the basophil cells of the anterior pituitary. It is released in response to a hypothalamic releasing factor. It is responsible for the growth and development of the follicle in the ovary. In the male, FSH and testosterone promote spermatogenesis in the testis. With LH, FSH greatly enhances estrogen secretion by the ovary.

SYNONYMS: *Gametokinetic Hormone, Follicle-Ripening Hormone, Prolan A, Thylakentrin.*

ABBREVIATIONS: FSH, FRH.

GASTROINTESTINAL HORMONES

Gastrointestinal hormones are protein substances extractable from the mucosa of some part of the gastrointestinal tract that, after entering the bloodstream, influence the activity of an organ of digestion. Historically, the word *hormone* was coined in 1904 in connection with the discovery of secretin. Secretin, gastrin, and pancreozymin-cholecystokinin are well-recognized. Secretin stimulates the flow of water and bicarbonate from the pancreas, the flow of bile from the liver, and the release of insulin. There are some similarities in the structure of glucagon and secretin. Gastrin stimulates or inhibits gastric secretion; it also stimulates secretion of pancreatic enzymes. Pancreozymin-cholecystokinin (PZ-CCK) causes secretion of amylase, trypsinogen, and lipase from the pancreas and causes contraction of the gallbladder.

GLUCAGON

Glucagon is a polypeptide hormone of known structure secreted by the alpha cells of the islets of Langerhans in the pancreas. It is released as a response to hypoglycemia to maintain normal blood sugar levels. Glucagon stimulates hepatic glycogenolysis and participates in gluconeogenesis. Glucagon is catabolic and lipolytic.

GONADOTROPINS

Gonadotropins are water-soluble proteins secreted by the anterior lobe of the pituitary. The pituitary secretes follicle-stimulating hormone, luteinizing hormone, and prolactin. The first two are glycoproteins. The placenta of certain species, including man, secretes chorionic gonadotropin; it is also a glycoprotein and in its biologic actions resembles LH. The gonadotropin of pregnant mares, which is present in serum but not in urine, resembles FSH in its biologic actions. The three glycoproteins— LH, FSH, and HCG—along with a fourth glycoprotein, TSH, all have two carbohydrate-containing subunits called α and β subunits, which are chemically dissimilar. In each hormone it is only the β subunit that determines the physiologic specificity of the entire molecule, although both subunits, bound together, are necessary for full hormonal activity. The α subunits may be interchanged from one hormone to another without loss of the hormone's physiologic specificity.

SYNONYMS: *Gonadotrophic Hormones, Gonadotrophins.*

HUMAN PLACENTAL LACTOGEN

Human placental lactogen is a protein produced by the syncytiotrophoblast of the placenta. Human placental lactogen is quite similar in amino acid composition and sequence to growth hormone. It has considerable lactogenic activity and relatively weak somatotropic activity. It has luteotropic activity in the rat, but whether this effect occurs in man is not known.

ABBREVIATION: HPL.

17-HYDROXYCORTICOIDS

The measurement of 17-hydroxycorticoids in plasma or urine affords an index of adrenal cortical activity. Chemical reactions characteristic of certain functional groups present in corticosteroids have been developed. Corticosteroids with a 17-hydroxyl group and with 20-ketone, 21-hydroxyl (α-ketol) groups react with phenylhydrazine in alcoholic sulfuric acid to yield yellow products, the so-called *Porter-Silber chromogens.* This reaction has been widely used to measure certain urinary and plasma corticosteroids, including cortisol, cortisone, 11-deoxycortisol, and their metabolites. In plasma, cortisol and small amounts of unconjugated dehydrocortisol represent most of the 17-hydroxycorticosteroids measured.

17-HYDROXYPROGESTERONE

17-Hydroxyprogesterone is a C_{21} steroid that is primarily an intermediate in the biosynthesis of corticosteroids, androgens, and estrogens. In congenital adrenal hyperplasia caused by 21-hydroxylase deficiency, the normal pathway to cortisol and aldosterone is shifted to an increased production of androgen and 17-OH-progesterone. Pregnanetriol, the reduced metabolite of 17α-hydroxyprogesterone, is increased in the urine as are the 17-ketosteroids.

CHEMICAL NAME: 4-Pregnen-17α-ol-3,20-dione.

HYPOTHALAMIC RELEASING FACTORS

Hypothalamic releasing factors are low molecular weight polypeptides released from the median eminence of the hypothalamus. They exert direct control of anterior pituitary secretion. The releasing factors are corticotropin-releasing factor (CRF), thyrotropin-releasing factor (TRF), growth hormone-releasing factor (GRF, SRF), follicle-stimulating hormone-releasing factor (FSHRF), and luteinizing hormone-releasing factor (LRF). A factor that inhibits luteotropic hormone secretion, prolactin-inhibiting factor (PIF), has also been extracted.

INSULIN

Insulin is a protein hormone of known structure synthesized and released by the beta cells of the islets of Langerhans of the pancreas. It is essential for the regulation of carbohydrate metabolism and also affects fat and protein metabolism. Insulin increases glycogenesis, oxidation of sugar, lipogenesis, and decreases protein depletion, lipolysis, and ketogenesis. Diabetes mellitus is the result of a decreased physiologic effect of insulin.

17-KETOSTEROIDS

This term generally is used to refer to neutral C_{19} steroids with a ketone group at C-17. The principal 17-ketosteroids are androsterone, etiocholanolone, dehydroepiandrosterone, and the 11-oxygenated androsterones and etiocholanolones. These steroids are the metabolic end products of a variety of hormones of the ovary, testis, and adrenal. Phenolic 17-ketosteroids, such as estrone, can be separated from neutral 17-ketosteroids by an alkali partition and are not included in this group.

LUTEINIZING HORMONE

Luteinizing hormone (LH) is a glycoprotein secreted by the basophil cells of the anterior pituitary. Its secretion is controlled by a hypothalamic releasing factor. In the male, it stimulates synthesis and the secretion of testosterone by the interstitial tissue of the testis. In the female, LH stimulates rupture of the follicle with resultant ovulation and the formation of the corpus luteum and progesterone secretion. Together with FSH, it stimulates estrogen formation. The ovulatory complex of gonadotropin appears to be comprised of both LH and FSH.

SYNONYMS: *Interstitial Cell-Stimulating Hormone, Prolan B, Metakentrin.*

ABBREVIATIONS: LH, ICSH.

MELANOCYTE-STIMULATING HORMONE

Melanocyte-stimulating hormone (MSH) is a polypeptide secreted by the pars intermedia of the pituitary in lower vertebrates and by certain basophils of the human pituitary in which a discrete intermediate lobe is not present. Part of its amino acid sequence is common to both ACTH and MSH. MSH causes expansion of the chromatophores in the skin and, in cold-blooded animals, it causes adaptation of the skin color to the environment. The levels of MSH increase in pregnancy and in Addison's disease.

ABBREVIATION: MSH.

MINERALOCORTICOID

Mineralocorticoid is a term applied to the C_{21} steroids of the adrenal cortex that cause sodium retention and potassium excretion. Aldosterone is the principal mineralocorticoid, followed by deoxycorticosterone and corticosterone. Several synthetic compounds such as 9α-fluorohydrocortisone and deoxycorticosterone acetate (DOCA) have high sodium-retaining activity.

NOREPINEPHRINE

Norepinephrine is a catecholamine formed by hydroxylation and decarboxylation of the essential amino acid, phenylalanine. It is released into the circulation primarily from adrenergic nerve endings, and small amounts are released from the adrenal medulla. Its effects mimic the action of adrenergic nervous discharge. In contrast to epinephrine, norepinephrine has relatively little effect on carbohydrate metabolism and oxygen consumption and will not cause relaxation of the uterus. However, both the catecholamines have a profound lipid-mobilizing activity.

SYNONYM: *Noradrenaline.*

CHEMICAL NAME: L-1-(3,4-Dihydroxyphenyl)-2-aminoethanol.

OXYTOCIN

Oxytocin is an octapeptide of known structure. It and vasopressin are synthesized in the supraoptic and paraventricular nuclei of the hypothalamus. These hormones, bound to a protein, travel down the axons to the neurohypophysis, or posterior lobe of the pituitary, where they are stored until released. Oxytocin stimulates contraction of smooth muscle of the uterus, milk ejection from the breast, and has been postulated to facilitate sperm transport in the nongravid uterus. A neurogenic reflex is responsible for the release of oxytocin by suckling and probably by labor. Oxytocin has some weak activity similar to that of vasopressin— that is, it can cause antidiuresis and vasoconstriction.

PARATHYROID HORMONE

Parathyroid hormone (PTH) is a polypeptide hormone, released from the parathyroid gland, that directly affects calcium and phosphate. It is released in response to lowered circulatory calcium levels. It mobilizes bone calcium by stimulating the small intestinal absorption of calcium, and by elevating the renal threshold of calcium. Parathyroid hormone causes phosphaturia by a change in tubular rather than glomerular function in the kidney. Calcium homeostasis involves a complex interrelationship between PTH, thyrocalcitonin and vitamin D.

SYNONYM: *Parathormone.*

ABBREVIATION: PTH.

PREGNANEDIOL

Pregnanediol, a C_{21} steroid, is the reduction product of the metabolism of progesterone and also of deoxycorticosterone. Although not a unique metabolite of progesterone, it is a good measure of progesterone production. It has proven useful in studying abnormalities of menstruation and fertility, and in studying abortion early in pregnancy and placental function in late pregnancy.

CHEMICAL NAME: 5β-Pregnan-3α,20α-diol.

PREGNANETRIOL

Pregnanetriol, a C_{21} steroid, is the reduction product of the metabolism of 17α-hydroxyprogesterone and 17α-hydroxypregnenolone. It may be markedly elevated in some forms of congenital adrenal hyperplasia of the 21-hydroxylase deficiency type.

CHEMICAL NAME: 5β-Pregnan-3α,17α,20α-triol.

PROGESTERONE

Progesterone is a C_{21} steroid hormone formed in the follicle, corpus luteum, adrenal cortex, and placenta. It is an important intermediate in the biosynthesis of steroid hormones (corticoids, androgens, and estrogens). Progesterone, with estrogen, is necessary for the normal secretory function of the endometrium, for decidua formation, and for gestation. Together with estrogen and other hormones, it causes growth of the breast and maintains lactation. It causes some increase in mitotic activity. Progesterone is weakly catabolic and causes increased sodium excretion.

SYNONYM: *Corpus Luteum Hormone.*
CHEMICAL NAME: 4-Pregnen-3,20-dione.

PROGESTINS

Progestins are compounds that are necessary for gestation. Naturally occurring progestins include progesterone, 4-pregnen-20α-ol-3-one, and 4-pregnen-20β-ol-3-one. There are several synthetic compounds with marked progestational activity, such as medroxyprogesterone acetate (Provera), norethynodrel (Enovid), and norethindrone (Norlutin).

SYNONYM: *Gestagens.*

PROLACTIN

Prolactin is a protein hormone formed in the eosinophil cells of the anterior pituitary. It has luteotropic activity in several species (rat, mouse, ferret) but apparently not in the human. With other hormones, it causes development of the mammary glands, milk formation, and secretion. Its role in the human male is not well defined.

SYNONYMS: *Luteotrophic Hormone, Luteotrophin, Mammotrophin, Lactogenic Hormone, Galactopoietic Hormone, Luteotropic Hormone, Luteotropin, Mammotropin.*
ABBREVIATIONS: PL, LTH.

PROSTAGLANDINS

Prostaglandins are cyclic, oxygenated, C_{20} fatty acids based on the prostanoic acid skeleton; two hydrocarbon chains are attached to two neighboring carbon atoms of a cyclopentane ring. Whether they are true hormones is debatable. They are found in all tissues so far examined and are readily released. They exhibit a broad spectrum of pharmacologic activity in such fields as reproduction, central nervous system, circulation, and renal physiology. They may either stimulate or inhibit smooth-muscle activity and so may play a role in normal uterine physiology. In some species, prostaglandins are luteolytic.

RELAXIN

Relaxin is a polypeptide secreted by the ovary. It relaxes the ligaments of the pubic symphysis and softens the cervix, facilitating delivery of the fetus. It is of major importance in some species, such as the guinea pig and mouse, but its role in man is not clear.

SOMATOTROPIN

Somatotropin (STH) is a protein hormone of known structure formed by the eosinophil cells of the anterior pituitary. Growth hormone causes body growth by promoting the deposition of protein, carbohydrate, and water, and the loss of fat. It stimulates protein synthesis and decreases carbohydrate oxidation. STH promotes lipolysis in fat deposits and inhibits sugar breakdown in muscle. It has a diabetogenic effect and is antagonistic to insulin. A primary site of action of STH is the epiphysial cartilage.

SYNONYMS: *Somatotrophic Hormone, Growth Hormone, Chondrotrophic Hormone, Somatotropic Hormone, Chondrotropic Hormone, Somatotrophin.*

ABBREVIATIONS: STH, GH.

TESTOSTERONE
Testosterone is a C_{19} steroid hormone synthesized in the Leydig cells of the testis, adrenal cortex, and ovary. It develops and maintains the function of male secondary sex structures. It is anabolic.

CHEMICAL NAME: 4-Androsten-17β-ol-3-one.

TETRAHYDROCORTISOL
Tetrahydrocortisol is a major metabolite of cortisol; it is formed by reduction of the A ring of the steroid nucleus. Further reduction of the C-20 ketone group results in cortol. These are urinary end products of cortisol metabolism. Cortisone yields comparable end products. (Some of the C_{21} compounds lose their 2-carbon side chain to give C_{19} 17-ketosteroids).

CHEMICAL NAME: Pregnan-3α,11β,17α,21-tetraol-20-one.

THYROCALCITONIN
Thyrocalcitonin is a polypeptide hormone secreted by the thyroid (and perhaps by the parathyroid) gland in response to hypercalcemia. It lowers plasma calcium and phosphate. Its primary action is to inhibit calcium resorption from bone. It may cause deposition of calcium in bone.

ABBREVIATION: TCT.

THYROID-STIMULATING HORMONE
Thyroid-stimulating hormone (TSH) is a glycoprotein formed and released from a specific basophil cell of the anterior lobe of the pituitary. It maintains thyroid function. This hormone is secreted through stimulation of the pituitary by a hypothalamic thyrotropin-releasing factor (TRF). Another thyroid stimulator of nonpituitary source is the so-called *long-acting thyroid stimulator (LATS)*. It appears to be an antibody that can mimic TSH action and is often present in hyperthyroidism.

ABBREVIATION: TSH.

THYROXINE
Thyroxine, an iodinated amino acid, is a hormone of the thyroid gland. With triiodothyronine, it regulates energy metabolism by controlling the rate of oxygen utilization of most cells in the body. The thyroid

hormones, with growth hormone, are essential for normal growth in the early stages of life of man and many animals, and for the normal maturation of bone. They have a marked effect on the metamorphosis of amphibian larvae. The thyroid hormones exist in different forms in the gland and in the blood. In the gland they are integral units of the peptide chain of thyroglobulin, whereas in the blood they are attached to certain serum proteins. Thyroxine is bound much more strongly than triiodothyronine to plasma proteins (alpha globulin, albumin, and prealbumin).

ABBREVIATION: T_4.

CHEMICAL NAME: 3,5,3'5'-Tetraiodothyronine.

TRIIODOTHYRONINE

Triiodothyronine, an iodinated amino acid, is a hormone of the thyroid gland; it differs from thyroxine by lacking the 5'-iodine molecule. In the blood, it is weakly bound to alpha globulin and albumin and not bound to thyroxine-binding prealbumin. It is about four times more potent than thyroxine. Because of this and its faster turnover, triiodothyronine accounts for about half the biologically effective secreted hormones of the thyroid.

ABBREVIATION: T_3.

CHEMICAL NAME: 3,5,3'-Triiodothyronine.

VASOPRESSIN

Vasopressin is an octapeptide. It is formed in the supraoptic and paraventricular nuclei of the hypothalamus. Bound to a carrier protein, it travels down the axons to the posterior lobe of the pituitary, where it is stored until released. Vasopressin inhibits diuresis by increasing the capacity of the distal tubules of the kidney to reabsorb water. The release of vasopressin by the posterior pituitary is controlled by osmoreceptors in the hypothalamus. These receptors react to changes in the total osmotic concentration of electrolytes in the extracellular fluid. Vasopressin is also released by stress. It causes vasoconstriction of peripheral vessels and has some weak activity, similar to that of oxytocin—that is, it can cause milk ejection and uterine contraction.

SYNONYM: *Antidiuretic Hormone*.

ABBREVIATION: ADH.

Enzymes

ENZYME
An enzyme is a complex protein of biologic origin that catalyzes biochemical reactions. The catalytic activity of many enzymes depends on the presence of a cofactor, which may be a coenzyme, a prosthetic group, or a metal ion that may or may not be dissociable from the protein moiety.

COENZYME
A coenzyme is a nonprotein cofactor that, in association with certain enzymes, acts as a carrier of a particular group and is therefore part of the catalytic mechanism. The principal coenzyme carriers of hydrogen in tissues are NAD^+ and $NADP^+$; some enzymes require either lipate, glutathione, or the cytochromes. Coenzyme A acts as an acyl carrier and adenosine diphosphate (ADP) as a carrier of phosphate. Other cofactors such as the prosthetic group, which are nonprotein molecules, are distinguished from coenzymes in that they are firmly bound parts of an enzyme. Flavin-adenine dinucleotide (FAD), pyridoxal phosphate, thiamine pyrophosphate, and biotin are examples of prosthetic cofactors.

ADENOSINE TRIPHOSPHATASE
Adenosine triphosphatase, an enzyme found in most tissues, is responsible for the hydrolysis of the terminal high-energy phosphate bond of adenosine triphosphate, a sequence essential to muscle contraction, transport across membranes, and production of intermediates for metabolic action. The enzyme requires Mg^{++} for activity.
E.C. 3.6.1.3. ATP phosphohydrolase.

ALKALINE PHOSPHATASE
Alkaline phosphatase catalyzes the hydrolysis of several phosphate esters to yield orthophosphate and an alcohol. Having an alkaline pH optimum, this enzyme apparently depends on ovarian steroids for maximum activity in some hormone-responsive tissues. Alkaline phosphatase is believed to be involved in the secretory changes of postovulatory uterine metabolism.
E.C. 3.1.3.1. Orthophosphoric monoester phosphohydrolase.

AROMATIC AMINO ACID DECARBOXYLASE
Aromatic amino acid decarboxylase is a nonspecific enzyme that catalyzes the decarboxylation of a variety of aromatic amino acids to produce

237

biologically active amines—for example, histidine to histamine, 5-hydroxy-tryptophan to serotonin, and DOPA to dopamine. The activity of this enzyme is markedly augmented in uterine tissues by estradiol.

E.C. 4.1.1.28. Hydroxytryptophan decarboxylase.

CARBONIC ANHYDRASE

Carbonic anhydrase is an enzyme requiring Zn^{++} for activity. It catalyzes both the hydration of CO_2 and the dehydration of $H_2CO_{3,}$ with equilibrium favoring H_2CO_3 formation. This enzyme system facilitates the conversion of CO_2 to bicarbonate in the erythrocyte for transport of CO_2 from the periphery to the lung. In the endometrium, the activity of this enzyme is hormonally regulated and is important in nidation. `

E.C 4.2.1.1. Carbonate hydrolyase.

FRUCTOSE–1,6–DIPHOSPHATASE

Fructose-1,6-diphosphatase is an enzyme of glycolysis controlling the reversible hydrolysis of fructose-1,6-diphosphate to fructose-6-phosphate. This is a key enzyme in the synthesis of glycogen and the production of glucose from triose phosphates.

E.C. 3.1.3.11. D-Fructose-1,6-diphosphate 1-phosphohydrolase.

GLUCOKINASE

Glucokinase is a specific phosphorylation enzyme for glucose found in the liver and muscle. It catalyzes the formation of glucose-6-phosphate from glucose, in which one molecule of adenosine triphosphate is used.

E.C. 2.7.1.2. ATP: D-Glucose-6-phosphotransferase.

GLUCOSE–6–PHOSPHATASE

Glucose-6-phosphatase is a microsomal enzyme catalyzing the hydrolysis of glucose-6-phosphate to glucose and inorganic phosphate. This enzyme is absent from muscle and adipose tissue but represents the final sequence of reverse glycolysis found in endometrium, liver, kidney, and intestinal mucosa.

E.C. 3.1.3.9. D-Glucose-6-phosphate phosphohydrolase.

GLUCOSE–6–PHOSPHATE DEHYDROGENASE

Glucose-6-phosphate dehydrogenase is an important rate-limiting enzyme that initiates carbohydrate metabolism through the hexose monophosphate shunt, the metabolic pathway leading to the generation of NADPH, which is necessary for reductive processes in the synthesis of fatty acids. NADPH is also necessary for the multiple hydroxylase reactions in steroid biosynthesis, and it provides reducing equivalents for nucleotide synthesis. Glucose-6-phosphate dehydrogenase, a soluble enzyme, catalyzes the oxidations of glucose-6-phosphate by $NADP^+$ to yield 6-phosphoglucolactone.

E.C. 1.1.1.49. D-Glucose-6-phosphate: $NADP^+$ oxidoreductase.

β–GLUCURONIDASE

β-Glucuronidase is a hydrolytic enzyme with high activity in the liver, spleen, endometrium, breast, adrenal glands, and testes. It catalyzes the hydrolysis of the β-D-glycosidic bond of certain glucuronidic acids and causes the release of active hormones from glucuronide conjugates in the tissues. Serum β-glucuronidase levels are elevated during estrogen administration and the last trimester of pregnancy, but they return to normal by the fifth postpartum day.

E.C. 3.2.1.31. β-D-Glucuronide glucuronhydrolase.

GLYCOGEN PHOSPHORYLASE

Glycogen phosphorylase is the rate-limiting enzyme of glycogen breakdown. It exists in two interconvertible forms: active phosphorylase a, and inactive phosphorylase b. The inactive form depends on the cofactor 5'-AMP for full activity. This enzyme system catalyzes glycogenolysis through hydrolysis of α-1-4 glucosidic bonds, and the activity of the individual forms are a function of the 5'-AMP/ATP ratio present in the tissue. Interconversion of the two forms depends primarily on hormonal regulation. In the human endometrium, where enzyme activity is maximal during the secretory phase of the ovulatory cycle, progesterone appears to be a regulatory hormone.

E.C. 2.4.1.1. α-1,4-Glucan: orthophosphate glucosyltransferase.

GLYCOGEN SYNTHETASE

Glycogen synthetase is the rate-limiting enzyme of glycogen synthesis that exists in two interconvertible forms: an independent and a dependent form. The dependent form is active only in the presence of glucose-6-phosphate. The interconversion of these forms occurs in the presence of ATP, Mg^{++}, and a kinase. Glycogen synthetase catalyzes the formation of α-1,4 bonds, linking glucose from uridine diphosphate-glucose (UDP) to a preexisting glycogen molecule. The enzyme is stimulated by estrogen in human endometrium and can be found in high levels during the early secretory phase of the ovulatory cycle.

E.C. 2.4.1.11. UDP glucose:α-1,4-Glucan α-2-4-glucosyltransferase.

HEXOKINASE

Hexokinase is a nonspecific phosphorylation enzyme found in muscle, brain, uterus, and adipose tissue. It catalyzes the phosphorylation of hexoses to give the corresponding 6-phosphates in the presence of adenosine triphosphate and Mg^{++}. This enzyme is the initial phosphorylation enzyme in glycolysis, and it depends on estradiol for maximal activity in uterine tissue.

E.C. 2.7.1.1. ATP: D-Hexose 6-phosphotransferase.

HISTAMINASE

Histaminase catalyzes the conversion of histamine to its corresponding aldehyde and ammonia. It is found in most tissues and requires the cofactor pyridoxal phosphate for activity. Some evidence indicates that histaminase and diamine oxidase may be two distinct enzymes.

E.C. 1.4.3.6. Diamine: Oxygen oxidoreductase.

SYNONYM: *Diamine oxidase.*

HISTIDINE DECARBOXYLASE

Histidine decarboxylase is found in stomach, kidney, and liver, with smaller concentrations in the ovary and uterus. It is influenced by ovarian hormones, and it catalyzes the decarboxylation of histidine to form histamine.

E.C. 4.1.1.22. L-Histine carboxylase.

HYDROXYLASES

Hydroxylations of the steroid molecule occur at almost all available carbon atoms on the molecule. The steroid hydroxylases belong to a class of enzymes classified as mixed-function oxidases. These enzymes in the presence of NADPH catalyze the introduction of one atom of molecular oxygen into the substrate, while the other is reduced to water. The hemoprotein cytochrome P-450 is involved in the activation of the molecular oxygen. Also, the participation of the flavoprotein adrenodoxin reductase and the nonheme iron protein adrenodoxin permits electron transfer from NADPH to cytochrome P-450.

11β–HYDROXYLASE

11β-Hydroxylase is found principally in adrenocortical mitochondria and is responsible for 11β-hydroxylation in steroid biosynthesis, yielding corticosterone from 11-deoxycorticosterone and cortisol from 11-deoxycortisol. The enzyme is a true hydroxylase, requiring NADPH, adrenodoxin, and cytochrome P-450 for activity.

E.C. 1.99.1.7. Steroid 11β-hydroxylase.

16α–HYDROXYLASE

16α-Hydroxylase is a microsomal enzyme that catalyzes the hydroxylation of estradiol-17β at position 16 to yield estriol, and dehydroepiandrosterone to 16α-hydroxydehydroepiandrosterone. The enzyme is located principally in the liver, and it requires NADPH and activated oxygen for activity.

E.C. 1.99.1.-. Steroid 16α-hydroxylase.

17α–HYDROXYLASE

17α-Hydroxylase is a microsomal enzyme located in the adrenal gland, ovary, and testis; it requires NADPH and activated molecular oxygen for activity. The enzyme catalyzes 17α-hydroxylation of pregnenolone and progesterone to yield 17α-hydroxypregnenolone and 17α-hydroxyprogesterone, both of which are important intermediates in steroid biosynthesis.

E.C. 1.99.1.9. Steroid 17α-hydroxylase.

19–HYDROXYLASE

19-Hydroxylase is located in all steroid-producing tissues and catalyzes an obligatory step in the biosynthesis of estrogens from androgens—the 19-hydroxylation of androstenedione to 19-hydroxyandrostenedione.

E.C. 1.99.1.10. Steroid 19-hydroxylase.

21–HYDROXYLASE

21-Hydroxylase is a microsomal enzyme located in the adrenal cortex, and it is responsible for the 21-hydroxylation of progesterone to deoxycorticosterone and 17α-hydroxyprogesterone to 17α-hydroxydeoxycorticosterone. 21–hydroxylase is an example of a mixed-function oxidase requiring the NADPH-cytochrome P-450 system for activity.

E.C. 1.99.1.11. Steroid 21-hydroxylase.

Δ^5–3β–HYDROXYSTEROID DEHYDROGENASE

Δ^5-3β-Hydroxysteroid dehydrogenase is a microsomal enzyme present in adrenal, ovarian, testicular, and placental tissues. Utilizing NAD^+, this enzyme catalyzes the conversion of Δ^5-3β-hydroxysteroid to a Δ^4-3-ketosteroid. Pregnenolone is oxidized to progesterone, 17α-hydroxypregnenolone to 17α-hydroxyprogesterone, and dehydroepiandrosterone to androstenedione. It has been postulated that this enzyme catalyzes two steps: one, the shift of the carbon 5-6 double bond to the carbon 4-5 position; and the other step, the oxidation of the hydroxyl group at carbon 3 to ketone.

E.C. 1.1.1.-.

ISOCITRIC DEHYDROGENASE

Isocitric dehydrogenase is an enzyme of the citric acid cycle catalyzing the decarboxylation of isocitrate to α-ketoglutarate in the presence of Mn^{++} and a nucleotide electron acceptor. Animal tissues contain two isocitric dehydrogenases, a NAD^+-dependent enzyme located intramitochondrially, and a $NADP^+$-specific enzyme found extramitochrondrially. The $NADP^+$-linked dehydrogenase of the endometrium and placenta is sensitive to estradiol and has been associated with the transhydrogenation reaction of these tissues.

E.C. 1.1.1.41. Ls-Isocitrate: NAD^+ oxidoreductase (decarboxylating).

E.C. 1.1.1.42. Ls-Isocitrate: $NADP^+$ oxidoreductase (decarboxylating).

LACTIC DEHYDROGENASE

Lactic dehydrogenase, an enzyme of the glycolytic pathway, catalyzes the reduction of pyruvate to lactate in the presence of NADH. The enzyme belongs to a class of metalloenzymes, in which an atom of zinc is an integral part of the enzyme-active center. Lactic dehydrogenase is a tetrameric molecule made up of four subunits from two parent molecular types, M and H. The enzyme has been resolved into five isoenzymic forms.

E.C. 1.1.1.27. L-Lactate: NAD^+ oxidoreductase.

MALATE DEHYDROGENASE

Malate dehydrogenase is an enzyme of the citric acid cycle and catalyzes the reversible reaction of L-malate to oxaloacetate in the presence of the coenzyme NAD^+. This enzyme is stimulated by estradiol-17β in the endometrium. This enzyme is located both intra- and extramitochondrially, catalyzing the oxidative decarboxylation of L-malate to pyruvate with the production of NADPH and CO_2, and the decarboxylation of oxaloacetate to pyruvate. The cofactors $NADPH^+$, biotin, and Mn^{++} are required for maximum activity.

E.C. 1.1.1.37. L-Malate: NAD^+ oxidoreductase.

E.C. 1.1.1.40. L-Malate: $NADP^+$ oxidoreductase (decarboxylating).

NICOTINAMIDE–ADENINE DINUCLEOTIDE (NAD$^+$)

Nicotinamide-adenine dinucleotide is a coenzyme of respiration. It functions as an electron acceptor from substrates in biologic oxidation reactions.

SYNONYM: *Diphosphopyridine nucleotide (DPN)*.

NICOTINAMIDE–ADENINE DINUCLEOTIDE PHOSPHATE (NADP$^+$)

Nicotinamide-adenine dinucleotide phosphate is a respiratory coenzyme. It functions as an electron acceptor from substrates in biologic oxidation reactions. It differs from NAD^+ in that it contains a third molecule of phosphate at carbon 2 of the ribose moiety of the adenosine portion of the molecule. Nicotinamide-adenine dinucleotide phosphate generally participates in reductive biosynthetic reactions and is generated principally in the pentose shunt pathway.

SYNONYM: *Triphosphopyridine nucleotide (TPN)*.

NICOTINAMIDE–ADENINE DINUCLEOTIDE, REDUCED (NADH)

This reduced coenzyme is an important cofactor in the reductive processes of fatty acid metabolism and is essential to steroid biosynthesis.

NICOTINAMIDE–ADENINE DINUCLEOTIDE PHOSPHATE, REDUCED (NADPH)

NADPH is generated primarily by the hexose monophosphate shunt, although malate dehydrogenase can augment the NADPH pool under certain physiologic conditions.

ORNITHINE DECARBOXYLASE

Ornithine decarboxylase catalyzes the conversion of ornithine to putrescine. Estrogen has a direct effect on chick oviduct tissue, promoting a rapid increase in the activity of this enzyme with elevated levels occurring at late proestrus. It is the first example of a completely in vitro enzyme response and may represent an early event in tissue in which growth is induced.

E.C. 4.1.1.17. L-Ornithine carboxylase.

PHOSPHOENOL PYRUVATE CARBOXYLASE

Phosphoenol pyruvate carboxylase is an enzyme of reverse glycolysis that catalyzes the formation of phosphoenol pyruvate from oxaloacetate in the presence of inosine triphosphate (ITP) or guanosine triphosphate (GTP) and Mg^{++} with the release of CO_2.

E.C. 4.1.1.32. GTP: Oxaloacetate carboxylase (transphosphorylating).

PHOSPHOFRUCTOKINASE

Phosphofructokinase, an enzyme of the glycolytic pathway, catalyzes the phosphorylation of fructose-6-phosphate to fructose-1,6-diphosphate in the presence of ATP and Mg^{++}. This enzyme controls the rate of glucose-6-phosphate utilization. It is greatly augmented in uterine tissue by estradiol administration.

E.C. 2.7.1.11. ATP: D-Fructose-6-phosphate 1-phosphotransferase.

PREGNENOLONE SYNTHETASE

Pregnenolone synthetase catalyzes the scission of the side chain of 20α, 22R-dihydroxycholesterol with the formation of pregnenolone and isocaproic acid. The enzyme is present in steroid-producing tissues and requires NADPH.

SYNONYM: *20α, $22R$-C_{27}-Desmolase.*

17α, 20-C_{21}-Desmolase

This enzyme catalyzes the cleavage of the side chain from C_{21} steroids to yield C_{19} steroids—for example, 17α-hydroxyprogesterone in the presence of NADPH and oxygen yields androstenedione, an intermediate in estrogen biosynthesis.

PYRUVATE CARBOXYLASE

Pyruvate carboxylase is a mitochondrial enzyme and catalyzes the carboxylation of pyruvic acid to give rise to oxaloacetate in the presence of adenosine triphosphate, Mg^{++}, and its prosthetic group, biotin. The enzyme has an absolute requirement for acetyl-CoA, which assures oxaloacetate formation in lieu of increased citric acid cycle activity.

E.C. 6.4.1.1. Pyruvate: Carbon-dioxide ligase (ADP).

SUCCINATE DEHYDROGENASE

Succinate dehydrogenase, an enzyme of the citric acid cycle and localized in the mitochondria, catalyzes the oxidation of succinic acid to fumaric acid in the presence of flavin-adenine dinucleotide. This enzyme catalyzes the only dehydrogenation step in the citric acid cycle, which involves the direct transfer of hydrogen to a flavoprotein without the participation of NAD^+. Succinate dehydrogenase is a component of the electron transport system.

E.C. 1.3.99.1. Succinate: FAD Oxidoreductase.

Menopause

MENOPAUSE
Menopause is the transitional phase in a woman's life when menstrual function ceases. It may be natural, premature, or artificial, and often is attended by a complex imbalance of the glandular and autonomic nervous systems.

SYNONYMS: *Climacteric, Change of Life.*

Artificial Menopause
Artificial menopause is the abrupt termination of ovarian function by surgical castration, x-irradiation of the ovaries, or following radium implantation in the uterus.

Natural Menopause
Natural menopause is the result of declining ovarian function due to aging of the ovaries and usually occurs between 40 and 50 years of age.

Premature Menopause
Premature menopause is the cessation of ovarian function before the age of 40. It may be due simply to premature aging of the ovaries or may follow prolonged lactation, debilitating diseases, or infectious processes.

SYNONYM: *Climacterium Praecox.*

COMEDOMASTITIS
Comedomastitis is a condition, generally in elderly women, in which it feels as if there were a mass of worms beneath the areola. Toothpaste-like debris can be expressed from the retracted nipple. It results from inspissation of desquamated debris. Comedomastitis is sometimes difficult to distinguish from comedocarcinoma.

SYNONYMS: *Ductule Ectasia, Mammary Duct Ectasia.*

ENDOMETRITIS, SENILE
Senile endometritis is an infection superimposed on postmenopausal endometrial atrophy. The endometrium is thin. Patches of squamous epithelium replace the normal columnar epithelium, and occasionally the entire endometrial surface is covered by stratified epithelium.

FISSURE, VULVAR
A vulvar fissure is a split in the mucous membrane or skin of the vulva, usually in natural folds.

HYPERPLASIA, POSTMENOPAUSAL ENDOMETRIAL

Postmenopausal endometrial hyperplasia is characterized by variations in the cellular activity of the endothelium. It is caused by estrogen stimulation, generally from extragenital sources. Various forms of hyperplasia may be present.

MASTITIS, PLASMA CELL

Plasma cell mastitis is an inflammatory condition of the breast, usually affecting multiparas approaching menopause. Stasis and inspissation are present, making this a chemical rather than a bacterial inflammation. Induration of the mass is questionable. The microscopic appearance is similar to that in tuberculosis. However, polymorphonuclear leukocytes and plasma cells are present. No caseation or bacilli can be observed. The lesion is very radiosensitive.

MASTODYNIA

Mastodynia is breast pain. In the young, it is associated with areas of fibrosis and small cyst formation. In menopausal and obese women, it is due to pendulous breasts.

SYNONYMS: *Mastalgia, Mammary Neuralgia, Mazodynia, Mammalgia.*

MENOPAUSAL SYNDROME

The menopausal syndrome is characterized by symptomatic, psychosomatic, and psychoneurotic manifestations that are experienced by some women during the climacteric period. Symptoms include hot flashes, chills, sweats, headache, nervousness, irritability, and depression. Other features may consist of palpitation, dizziness, and gastrointestinal symptoms with epigastric reference. The symptoms are transient, recurrent, and mild to severe. Although the syndrome may be induced by oophorectomy or irradiation, the cause is commonly attributed to gradual aging of the ovaries with hypofunction. Although most women experience menopause by the age of 50, some are unaware of any symptoms inasmuch as significant amounts of estrogen continue to be produced after the menopause. The normal source of such estrogen is the adrenal cortex, which apparently continues throughout life to produce amounts adequate for metabolic requirements.

SYNONYM: *Climacteric Syndrome.*

METAPLASIA, ENDOMETRIAL SQUAMOUS

Endometrial squamous metaplasia is the replacement of endometrial columnar epithelium by squamous epithelium. This is an uncommon phenomenon and generally occurs in elderly patients. It may result in squamous cell carcinoma.

SYNONYM: *Ichthyosis Uteri.*

OSTEOPOROSIS

Osteoporosis is an abnormal softening, porousness, or rarefaction of bone. It is the end result of any one of many conditions, and depends on a long, sustained imbalance between rates of bone formation and bone resorption in favor of resorptive activity. Among the recognized causes are adrenal hyperfunction, hyperparathyroidism, hyperthyroidism, long-standing hypogonadism, prolonged calcium deficiency, and prolonged immobilization. The incidence of osteoporosis rises sharply in the sixth decade in women and in the seventh decade in men.

POSTMENOPAUSAL MUSCULAR DYSTROPHY SYNDROME

The postmenopausal muscular dystrophy syndrome is characterized by progressive weakness of the muscles of the hip and shoulder girdle. It occurs in women after menopause. The onset may be slow or rapid. The lower extremities are usually more severely affected than the upper ones. The patient experiences difficulty in climbing stairs, rising from a chair, or in reaching above her head. A waddling gait may be seen later, with complete inability to ascend stairs. Falls occur frequently. The face, hands, and feet remain unaffected. There is no dysphagia or change in vision. No atrophy of the affected muscles occurs. The cause is not known. There is no evidence of a thyroid myopathy. The slight creatinuria does not indicate an extensive or general muscular disorder. Diagnosis is confirmed by a biopsy that reveals patchy degeneration or necrosis of individual muscle fibers.

VAGINITIS, ATROPHIC

Atrophic vaginitis is a relatively frequent inflammation of the vaginal mucosa in postmenopausal women when estrogen levels fall below physiologic levels. The vaginal infection generally produces burning, itching, soreness, and in some patients, vaginal bleeding. The epithelium is thin, and may be ulcerated and subject to minimal bleeding.

SYNONYM: *Senile Vaginitis.*

Sterility and Infertility

INFERTILITY, FEMALE

Female infertility is diminished or absent fertility. It does not imply the existence of as positive or irreversible a condition as sterility. Infertility indicates adequate anatomic structures and equivocal function, with the possibility of pregnancy that may or may not proceed to term.

SYNONYM: *Relative Sterility.*

Primary Infertility

Primary infertility is infertility ascribed to patients who have never conceived.

Secondary Infertility

Secondary infertility is infertility occurring in patients who have previously conceived.

INFERTILITY, MALE

Male infertility is diminished or absent fertility. It does not imply the existence of as positive or irreversible a condition as sterility.

STERILITY, FEMALE

Female sterility is the inability of the female to conceive. It signifies inability to conceive due to inadequacy in structure or function of the genital organs.

SYNONYM: *Absolute Sterility.*

STERILITY, MALE

Male sterility is the inability of the male to fertilize the ovum. It may or may not be associated with impotence.

Aspermatogenic Sterility

Aspermatogenic sterility is sterility due to a failure to produce living spermatozoa.

Dysspermatogenic Sterility

Dysspermatogenic sterility is sterility due to some abnormality in production of spermatozoa.

Normospermatogenic Sterility

Normospermatogenic sterility is sterility due to some cause other than failure to produce live, normal spermatozoa.

AGGLUTINATION, SPERM
Sperm agglutination is immobilization of the sperm due to occlusion of the vas deferens or previous orchitis. The occlusion results in the production of unknown antibodies by the reticuloendothelial system, which in turn immobilize or agglutinate the sperm at the time of ejaculation.

ASPERMIA
Aspermia is the absence of seminal fluid during ejaculation.

AZOOSPERMIA
Azoospermia is the lack of spermatozoa in the semen.

BIOPSY, TESTICULAR
Testicular biopsy is the removal and examination, usually microscopic, of tissue from the testis for purposes of diagnosis.

FERTILITY
Fertility is the ability to produce young.

HEMOSPERMIA
Hemospermia is the presence of blood in the seminal fluid.
SYNONYM: *Hematospermia.*

Hemospermia Spuria
Hemospermia spuria is a condition in which there is an admixture of blood and seminal fluid occurring in the prostatic urethra.

Hemospermia Vera
Hemospermia vera is a condition in which there is an admixture of blood and seminal fluid occurring in the seminal vesicles.

INSEMINATION
Insemination is the introduction of semen into the vagina.
SYNONYM: *Semination.*

INSEMINATION, ARTIFICIAL
Artificial insemination is the introduction of semen into the vagina by artificial means. Concentrated semen, used in the process of artificial insemination, may be obtained by the split ejaculate, centrifugation, environmental temperature reduction, or filter methods.

Heterologous Insemination
Heterologous insemination is artificial insemination with semen from one who is not the woman's husband.
SYNONYM: *Donor Insemination.*
ABBREVIATION: AID.

Homologous Insemination
Homologous insemination is artificial insemination with the husband's semen.
ABBREVIATION: AIH.

MANN TEST

The Mann test is the insertion of a specially constructed rubber balloon filled with an opaque substance into the uterus to test the competency of the cervix.

SYNONYM: *Balloon Test for Cervical Incompetency.*

NECROSPERMIA

Necrospermia is a condition in which the semen contains a high percentage of nonmotile sperm.

OLIGOSPERMIA

Oligospermia is a deficiency in the number of spermatozoa in the semen.

POLYSPERMIA

Polyspermia is the excessive secretion of semen.

POSTCOITAL SEMEN TEST

The postcoital semen test is the histologic examination of the semen from the vaginal pool and endocervix soon after intercourse. Failure to observe sperm from these locations may mean aspermia, hostile endocervical secretion, local inflammation, or immunologic reaction to the cervical secretion.

SYNONYMS: *Sims' Test, Huhner Test.*

RUBIN TEST

The Rubin test determines the patency of the fallopian tubes; it is made by transuterine insufflation with carbon dioxide. If the tubes are patent, the gas enters the peritoneal cavity and may be demonstrated fluoroscopically or roentgenographically. This subphrenic pneumoperitoneum causes pain in both shoulders of the patient. The tubes are patent if the manometer registers not more than 100 mm Hg; there is stenosis or stricture, but not complete occlusion if the manometer registers between 120 and 130 mm Hg; the tubes are completely occluded if it rises to 200 mm Hg.

SEMEN, CONCENTRATION OF

Concentration of semen is a procedure by which seminal fluid is condensed into a more potent form. There are four methods: centrifugation, environmental temperature reduction, the filter, and split-ejaculate methods.

Centrifugation Method

Centrifugation is a method of semen concentration in which the seminal fluid is centrifuged for 10 minutes.

Environmental Temperature Reduction Method

Environmental temperature reduction is a method of semen concentration in which the temperature of the seminal fluid is lowered. Decantation of the supernatant fluid results in a concentrated specimen.

Filter Method

The filter method is a method of semen concentration by use of a millipore filter.

Split-Ejaculate Method

The split-ejaculate method is a method of semen concentration by which only the first portion of the ejaculated semen is collected.

SEMEN, NONLIQUEFACTION OF

Nonliquefaction of semen is failure of the seminal fluid to change its viscosity. Normally, the fluid becomes liquefied in 15 to 20 minutes. The addition of 1 cc of 5 per cent α-amylase solution into the vagina after intercourse generally increases liquefaction.

SPERMATEMPHRAXIS

Spermatemphraxis is an impediment to the discharge of semen.

SPERMATOLYSIN

Spermatolysin is a specific lysin formed in the female body in response to a sensitivity to spermatozoa.

SPERMATOLYSIS

Spermatolysis is destruction with dissolution of the spermatozoa.

SPERMATORRHEA

Spermatorrhea is an involuntary discharge of semen without orgasm.

SPERMATOSCHESIS

Spermatoschesis is nonsecretion of semen.

SPERMATURIA

Spermaturia is discharge of seminal fluid with the passage of urine.
SYNONYM: *Seminuria.*

SPERMOTOXIN

Spermotoxin is a toxin destructive to spermatozoa. It is an antibody produced by injecting an animal with spermatozoa.

SECTION 5: SELECTED GYNECOLOGIC TOPICS

Endocrinology

ACHARD-THIERS SYNDROME

The Achard-Thiers syndrome is a rare syndrome characterized by diabetes mellitus, hirsutism, and hypertension in women. It is seen predominantly in middle-aged and elderly females. Conspicuous clinical characteristics are a masculine type of hypertrichosis of the face, voice changes, hypertrophy of the clitoris, and a masculine type of body build. Recessive function of sexual organs includes irregular or absent menstruation and atrophy of the breasts. Obesity of the trunk, striae, acne, hypertension, and occasionally osteoporosis may be evident. Carbohydrate tolerance is decreased. The cause of the symptom complex is as yet uncertain, although it is thought to be associated with adrenal cortical dysfunction.

SYNONYM: *Diabetic-Bearded Women Syndrome.*

ACNE VULGARIS

Acne vulgaris is an inflammatory skin disease of the sebaceous glands occurring on the face, back, chest, or neck. It is often stimulated by the action of androgen on the sebaceous glands. In the female, acne generally develops during puberty when ovarian function becomes sufficient to produce menstrual cycles but the ratio of estrogen to androgen has not become optimal. It appears more often in the female with irregular periods, quite regularly in association with androgenic syndromes.

ACROMEGALOGIGANTISM

Acromegalogigantism is a disease characterized by disproportionate growth of the extremities together with the other signs of acromegaly. It occurs before epiphysial closure.

ACROMEGALY

Acromegaly is characterized by heavy bone and soft tissue facial features, prognathism, marked enlargement of hands and feet, and some enlargement of the forearms and other bones. Many tissues and organs share in the hypertrophic changes. External genitalia are rarely affected. Morphologic findings in the gonads are variable, although generally the ovaries become inactive. Occasionally, however, pregnancy may occur. A decrease in libido and potentia eventually ensues. Headache and visual disturbance are common symptoms, a sequel of the causative pituitary tumor. The syndrome is due to an excessive secretion of the growth hormone of the anterior portion of the pituitary gland, usually from a chromophil (eosinophilic) adenoma. If the hyperplasia and hypersecretion begin before puberty, gigantism ensues.

SYNONYMS: *Eosinophilic Adenoma Syndrome, Marie's Syndrome.*

ADRENAL HYPERPLASIA, ACQUIRED

Acquired adrenal hyperplasia denotes increased function of the adrenal cortex in a previously normal individual. It is usually associated with bilateral hypertrophy of the adrenal glands. A variety of syndromes may result, depending on which hormones are secreted in excess, such as Cushing's syndrome (glucocorticoids), adrenogenital syndrome (androgens), and hyperaldosteronism (mineralocorticoids).

ADRENOCORTICAL INSUFFICIENCY

Adrenocortical insufficiency includes the well-known clinical picture that results from partial or complete loss of function of the adrenal cortex. It occurs as a primary disorder (*Addison's disease*), but may in a small percentage of cases be secondary to pituitary deficiency. Symptoms, often insidious, include weakness, asthenia, and gastrointestinal manifestations. Anemia, arterial hypotension, decreased metabolic rate, hypoglycemia, decreased serum sodium and chloride, and increased serum potassium are supporting diagnostic indications. In primary adrenal failure, pigmentary changes of external genitalia and mucous membranes frequently parallel the degree of hormonal deficiency. The characteristic pigmentation of the skin and mucous membranes is not present in adrenal failure secondary to pituitary insufficiency (*Simmonds' disease, Sheehan's syndrome*). Stress, trauma, or surgery may precipitate a crisis that threatens life. In Addison's disease, the urinary 17-hydroxycorticosteroids and 17-ketosteroids, and the plasma cortisol are very low and fail to increase following adrenocorticotropic hormone stimulation, whereas there is a significant increase in secondary adrenal failure.

ADRENOGENITAL SYNDROME

The adrenogenital syndrome in women is characterized by an increased secretion of adrenal androgens, resulting in virilization. A recessively transmitted hereditary type may begin in utero. Usual symptoms include signs of defeminization, premature growth of pubic and axillary hair, hirsutism, excessive muscular development, short stature in the adult, amenorrhea, and a masculine voice. In female infants, varying degrees of abnormalities and ambiguity of the external genitalia are evident. In childhood, the syndrome is usually due to hyperplasia of the adrenal cortex with excess secretion of androgens resulting from a congenital defect of steroidogenesis, of which several types have been described. The urinary 17-ketosteroids and pregnanetriol are generally elevated. The plasma cortisol levels may be low, particularly in the salt-losing types. Sudden death in the newborn may occur due to cortisol deficiency. Onset of the syndrome during childhood may be due to a functioning adrenal tumor or virilizing tumor of the ovary. Virilizing adrenal hyperplasia may also have its onset at puberty or soon thereafter.

SYNONYMS: *Adrenal Virilism Syndrome, Congenital Virilizing Adrenocortical Hyperplasia Syndrome.*

AHUMADA-DEL CASTILLO SYNDROME

The Ahumada-Del Castillo syndrome is a triad of amenorrhea, low gonadotropin secretion, and galactorrhea unrelated to pregnancy.

ALBRIGHT'S SYNDROME

Albright's syndrome is a rare syndrome characterized by dysplasia of bone, brown-pigmented areas of the skin, and sexual and somatic precocity in females. The syndrome usually occurs in children or young adults. The multiple bone lesions are characterized by fibrous dysplastic replacement of the medullary structure. Pelvic bones and the lower extremities are most often affected. These lesions may not be recognized until a pathologic fracture occurs in childhood or early adult life. The degree of pigmentation often parallels the extent of skeletal involvement. These cafe-au-lait spots occur more often on the same side as the bone lesion and are found most frequently on the scalp, back of the neck, upper spine, the sacrum, and thighs. Oral pigmentation has also been reported. Associated endocrine features consist of unusual sexual precocity with early menarche, enlargement of breasts, and the development of adolescent external genitalia. Sterility is not a later factor. Normal 17-ketosteroid values rule out an adrenocortical tumor. Urinary follicle-stimulating hormone excretion, serum calcium, and serum phosphorus values are also normal. Serum phosphatase is often elevated. The bone changes are usually progressive until growth ceases. Treatment of fractures and orthopedic correction of deformities may be necessary.

SYNONYMS: *Albright-McCune-Sternberg Syndrome, McCune-Albright Syndrome, Polyostotic Fibrous Dysplasia, Wright's Syndrome, Osteitis Fibrosa Disseminata.*

ALOPECIA

Alopecia is the absence of skin hair from areas in which it is normally present.

ANOREXIA NERVOSA

Anorexia nervosa is the development of cachexia due to psychogenic disturbance in eating habits after previous good health. There are generally amenorrhea, nervousness, hypotension, and emotional disturbances. It may be differentiated from pituitary cachexia (Simmonds' disease) in that there is no organic lesion of the pituitary, and thyroid and adrenal function are not markedly depressed.

CHIARI-FROMMEL SYNDROME

The Chiari-Frommel syndrome is a condition characterized by persistent postpartum amenorrhea and galactorrhea, and atrophy of the uterus and ovaries probably due to hypothalamic dysfunction. The diagnosis is generally entertained in women who have amenorrhea and lactation for more than a year following delivery or cessation of nursing, and in whom no organic lesion of the central nervous system can be demonstrated by appropriate studies. Gonadotropins and estrogens are markedly diminished. Other endocrine studies are generally normal. Spontaneous recovery may occur after prolonged intervals. Recurrence may be noted after subsequent pregnancies.

SYNONYMS: *Frommel's Disease, Persistent Postpartum Amenorrhea-Galactorrhea Syndrome.*

CONGENITAL ADRENAL HYPERPLASIA SYNDROME

The congenital adrenal hyperplasia syndrome is a genetic disorder of steroid metabolism resulting in virilization in both sexes. In the female child, the external genitalia are often ambiguous. The syndrome is generally characterized by elevated urinary 17-ketosteroids and pregnanetriol, progressive virilization, and large amounts of abnormal adrenal steroids in the urine. There are several forms of the syndrome, including uncomplicated or compensate, C_{21} hydroxylase deficiency; salt-losing, C_{21} hydroxylase deficiency; a hypertensive type (a relatively rare form) due to C_{11} hydroxylation defect; 3β-hydroxysteroid dehydrogenase deficiency. The synthesis of cortisol is blocked by lack of a different enzyme for each of the four forms.

SYNONYMS: *Congenital Adrenogenital Syndrome, Virilizing Adrenal Hyperplasia.*

CONSTITUTIONAL PRECOCITY

Constitutional precocity is a form of sexual precocity that results from the early release of gonadotropin. This release is presumably the result of accelerated organization of the hypothalamic mechanisms that control secretion of pituitary gonadotropins. The condition may be genetically carried, but a familial incidence occurs in less than 10 per cent of cases. The condition is much more common in girls than in boys. It may occur at any time before puberty. The diagnosis is established by ruling out organic lesions of the central nervous system or functioning tumors of the ovary or adrenal gland as the cause for the early sexual development. In rare instances, hypothyroidism may initiate the condition.

SYNONYMS: *Constitutional Precocious Puberty, Idiopathic Sexual Precocity.*

CUSHING'S SYNDROME

Cushing's syndrome is a condition resulting from excess secretion of the adrenal cortical hormones, particularly the glucocorticoids (cortisol group). It is characterized clinically by a truncal type of obesity with relatively thin extremities, rounding and plethora of the face, well-marked purplish striae, thinning of the skin with easy bruising, slight to marked hirsutism, hypertension, and amenorrhea. Later complications include osteoporosis, crush fractures of the vertebrae, and diabetes. The condition may result from bilateral adrenal hyperplasia or benign or malignant tumors of the adrenal cortex. In some instances, there may be a baso-philic adenoma of the pituitary (Cushing's disease). In rare instances, the syndrome may result from adrenocorticotropic hormone-secreting tumors of the ovary or nonendocrine structures. The diagnosis is con-firmed by the findings of an elevated plasma cortisol with absence of diurnal variation. In hyperplasia cases, the plasma and urinary corticos-teroids are suppressed by dexamethasone and increased by adrenocorti-cotropic hormone stimulation, and adrenal tumors are generally autonomous.

DEFEMINIZATION
Defeminization is the relative loss of the female sexual characteristics.

DIABETES INSIPIDUS
Diabetes insipidus is a disease of the posterior pituitary gland or hypothalamus resulting in an inadequate secretion of neurohypophysial antidiuretic hormone (ADH). The deficiency causes the production of large volumes of dilute urine owing to the defect in ability of the renal tubule to reabsorb filtered water.

EDEMA, IDIOPATHIC
Idiopathic edema is a condition occurring predominantly in women and is characterized by general fluid retention in the absence of cardiac, kidney, or liver disorder. The cause of the condition is not known, but it appears to be associated with a dysfunction of the angiotensin, renin, aldosterone mechanism. Other hormonal and psychogenic factors may play a role.

FORBES-ALBRIGHT SYNDROME
Forbes-Albright syndrome is a combination of galactorrhea with amen-orrhea and low urinary follicle-stimulating hormone (FSH), unassoci-ated with recent pregnancy or with acromegaly. Overproduction of prolactin is a suspected etiologic factor. Pituitary tumors are frequently associated.
SYNONYM: *Argonz-Del Castillo Syndrome.*

FRÖHLICH'S SYNDROME
Fröhlich's syndrome is a syndrome resulting from a hypothalamic or pituitary lesion accompanied by obvious physical characteristics, includ-ing obesity and retarded sexual development. In the female, menstrua-tion fails to appear at puberty or may cease in the postpubertal period. In the male, the voice remains high-pitched, the testes remain unde-scended, facial hair is absent, and there is a feminine pubic line. The neurologic and other endocrine manifestations depend on the site and extent of the lesion. Roentgenographic studies may show enlargement or destruction of the sella turcica or suprasellar calcification, suggesting a craniopharyngioma. Other pituitary effects include polyuria, poly-

dypsia, increased sugar tolerance, and reduction or absence of urinary gonadotropins. The most typical form of Fröhlich's syndrome arises from Rathke-pouch tumors or craniopharyngiomas. Chromophobe adenomas, trauma, and inflammatory lesions may also be a cause.

SYNONYMS: *Adiposogenital Dystrophy Syndrome, Dystrophia Adiposogenitalis Syndrome, Neuropituitary Dystrophy Syndrome, Pituitary Infantilism of Adults, Cerebral Adiposity Syndrome.*

GALACTORRHEA SYNDROMES

Several galactorrhea syndromes are now recognized, depending on the underlying etiologic factor. The galactorrhea varies from extrusion of a few drops of whitish secretion to an abundant and spontaneous flow of milk. Usually, but not invariably, there is an associated amenorrhea or menstrual dysfunction. In some instances, the galactorrhea and amenorrhea may be a persistence of the postpartum state; in others they are nonpuerperal. Some cases are due to dysfunction; others may be associated with organic lesions, particularly of the central nervous system and pituitary; still others may be of iatrogenic origin. The following classification is based on the etiologic factors:

Dysfunctional.
1. Chiari-Frommel syndrome. Persistent postpartum amenorrhea and galactorrhea.
2. Ahumada-Del Castillo syndrome. Nonpuerperal.
3. Hypothyroidism.

Associated with an organic lesion of the central nervous system.
1. Forbes-Albright syndrome. Most of these patients have a chromophobe adenoma.
2. Acromegaly.
3. Extrasellar lesions, such as craniopharyngiomas, meningiomas, and sarcoidosis.

Local lesions involving chest wall, such as post-thoracotomy lesions, and Herpes zoster.

Iatrogenic.

Psychopharmacologic drugs such as reserpine, chlorpromazine, and methyldopa.

Hormonal. Following the use of oral contraceptives.

GORDAN-OVERSTREET SYNDROME

The Gordan-Overstreet syndrome is a syndrome that presents the characteristics of Turner's syndrome with virilization that apparently arises from secreting epithelioid cells of the dysgenetic gonad. Evidence of androgenic activity is seen in hirsutism and hypertrophy of the clitoris. Prominent masculinity may be proved by skin biopsy or smears from buccal mucous membranes.

SYNONYM: *Androgenicity-Gonadal Dysgenesis Syndrome.*

HERMAPHRODITISM

Hermaphroditism is a variable genetic disturbance in patients who have both ovarian and testicular tissue. Unilateral or bilateral ovotestes are common. When an ovary is present on one side and a testis on the other, the corresponding genital ducts tend to differentiate in a manner consistent with the sex of the gonad. When ovotestes are present, fusion of the paramesonephric ducts is common. Abnormal sex chromosome complexes may be present.

HIRSUTISM, IDIOPATHIC

Idiopathic hirsutism is the presence of excessive facial and body hair with little or no other virilization in a normally feminized woman. These women generally have a racial or genetic tendency to hirsutism. The 17-ketosteroids and plasma testosterone levels are within the normal range, and there is no evidence of an endocrine dysfunction to account for the hirsutism.

HIRSUTISM SYNDROMES

Excessive hair growth on the face or body in women may occur on a genetic, racial, or constitutional basis. Idiopathic hypertrichosis may occur at puberty, during or immediately after pregnancy, following the menopause, after severe burns, and during starvation and stress. Hirsutism of varying degree is noted in association with the following syndromes: adrenogenital syndrome, Cushing's syndrome, masculinizing tumors of the ovary, polycystic ovarian disease, hyperthecosis of the ovary, Achard-Thiers syndrome, and cretinism.

HUTCHINSON-GILFORD SYNDROME

The Hutchinson-Gilford syndrome is characterized by infantilism, facial and pubic alopecia, and premature aging. The syndrome does not appear to be familial or hereditary, and either sex may be affected. Clinically, there is no abnormality at birth, but there follows a failure to gain weight, limitation of growth, and loss of hair. Dwarfism gradually develops. The appearance of these patients is characteristic and has been described as that of premature old age. There is a small face, projecting eyes, beaked nose, and receding chin. Scalp veins are prominent, and the lower jaw is micrognathic with crowded and irregular teeth. There may be a high, arched palate, marked baldness, absence of eyebrows and lashes, marked atrophy and inelasticity of the skin, and absence of subcutaneous fat except in the pubic region. The chest is narrow, the abdomen protrudes, and the fingernails may show trophic changes or may be absent. Until puberty the genitalia are normal, but thereafter little sexual maturation occurs. The muscles are poorly developed, and the limbs are thin. The cause of this syndrome is not known.

SYNONYMS: *Progeria Syndrome, Premature Senility Syndrome, Gilford's Syndrome, Senilism Syndrome.*

HYPERGONADOTROPIC HYPOGONADISM, FEMALE

Female hypergonadotropic hypogonadism is failure of the ovaries to respond to gonadotropins. It is characterized by diminished estrogen secretion and elevated gonadotropins in the blood and urine. The clinical manifestations depend on the period of life during which this occurs. It may result from a genetic abnormality of the ovary such as Turner's syndrome or other types of gonadal dysgenesis, or it may result from acquired ovarian failure during childhood, such as destructive lesions of the ovary due to tumor, inflammation, or radiation. It may also occur after puberty owing to organic or functional lesions that destroy ovarian tissue or inhibit ovarian response. Occasionally, neurologic or psychogenic factors inhibit the response of the ovary. It occurs physiologically at the climacteric.

HYPERTHYROIDISM

Hyperthyroidism is a disorder caused by an increase above normal in the circulating thyroid hormone. It may result from increased secretory activity of the thyroid gland or from the administration of thyroid hormones. The clinical symptoms include nervousness, restlessness, tachycardia, excessive sweating, tremor, and loss of weight in spite of increased appetite. In *Graves' disease,* there is diffuse enlargement of the thyroid gland, often associated with ophthalmopathy characterized by exophthalmos and stare. In *Plummer's disease,* the patient has a toxic nodular goiter usually without ophthalmopathy. Hyperthyroidism is commonly but not invariably associated with a change in the menstrual pattern. There is usually a decrease in frequency, duration, and amount of menstrual flow, and in severe cases amenorrhea may occur. Hyperthyroidism may be associated with pregnancy, although fertility is moderately reduced in severe cases. Hyperthyroidism is associated with an increase in the basal metabolic rate, and an increase in the protein-bound iodine, thyroxine, triiodothyronine, and radioactive iodine uptake.

SYNONYM: *Thyrotoxicosis.*

HYPOGONADISM, FEMALE

Female hypogonadism is a condition caused by failure of the ovaries to function due to an intrinsic or acquired defect, failure to respond to the pituitary gonadotropins, or failure of the pituitary gland to secrete gonadotropins in sufficient amounts to stimulate the ovaries.

HYPOGONADOTROPIC HYPOGONADISM

Hypogonadotropic hypogonadism is failure of the pituitary to secrete gonadotropins. Failure may result from neoplasm, hemorrhage, infection of the gland, or anatomic or functional disease either of the hypothalamic centers or the anterior pituitary lobe. The clinical manifestations depend on the period of life in which the condition occurs, the underlying cause, and whether other pituitary hormones are diminished. If only the gonadotropins are involved, the condition is referred to as an isolated hypogonadotropism. If it occurs in childhood, it may result in pituitary or

hypogonadotropic eunuchoidism, or hypogonadotropic primary amenorrhea.

HYPOPARATHYROIDISM SYNDROME

The hypoparathyroidism syndrome results in chronic hypocalcemia
with varied and widespread neuromuscular effects. It may be classified
etiologically under three headings: postoperative (following thyroidectomy), idiopathic, and following organic lesions of the parathyroids.
Postoperative hypoparathyroidism is by far the most common variety.
Symptoms of the idiopathic variety may be varied and vague; mild cases
of this syndrome may not be recognized for many years, sometimes
decades. Characteristic symptoms include fatigue, muscular weakness,
paresthesias and cramps of the extremities, tetany, muscular hyperexcitability, and laryngeal stridor. Tetany is the outstanding clinical manifestation of hypoparathyroidism; it may be latent or manifest. Other
manifestations include delayed and defective dentition, trophic nail
changes, and cataracts. Personality changes, mental retardation, attacks
of unconsciousness, and general convulsions may be present. Because
convulsive manifestations are accompanied by an epileptic encephalographic pattern, it has been postulated that hypocalcemia precipitates
convulsive seizures in susceptible individuals. Idiopathic hypoparathyroidism is thus often misdiagnosed as epilepsy. The diagnosis of idiopathic tetany depends chiefly on differentiating it from other forms of
tetany. Diagnostic criteria include: low serum calcium level, elevated
serum inorganic phosphorus level, chronic latent tetany, the absence of
severe renal insufficiency, and normal roentgenograms of bone. Electrocardiographic changes often show a prolongation of the QT interval.

HYPOPITUITARISM

Hypopituitarism is a condition due to pathologically diminished activity
of the hypophysis.

HYPOPITUITARISM SYNDROMES

Several syndromes may result from a deficiency of the anterior pituitary gland, depending on the number of hormones involved, the period
of life at which the condition occurs, and the nature of the underlying
lesion. The term *panhypopituitarism* is generally used to indicate complete or nearly complete loss of adenohypophysial function. The resulting
condition is often described under the terms of *Simmonds-Sheehan disease, Simmonds' syndrome, Sheehan's syndrome,* and *pituitary cachexia.*
Panhypopituitarism is characterized by a chronic progressive endocrine
deficiency with widespread disturbance of tissue and organ function resulting from failure of hormone production by the anterior lobe of the
pituitary gland. The syndrome occurs more commonly in females. The
symptoms are manifold and include asthenia, hypotension, anemia, progressive weight loss that may progress to severe cachexia, and decreased
sexual function associated with atrophy of the genital organs. Clinical
features also include loss of axillary and pubic hair, atrophic changes in

the skin, markedly decreased metabolic rate with hypothermia, and in women, amenorrhea and failure of lactation. The syndrome is caused by the destruction of the anterior lobe of the pituitary gland. Pathologic lesions include postpartum necrosis of the pituitary, usually associated with severe hemorrhage at the time of delivery, spontaneous atrophy and fibrosis, destruction by chromophobe adenoma, and traumatic injuries. Similar effects may follow excessive radiation or surgical removal. Hypopituitarism in childhood may be associated with dwarfism and sexual infantilism. *Pituitary dwarfism* may be associated with a detectable lesion in the pituitary or parasellar regions or may be due to a genetic deficiency of growth hormones and gonadotropic hormones.

HYPOTHALAMIC PRECOCITY

Hypothalamic precocity is due to neoplasms that damage the hypothalamic centers inhibiting gonadotropin release. This condition results in increased somatic growth, premature maturation of secondary sex characteristics in both sexes, and early development of the genital structures. It may be associated with hydrocephalus and encephalitis. Hamartomas, pinealomas, and craniopharyngiomas may cause the condition.

SYNONYM: *Neurogenic Precocity.*

HYPOTHYROIDISM

In hypothyroidism occurring during the childbearing age, there is often excessive uterine bleeding including both menorrhagia and metrorrhagia. Frankly hypothyroid women may also be amenorrheic and are often anovulatory. The incidence of abortion, prematurity, and stillborn infants is increased in proportion to the severity of the hypothyroidism. Occasionally, living and viable children are born to nontreated myxedematous mothers. The children are euthyroid, but may exhibit various anomalies. *Cretinism* is the term applied to severely hypothyroid children, and may be due to congenital absence of the thyroid gland or hypoplasia of unknown origin. *Endemic cretinism* occurs in the population of endemic goiter belts, but *sporadic cretinism* may occur outside such areas. Hypothyroidism is characterized by diminished protein-bound iodine, decreased thyroxine, diminished triiodothyronine uptake, and diminished radioactive iodine uptake. Cholesterol levels are elevated.

KLINEFELTER'S SYNDROME

Klinefelter's syndrome, which occurs in the male, is characterized by small testes of firm consistency, spermatogenic failure with normal or impaired Leydig-cell function, gynecomastia, and high urinary follicle-stimulating hormone levels. In its true form this syndrome is a type of gonadal dysgenesis and is associated with chromosomal aberration. Most of these patients are sex chromatin-positive and on chromosomal analysis have 47 chromosomes with an XXY karyotype. Other patterns of chromosomal aberration may be present such as XXXXY, XXYY, XXXY, and a variety of mosaic patterns. Some patients with the clinical manifestations of this condition are sex chromatin-negative with an XY karyotype, and are sometimes referred to as "sex chromatin-negative Klinefelter" patients. It is not known at present whether these patients also have a genetic defect or if the disorder results from a postnatal testicular lesion.

SYNONYMS: *Klinefelter-Reifenstein-Albright Syndrome, Gynecomastia-Aspermatogenesis Syndrome, XXY Sex Chromosome Constitution, Seminiferous Tubule Dysgenesis.*

LAUNOIS-CLÉRET SYNDROME

The Launois-Cléret syndrome is characterized by obesity and lack of development of internal or external genitalia in children. The general and endocrinopathic features of this hypophysial dystrophy are essentially similar to those of Fröhlich's syndrome.

SYNONYM: *Hypophysial-Adiposogenital Syndrome.*

LAURENCE-MOON-BIEDL SYNDROME

The Laurence-Moon-Biedl syndrome is an autosomal recessive congenital disorder of childhood characterized by obesity, retinal degeneration, genital hypoplasia, polydactylism, and mental retardation. The complete syndrome is seldom observed in the same person, but the characteristics are often scattered among the siblings of one family or generation. Members of these families have an increased number of abortions and early deaths. In addition to the cardinal features, acrocephaly, syndactyly, dwarfism, atresia ani, deafness, mongolian facies, and dental anomalies may be present. The ophthalmic abnormalities are numerous. Retinal degeneration with varying degrees of pigmentary changes is the chief ocular defect. Microphthalmos, cataracts, macular atrophy, convergent strabismus, hemeralopia, and nystagmus may be present. If the patient reaches adulthood, there may be an absence of body hair and other physical signs of anterior pituitary deficiency. Underdevelopment of the breasts and amenorrhea are present in the female; pseudogynecomastia, impotence, aleydigism, and azoospermia are present in the male.

SYNONYMS: *Laurence-Moon Syndrome, Biedl-Bardet Syndrome, Laurence-Moon-Bardet-Biedl Syndrome.*

LYMPHOCYTIC THYROIDITIS

Lymphocytic thyroiditis is a chronic inflammatory condition of the thyroid, secondary to tissue destruction caused by an antigen-antibody interaction. Clinically, the patient exhibits a diffuse goiter or enlargement of the gland accompanied or followed by hypothyroidism.

SYNONYM: *Hashimoto's Disease.*

MYXEDEMA

Myxedema is a condition that develops in severe cases of hypothyroidism and is characterized by boggy swelling of the face and hands, resulting from an accumulation of extracellular fluid. A characteristic feature of myxedema is the presence of an excess of mucus in the corium. Myxedema is firm and does not pit on pressure.

SYNONYM: *Gull's Disease.*

OSTEOPOROSIS

Osteoporosis is an abnormal softening, porousness, or rarefaction of bone. It is the end result of any one of many conditions, and depends on a long, sustained imbalance between rates of bone formation and bone resorption in favor of resorptive activity. Among the recognized causes are adrenal hyperfunction, hyperparathyroidism, hyperthyroidism, long-standing hypogonadism, prolonged calcium deficiency, and prolonged immobilization. The incidence of osteoporosis rises sharply in the sixth decade in women and in the seventh decade in men.

POLYCYSTIC OVARIAN DISEASE

Polycystic ovarian disease is an entity associated with polycystic ovaries and clinical symptoms and signs such as oligomenorrhea, anovulation, infertility, and hirsutism. Grossly, the ovaries are enlarged and oyster gray, with a firm, smooth cortex indicating no evidence of ovulation or corpus luteum formation. The tunica albuginea is thickened, tough, and fibrous. Many trapped follicles in all stages of development are present underneath the tunica albuginea. Microscopically, multiple cysts are present in the cortex without corpus luteum formation. Marked hyperplasia of the theca interna of the atretic follicles is frequent. Urinary 17-ketosteroids and plasma testosterone levels are usually normal or slightly elevated. Gonadotropin levels vary. The condition is associated with a defect in ovarian steroidogenesis favoring the production of androgenic steroids at the expense of the estrogens. The underlying cause is not known. A relative enzyme deficiency in the ovary has been postulated. In the differential diagnosis, it is important to rule out other conditions that may be associated with bilateral cystic ovaries and hirsutism, including adrenogenital syndrome, Cushing's syndrome, and pituitary or hypothalamic lesions.

SYNONYMS: *Stein-Leventhal Syndrome, Stein's Syndrome, Bilateral Polycystic Ovarian Syndrome, Sclerocystic Disease of the Ovaries.*

POSTPARTUM PITUITARY NECROSIS SYNDROME

The postpartum pituitary necrosis syndrome is due to postpartum thrombosis of sinuses and ischemic infarction and necrosis of the pituitary gland, usually as a result of obstetric hemorrhage and shock that occur at term. If both the anterior and posterior lobes are involved and the gonadotropins, thyrotropin, and corticotropin are all absent, the appropriate descriptive term is *panhypopituitarism.* These deficiences indicate secondary atrophy and failure of the adrenal cortices, the thyroid, and the ovaries. Excretion of corticoids in the urine is reduced. The resulting symptoms appear insidiously, and usually after several months. Symptoms of multiglandular deficiency are variable. Some patients exhibit the characteristics of myxedema. There is pallor, asthenia, apathy, atrophy of the breasts with loss of areolar pigment, inhibition of lactation, loss of pubic and axillary hair, and genital atrophy. Amenorrhea may be temporary or permanent; rarely some women continue to menstruate indefinitely. Lipemia and xanthomatosis are sometimes present. Diabetes mellitus, if present, vanishes. Hypoglycemia is usually found and may be sufficiently severe to produce coma. A flat glucose tolerance curve and extreme sensitivity to insulin may be demonstrated.

SYNONYMS: *Sheehan's Syndrome, Postpartum Panhypopituitary Syndrome.*

PREMENSTRUAL TENSION SYNDROME

The premenstrual tension syndrome occurs during the second half of the menstrual cycle and may consist of variable combinations of the following symptoms: painful swelling of the breasts, abdominal bloating and discomfort, headache, nausea, vomiting, fatigue, swelling of the subcutaneous tissues, and nervous and emotional instability. There may also be excessive thirst, increased appetite, hypersomnia, dizziness, and palpitation. Most often the condition occurs during the final week of the menstrual cycle and ends soon after the onset of menses. Although the cause for the premenstrual tension syndrome is not known, it is believed to be associated with the cyclic fluctuation of the ovarian hormones.

SYNONYM: *Premenstrual Syndrome.*

PRIMARY ALDOSTERONISM

Primary aldosteronism is a condition associated with arterial hypertension and potassium wasting caused by an adrenocortical tumor secreting an excess of aldosterone only. Symptoms and signs include hypertension, headache, polyuria, polydipsia, muscular weakness, paresthesias, and periodic paralysis. A tentative diagnosis is supported by the triad of resting hypertension, low serum potassium, and failure of urine concentration after the administration of antidiuretic hormone. The definitive diagnosis is made on the basis of a low level of renin in the plasma and elevated aldosterone levels on a normal salt intake. Removal of the aldosterone-secreting tumor yields an excellent prognosis in a high percentage of cases. Excessive secretion of aldosterone may occur also in certain edematous states, during salt deprivation, or in malignant hypertension and is referred to as *secondary hyperaldosteronism.*

SYNONYM: *Conn's Syndrome.*

PRIMARY HYPERPARATHYROIDISM

Primary hyperparathyroidism is characterized by a disturbance of the metabolism of bone with general demineralization due to excessive secretion of parathyroid hormones in association with hyperplasia or tumor of the parathyroid glands. Manifestations of hyperparathyroidism are commonly seen and occur most frequently between 20 and 60 years of age. Females are more commonly affected in an approximate ratio of two to one. Symptoms, usually of long duration, relate to the skeletal, gastrointestinal, and renal systems. Muscle weakness, bone pain, tenderness, and fractures are common. Nausea, vomiting, anorexia, polyuria, polydipsia, and weight loss are other characteristics. Metabolic manifestations include hypercalcemia, increased serum phosphatase, hypophosphatemia, and hypercalciuria. Local pathologic characteristics include renal calculi and nephrocalcinosis in tubules, osteomalacia, bone cysts, and general decalcification. Differential diagnosis should exclude the presence of other causes of osteoporosis and osteomalacia.

PSEUDOHERMAPHRODITISM

Pseudohermaphroditism is a condition in which a person is distinctly one sex, possessing either testes or ovaries, but there is ambiguity or contradiction in the morphologic appearance of the other genital structures. If testes are present, the person is referred to as a male pseudohermaphrodite; if ovaries are present, the term female pseudohermaphrodite is used.

RACINE'S SYNDROME

Racine's syndrome is characterized by glandular abnormalities that may occur prior to menstruation, including swelling of the salivary glands and the breast tissues. Enlargement of the salivary glands occurs four to five days premenstrually and subsides with the onset of flow.

SYNONYM: *Premenstrual Salivary Syndrome.*

SECONDARY HYPERPARATHYROIDISM

Secondary hyperparathyroidism is a state of hyperparathyroidism in which parathyroid hyperplasia may occur. It may be noted in association with the following conditions: chronic glomerulonephritis; true rickets and osteomalacia; pregnancy; certain cases of senile osteoporosis, multiple myeloma, Cushing's syndrome, acromegaly, metastatic malignancy involving the skeleton, osteogenesis imperfecta; and steatorrhea (sprue, celiac disease).

SEXUAL PRECOCITY

Sexual precocity is a condition characterized by early sexual maturation before the age of 8 in girls and 10 in boys. The precocity may be either isosexual or heterosexual. It is generally accompanied by early somatic development.

SYNONYM: *Precocious Puberty.*

Heterosexual Precocity

Heterosexual precocity is virilization of the female or feminization of the male in childhood. It may result from a functioning tumor of the gonad, hyperplasia or tumor of the adrenal gland, or the administration of sex hormones.

Isosexual Precocity

Isosexual precocity is early maturation in the pattern normal for the patient's sex. Isoprecocity in either sex may be due to premature stimulation of the gonads by gonadotropin, autonomous release of sex steroids by the gonad or adrenal cortex (often from neoplasm), or unusual sensitivity of the sexual tissues to the normal hormone levels. The physical growth is usually accelerated.

SIMMONDS' SYNDROME

Simmonds' syndrome is characterized by a chronic, progressive endocrine deficiency with widespread disturbance of tissue and organ function resulting from failure of hormone production of the anterior lobe of the pituitary gland. The clinical features are associated with destruction of the anterior lobe. The syndrome occurs more commonly in females. The symptoms are manifold and include asthenia, progressive weight loss, often to the point of emaciation, and decreased sexual function associated with atrophy of the genital organs. There is absence of lactation and amenorrhea in women. Clinical features include loss of axillary and pubic hair, loss of beard in men, atrophic changes in the skin that give the appearance of premature aging, and a markedly decreased metabolic rate with hypothermia, bradycardia, and hypotonia. Hypoglycemia and extreme sensitivity to insulin are characteristic. Protein reserves are diminished. Gastrointestinal disorders, anemia, and achlorhydria are frequently present. Many of the symptoms are obviously related to hypofunction of the thyroid, parathyroid, and adrenal glands. Psychic changes also occur, and may show less response to treatment than do the somatic manifestations. The syndrome is caused by destruction of the anterior lobe of the hypophysis. Pathologic lesions include spontaneous atrophy and fibrosis, tumors, granulomas, and trauma. Similar effects follow excessive radiation or surgical removal.

SYNONYMS: *Pituitary Cachexia, Simmonds' Disease.*

TESTICULAR FEMINIZATION SYNDROME

The testicular feminization syndrome is a genetic type of male pseudohermaphroditism that occurs in phenotypic females with well-developed breasts and other female sex characteristics but with a paucity of pubic and axillary hair. These patients are generally first seen by the physician because of primary amenorrhea. On pelvic examination, it is noted that pubic hair is sparse or absent, the external genitalia are otherwise usually normal, but the vagina ends in a blind pouch. The uterus and fallopian tubes are absent or rudimentary; the internal ducts are usually predominantly male. The bilateral testes are usually cryptorchid but may descend and in some cases are found as the sole content of inguinal hernias. The gonadal tissue is histologically similar to that of undescended testes. Tubular adenomas are often present and occasionally malignant tumors. Studies indicate that the testes produce both estrogen and androgen. It appears, however, that in these patients there is a genetic target-organ unresponsiveness to androgen, thus accounting for the lack of development of the male genitalia and the lack of pubic and axillary hair. This condition appears to be transmitted by a sex-limited recessive or sex-limited dominant gene.

SYNONYMS: *Syndrome of Feminizing Testes, Male Pseudohermaphroditism, Syndrome of Hairless Women, Goldberg-Maxwell Syndrome, Androgynoidism.*

THYROID-ADRENOCORTICAL INSUFFICIENCY SYNDROME

The thyroid-adrenocortical insufficiency syndrome is a combination of adrenocortical insufficiency (Addison's disease) and chronic thyroiditis, XO karyotype. In some instances, a few follicles or epithelioid tissue may also coexist. There is some overlay in the early symptomatic period; however, the symptomatology, clinical observations, and laboratory findings permit ready differentiation in advanced stages. There is usually a lowered basal metabolic rate in both conditions. Thyroid insufficiency may be proved by the finding of decreased plasma protein-bound iodine and a low thyroidal radioactive iodine (^{131}I) uptake. Adrenocortical insufficiency may be confirmed by decreased serum sodium, increased potassium, and decreased plasma cortisol levels. With occasional exceptions, the adrenal disorder occurs first and thyroid insufficiency appears subsequently. Antiadrenal and antithyroid bodies are increased in these cases, and the condition is now thought to be the result of an autoimmunity process.

SYNONYM: *Schmidt's (M.B.) Syndrome.*

TIMME'S SYNDROME

Timme's syndrome is characterized by ovarian and adrenal insufficiency with compensatory hypopituitarism.

TURNER'S SYNDROME

Turner's syndrome is a genetic abnormality occurring in phenotypic females characterized by dwarfism, sexual infantilism, webbing of the neck, and cubitus valgus. These persons have rudimentary gonads consisting of streaks of connective tissue devoid of germ cells. Most of these persons are sex chromatin-negative, and have 45 chromosomes with an XO karyotype. In some instances, a few follicles or epithelioid tissue may be present in the streak gonad. Many variations of the syndrome have been described and are grouped under the general term *gonadal dysgenesis.* A large variety of other associated somatic stigmata has been noted, including an underdeveloped mandible; a high arched palate; a broad shieldlike chest with widely spaced, immature nipples; large, dark, elevated moles on the face and neck; low-set ears; a low posterior hairline, and many others. When none of the somatic stigmata are present, the condition may be referred to as *pure gonadal dysgenesis.* If a testis is present on one side and a streak gonad on the other with both wolffian and müllerian gonadal accessories, the term *male Turner syndrome* is used to describe phenotypic males with short stature, webbed neck, and hypoplastic testes. Many types of chromosomal aberrations have been found in patients with gonadal dysgenesis, including a variety of mosaic patterns such as XO/XX, XO/XXX, XO/XX/XXX, and XO/XY, and structural defects of the X and Y chromosomes. Hormonal assays in Turner's syndrome and its variants show markedly elevated urinary gonadotropins, very low estrogen levels, and normal or moderately diminished 17-ketosteroid levels.

SYNONYMS: *Turner-Albright Syndrome, Turner-Varny Syndrome, Gonadal Dysgenesis, Ovarian-Short Stature Syndrome, Gonadal Agenesis, Genital Dwarfism Syndrome, Pterygonuchal Infantilism Syndrome, Ovarian Agenesis, Ovarian Dwarfism, Ovarian Aplasia, Congenitally Absent Ovaries Syndrome, Rudimentary Ovary Syndrome, Morgagni-Turner Syndrome, Morgagni-Turner-Albright Syndrome, Shereshevskii-Turner Syndrome, Primary Ovarian Insufficiency, Pseudonuchal Infantilism, XO Sex Chromosome Constitution, XO Syndrome.*

VIRILIZATION

Virilization is the development of male secondary sex characteristics in the female due to stimulation of the responsive tissues by excessive androgen. The increased androgen produces increased facial and body hair, a male alopecia pattern in some, increased sebaceous gland secretion, enlarged clitoris, deepening of the voice, defeminization in the adult female, amenorrhea, and ovarian failure. The source of androgen is generally the adrenal cortex, but the ovary may also produce the hormone.

SECTION 5: SELECTED GYNECOLOGIC TOPICS

Syndromes

ABRUPTIO PLACENTAE SYNDROME

The abruptio placentae syndrome is a syndrome characterized by the abnormal separation of a normally implanted placenta, hypofibrino-genemia, hemorrhage, and shock. The incidence varies from 1 in 85 to 1 in 250 deliveries. The onset of symptoms is subacute or abrupt and consists of severe abdominal pain caused by tetanic contractions of the uterus, marked vaginal hemorrhage from incoagulable blood, and beginning shock. Abruptio placentae is the most widely recognized complication of hypofibrinogenemia. Clinical symptoms occur at a level below 150 mg per 100 cc of plasma fibrinogen concentration, with a critical level at 90 mg or below. The degree of defibrination is coincident with and apparently directly proportional to the severity of the placental abruption. The placenta often shows either many infarcts or a large retroplacental hematoma. Uterine infiltration of suffused blood is sometimes found, a so-called Couvelaire uterus. The cause of the syndrome may be hypertensive disorders of pregnancy, chronic glomerulonephritis, chronic vascular disease, or trauma. Differential diagnosis should exclude placenta previa, in which the bleeding is painless and tetanic contractions of the uterus and fibrinogen depression are absent; and a ruptured uterus, in which pain is localized at the site of the rupture.

ACHARD-THIERS SYNDROME

The Achard-Thiers syndrome is a rare syndrome characterized by diabetes mellitus, hirsutism, and hypertension in women. It is seen predominantly in middle-aged and elderly females. Conspicuous clinical characteristics are a masculine type of hypertrichosis of the face, voice changes, hypertrophy of the clitoris, and a masculine type of body build. Recessive function of sexual organs includes irregular or absent menstruation and atrophy of the breasts. Obesity of the trunk, striae, acne, hypertension, and occasionally osteoporosis may be evident. Carbohydrate tolerance is decreased. The cause of the symptom complex is as yet uncertain, although it is thought to be associated with adrenal cortical dysfunction.

SYNONYM: *Diabetic-Bearded Women Syndrome.*

ACROMEGALY

Acromegaly is characterized by heavy bone and soft tissue facial features, prognathism, marked enlargement of hands and feet, and some enlargement of the forearms and other bones. Many tissues and organs share in the hypertrophic changes. External genitalia are rarely affected.

Morphologic findings in the gonads are variable, although generally the ovaries become inactive. Occasionally, however, pregnancy may occur. A decrease in libido and potentia eventually ensues. Headache and visual disturbance are common symptoms, a sequel of the causative pituitary tumor. The syndrome is due to an excessive secretion of the growth hormone of the anterior portion of the pituitary gland, usually from a chromophil (eosinophilic) adenoma. If the hyperplasia and hypersecretion begin before puberty, gigantism ensues.

SYNONYMS: *Eosinophilic Adenoma Syndrome, Marie's Syndrome.*

ADRENOCORTICAL INSUFFICIENCY

Adrenocortical insufficiency includes the well-known clinical picture that results from partial or complete loss of function of the adrenal cortex. It occurs as a primary disorder (*Addison's disease*), but may in a small percentage of cases be secondary to pituitary deficiency. Symptoms, often insidious, include weakness, asthenia, and gastrointestinal manifestations. Anemia, arterial hypotension, decreased metabolic rate, hypoglycemia, decreased serum sodium and chloride, and an increased serum potassium are supporting diagnostic indications. In primary adrenal failure, pigmentary changes of external genitalia and mucous membranes frequently parallel the degree of hormonal deficiency. The characteristic pigmentation of the skin and mucous membranes is not present in adrenal failure secondary to pituitary insufficiency (*Simmonds' disease, Sheehan's syndrome*). Stress, trauma, or surgery may precipitate a crisis that threatens life. In Addison's disease, the urinary 17-hydroxycorticosteroids and 17-ketosteroids, and the plasma cortisol are very low and fail to increase following adrenocorticotropic hormone stimulation, whereas there is a significant increase in secondary adrenal failure.

ADRENOGENITAL SYNDROME

The adrenogenital syndrome in women is characterized by an increased secretion of adrenal androgens, resulting in virilization. A recessively transmitted hereditary type may begin in utero. Usual symptoms include signs of defeminization, premature growth of pubic and axillary hair, hirsutism, excessive muscular development, short stature in the adult, amenorrhea, and a masculine voice. In female infants, varying degrees of abnormalities and ambiguity of the external genitalia are evident. In childhood the syndrome is usually due to hyperplasia of the adrenal cortex with excess secretion of androgens resulting from a congenital defect of steroidogenesis, of which several types have been described. The urinary 17-ketosteroids and pregnanetriol are generally elevated. The plasma cortisol levels may be low, particularly in the salt-losing types. Sudden death in the newborn may occur due to cortisol deficiency. Onset of the syndrome during childhood may be due to a functioning adrenal tumor or virilizing tumor of the ovary. Virilizing adrenal hyperplasia may also have its onset at puberty or soon thereafter.

SYNONYMS: *Adrenal Virilism Syndrome, Congenital Virilizing Adrenocortical Hyperplasia Syndrome.*

AHUMADA-DEL CASTILLO SYNDROME

The Ahumada-Del Castillo syndrome is a triad of amenorrhea, low gonadotropin secretion, and galactorrhea unrelated to pregnancy.

ALBRIGHT'S SYNDROME

Albright's syndrome is a rare syndrome characterized by dysplasia of bone, brown-pigmented areas of the skin, and sexual and somatic precocity in females. The syndrome usually occurs in children or young adults. The multiple bone lesions are characterized by a fibrous dysplastic replacement of the medullary structure. Pelvic bones and the lower extremities are most often affected. These lesions may not be recognized until a pathologic fracture occurs in childhood or early adult life. The degree of pigmentation often parallels the extent of skeletal involvement. These cafe-au-lait spots occur more often on the same side as the bone lesion and are found most frequently on the scalp, back of the neck, upper spine, the sacrum, and thighs. Oral pigmentation has also been reported. Associated endocrine features consist of unusual sexual precocity with early menarche, enlargement of breasts, and the development of adolescent external genitalia. Sterility is not a later factor. Normal 17-ketosteroid values rule out an adrenocortical tumor. Urinary follicle-stimulating hormone excretion, serum calcium, and serum phosphorus values are also normal. Serum phosphatase is often elevated. The bone changes are usually progressive until growth ceases. Treatment of fractures and orthopedic correction of deformities may be necessary.

SYNONYMS: *Albright-McCune-Sternberg Syndrome, McCune-Albright Syndrome, Polyostotic Fibrous Dysplasia, Wright's Syndrome, Osteitis Fibrosa Disseminata.*

AMNIOTIC FLUID SYNDROME

The amniotic fluid syndrome is caused by the sudden intravenous infusion of a large volume of amniotic fluid, which causes pulmonary edema and pulmonary embolic phenomena. Clinically, cardiopulmonary distress, obstetric shock, and sometimes sudden death occur. The postulated factors consist of defibrination, massive fibrin embolism, and embolization from the particulate material contained in the amniotic fluid. Laboratory studies usually reveal a depression of fibrinogen, characteristic of defibrination with hemorrhagic phenomena, and evidence of a fibrinogen-fibrin conversion syndrome. The embolic syndrome is the result of a break in the wall of a blood vessel. It occurs during long labors, in traumatic births (forceps operation), in the dead fetus syndrome, in elderly women, and with large fetuses. The syndrome should be differentiated from other causes of sudden death, including massive intraabdominal hemorrhage from a ruptured uterine vein. The course is rapid, and the prognosis is always serious with survival in doubt.

ANGIECTID SYNDROME

The angiectid syndrome is characterized by a type of superficial venous lesion that appears during the first trimester of pregnancy. These vascular abnormalities occur on the posterior thigh and calf areas and consist of small, intradermal, raised, sharply circumscribed clumps of blood vessels. The areas are tender, have increased local temperature, and may be painful. They are not related in any way to thrombophlebitis or to the commonplace saphenous varicosities of pregnancy. A distinct etiologic relationship exists between these lesions and the level of female sex hormones, more particularly with variations in the titers of serum estrogen and urinary pregnanediol. Patients with the most painful lesions show the greatest degree of estrogen or pregnanediol deficiency. After a few weeks, the lesions sometimes disappear spontaneously, but they usually continue longer, often throughout pregnancy and for a few weeks postpartum.

ASHERMANN SYNDROME

The Ashermann syndrome is a condition of intrauterine adhesions and infection generally created by frequent and vigorous curettage. The endometrial cavity is practically obliterated and amenorrhea is a persistent sign.

SYNONYM: *Traumatic Intrauterine Synechiae.*

BAR'S SYNDROME

Bar's syndrome is characterized by pain in the region of the gallbladder, ureters, or appendix, and is accompanied by fever and bacteriuria. The bacilli may invade the circulation and become localized in organs of predilection. This syndrome is observed most often during pregnancy; it is perhaps related to constipation. If present during the puerperium, the syndrome may simulate puerperal infection.

SYNONYM: *Colibacillose Gravidique.*

BILIRUBIN ENCEPHALOPATHY SYNDROME

Bilirubin encephalopathy syndrome is characterized by damage to the central nervous system from the toxic effects of bilirubin on cerebral tissues. The syndrome follows an attack of icterus gravis neonatorum. A rare recessive gene is thought responsible. Clinical manifestations may include a slowing of mental development, an intention tremor, progressive slurring of speech, and perhaps later a disturbance in gait. Among the suspected causes of this syndrome are: incompatibility of the blood of the parents, and diminished capacity of the hepatic cells to metabolize and excrete bilirubin. The syndrome may be differentiated from the neurologic features of kernicterus, a closely related condition, in which deposition of pathologic amounts of biliary pigment is limited essentially to the basal nuclei.

CHIARI-FROMMEL SYNDROME

The Chiari-Frommel syndrome is a condition characterized by persistent postpartum amenorrhea and galactorrhea, and atrophy of the uterus and ovaries probably due to hypothalamic dysfunction. The diagnosis is generally entertained in women who have amenorrhea and lactation for more than a year following delivery or cessation of nursing, and in whom no organic lesion of the central nervous system can be demonstrated by appropriate studies. Gonadotropins and estrogens are markedly diminished. Other endocrine studies are generally normal. Spontaneous recovery may occur after prolonged intervals. Recurrence may be noted after subsequent pregnancies.

SYNONYMS: *Frommel's Disease, Persistent Postpartum Amenorrhea-Galactorrhea Syndrome.*

CONGENITAL ADRENAL HYPERPLASIA SYNDROME

The congenital adrenal hyperplasia syndrome is a genetic disorder of steroid metabolism resulting in virilization in both sexes. In the female child, the external genitalia are often ambiguous. The syndrome is generally characterized by elevated urinary 17-ketosteroids and pregnanetriol, progressive virilization, and large amounts of abnormal adrenal steroids in the urine. There are several forms of the syndrome, including uncomplicated or compensate C_{21} hydroxylase deficiency; salt-losing C_{21} hydroxylase deficiency; a hypertensive type (a relatively rare form) due to a C_{11} hydroxylation defect; and 3β-hydroxysteroid dehydrogenase deficiency. The synthesis of cortisol is blocked by lack of a different enzyme for each of the four forms.

SYNONYMS: *Congenital Adrenogenital Syndrome, Virilizing Adrenal Hyperplasia.*

CONSUMPTIVE COAGULOPATHY SYNDROME

Consumptive coagulopathy syndrome is characterized by severe depletion of fibrinogen and reduction of platelet number in patients undergoing termination of pregnancy by infusion of hypertonic intraamniotic salt between the 16th and 20th week of gestation. Fibrinolysis breakdown products increase and Factor V decreases consecutively. Antithrombin III, alpha-2-macroglobulin, and plasminogen remain unchanged. The decreased values return to normal 12 to 24 hours after expulsion of the fetus. There is no evidence of fibrin deposition in the microcirculation as evidenced by unchanged values of plasma hemoglobin. Although the coagulopathy is self-limited, it may provide a potential danger of serious bleeding complications in some patients.

CORPUS LUTEIN DEFICIENCY SYNDROME

Corpus lutein deficiency syndrome is a syndrome of insufficient luteinization in the ovaries. Symptoms include fatigue regardless of effort or rest, nervousness, irritability, depression, and emotional instability with weeping at the slightest provocation. Irregular menses, dysmenorrhea, ovulation pains, premenstrual headaches, and partial or total frigidity are often present. Functional disturbances include tachycardia and palpitation, dyspnea, dermographia, elevated blood pressure, and blotchy flushing over the face, neck, and chest. Fibrocystic degeneration in breast tissue may be found. The disorder is frequently the cause of relative sterility and early abortion. The cause is not known. Postulated causative factors are polycystic ovaritis and inhibition of ovarian function preceding menopause.

CUSHING'S SYNDROME

Cushing's syndrome is a condition resulting from excess secretion of the adrenal cortical hormones, particularly the glucocorticoids (cortisol group). It is characterized clinically by a truncal type of obesity with relatively thin extremities, rounding and plethora of the face, well-marked purplish striae, thinning of the skin with easy bruising, slight to marked hirsutism, hypertension, and amenorrhea. Later complications include osteoporosis, crush fractures of the vertebrae, and diabetes. The condition may result from bilateral adrenal hyperplasia or benign or malignant tumors of the adrenal cortex. In some instances, there may be a basophilic adenoma of the pituitary (Cushing's disease). In rare instances, the syndrome may result from adrenocorticotropic hormone-secreting tumors of the ovary or nonendocrine structures. The diagnosis is confirmed by the findings of an elevated plasma cortisol with absence of diurnal variation. In hyperplasia cases, the plasma and urinary corticosteroids are suppressed by dexamethasone and increased by adrenocorticotropic hormone stimulation and adrenal tumors are generally autonomous.

DEAD FETUS SYNDROME

The dead fetus syndrome is characterized by the lengthy intrauterine retention of a dead fetus associated with hemorrhage of incoagulable blood. Decreased fibrinogen values between 250 and 150 mg per 100 cc of plasma concentration have been observed in this syndrome, although frank hemorrhage seldom occurs until the level reaches 90 mg or less. Few accompanying symptoms may be present before onset of the hemorrhage aside from persistent tachycardia, which is almost a constant feature. The syndrome is not always associated with Rh incompatibility inasmuch as Rh-positive patients with a negative Coombs test have been observed. Fibrinogen depression usually develops in chronic fashion. Defibrination may become apparent weeks before the onset of labor. Although fibrinogen recovery begins with the emptying of the uterus, low values may continue. The optimum time for interrupting the pregnancy in the dead fetus syndrome depends on the level of fibrinogen recovery after transfusion or the administration of fibrinogen.

DORSALGIA-GYNECOLOGIC SYNDROME

The dorsalgia-gynecologic syndrome is characterized by thoracic and lumbosacral pain in women with functional gynecologic disorders. The thoracic pain is unilateral with radicular reference. It varies from a dull ache to a paroxysmal lancinating pain. Roentgenography reveals flattening of the thoracic vertebrae, with a squamous aspect of the cartilage. Hemisacralization or sacralization of the fifth lumbar vertebra is frequently observed. The functional endocrine disturbance includes menstrual abnormality and painful breasts.

DYSTOCIA-DYSTROPHIA SYNDROME

The dystocia-dystrophia syndrome is a syndrome that concerns the improbability of normal vaginal birth of an overmature fetus, the head of which does not engage and the position of which is occiput posterior.

Both fetal and maternal dystocia contribute to the failure of normal events. As a rule the mother has conceived for the first time rather late in life, or perhaps has had previous unsuccessful pregnancies. In body habitus, she is heavyset, with girdle obesity; has a masculine type of pelvis, small cervix, and narrow, rigid vagina; and exhibits other signs of dystrophia adiposogenitalis. The pelvic measurements are decreased. Pregnancy is prolonged, and there is disproportion between the fetal head and the maternal pelvis. The fetal head is not engaged when labor begins, the membranes rupture prematurely, and uterine contractions are weak, resulting in a protracted first stage of labor.

FEMALE PROSTATIC OBSTRUCTING SYNDROME

The female prostatic obstructing syndrome is characterized by bladder irritation, a sense of obstruction, difficulty in voiding, and at times complete urinary retention. The most common symptom is bladder irritation with difficulty in voiding. The urine may be clear or show marked pyuria that originates from the posterior part of the urethra. Urine from the kidney is clear. Cystoscopy reveals a normal bladder mucosa. Cystography reveals a filling defect in the region of the internal orifice. In most instances, there is fibromuscular hypertrophy with fibrous hyperplasia producing collarets and cicatricial contractions.

FETAL ASPIRATION SYNDROME

The fetal aspiration syndrome is characterized by aspiration of the amniotic sac contents by the fetus. It may occur at term, but it is often associated with post-term infants. This neonatal distress syndrome ensues when the demands of the fetus for food and oxygen outgrow placental capacity. Aside from malnutrition, there is yellow staining of skin and nails and aspiration of meconium and keratinized squamous cells into distal bronchi. Symptoms are not pathognomonic. Pulmonary findings, often complicated by focal hemorrhage or pneumonia, include hyperresonance, loud breath sounds, and coarse rales. Roentgenographic findings of this syndrome are fairly characteristic with coarse and irregular streaks of interstitial markings and areas of focal irregularities of aeration. By contrast, the roentgenographic pattern in hyaline membrane disease shows a fine, diffuse miliary or stippled increase in density. As a rule, pulmonary features show evidence of clearing within 24 hours. The condition is much less frequent and hazardous than hyaline membrane disease.

FIBRINOGEN-FIBRIN CONVERSION SYNDROME

The fibrinogen-fibrin conversion syndrome is characterized by a degree of hypofibrinogenemia that causes incoagulable blood. It is a factor in three obstetric complications: abruptio placentae, amniotic fluid syndrome, and prolonged retention of a dead fetus in an Rh-isosensitized mother. The failure of coagulation, which relates to fibrinogen-fibrin conversion, may also occur in Sheehan's syndrome, bilateral renal cortical necrosis, hemolytic blood reactions, and surgical or accidental trauma.

Clinically, this syndrome has two pathologic potentialities—embolism and hemorrhage. Decreasing fibrinogen values, determined by serial blood studies, indicate the degree of depletion due to intravascular conversion of fibrinogen to fibrin. Hyperthromboplastinemia, with its defibrinating influence, is one accepted cause. Blood incoagulability occurs when fibrinogenopenia reaches a critical level of 90 mg per 100 cc. If a seriously depressed level is reached suddenly, embolic phenomena may predominate, or hemorrhage and embolic manifestations may occur. Shock is a common sequel to either state. Other accompanying abnormalities include decreased Ac-globulin, prothrombin, and platelets. The onset of the syndrome may not depend on placental separation. If decreasing fibrinogen blood values continue to drop downward from 150 mg per 100 cc to the critical level, pregnancy should be terminated.

SYNONYMS: *Acquired Afibrinogenemia, Defibrination Syndrome.*

FITZ-HUGH SYNDROME

The Fitz-Hugh syndrome consists of pain in the right upper quadrant of the abdomen occurring in young women during gonococcic pelvic inflammatory disease. Since the advent of antibiotic therapy, this complication is less often encountered. After the onset of acute pelvic inflammatory disease, pain and tenderness may develop in the right upper quadrant. Additional symptoms may include nausea and vomiting, chills, fever, sweats, and headache. The route of spread of the infection from the pelvis is thought to be through the retroperitoneal lymphatic channels.

SYNONYMS: *Fitz-Hugh-Curtis Syndrome, Subcostal Syndrome of Stajano, Gonococcic Peritonitis of Upper Abdomen.*

FORBES-ALBRIGHT SYNDROME

Forbes-Albright syndrome is a combination of galactorrhea with amenorrhea and low urinary follicle-stimulating hormone (FSH), unassociated with recent pregnancy or with acromegaly. Overproduction of prolactin is a suspected etiologic factor. Pituitary tumors are frequently associated.

SYNONYM: *Argonz-Del Castillo Syndrome.*

FOX-FORDYCE SYNDROME

The Fox-Fordyce syndrome is characterized by a rare, chronic, lichenoid eruption involving the nipple areas, axillae, and pubic and sternal regions. The eruption consists of dry papules, a result of obstruction at the orifice of hair follicles; the apocrine glands are therefore distended. Pruritus is intense and sometimes almost intolerable. The condition occurs mostly in females.

SYNONYM: *Fox-Fordyce Disease.*

FRÖHLICH'S SYNDROME

Fröhlich's syndrome is a syndrome resulting from a hypothalamic or pituitary lesion accompanied by obvious physical characteristics, including obesity and retarded sexual development. In the female, menstruation fails to appear at puberty or may cease in the postpubertal period. In the male, the voice remains high-pitched, the testes remain undescended, facial hair is absent, and there is a feminine pubic line. The neurologic and other endocrine manifestations depend on the site and extent of the lesion. Roentgenographic studies may show enlargement or destruction of the sella turcica or suprasellar calcification, suggesting a craniopharyngioma. Other pituitary effects include polyuria, polydypsia, increased sugar tolerance, and reduction or absence of urinary gonadotropins. The most typical form of Fröhlich's syndrome arises from Rathke-pouch tumors or craniopharyngiomas. Chromophobe adenomas, trauma, and inflammatory lesions may also be a cause.

SYNONYMS: *Adiposogenital Dystrophy Syndrome, Dystrophia Adiposogenitalis Syndrome, Neuropituitary Dystrophy Syndrome, Pituitary Infantilism of Adults, Cerebral Adiposity Syndrome.*

GALACTORRHEA SYNDROMES

Several galactorrhea syndromes are now recognized, depending on the underlying etiologic factor. The galactorrhea varies from extrusion of a few drops of whitish secretion to an abundant and spontaneous flow of milk. Usually, but not invariably, there is an associated amenorrhea or menstrual dysfunction. In some instances, the galactorrhea and amenorrhea may be a persistence of the postpartum state; in others they are nonpuerperal. Some cases are due to dysfunction; others may be associated with organic lesions, particularly of the central nervous system and pituitary; still others may be of iatrogenic origin. The following classification is based on the etiologic factors:

Dysfunctional.
1. Chiari-Frommel syndrome. Persistent postpartum amenorrhea and galactorrhea.
2. Ahumada-Del Castillo syndrome. Nonpuerperal.
3. Hypothyroidism.
Associated with an organic lesion of the central nervous system.
1. Forbes-Albright syndrome. Most of these patients have a chromophobe adenoma.
2. Acromegaly.
3. Extrasellar lesions, such as craniopharyngiomas, meningiomas, and sarcoidosis.
Local lesions involving chest wall, such as post-thoracotomy lesions, and Herpes zoster.
Iatrogenic.
Psychopharmacologic drugs such as reserpine, chlorpromazine, and methyldopa.
Hormonal. Following the use of the oral contraceptives.

GORDAN-OVERSTREET SYNDROME

The Gordan-Overstreet syndrome is a syndrome that presents the characteristics of Turner's syndrome with virilization that apparently arises from secreting epithelioid cells of the dysgenetic gonad. Evidence of androgenic activity is seen in hirsutism and hypertrophy of the clitoris. Predominant masculinity may be proved by skin biopsy or smears from buccal mucous membranes.

SYNONYM: *Androgenicity-Gonadal Dysgenesis Syndrome.*

GUILLAIN-BARRÉ SYNDROME

The Guillain-Barré syndrome is characterized by multiple peripheral nerve involvement, chiefly at the extremities, plus cranial nerve implication, usually of both facial nerves. Microscopically the cerebrospinal fluid exhibits few or no cells, and it has a high protein content that rises as the disease progresses. The patient tends to recover spontaneously.

SYNONYMS: *Landry-Guillain-Barré Syndrome, Guillain-Barré-Strohl Syndrome, Landry's Paralysis, Primary Infectious Polyneuritis, Radicular Neuritis, Acute Polyradiculitis, Motoneuronitis, Myeloradiculitis, Polyradiculoneuritis, Acute Infectious Polyneuritis, Infectious Neuronitis, Polyneuritis with Facial Diplegia, Neuritis with Albuminocytologic Dissociation.*

HERPES GESTATIONIS SYNDROME

The herpes gestationis syndrome is a relatively rare exanthema that occurs as a complication of the latter half of pregnancy or during the early phase of the puerperium. The condition occurs most commonly in women 30 to 35 years old. Symptoms include fever, malaise, dyspnea, burning sensation, neuralgic pains, and intense pruritus. The cutaneous lesions consist of bullae and vesicles that are present over the chest, abdomen, and extremities. The syndrome may occur with each gestation or during every second or third pregnancy. Exacerbations are likely, even during treatment. Recurrences may occasionally extend into the puerperium as episodes of severe pruritus, prior to the first few menstrual periods. These episodes are called *herpes menstrualis recidivans.* The higher incidence of erythroblastosis fetalis, spontaneous abortions, monstrosities, and stillborn infants among women who seem predisposed to herpes gestationis may be an expression of Rh incompatibility or isosensitization.

SYNONYMS: *Duhring's Disease, Brocq-Duhring Disease, Dermatitis Herpetiformis, Dermatitis Multiformis, Dermatitis Neurotica, Dermatitis Polymorpha Dolorosa, Dermatitis Pruriginosa, Dermatitis Trophoneurotica, Herpes Circinatus Bullosus, Hydroa Herpetiformis, Hydroa Pruriginosa, Pemphigus Circinatus, Fetal Anomaly Syndrome, Dermatitis Herpetiformis Gestationis Syndrome, Hydroa Gravidarum, Pemphigus Pruriginosus, Prurigo Gestationis Syndrome.*

HIRSUTISM SYNDROMES

Excessive hair growth on the face or body in women may occur on a genetic, racial, or constitutional basis. Idiopathic hypertrichosis may occur at puberty, during or immediately after pregnancy, following the menopause, after severe burns, and during starvation and stress. Hirsutism of varying degree is noted in association with the following syndromes: adrenogenital syndrome, Cushing's syndrome, masculinizing tumors of the ovary, polycystic ovarian disease, hyperthecosis of the ovary, Achard-Thiers syndrome, and cretinism.

HUTCHINSON-GILFORD SYNDROME

The Hutchinson-Gilford syndrome is characterized by infantilism, facial and pubic alopecia, and premature aging. The syndrome does not appear to be familial or hereditary, and either sex may be affected. Clinically, there is no abnormality at birth, but there follows a failure to gain weight, limitation of growth, and loss of hair. Dwarfism gradually develops. The appearance of these patients is characteristic and has been described as that of premature old age. There is a small face, projecting eyes, beaked nose, and receding chin. Scalp veins are prominent, and the lower jaw is micrognathic with crowded and irregular teeth. There may be a high, arched palate, marked baldness, absence of eyebrows and lashes, marked atrophy and inelasticity of the skin, and absence of subcutaneous fat except in the pubic region. The chest is narrow, the abdomen protrudes, and the fingernails may show trophic changes or may be absent. Until puberty the genitalia are normal, but thereafter little sexual maturation occurs. The muscles are poorly developed, and the limbs are thin. The cause of this syndrome is not known.

SYNONYMS: *Progeria Syndrome, Premature Senility Syndrome, Gilford's Syndrome, Senilism Syndrome.*

HYPOPARATHYROIDISM SYNDROME

The hypoparathyroidism syndrome results in chronic hypocalcemia with varied and widespread neuromuscular effects. It may be classified etiologically under three headings: postoperative (following thyroidectomy), idiopathic, and following organic lesions of the parathyroids. Postoperative hypoparathyroidism is by far the most common variety. Symptoms of the idiopathic variety may be varied and vague; mild cases of this syndrome may not be recognized for many years, sometimes decades. Characteristic symptoms include fatigue, muscular weakness, paresthesia and cramps of extremities, tetany, muscular hyperexcitability, and laryngeal stridor. Tetany is the outstanding clinical manifestation of hypoparathyroidism; it may be latent or manifest. Other manifestations include delayed and defective dentition, trophic nail changes, and cataracts. Personality changes, mental retardation, attacks of unconsciousness, and general convulsions may be present. Because convulsive manifestations are accompanied by an epileptic encephalographic pattern, it has been postulated that hypocalcemia precipitates convulsive seizures in susceptible individuals. Idiopathic hypoparathyroidism is thus often misdiagnosed as epilepsy. The diagnosis of idiopathic tetany depends chiefly on differentiating it from other forms of tetany. Diagnostic criteria include: low serum calcium level, elevated serum inorganic phosphorus level, chronic latent tetany, the absence of severe renal insufficiency, and normal roentgenograms of bone. Electrocardiographic changes often show a prolongation of the QT interval.

HYPOPITUITARISM SYNDROMES

Several syndromes may result from a deficiency of the anterior pituitary gland, depending on the number of hormones involved, the period of life at which the condition occurs, and the nature of the underlying lesion. The term *panhypopituitarism* is generally used to indicate complete or nearly complete loss of adenohypophysial function. The resulting condition is often described under the terms of *Simmonds-Sheehan disease, Simmonds' syndrome, Sheehan's syndrome, and pituitary cachexia.* Panhypopituitarism is characterized by a chronic progressive endocrine deficiency, with widespread disturbance of tissue and organ function resulting from failure of hormone production by the anterior lobe of the pituitary gland. The syndrome occurs more commonly in females. The symptoms are manifold and include asthenia, hypotension, anemia, progressive weight loss that may progress to severe cachexia, and decreased sexual function associated with atrophy of the genital organs. Clinical features also include loss of axillary and pubic hair, atrophic changes in the skin, markedly decreased metabolic rate with hypothermia, and in women, amenorrhea and failure of lactation. The syndrome is caused by destruction of the anterior lobe of the pituitary gland. Pathologic lesions include postpartum necrosis of the pituitary, usually associated with severe hemorrhage at the time of delivery, spontaneous atrophy and fibrosis, destruction by chromophobe adenoma, and traumatic injuries. Similar effects may follow excessive radiation or surgical removal. Hypopituitarism in childhood may be associated with dwarfism and sexual infantilism. *Pituitary dwarfism* may be associated with a detectable lesion in the pituitary or parasellar regions or may be due to a genetic deficiency of growth hormones and gonadotropic hormones.

LAUNOIS-CLÉRET SYNDROME

The Launois-Cléret syndrome is characterized by obesity and lack of development of internal or external genitalia in children. The general and endocrinopathic features of this hypophysial dystrophy are essentially similar to those of Fröhlich's syndrome.

SYNONYM: *Hypophysial-Adiposogenital Syndrome.*

MATERNAL OBESITY SYNDROME

The maternal obesity syndrome is a syndrome characterized by rapid and excessive gain in weight during pregnancy or after childbirth. Related endocrine factors include the large baby-diabetic syndrome, frank diabetes, a diabetic glucose tolerance curve, and the features of Cushing's syndrome.

MATERNAL SYNDROME

The maternal syndrome is characterized by general pruritus, ankle edema, a sudden marked gain in weight, polyhydramnios, and impending fetal death due to isoimmunization. In addition to the essential features, there may be albuminuria and hypertension. Insofar as can be determined, the fetus remains alive until the onset of the syndrome, which is usually prior to the 36th week of pregnancy. Fetal death varies from 2 to 21 days after the onset of symptoms in the mother. The syndrome does not subside until pregnancy is terminated. The etiologic agent is thought to be the severely affected erythroblastotic fetus or its placenta.

MEIGS' SYNDROME

Meigs' syndrome is characterized by an ovarian tumor, usually a fibroma, which is accompanied by ascites and hydrothorax. The clinical symptoms relate directly to the degree of ascites and hydrothorax. The amount of fluid in the abdomen does not necessarily determine the amount to be found in the chest and vice versa. The clear yellow transudate from each cavity yields a similar chemical analysis. Experiments with particles of carbon have shown a rapid and irreversible passage of the ascitic fluid into the thoracic cavity. It is generally agreed that the fluid originates from the ovarian tumor. The tumor in most instances has the gross appearance of a benign, solid fibroma.

synonyms: *Demons-Meigs Syndrome, Ovarian-Ascites-Pleural Effusion Syndrome, Meigs-Coss Syndrome.*

MENOPAUSAL SYNDROME

The menopausal syndrome is characterized by symptomatic, psychosomatic, and psychoneurotic manifestations that are experienced by some women during the climacteric period. Symptoms include hot flashes, chills, sweats, headache, nervousness, irritability, and depression. Other features may consist of palpitation, dizziness, and gastrointestinal symptoms with epigastric reference. The symptoms are transient, recurrent, and mild to severe. Although the syndrome may be induced by oophorectomy or irradiation, the cause is commonly attributed to gradual aging of the ovaries with hypofunction. Although most women experience menopause by the age of 50, some are unaware of any symptoms inasmuch as significant amounts of estrogen continue to be produced after the menopause. The normal source of such estrogen is the adrenal cortex, which apparently continues throughout life to produce amounts adequate for metabolic requirements.

synonym: *Climacteric Syndrome.*

NEPHROTIC SYNDROME

Nephrotic syndrome results from many underlying diseases such as glomerulonephritis, lupus nephritis, diabetic nephropathy, and amyloidosis. Edema, massive proteinuria, hypoalbuminemia, and increased blood cholesterol levels are clinically evident.

synonyms: *Epstein's Syndrome, Idiopathic Nephrotic Syndrome.*

PAXSON'S SYNDROME

Paxson's syndrome is a syndrome that may occur as a result of obstetric and gynecologic complications. The features include primary injury to tissue; the presence or absence of shock; suppression of urine with urinary casts and leukocytes; and elevation of blood urea nitrogen, which attains its maximum increase between the fifth and ninth days. The syndrome occurs in three obstetric and gynecologic conditions: placental separation with retroplacental hematoma, ruptured uterus, and hemorrhagic twisted ovarian cyst. It is believed that bloody infiltration into any type of cellular tissue may be responsible for the elaboration of toxic metabolites with resulting renal damage. Thus, this syndrome should be suspected in any severe gynecologic hemorrhagic condition.

SYNONYMS: *Paxson's Crush Syndrome, Obstetric-Gynecologic-Crush Syndrome.*

PLACENTAL HEMANGIOMA SYNDROME

The placental hemangioma syndrome is characterized by placental hemangiomas, polyhydramnios, prematurity, an increased incidence of stillborn infants, and a variety of major congenital abnormalities. Other features consist of antepartum hemorrhage and premature rupture of the membranes. Placental hemangiomas appear to be the primary pathologic feature. These tumors are benign and single or multiple, and they may vary in size. They occur as an elevation on the fetal or maternal surface of the placenta, or occasionally may be attached to the umbilical cord. Large tumors near the cord are most likely to cause symptoms. Polyhydramnios is present in about a third of the cases.

PLUMMER-VINSON SYNDROME

The Plummer-Vinson syndrome is characterized by dysphagia, atrophic changes in the buccal, glossopharyngeal, and esophageal mucous membranes, spoon-shaped nails, and a microcytic, hypochromic anemia. The condition occurs predominantly in middle-aged women, rarely in the male. Anemia is usually present; if not, sideropenia (decreased plasma iron) is normally found. In addition to the symptoms characteristic of chronic anemia, there may be a dry mouth and pharynx and a sensation of nasal obstruction, which may be present a number of years before the onset of the anemia. Dysphagia, often called sideropenic dysphagia, is the most conspicuous symptom. Clinical manifestations often include stomatitis, glossitis, cheilitis, hypochlorhydria or achlorhydria, splenomegaly, and the characteristic spoon-shaped brittle nails.

SYNONYMS: *Paterson's Syndrome, Kelly-Paterson Syndrome, Sideropenic Dysphagia Syndrome, Sideropenic Nasopharyngopathy Syndrome, Waldenström-Kjellberg Syndrome.*

POLYCYSTIC OVARIAN DISEASE

Polycystic ovarian disease is an entity associated with polycystic ovaries and clinical symptoms and signs such as oligomenorrhea, anovulation, infertility, and hirsutism. Grossly, the ovaries are enlarged and oyster gray, and they have a firm, smooth cortex indicating no evidence of ovulation or corpus luteum formation. The tunica albuginea is thickened, tough, and fibrous. Many trapped follicles in all stages of development are present underneath the tunica albuginea. Microscopically, multiple cysts are present in the cortex without corpus luteum formation. Marked hyperplasia of the theca interna of the atretic follicles is frequent. Urinary 17-ketosteroids and plasma testosterone levels are usually normal or slightly elevated. Gonadotropin levels vary. The condition is associated with a defect in ovarian steroidogenesis favoring the production of androgenic steroids at the expense of the estrogens. The underlying cause is not known. A relative enzyme deficiency in the ovary has been postulated. In the differential diagnosis, it is important to rule out other conditions that may be associated with bilateral cystic ovaries and hirsutism, including adrenogenital syndrome, Cushing's syndrome, and pituitary or hypothalamic lesions.

SYNONYMS: *Stein-Leventhal Syndrome, Stein's Syndrome, Bilateral Polycystic Ovarian Syndrome, Sclerocystic Disease of the Ovaries.*

POSTMATURITY SYNDROME

The postmaturity syndrome is characterized by a prolonged gestation period, sometimes an enlarged fetus, diminished placental capacity to supply food and oxygen, and cutaneous and nutritional changes in the newborn infant.

SYNONYMS: *Ballantyne-Runge Syndrome, Ballantyne's Syndrome, Clifford's Syndrome, Runge's Syndrome, Dysmaturity Syndrome, Placental Dysfunction Syndrome, Prolonged Gestation Syndrome, Placental Insufficiency Syndrome.*

POSTMENOPAUSAL MUSCULAR DYSTROPHY SYNDROME

The postmenopausal muscular dystrophy syndrome is characterized by progressive weakness of the muscles of the hip and shoulder girdle. It occurs in women after menopause. The onset may be slow or rapid. The lower extremities are usually more severely affected than the upper ones. The patient experiences difficulty in climbing stairs, rising from a chair, or in reaching above her head. A waddling gait may be seen later, with complete inability to ascend stairs. Falls occur frequently. The face, hands, and feet remain unaffected. There is no dysphagia or change in vision. No atrophy of the affected muscles occurs. The cause is not known. There is no evidence of a thyroid myopathy. The slight creatinuria does not indicate an extensive or general muscular disorder. Diagnosis is confirmed by a biopsy that reveals patchy degeneration or necrosis of individual muscle fibers.

POSTPARTUM PITUITARY NECROSIS SYNDROME

The postpartum pituitary necrosis syndrome is due to postpartum thrombosis of sinuses, and ischemic infarction and necrosis of the pituitary gland, usually as a result of obstetric hemorrhage and shock that occur at term. If both the anterior and posterior lobes are involved and the gonadotropins, thyrotropin, and corticotropin are all absent, the appropriate descriptive term is *panhypopituitarism*. These deficiencies indicate secondary atrophy and failure of the adrenal cortices, the thyroid, and the ovaries. Excretion of corticoids in the urine is reduced. The resulting symptoms appear insidiously, and usually after several months. Symptoms of the multiglandular deficiency are variable. Some patients exhibit the characteristics of myxedema. There is pallor, asthenia, apathy, atrophy of the breasts with loss of areolar pigment, inhibition of lactation, loss of pubic and axillary hair, and genital atrophy. Amenorrhea may be temporary or permanent; rarely some women continue to menstruate indefinitely. Lipemia and xanthomatosis are sometimes present. Diabetes mellitus, if present, vanishes. Hypoglycemia is usually found and may be sufficiently severe to produce coma. A flat glucose tolerance curve and extreme sensitivity to insulin may be demonstrated.

SYNONYMS: *Sheehan's Syndrome, Postpartum Panhypopituitary Syndrome.*

POSTPHLEBITIC SYNDROME

The postphlebitic syndrome is characterized by progressive development of venous insufficiency, caused by thrombosis of the deep venous system of the lower extremities and the pelvis. The syndrome becomes manifest, clinically, when the thrombosis has extended into the superficial veins of the legs. Clinical features follow a definite sequence and consist of varicosities, edema, induration, stasis dermatitis, pigmentation especially above the medial malleolus, and perhaps ulceration.

SYNONYMS: *Postthrombotic Syndrome, Venous-Ulcer Leg Syndrome.*

POSTRUBELLA SYNDROME

The postrubella syndrome is a syndrome characterized by a high incidence of congenital malformations and defects in the human fetus caused by maternal rubella during the first three months of gestation. The defects and malformations consist of microcephaly, severe mental deficiency, bilateral congenital cataract with blindness, complete or partial deafness, congenital malformation of the heart, such as atrial septal defect or patent ductus arteriosus, feeding difficulties, retarded physical development, and many other anomalies.

SYNONYM: *Gregg's Syndrome.*

PREMENSTRUAL TENSION SYNDROME

The premenstrual tension syndrome occurs during the second half of the menstrual cycle and may consist of variable combinations of the following symptoms: painful swelling of the breasts, abdominal bloating and discomfort, headache, nausea, vomiting, fatigue, swelling of the subcutaneous tissues, and nervous and emotional instability. There may also be excessive thirst, increased appetite, hypersomnia, dizziness, and palpitation. Most often the condition occurs during the final week of the menstrual cycle and ends soon after the onset of menses. Although

the cause for the premenstrual tension syndrome is not known, it is believed to be associated with the cyclic fluctuation of the ovarian hormones.
SYNONYM: *Premenstrual Syndrome.*

PRIMARY ALDOSTERONISM

Primary aldosteronism is a condition associated with arterial hypertension and potassium wasting caused by an adrenocortical tumor secreting an excess of aldosterone only. Symptoms and signs include hypertension, headache, polyuria, polydipsia, muscular weakness, paresthesias, and periodic paralysis. A tentative diagnosis is supported by the triad of resting hypertension, low serum potassium, and failure of urine concentration after the administration of antidiuretic hormone. The definitive diagnosis is made on the basis of a low level of renin in the plasma and elevated aldosterone levels on a normal salt intake. Removal of the aldosterone-secreting tumor yields an excellent prognosis in a high percentage of cases. Excessive secretion of aldosterone may occur also in certain edematous states, during salt deprivation, or in malignant hypertension, and is referred to as *secondary hyperaldosteronism.*
SYNONYM: *Conn's Syndrome.*

RACINE'S SYNDROME

Racine's syndrome is characterized by glandular abnormalities that may occur prior to menstruation, including swelling of the salivary glands and the breast tissues. Enlargement of the salivary glands occurs four to five days premenstrually and subsides with the onset of flow.
SYNONYM: *Premenstrual Salivary Syndrome.*

RÉNON-DELILLE SYNDROME

The Rénon-Delille syndrome is a syndrome characterized by a combination of thyroid-ovarian deficiency and associated hypophysial hyperactivity manifested as acromegaly. Clinical features include hypotension, tachycardia, hyperhidrosis, intolerance to heat, insomnia, and oliguria.

RESIDUAL OVARY SYNDROME

The residual ovary syndrome is characterized by the development of a pelvic mass, pelvic pain, and occasionally dyspareunia following hysterectomy without removal of both ovaries.

SIMMONDS' SYNDROME

Simmonds' syndrome is characterized by a chronic, progressive endocrine deficiency with widespread disturbance of tissue and organ function resulting from failure of hormone production of the anterior lobe of the pituitary gland. The clinical features are associated with destruction of the anterior lobe. The syndrome occurs more commonly in females. The symptoms are manifold and include asthenia, progressive weight loss, often to the point of emaciation, and decreased sexual function associated with atrophy of the genital organs. There is absence of lactation and amenorrhea in women. Clinical features include loss of axillary and pubic hair, loss of beard in men, atrophic changes in the skin that give the appearance of premature aging, and a markedly decreased metabolic rate with hypothermia, bradycardia, and hypotonia. Hypoglycemia and extreme sensitivity to insulin are characteristic. Protein reserves are diminished. Gastrointestinal disorders, anemia, and achlorhydria are frequently present. Many of the symptoms are obviously related to hypofunction of the thyroid, parathyroid, and adrenal glands. Psychic changes also occur, and may show less response to treatment than do the somatic manifestations. The syndrome is caused by destruction of the anterior lobe of the hypophysis. Pathologic lesions include spontaneous atrophy and fibrosis, tumor, granulomas, and trauma. Similar effects follow excessive radiation or surgical removal.

SYNONYMS: *Pituitary Cachexia, Simmonds' Disease.*

STEWART-TREVES SYNDROME

The Stewart-Treves syndrome is characterized by the late development of an angiosarcoma in an edematous upper extremity after radical breast surgery. The condition occurs in women between 44 and 68 years of age with no history of delayed healing, postoperative infection, or thrombosis. Postmastectomy edema usually appears in the arm on the operated side within a year and gradually spreads to involve the hand and fingers. Other manifestations include minor atrophy of the skin, hyperkeratoses, spontaneous telangiectasia, and febrile bouts with true erysipelas or erysipeloid changes. After an interval of 6 to 24 years, there appears a single, purplish red, subdermal, slightly raised, macular or polypoid lesion in the skin of the arm or antecubital area. Later, additional lesions develop on the forearm, hand, and thorax with all stages of ulceration, discharge, and healing. The lesions do not resemble the cutaneous nodules of recurrent mammary cancer and are distinct from the early mammary lesion. It is suggested that the syndrome is probably due to a systemic carcinogenic factor. Differential diagnosis should exclude metastatic carcinoma and Kaposi's sarcoma.

SYNONYM: *Postmastectomy Lymphangiosarcoma Syndrome.*

THYROID-ADRENOCORTICAL INSUFFICIENCY SYNDROME

The thyroid-adrenocortical insufficiency syndrome is a combination of adrenocortical insufficiency (Addison's disease) and chronic thyroiditis, with lymphocytic infiltration of the thyroid gland. Diabetes mellitus may also coexist. There is some overlay in the early symptomatic period; however, the symptomatology, clinical observations, and laboratory findings permit ready differentiation in advanced stages. There is usually a lowered basal metabolic rate in both conditions. Thyroid insufficiency may be proved by the finding of decreased plasma protein-bound iodine and a low thyroidal radioactive iodine (^{131}I) uptake. Adrenocortical insufficiency may be confirmed by decreased serum sodium, increased potassium, and decreased plasma cortisol levels. With occasional exceptions, the adrenal disorder occurs first and thyroid insufficiency appears subsequently. Antiadrenal and antithyroid bodies are increased in these cases, and the condition is now thought to be the result of an auto-immunity process.

SYNONYM: *Schmidt's* (*M.B.*) *Syndrome.*

TIMME'S SYNDROME

Timme's syndrome is characterized by ovarian and adrenal insufficiency with compensatory hypopituitarism.

YOUNG'S SYNDROME

Young's syndrome is characterized by hyperlactation, rapid weight gain during pregnancy, and the birth of a living child weighing more than 4000 gm or termination of pregnancy because of fetal or previous neonatal mortality. In addition, there is a late onset, often after meno-pause, of diabetes mellitus. A definite hereditary tendency prevails.

SYNONYM: *Somatotrophic Hormone Syndrome.*

Section 6: *Physiology of Reproduction*

Menstruation

MENSTRUATION

Menstruation is a cyclic, physiologic discharge of blood, mucus, and cellular debris from the uterine mucosa. Menstruation is the result of hormonal changes produced on the endometrium by the interaction of the ovaries and the anterior pituitary gland.

SYNONYM: *Menses.*

MENSTRUAL CYCLE

The menstrual cycle is the period extending from the onset of one normal menstrual period to the onset of the next normal period, generally 21 to 37 days. Histologic and biochemical events occur in the endometrium. They are characterized by endometrial growth, metabolism, secretion of essential nutrient substances, and regression. These endometrial functions are produced by the cyclic stimulation of estrogen and progesterone. The histologic changes in the endometrium are divided into the postmenstrual, proliferative, secretory, premenstrual, and menstrual phases:

Postmenstrual Phase

The postmenstrual phase is the phase that includes the four to five days following the menstrual phase. The endometrium is thin, measuring ordinarily only 1 or 2 mm in thickness. The surface epithelium and the epithelium lining the glands is of cuboidal type. The endometrial glands are straight, narrow, and collapsed; the stroma is dense and compact.

Proliferative Phase

The proliferative phase is the growth phase of the endometrium. The endometrium is stimulated by estrogen. The endometrial glands are straight and short, and the glandular epithelium is cuboidal and shows no evidence of secretory activity. The stromal cells multiply, and the spiral arteries begin to grow.

SYNONYMS: *Preovulatory Phase, Follicular Phase.*

Secretory Phase

The secretory phase is the postovulatory phase of the endometrium. The endometrium is stimulated by estrogen and progesterone. The endometrial glands are long and tortuous. The glandular epithelium is columnar and filled with secretion. The stromal cells are large, and the spiral arteries are long and tortuous.

SYNONYMS: *Postovulatory Phase, Progestational Phase, Progravid Endometrium, Luteal Phase.*

Premenstrual Phase

The premenstrual phase is the phase that includes the two to three days prior to the menstrual phase and corresponds to the regression of the corpus luteum. The chief histologic characteristic of this phase is infiltration of the stroma by polymorphonuclear or mononuclear leukocytes, producing a pseudoinflammatory appearance. Concurrently, the reticular framework of the stroma in the superficial zone disintegrates. As a result of the loss of tissue fluid and secretion, the thickness of the endometrium often decreases significantly during the two days before the menstrual phase. In the process of reduction, the glands and arteries collapse.

Menstrual Phase

The menstrual phase is the period of desquamation of the endometrium. There are increased numbers of polymorphonuclear leukocytes, plasmatocytes, and other wandering blood cells in the tissue.
SYNONYM: *Bleeding Phase.*

ADRENARCHE

Adrenarche is augmentation of adrenal cortex function, involving both androgens and glucocorticoids. This physiologic change occurs at approximately the age of eight years.

AMENORRHEA

Amenorrhea is the absence of menstruation. It may be primary or secondary, physiologic or pathologic. It is a subjective, but not a reliable, sign of pregnancy.
SYNONYM: *Menostasis.*

AMENORRHEA, PATHOLOGIC

Pathologic amenorrhea is the cessation of menstruation at any time after the menarche, other than during pregnancy and lactation, and before the menopause. It can be either primary or secondary and caused by any of the following factors: congenital abnormalities, central nervous system lesions, systemic conditions, ovarian disturbances, and uterine trauma.

AMENORRHEA, PHYSIOLOGIC

Physiologic amenorrhea is the normal absence of menstruation before the menarche, during pregnancy and lactation, and after the menopause.

Primary Physiologic Amenorrhea

Primary physiologic amenorrhea is lack of the menarche in a woman at least 18 years of age.

Secondary Physiologic Amenorrhea

Secondary physiologic amenorrhea is the cessation of menstruation for at least three months in a woman who has previously had her menarche.

ANOVULAR MENSTRUATION
Anovular menstruation is menstrual bleeding without discharge of an ovum.

SYNONYMS: *Anovulational Menstruation, Nonovulational Menstruation.*

CERVICAL MUCUS ARBORIZATION
Cervical mucus arborization is the specific palm-leaf pattern created by the drying and resulting crystallization of cervical mucus due to electrolyte action on protein. It occurs in the proliferative phase of the menstrual cycle.

SYNONYM: *Ferning.*

CRYPTOMENORRHEA
Cryptomenorrhea is the occurrence of menstrual symptoms without menstrual bleeding.

DECIDUATION
Deciduation is the shedding of the endometrial tissue during menstruation.

DYSMENORRHEA
Dysmenorrhea is a symptom characterized by painful menstruation. It is not a disease entity.

SYNONYM: *Menorrhalgia.*

Mechanical Dysmenorrhea
Mechanical dysmenorrhea is menstrual pain due to cervical stenosis or other obstruction to the menstrual flow.

SYNONYM: *Obstructive Dysmenorrhea.*

Primary Dysmenorrhea
Primary dysmenorrhea is menstrual pain observed in the absence of any noteworthy pelvic lesion and is due to factors intrinsic in the uterus itself.

SYNONYMS: *Essential Dysmenorrhea, Functional Dysmenorrhea, Intrinsic Dysmenorrhea.*

Secondary Dysmenorrhea
Secondary dysmenorrhea is menstrual pain caused by demonstrable pelvic disease.

EMMENAGOGUE
An emmenagogue is an agent that induces or increases menstruation.

ENTEROMENIA
Enteromenia is vicarious menstruation from the intestine.

GASTROMENIA
Gastromenia is a gastric hemorrhage occurring as a form of vicarious menstruation.

HELCOMENIA

Helcomenia is vicarious menstruation involving an ulcer.

HEMATOCOLPOS

Hematocolpos is an accumulation of menstrual blood in the vagina resulting from an imperforate hymen or other obstruction.

SYNONYM: *Retained Menstruation.*

HYPOMENORRHEA

Hypomenorrhea is a diminution in the amount of the flow or a shortening of the duration of menstruation.

MASTOMENIA

Mastomenia is vicarious menstruation from the breast.

MENARCHE

The menarche is the appearance of the first menstrual period.

MENOLIPSIS

Menolipsis is temporary cessation of menstruation.

MENOMETRORRHAGIA

Menometrorrhagia is irregular or excessive bleeding during menstruation and between menstrual periods. This is a symptom, not an acceptable diagnosis.

MENOPAUSE

Menopause is the transitional phase in a woman's life when menstrual function ceases. It may be natural, premature, or artificial, and often is attended by a complex imbalance of the glandular and autonomic nervous systems.

SYNONYMS: *Climacteric, Change of Life.*

MENOPHANIA

Menophania is the first sign of menses at puberty.

MENORRHAGIA

Menorrhagia is excessive or prolonged menstrual bleeding. It is a sign of a disease process.

MENORRHEA

Menorrhea is normal menstruation.

MENOSCHESIS

Menoschesis is suppression of menstruation.

SYNONYM: *Ischomenia.*

MENOSEPSIS

Menosepsis is septic poisoning due to the absorption of material from a retained menstrual discharge.

MENOSTAXIS
Menostaxis is an unduly prolonged menstrual flow.

MENOURIA
Menouria is menstruation from the urinary bladder as a result of a vesicouterine fistula.

MENOXENIA
Menoxenia is any abnormality of menstruation.

MENSTRUAL MOLIMEN
Menstrual molimen is a term used to designate the unpleasant symptoms that may be experienced during the menstrual cycle.

MITTELSCHMERZ
Mittelschmerz is intermenstrual pain in the lower abdomen generally associated with ovulation.

MYELOMENIA
Myelomenia is a spinal hemorrhage occurring as a form of vicarious menstruation.

OLIGOMENORRHEA
Oligomenorrhea is a reduction in the frequency of menstruation. An interval between the cycles of longer than 38 days but less than three months indicates oligomenorrhea.

OVULATION
Ovulation is the expulsion of a female germ cell from a ruptured graafian follicle.

PARAMENIA
Paramenia is any disorder or irregularity of menstruation.

PREMENSTRUAL SWELLING
Premenstrual swelling is general edema or the accumulation of body fluids during the secretory phase of the menstrual cycle.

PREMENSTRUAL TENSION
Premenstrual tension is a condition characterized by increased nervousness, irritability, emotional instability, depression, frequent headaches, general edema, and nostalgia. Premenstrual tension occurs periodically and cyclically in the seven to ten days preceding menstruation, but it usually disappears a few hours after onset of the menstrual flow.

PREMENSTRUAL TENSION SYNDROME
The premenstrual tension syndrome occurs during the second half of the menstrual cycle and may consist of variable combinations of the following symptoms: painful swelling of the breasts, abdominal bloating and discomfort, headache, nausea, vomiting, fatigue, swelling of the

subcutaneous tissues, and nervous and emotional instability. There may also be excessive thirst, increased appetite, hypersomnia, dizziness, and palpitation. Most often the condition occurs during the final week of the menstrual cycle and ends soon after the onset of menses. Although the cause for the premenstrual tension syndrome is not known, it is believed to be associated with the cyclic fluctuation of the ovarian hormones.

SYNONYM: *Premenstrual Syndrome.*

PROCTOMENIA
Proctomenia is vicarious menstruation involving the rectum.

PUBERTY
Puberty is the period when a person becomes sexually mature. The reproductive organs become functional and secondary sex characteristics are developed.

RACINE'S SYNDROME
Racine's syndrome is characterized by glandular abnormalities that may occur prior to menstruation, including swelling of the salivary glands and the breast tissues. Enlargement of the salivary glands occurs four to five days premenstrually and subsides with the onset of flow.

SYNONYM: *Premenstrual Salivary Syndrome.*

RETROGRADE MENSTRUATION
Retrograde menstruation is a flow of menstrual blood through the fallopian tubes. It may give rise to endometriosis.

SPINNBARKEIT
Spinnbarkeit is a term used to denote cervical mucus of decreased viscosity. It is indicative of ovulation in some women.

STETHOMENIA
Stethomenia is hemoptysis occurring as a form of vicarious menstruation.

STOMATOMENIA
Stomatomenia is bleeding from the gums as a form of vicarious menstruation.

SYNONYM: *Stomenorrhagia.*

SUPPLEMENTARY MENSTRUATION
Supplementary menstruation is bleeding from the umbilicus, urinary tract, or other areas. It is generally associated with endometriosis.

VICARIOUS MENSTRUATION
Vicarious menstruation is bleeding from any surface other than the mucous membrane of the uterine cavity. It occurs periodically at the time when normal menstruation should take place.

SYNONYMS: *Menoplania, Xenomenia, Atopomenorrhea.*

Male Reproductive System

BULBOURETHRAL GLAND

The bulbourethral gland is one of the two small, compound, racemose glands lying side by side along the membranous urethra just above the bulb of the corpus spongiosum. It secretes a substance through a small duct into the spongy portion of the urethra.

SYNONYMS: *Cowper's Gland, Méry's Gland, Glandula Bulbourethralis* (NA).

CORPUS CAVERNOSUM OF PENIS

The corpus cavernosum of the penis is one of two columns of erectile tissue lying side by side on the dorsum of the penis. The columns are separated posteriorly, forming the crura penis, and they are attached to the inner portion of the arch of the pubis.

SYNONYM: *Corpus Cavernosum Penis* (NA).

CORPUS SPONGIOSUM OF PENIS

The corpus spongiosum of the penis is the spongy body of the penis. It is the median column of erectile tissue located between and below the two corpora cavernosa of the penis. It is traversed by the urethra.

SYNONYM: *Corpus Spongiosum Penis* (NA).

DUCT, EJACULATORY

The ejaculatory duct is the duct formed by the union of the vas deferens and the excretory duct of the seminal vesicle. The ejaculatory duct opens into the prostatic urethra.

SYNONYM: *Ductus Ejaculatorius* (NA).

EJACULATION OF SEMEN

The ejaculation of semen is the ejection of seminal fluid during male orgasm.

EPIDIDYMIS

The epididymis is a long, narrow, flattened structure consisting of a central portion or body; an upper enlarged extremity, the head; and a lower pointed extremity, the tail, which is continuous with the vas deferens. The epididymis lies on the lateral edge of the posterior border of the testis.

SYNONYM: *Epididymis* (NA).

EPIDIDYMIS, DUCTS OF

The ducts of the epididymis are convoluted single tubules that lead from the efferent ducts of the testis to the vas deferens.

SYNONYM: *Ductus Epididymis* (NA).

PENIS

The penis is the male copulatory organ, generally cylindrical, consisting of a terminal enlargement or glans, body, and root.

SYNONYM: *Penis* (NA).

Glans Penis

The glans penis is the head or distal end of the penis, which contains erectile tissue. It is hooded by the prepuce unless circumcised. The glans has sense receptors that become stimulated during coitus.

SYNONYM: *Glans Penis* (NA).

Penile Body

The penile body consists of erectile tissue arranged in three columns, the two corpora cavernosa and the corpus spongiosum, sheathed in connective tissue. The lower and central one, the corpus spongiosum, is traversed by the urethra.

SYNONYM: *Corpus Penis* (NA).

Penile Root

The penile root consists of a urethral bulb (corpus spongiosum) and the corpora cavernosa. It is attached to the medial border of the inferior ramus of the pubis by the separately formed crura.

SYNONYM: *Radix Penis* (NA).

PREPUCE OF PENIS

The prepuce of the penis is the foreskin that hoods the glans penis unless it has been removed by circumcision.

SYNONYM: *Preputium* (NA).

PROSTATE

The prostate is a chestnut-shaped body, partly muscular and partly glandular, that surrounds the beginning of the male urethra. It consists of two lateral lobes that are practically fused posteriorly and are connected anteriorly by an isthmus, and a middle lobe lying above and between the ejaculatory ducts. The prostate secretes a milky fluid that is discharged into the urethra at the time of the emission of the semen, mixing with this secretion.

SYNONYM: *Prostata* (NA).

SCROTUM

The scrotum is a musculocutaneous sac containing the testes.

SYNONYM: *Scrotum* (NA).

SEMEN
Semen is a thick, yellowish white, viscid fluid containing spermatozoa. It is a mixture of the secretions of the testes, seminal vesicles, prostate, and bulbourethral glands.

SEMINIFEROUS TUBULES, CONVOLUTED
The convoluted seminiferous tubules are testicular elements in which spermatozoa develop.
SYNONYM: *Tubuli Seminiferi Contorti* (NA).

SEMINIFEROUS TUBULES, STRAIGHT
The straight seminiferous tubules are continuations of the convoluted tubules and form the rete testis.
SYNONYM: *Tubuli Seminiferi Recti* (NA).

SERTOLI CELLS
Sertoli cells are cells in the testicular tubules in which the spermatids become embedded. They furnish nutrition to the developing spermatids.
SYNONYMS: *Sustentacular Cells, Nurse Cells, Foot Cells, Trophocytes.*

SPERMATID
A spermatid is a male sex cell. It is derived from a secondary spermatocyte by mitotic division and develops into a spermatozoon by reduction in cytoplasm and formation of a tail.

SPERMATIN
Spermatin is an albuminous material in the seminal fluid.

SPERMATOCYTE, PRIMARY
A primary spermatocyte is a male sex cell containing 46 chromosomes. It is derived from a spermatogonium and becomes converted into a secondary spermatocyte by the first meiotic division.

SPERMATOCYTE, SECONDARY
A secondary spermatocyte is a male sex cell containing 23 chromosomes. It is derived by meiotic division from a primary spermatocyte.

SPERMATOGENESIS
Spermatogenesis is the process of development of the male germ cell.

SPERMATOGONIUM
A spermatogonium is one of the undifferentiated male sex cells that remain in the testis and from which mature sperm cells are derived.

SPERMATOZOON
A spermatozoon is a mature microgamete, or male sex cell. It is derived from a spermatid in the testis, stored in the epididymis, and ejaculated in the semen. It conveys paternal inheritance to the offspring.

TESTIS
The testis is one of the two male reproductive glands located in the cavity of the scrotum.

SYNONYM: *Testis* (NA).

TESTIS, EFFERENT DUCTS OF
The efferent ducts of the testis are small ducts that convey spermatozoa from the rete testis to the single duct of the epididymis.

SYNONYM: *Ductuli Efferentes Testis* (NA).

URETHRA, MALE
The male urethra is a canal about 22 cm in length extending from the bladder to an opening at the extremity of the glans penis. It gives passage to semen and to urine.

SYNONYM: *Urethra Masculina* (NA).

VAS DEFERENS
The vas deferens is the excretory duct of the testis, extending from the epididymis to the prostatic urethra, where it terminates at the ejaculatory duct.

SYNONYMS: *Duct of Testis, Ductus Deferens* (NA).

VESICLE, SEMINAL
The seminal vesicle is one of two folded, sacculated, glandular structures which is a diverticulum of the vas deferens. Its secretion is one of the components of semen.

SYNONYM: *Vesicula Seminalis* (NA).

Gametogenesis and Fertilization

GAMETOGENESIS
Gametogenesis is the process of formation and development of gametes or mature sex cells.

FERTILIZATION
Fertilization is the process that begins with the penetration of the secondary oocyte by the spermatozoon and is completed with the fusion of the male and female pronuclei.
SYNONYM: *Syngamy.*

BLASTOCYST
The blastocyst is a structure that results when fluid accumulates within the morula, producing a cavity with the inner cell mass at one pole. The wall of the blastocyst develops into the trophoblast.
SYNONYM: *Blastula.*

BLASTOMERE
A blastomere is any one of the cells produced by one of the early divisions of the zygote.
SYNONYM: *Cleavage Cell.*

CLEAVAGE
Cleavage is the process by which the zygote divides into blastomeres.
SYNONYM: *Segmentation.*

CONCEPTION
Conception is the implantation of the blastocyst. It is not synonymous with fertilization.
SYNONYM: *Implantation.*

CORONA RADIATA
The corona radiata is a layer of radially arranged granulosa cells that remains temporarily attached to the primary oocyte following its separation from the wall of the follicle. It is derived from part of the cumulus oophorus.

CUMULUS OOPHORUS
The cumulus oophorus is a mass of follicular or granulosa cells that surrounds the female germ cell.
SYNONYMS: *Cumulus Ovaricus, Cumulus Proligerus, Discus Proligerus, Cumulus Oophorus* (NA).

299

EMBRYONIC NIDUS

The embryonic nidus is the site where the blastocyst implants in the endometrium.

FERTILIZATION IN VITRO

Fertilization in vitro is the artificial fertilization of an ovum outside the female body.

FERTILIZATION IN VIVO

Fertilization in vivo is the fertilization of an ovum within the female body.

FOLLICLE

A follicle is a group of cells usually containing a fluid-filled cavity.

FOLLICULAR STIGMA

The follicular stigma is the site on the surface of the ovary where the graafian follicle ruptures to permit extrusion of its contents.

GAMETE

A gamete is a mature sex cell, either a secondary oocyte (macrogamete) or a spermatozoon (microgamete).

GONAD

A gonad is an organ that produces female or male sex cells and hormones.

GRAAFIAN FOLLICLE

The graafian follicle is an ovarian follicle possessing an antrum.

SYNONYMS: *Vesicular Follicle, Folliculus Oophorus Vesiculosus, Folliculi Ovarici Vesiculosi* (NA).

IMPLANTATION, CORTICAL

Cortical implantation is implantation of the blastocyst in the ovarian cortex, resulting in an ovarian pregnancy.

IMPLANTATION, ENDOMETRIAL

Endometrial implantation is the process by which the blastocyst adheres to, penetrates into, and obtains nutritional support from the endometrium.

IMPLANTATION, INTRAFOLLICULAR

Intrafollicular implantation is implantation of a blastocyst in the follicle or corpus luteum, resulting in an ovarian pregnancy.

IMPLANTATION, JUXTAFOLLICULAR

Juxtafollicular implantation is implantation of a blastocyst in the deeper ovarian stroma as a result of trophoblastic penetration. This results in an ovarian pregnancy.

INSEMINATION

Insemination is the introduction of semen into the vagina.

SYNONYM: *Semination.*

MEIOSIS

Meiosis is the process of germ cell division. One-half of each pair of chromosomes is removed in preparation for postfertilization replacement with a corresponding chromosome from a gamete of the other sex. In the female, the prophase of meiosis begins in fetal life and is not complete until penetration of the ovum by a spermatozoon. The first meiotic (maturation) division in the primary oocyte takes place at about the time of ovulation. It produces two cells, each with a haploid (23) number of chromosomes. One of the cells (secondary oocyte) receives all the cytoplasm and the other (first polar body) receives none. The chromosomes of the secondary oocyte previously produced in mitotic division, now separate (equation division) and produce two cells, each having a haploid number of chromosomes. One cell (ootid) receives all the cytoplasm, and the other (second polar body) receives none. In the male, meiosis begins after puberty, and each primary spermatocyte gives rise to four functional sperm cells.

SYNONYM: *Maturation Division.*

MITOSIS

Mitosis is a cell division. It provides identical numbers and types of chromosomes to all descendant cells.

MORULA

The morula is a solid mass of cells (usually 8 to 16) resulting from cleavage of the zygote.

OOCYTE, PRIMARY

A primary oocyte is a female germ cell derived from an oogonium. It contains a diploid number of chromosomes. The primary oocyte becomes converted into a secondary oocyte and first polar body by the first maturation (reduction) division.

OOCYTE, SECONDARY

A secondary oocyte is a female germ cell that contains a haploid number of chromosomes and is derived from a primary oocyte by the first maturation (reduction) division. The secondary oocyte becomes converted into an ootid and second polar body by a second maturation (equation) division following penetration of the secondary oocyte by a spermatozoon.

OOGENESIS

Oogenesis is the process of development of the female germ cell from the oogonium, through the stages of maturation division, to the formation of an ootid.

OOGONIUM

The oogonium is a primitive female germ cell containing a diploid number of chromosomes. It may reproduce itself by mitotic division, or may become a primary oocyte preparatory to undergoing meiotic division.

OOTID

An ootid is produced by the second maturation division from a secondary oocyte, a process thought to occur only after fertilization.

OVARIAN FOLLICLE

The ovarian follicle is a vascular body in the ovary that contains an ovum. It can either be a primordial follicle or a graafian follicle.

OVULATION

Ovulation is the expulsion of a female germ cell from a ruptured graafian follicle.

OVUM

Ovum is a general term referring to the female germ cell at any stage of development.

SYNONYM: *Ovum* (NA).

OVUM, MIGRATION OF

Migration of the ovum is the passage of the ovum from the ovarian follicle to the endometrium.

External Migration of Ovum

External migration of the ovum is the passage of the ovum from the ovarian follicle of one ovary to the opposite fallopian tube.

Internal Migration of Ovum

Internal migration of the ovum is the passage of the ovum from the ovarian follicle to and through the adjacent fallopian tube, across the uterine fundus internally, and up into the opposite fallopian tube.

PABULUM

Pabulum is a nutrient fluid secreted by the decidua.

PERIVITELLINE SPACE

The perivitelline space is the space between the plasma membrane of the female germ cell and the zona pellucida.

PLACENTATION

Placentation is the development of the placenta after attachment of the blastocyst to the uterine wall or other structures.

POLAR BODY I

The first polar body is a cell containing a haploid number of chromosomes, but no cytoplasm. It is derived from a primary oocyte at the time of the first maturation division.

POLAR BODY II
The second polar body is a cell containing a haploid number of chromosomes, but no cytoplasm. It is derived from the secondary oocyte at the time of the second maturation division.

PRIMORDIAL FOLLICLE
The primordial follicle is a young ovarian follicle before the formation of the antrum with its contained liquor folliculi.
SYNONYM: *Folliculi Ovarici Primarii* (NA).

PRIMORDIAL GERM CELL
A primordial germ cell is an undifferentiated sex cell possessing the potential of becoming either a male or female gamete. It is found only in the young embryo.

PRONUCLEUS
A pronucleus is either one of the two haploid chromosome groups within the ootid. It consists of the chromatin material derived by meiotic division from either a male or female germ cell.

Female Pronucleus
The female pronucleus is a reduced nucleus in the ootid formed during the second maturation division. It consists of 23 chromosomes.

Male Pronucleus
The male pronucleus is the head of the spermatozoon after penetration of the secondary oocyte. It consists of 23 chromosomes.

SERTOLI CELLS
Sertoli cells are cells in the testicular tubules in which the spermatids become embedded. They furnish nutrition to the developing spermatids.
SYNONYMS: *Sustentacular Cells, Nurse Cells, Foot Cells, Trophocytes.*

SPERMATID
A spermatid is a male sex cell. It is derived from a secondary spermatocyte by mitotic division and develops into a spermatozoon by reduction in cytoplasm and formation of a tail.

SPERMATOCYTE, PRIMARY
A primary spermatocyte is a male sex cell containing 46 chromosomes. It is derived from a spermatogonium and becomes converted into a secondary spermatocyte by the first meiotic division.

SPERMATOCYTE, SECONDARY
A secondary spermatocyte is a male sex cell containing 23 chromosomes. It is derived by meiotic division from a primary spermatocyte.

SPERMATOGENESIS
Spermatogenesis is the process of development of the male germ cell.

SPERMATOGONIUM

A spermatogonium is one of the undifferentiated male sex cells that remains in the testis and from which mature sperm cells are derived.

SPERMATOZOON

A spermatozoon is a mature microgamete, or male sex cell. It is derived from a spermatid in the testis, stored in the epididymis, and ejaculated in the semen. It conveys paternal inheritance to the offspring.

THECA CELLS

Theca cells are cells that surround the granulosa cells and form the outer part of the wall of an ovarian follicle.

THECA FOLLICULI

The theca folliculi is the outer layer of connective tissue which covers a graafian follicle. It is divided into a poorly defined outer layer, the theca externa, and a sharply demarcated inner layer, the theca interna.

Theca Externa

The theca externa is the layer of theca cells that forms the outer part of the wall of an ovarian follicle.

Theca Interna

The theca interna is the layer of theca cells lying between the granulosa cells and the theca externa.

TRANSPORT, OVUM

Ovum transport is the process by which the ovum is propelled from the ovary to the point of implantation or expulsion.

TRANSPORT, TUBAL

Tubal transport is the mechanism by which the ova and spermatozoa are transported through the fallopian tube.

ZONA PELLUCIDA

The zona pellucida is a clear, thick membrane that forms around the plasma membrane of the female germ cell and persists until the blastocyst is well developed.

SYNONYM: *Oolemma.*

ZYGOTE

The zygote is derived from an ootid after fusion of the male and female pronuclei. It possesses a diploid number of chromosomes.

SECTION 6: PHYSIOLOGY OF REPRODUCTION

Chromosomes

CHROMOSOMES
Chromosomes are deeply staining bodies in the nucleus of a cell that contain the hereditary material (genes) of an organism. The genes are arranged in linear order along the chromosomes, each gene having a precise location, known as the locus. After replication of chromosomes, the resulting chromosome pairs segregate so that each daughter cell receives a specific complement of hereditary material. The total chromosome number in man is 46. Females have 44 autosomes plus two X chromosomes; males have 44 autosomes plus an X and Y chromosome.

ACENTRIC CHROMOSOME
An acentric chromosome is a chromosome or chromosomal fragment without a centromere. It is the result of a translocation or deletion.

ACHROMATIN
Achromatin is the plasm of the cell, so called because of its weak staining property.

ACROCENTRIC CHROMOSOME
An acrocentric chromosome is a chromosome with the centromere near one end.

ANAPHASE LAG
Anaphase lag is slow movement or no movement of chromosomes during anaphase, resulting in failure of the chromosomes concerned to be included in one of the daughter cells.

ANEUPLOIDY
Aneuploidy is the state in which the cells have more or less than the basic number of chromosomes for the species in question—that is, the chromosome number is not an exact multiple of the haploid number.

AUTOSOME
An autosome is a non-sex-determining chromosome. There are 44 autosomes in man.

BIVALENT CHROMOSOME
A bivalent chromosome is a pair of homologous chromosomes (paternal and maternal) that are temporarily united during the pachytene stage of meiosis.

CENTROMERE
The centromere is the nonstaining primary constriction where the arms of a chromosome meet. It is a very constant feature of each chromosome and has an important role in the movements of chromosomes during cell division. The position of the centromere may be near one end of the chromosome (acrocentric), near the center (metacentric), or slightly eccentric (submetacentric). Terminal centromeres are called telocentric.
SYNONYM: *Kinetochore.*

CHROMATIDS
Chromatids are the two spiral filaments, held together at the centromere, that make up the chromosome and that separate and move toward opposite poles during cell division.

CHROMATIN
Chromatin is the portion of the cell nucleus that is readily stained and that forms a network of nuclear fibrils within the achromatin of a cell. It consists of deoxyribonucleic acid attached to a protein structure base and is the carrier of the genes.

CHROMOSOMAL ABERRATIONS
Chromosomal aberrations are abnormalities of number or structure of chromosomes. The phenotypic abnormalities that result from chromosomal aberration are due primarily to imbalance of genetic material.

CHROMOSOMAL MOSAIC
A chromosomal mosaic is an individual who has two or more cell populations derived from a single zygote. Each population has a different karyotype.

CHROMOSOME DELETION
Chromosome deletion is the loss of a portion of a chromosome. It may be terminal or involve loss of a segment between two breaks. If the deleted portion has a centromere it can replicate.

Deletion of Short Arm of Chromosome No. 4 (4p—)
Deletion of the short arm of chromosome No. 4 (4p—) is characterized by ocular hypertelorism, low-set ears, cleft lip and palate, preauricular dimple, midline scalp defects, mental retardation, short stature, seizures, sacral dimples, and a beaklike nose.

Deletion of Short Arm of Chromosome No. 18 (18p—)
Deletion of the short arm of chromosome No. 18 (18p—)is characterized by severe malformations of the midface and brain, cyclopia, cebocephaly, and severe mental retardation.

Deletion of Long Arm of Chromosome No. 18 (18q—)
Deletion of the long arm of chromosome No. 18 (18q—) is characterized by severe mental retardation, midfacial hypoplasia, absent labia minora, subacromial dimples, perioral subcutaneous nodules, cataracts, and growth failure.

CHROMOSOME ENDOREDUPLICATION

Chromosome endoreduplication is a form of polyploidy or polysomy caused by doubling of chromosomes without division, giving rise to a tetraploid condition.

CHROMOSOME INVERSION

Chromosome inversion is the chromosomal aberration that involves breakage of a chromosome followed by refusion of the fragments in such a way that a section of the chromosome is inverted. This results in reversal of the order of genes in a segment of the chromosome.

CHROMOSOME SATELLITE

A chromosome satellite is a small mass of condensed chromatin attached to the short arms of a human acrocentric chromosome by a relatively uncondensed stalk (secondary constriction).

CHROMOSOME SEGMENT DUPLICATION

Chromosome segment duplication is a chromosomal aberration due to the presence of an extra piece of chromosome. This extra piece may be a separate fragment or a duplication within a chromosome, or it may be attached to a nonhomologous chromosome (translocation).

DENVER CLASSIFICATION

The Denver classification is the standard system of nomenclature for human mitotic chromosomes on the basis of length. The chromosomes in man are classified as follows:

Group 1–3 (A) Large chromosomes with median centromeres.

Group 4–5 (B) Large chromosomes with submedian centromeres.

Group 6–12 (C) Medium-sized chromosomes with submedian centromeres. By common agreement the X chromosome is assigned to this group.

Group 13–15 (D) Medium-sized chromosomes with nearly terminal centromeres.

Group 16–18 (E) Rather short chromosomes with median or submedian centromeres.

Group 19–20 (F) Short chromosomes with median centromeres.

Group 21–22 (G) Very short acrocentric chromosomes. The Y chromosome is similar to these chromosomes.

DEOXYRIBONUCLEIC ACID

Deoxyribonucleic acid is a nucleic polymer composed of purine and pyrimidine bases with deoxyribose and phosphoric acid. The genetic code is stored in the deoxyribonucleic acid in the chromosomes of the cell nucleus. Deoxyribonucleic acid directs the production of polypeptides that combine to form proteins and enzymes. The link between deoxyribonucleic acid and polypeptide is ribonucleic acid.

SYNONYM: *Desoxyribonucleic Acid.*

ABBREVIATION: DNA.

DICENTRIC CHROMOSOME

A dicentric chromosome is a chromosome with two centromeres. It is an abnormality that may result from translocation.

DIPLOID CELL

A diploid cell is a cell containing one pair of homologous chromosomes. The diploid number in man is 46, each parent contributing 23 chromosomes, one of each kind.

DRUMSTICK

Drumstick refers to the sex chromatin of polymorphonuclear leukocytes of human blood. It appears as a drumstick-like appendage attached to the nucleus of the blood cell by a threadlike stalk.

EUPLOID CELL

A euploid cell is a cell with the normal complement of autosomes and sex chromosomes.

GENE

A gene is the functional unit of heredity. Each gene occupies a specific place or locus in a chromosome, is capable of reproducing itself exactly at each cell division, and is capable of directing the formation of an enzyme or other protein. The gene as a functional unit probably consists of a discrete segment of a giant deoxyribonucleic acid (DNA) molecule containing the proper number of purine (adenine and guanine) and pyrimidine (cytosine and thymine) bases in the correct sequence to code the sequence of amino acids needed to form a specific peptide.

GENOTYPE

The genotype is the fundamental hereditary constitution or assortment of genes of an individual.

HAPLOID CELL

A haploid cell is a cell that contains only one member of each pair of homologous chromosomes. The haploid number in man is 23.

HEMICHROMOSOME

A hemichromosome is the lateral half of a chromosome.

HEMIZYGOSITY

Hemizygosity is the state of having only one of a pair of genes that determines a particular trait. Males are normally hemizygous for genes on the X chromosome.

HOMOLOGOUS CHROMOSOME

A homologous chromosome is one member of a pair of chromosomes.

HYPERPLOIDY

Hyperploidy is the state of having more than the typical number of chromosomes in unbalanced sets.

IDIOGRAM
An idiogram is a diagrammatic representation of a karyotype.

ISOCHROMOSOME
An isochromosome is a chromosome that has two genetically identical arms. It results from a misdivision of the centromere at right angles to the chromosome axis.

KARYOTYPE
Karyotype is the term used to denote the chromosomes characteristic of an individual or of a cell line. It is usually represented as a systematized array of metaphase chromosomes of a single cell nucleus arranged in pairs in descending order of size and according to the position of the centromere.

LYON HYPOTHESIS
The Lyon hypothesis is a hypothesis that suggests that only one X chromosome per cell is active. The inactivated X is randomly determined early in embryonic life and can be either the maternal or paternal X in different cells of the same individual.

MEIOSIS
Meiosis is the process of germ cell division. Half of each pair of chromosomes is removed in preparation for postfertilization replacement with a corresponding chromosome from a gamete of the other sex. In the female, the prophase of meiosis begins in fetal life and is not complete until penetration of the ovum by a spermatozoon. The first meiotic (maturation) division in the primary oocyte takes place at about the time of ovulation. It produces two cells, each with a haploid (23) number of chromosomes. One of the cells (secondary oocyte) receives all the cytoplasm and the other (first polar body) receives none. The chromosomes of the secondary oocyte, previously produced in mitotic division, now separate (equation division) and produce two cells, each having a haploid number of chromosomes. One cell (ootid) receives all the cytoplasm, and the other (second polar body) receives none. In the male, meiosis begins after puberty, and each primary spermatocyte gives rise to four functional sperm cells.
SYNONYM: *Maturation Division.*

METACENTRIC CHROMOSOME
A metacentric chromosome is a chromosome with a centrally placed centromere that divides the chromosome into two arms of approximately equal length.

MITOSIS
Mitosis is a cell division. It provides identical numbers and types of chromosomes to all descendant cells.

MONOSOMY
Monosomy is the absence of one chromosome from a diploid cell (2N—1).

NONDISJUNCTION
Nondisjunction is failure of a pair of homologous chromosomes to disjoin in meiosis, leading to unequal distribution, so that one daughter cell has both and the other has neither chromosome of a pair.

PACHYTENE
Pachytene is a stage in meiosis during which the bivalent chromosomes are thickened and in close association.

PHENOTYPE
The phenotype is the expression of the hereditary constitution of an organism. It is potentially variable, reflecting the interaction between genotype and nongenetic environment.

PHILADELPHIA CHROMOSOME (Ph′)
The Philadelphia chromosome is a chromosomal aberration that is found in the leukocytes of patients with chronic granulocytic leukemia. It appears to be a deleted chromosome 21.

RIBONUCLEIC ACID
Ribonucleic acid is a polynucleotide containing the pentose sugar D-ribose. It is synthesized on a deoxyribonucleic acid template by direct transcription of the deoxyribonucleic acid code into a complementary ribonucleic acid code. Ribonucleic acid is contained mainly in the nucleolus and cytoplasm of the cell; the nucleus contains deoxyribonucleic acid. Three kinds of ribonucleic acid take part in protein synthesis: messenger RNA, transfer RNA, and ribosomal RNA.
ABBREVIATION: RNA.

RING CHROMOSOME
A ring chromosome results from two chromosome breaks, one on each side of the centromere, followed by fusion of the two ends of the centric fragment to form a ring.

SEX CHROMATIN
Sex chromatin refers to the mass of densely staining chromatin material found at the periphery of the nucleus in many interphase cells of the female. As a general rule, the number of masses of sex chromatin is one less than the number of X chromosomes. Each sex chromatin mass is formed by a single inactive X chromosome.
SYNONYM: Barr Body.

SEX CHROMOSOMES
Sex chromosomes are the chromosomes concerned with the determination of sex. In mammals they are an unequal pair, one X chromosome and one Y chromosome.

SUBMETACENTRIC CHROMOSOME
A submetacentric chromosome is a chromosome whose centromere is located somewhere between its end and midpoint.

TELOCENTRIC CHROMOSOME
A telocentric chromosome is a chromosome with a terminal centromere.

TETRAPLOID CELL
A tetraploid cell is a cell that has four times the haploid number of chromosomes.

TRANSLOCATION
Translocation is a chromosomal aberration in which there is interchange of material between two chromosomes. In reciprocal translocation, there is exchange of segments between nonhomologous chromosomes.

TRISOMY
Trisomy is the presence of three chromosomes of a kind in a cell instead of the normal pair.

X CHROMOSOME
The X chromosome is a sex chromosome. The human female has two identical X chromosomes; the human male has an X chromosome and a Y chromosome.

Y CHROMOSOME
The Y chromosome is one of the male sex chromosomes. Sex determination in man depends on the Y chromosome.

Fetal Membranes and Placenta

FETAL MEMBRANES

The fetal membranes consist of an outer chorionic and an inner amniotic membrane. They adhere to each other in the second and third trimesters and make up the wall of the amniotic sac.

PLACENTA

The placenta is the structure providing the principal means of communication between the mother and the fetus. It increases in size until the end of pregnancy, by which time it is a round or oval disk covering about one-fifth of the inner surface of the uterus. It is composed of villi containing vessels that carry fetal blood. The villi penetrate the maternal decidua and are bathed in maternal blood. The portion of the decidua basalis superior to Nitabuch's layer forms a thin covering on the maternal surface of the placenta. The fetal surface is composed of chorion to which the amnion is adherent. The placental chorion and the amnion form the amniotic sac. The placenta performs the functions of respiration, nutrition, and excretion, and secretes estrogen, progesterone, and other hormones.

SYNONYMS: *Afterbirth, Placenta* (NA).

AMNION

The amnion is a membrane composed of a layer of cuboidal cells with associated connective tissue. It forms the lining of the amniotic sac.

SYNONYM: *Amniotic Membrane.*

AMNION NODOSUM

The amnion nodosum are nodules in the amnion occurring most commonly in that part of the amnion in contact with the chorionic plate. They usually appear near the insertion of the cord as multiple, rounded or oval, opaque elevations that vary from less than 1 to 5 or 6 mm in diameter. Microscopically, they consist of typical stratified squamous epithelium, the upper layers of which are increasingly flattened and pale-staining toward the surface. They may become calcified and are common enough to be found as isolated nodules in about 60 per cent of placentas. The nodules occur in greater concentration in association with oligohydramnios and renal agenesis.

SYNONYMS: *Amniotic Caruncles, Squamous Metaplasia of Amnion.*

AMNIONITIS
Amnionitis is inflammation of the amnion. It is a manifestation of intrauterine infection, frequently associated with prolonged rupture of the membranes and long labor.

AMNIOTIC FLUID
Amniotic fluid is the fluid that surrounds the fetus. Its exact origin is disputed, but late in pregnancy it seems to be composed principally of fetal urine.

AMNIOTIC FOLD
The amniotic fold is a fold of amnion extending from the point of insertion of the umbilical cord to the yolk sac. It carries the vitelline duct.
SYNONYM: *Schultze's Fold.*

AMNIOTIC SAC
The amniotic sac is a baglike structure that contains the amniotic fluid and the fetus.
SYNONYM: *Bag of Waters.*

ANCHORING VILLI
The anchoring villi are villi that become intimately related to the maternal tissue. The connective tissue of the distal ends of the villi actually becomes adherent to the endometrial connective tissue.

BLASTOCYST
The blastocyst is a structure that results when fluid accumulates within the morula, producing a cavity with the inner cell mass at one pole. The wall of the blastocyst develops into the trophoblast.
SYNONYM: *Blastula.*

CAUL
The caul is the portion of the amniotic sac that may cover the fetal head at birth. It results from failure of the amniotic sac to rupture before birth.

CHORION
The chorion is composed of trophoblast and mesenchyme. It forms the outer wall of the amniotic sac.

CHORION FRONDOSUM
The chorion frondosum is the portion of the chorion that is in contact with the decidua basalis. The chorion frondosum and decidua basalis eventually form the placenta. The greatest growth of chorionic villi takes place in the chorion frondosum.

CHORION LAEVE
The chorion laeve is the portion of the chorion in contact with the decidua capsularis. The villi of the chorion laeve degenerate after the third month of pregnancy.

CHORIONIC PLATE

The chorionic plate is the portion of the chorion that is attached to the uterus. It is the primordium of the chorion frondosum.

CHORIONIC VILLI

The chorionic villi are slender branching projections of chorion. They contain capillaries and are the means by which all substances are exchanged between maternal and fetal circulation.

COTYLEDON

A cotyledon is a portion of the placenta composed of fetal and maternal elements.

CYTOTROPHOBLAST

The cytotrophoblast is composed of giant, multinucleated cells. It forms the innermost of two layers covering the early chorionic villi. These cells ordinarily disappear before midpregnancy.

SYNONYM: *Langhans' Cells.*

DECIDUA

The decidua is the endometrium during pregnancy. There are marked hypertrophic and secretory changes. Glands are more prominent with a marked saw-toothed appearance. The epithelium is low, pale-staining, and it actively secretes nutritive substances. The stromal cells are large and polygonal with a wide zone of cytoplasm. The spongy zone is hypertrophic. The basal layer has glands lined with nonsecretory cells.

SYNONYM: *Endometrium of Pregnancy.*

DECIDUA BASALIS

The decidua basalis is the area of endometrium on which the blastocyst implants.

SYNONYMS: *Decidua Serotina, Decidua Basalis* (NA).

DECIDUA CAPSULARIS

The decidua capsularis is the thin layer of endometrium covering the implanted blastocyst.

SYNONYMS: *Decidua Reflexa, Decidua Capsularis* (NA).

DECIDUA COMPACTA

The decidua compacta is the superficial portion of the decidua basalis. At the end of pregnancy, separation of the placenta from the uterine wall occurs in this layer.

DECIDUA POLYPOSA

Decidua polyposa is the appearance of polypoid projections on the surface of the decidua. It is caused by local hyperplasia of the decidua.

DECIDUA SPONGIOSA

The decidua spongiosa is the deep portion of the decidua basalis. It is attached to the myometrium.

DECIDUA VERA

The decidua vera is the endometrium that lines the entire uterine cavity except at the site of the implanted blastocyst.

SYNONYM: *Decidua Parietalis* (NA).

DECIDUAL CAST

A decidual cast is the entire decidua expelled from the uterus in a single piece.

DECIDUAL HYPERPLASIA

Decidual hyperplasia is abnormal thickening of the decidua. It may be diffuse or local.

DECIDUITIS

Deciduitis is inflammation of the decidua.

DESMOSOMES

Desmosomes are sites of adhesion in the trophoblast between individual cytotrophoblasts and the syncytium.

ECTOPIC DECIDUA

Ectopic decidua is a condition in which decidual cells arise from implants of endometrium in other parts of the body.

ENDOMETRITIS DECIDUA CYSTICA

Endometritis decidua cystica is a nodulated appearance of the decidua due to retention cysts. These cysts are the result of occlusion of the ducts.

FOREWATER

The forewater is the portion of the amniotic sac that pouches into the cervix in front of the presenting part.

GEMMULAE HOBOKENII

Gemmulae Hobokenii are gross dilatations on the outer surface of the umbilical arteries.

SYNONYM: *Noduli Hobokenii.*

HOFBAUER CELL

A Hofbauer cell is a mononuclear, wandering phagocyte found in the stroma of the chorionic villi.

INFLAMMATION OF CORD

Inflammation of the cord is an infection of the umbilical cord due to a variety of organisms. Leukocyte infiltration may occur in the substance of the cord.

KNOT OF UMBILICAL CORD

A knot of the umbilical cord is an entanglement of the umbilical cord that produces anoxia if it becomes taut.

316 PHYSIOLOGY OF REPRODUCTION

LACUNA

A lacuna is the space between the villi. It is bounded by the chorionic membrane on the fetal side and the decidua basalis on the maternal side.
SYNONYM: *Intervillous Space.*

MARGINAL SINUS

The marginal sinus is the lacuna at the edge of the placenta. The term was originally used to designate a circumferential venous channel into which all maternal blood was thought to flow prior to leaving the placenta. Many now doubt its functional significance.

NITABUCH'S LAYER

Nitabuch's layer is the zone of canalized fibrin between the tropho-blastic and decidual tissues.

NOURISHING VILLI

The nourishing villi are villi that lie free in the excavated spaces of the decidua basalis and absorb nutritional substances for embryonic and fetal growth.
SYNONYM: *Free Villi.*

OLIGOHYDRAMNIOS

Oligohydramnios is a deficiency in the amount of amniotic fluid.
SYNONYM: *Oligoamnios.*

PLACENTA, ACCESSORY

An accessory placenta is a mass of placental tissue, distinct from the main placenta, with or without a blood supply.

PLACENTA ACCRETA

Placenta accreta is a placenta of which a part or all is inseparable from the uterine wall. It is caused by partial or complete absence of the decidua basalis, especially of the spongy layer.

PLACENTA, ADHERENT

An adherent placenta is a placenta that fails to separate easily from the uterus after birth of the fetus.

PLACENTA, ANNULAR

An annular placenta is a placenta in a beltlike band encircling the interior of the uterus.
SYNONYM: *Zonary Placenta.*

PLACENTA, BATTLEDORE

A battledore placenta is a placenta with marginal attachment of the umbilical cord.
SYNONYM: *Marginal Insertion of Umbilical Cord.*

PLACENTA, BILOBATE

A bilobate placenta is a placenta composed of two parts, each with marginal insertion of vessels. The two parts are separated by membranes and are united only where the vessels leave the placenta to form the umbilical cord.

SYNONYM: *Duplex Placenta.*

PLACENTA, CIRCUMVALLATE

A circumvallate placenta is a placenta in which the peripheral portion of the chorion is turned inward forming a cufflike ring. The membranes are attached to the edge of the ring and overlie the peripheral portion of the placenta.

SYNONYM: *Placenta Nappiformis.*

PLACENTA EXTRACHORALES

Placenta extrachorales is a placenta in which there is limitation of the chorionic plate by a thin membranous fold at the edge of the plate.

PLACENTA, FENESTRATE

A fenestrate placenta is one in which there are areas of thinning. Sometimes placental tissue is entirely absent.

PLACENTA, FETAL

The fetal placenta is the portion of the placenta formed of chorion and containing fetal blood vessels.

SYNONYM: *Pars Fetalis* (NA).

PLACENTA, HORSESHOE

A horseshoe placenta is a long, curved placenta resembling a horseshoe in shape.

PLACENTA INCRETA

Placenta increta is a form of placenta accreta in which the chorionic villi invade the myometrium.

PLACENTA, MARGINAL

A marginal placenta is a placenta with a peripheral ring of fibrin and degenerated decidua on the surface of the chorionic plate.

SYNONYMS: *Placenta Marginata, Placenta Circummarginata.*

PLACENTA MEMBRANACEA

Placenta membranacea is a thin placenta occupying a greater than normal part of the chorion. It results from failure of a normal proportion of the chorion laeve to atrophy.

PLACENTA, MONOCHORIONIC MONOAMNIOTIC

A monochorionic monoamniotic placenta is a placenta with a single amnion and chorion occurring in a twin pregnancy.

PLACENTA, MULTILOBATE

A multilobate placenta is a placenta consisting of several lobes, usually variable in size, with blood vessels coming directly from the umbilical cord or from another lobe.

SYNONYMS: *Placenta Multipartita, Placenta Multiloba.*

PLACENTA PERCRETA

Placenta percreta is abnormal penetration of chorionic elements to the serosal layer of the uterus.

PLACENTA RENIFORMIS

Placenta reniformis is a kidney-shaped placenta.

PLACENTA, RETAINED

A retained placenta is a placenta that has not separated or been expelled within one hour after the completion of the second stage of labor.

PLACENTA, SEPTUPLEX

A septuplex placenta is a placenta that consists of seven small lobes.

PLACENTA SPURIA

Placenta spuria is an accessory lobe of placental tissue having no vascular connection with the main placenta.

PLACENTA, SUCCENTURIATE

A succenturiate placenta is a placenta having one or more lobes distal to its margin. Blood supply is by extension of placental vessels.

PLACENTA, TRAPPED

A trapped placenta is a placenta that is retained within the uterus, generally due to closure of the uterine cervix.

SYNONYM: *Incarcerated Placenta.*

PLACENTA, TRILOBATE

A trilobate placenta is a placenta composed of three parts, each with marginal insertion of vessels. The three parts are separated by membranes and are united only where the vessels leave the placenta to form the umbilical cord.

SYNONYMS: *Placenta Tripartita, Placenta Triplex.*

PLACENTA TRUFFÉE

Placenta truffée is a placenta with small, dark red infarcts suggesting truffles.

PLACENTA, TUBAL-CORNUAL

A tubal-cornual placenta is a placenta that has implanted in the cornual portion of the uterus near the insertion of the fallopian tube. It separates poorly and often has to be manually removed.

PLACENTA, VELAMENTOUS

A velamentous placenta is a placenta with the umbilical vessels attached to and spread out on the membranes and entering the placenta separately.

SYNONYMS: *Lobstein's Placenta, Placenta Velamentosa.*

PLACENTAL AGING

Placental aging is a process resulting in decreased placental activity. It is characterized, histologically, by deposition of fibrin around the villi, thickening of the basement membrane of the trophoblast and capillary endothelium, and focal ischemia with degeneration. Placental aging causes decreased secretion of the placental steroids and impaired transfer of material to and from the fetus.

PLACENTAL CYST

A placental cyst is a cyst formed on the fetal surface of the mature placenta. It varies in size from microscopic to 6 mm in diameter. There is a white infarct beneath the cyst, and it is generally lined with degenerative cytotrophoblastic cells. Occasionally, the cyst may contain a blighted ovum.

PLACENTAL INFARCTS

Placental infarcts are solid areas that may be present in the substance or on either surface of the placenta. They are of variable size and are usually composed of degenerating villi embedded in fibrin. The color of the infarcts changes from red to yellow-white with increasing placental age.

PLACENTAL MEMBRANE

The placental membrane is the semipermeable layer of tissue separating the maternal blood supply from the fetal blood supply.

SYNONYM: *Placental Barrier* (obsolete).

PLACENTAL MICROVILLI

Placental microvilli are minute slender processes that extend peripherally from the syncytiotrophoblast. They are visible only with the electron microscope.

PLACENTAL SECUNDINES

Placental secundines is a collective term referring to the placenta and fetal membranes.

PLACENTAL SEPTUM

A placental septum is a projection of decidual tissue forming a partial partition between cotyledons.

PLACENTAL SYNCYTIAL BUD

The placental syncytial bud is a small zone of proliferated syncytiotrophoblastic cells. Although the cells increase in number in late pregnancy, the number is extremely variable and is thought to change with the concentration of oxygen.

SYNONYMS: *Syncytial Knot, Syncytial Sprout.*

PLACENTAL TRANSFER
Placental transfer is the passage of gases, chemicals, or fluids from maternal to fetal circulation or the reverse.

PLACENTATION
Placentation is the development of the placenta after attachment of the blastocyst to the uterine wall or other structures.

PLACENTITIS
Placentitis is an inflammatory reaction, usually limited to the fetal surface of the placenta, involving especially the zone between the amnion and chorion. The inflammatory reaction may extend into the walls of the umbilical vessels. It may be responsible for fetal bacteremia or pneumonia.

SYNONYM: *Placuntitis.*

PRIMARY VILLI
Primary villi are early projections of the trophoblast that extend into the decidua. In the human, they establish the basic relationship of the placenta to the uterine decidua.

ROHR'S STRIA
Rohr's stria is an inconstant deposition of fibrin at the bottom of the lacuna and surrounding the anchoring villi. It occurs when the decidua is defective.

SUBCHORIAL SPACE
The subchorial space is the portion of the placenta just beneath the chorion.

SYNONYM: *Subchorial Lake.*

SYNCYTIOTROPHOBLAST
The syncytiotrophoblast is the outer layer of cells covering each chorionic villus and in contact with maternal blood or decidua.

SYNONYMS: *Plasmoditrophoblast, Syntrophoblast, Syncytial Trophoblast.*

TORSION OF UMBILICAL CORD
Torsion of the umbilical cord is a twisting of the umbilical cord, which is created by violent fetal movement, causing fetal anoxia and death.

TROPHOBLAST
The trophoblast is the nonfetal part of the implanted blastocyst. It originates from the peripheral cells of the blastocyst. In this early stage, the trophoblast is believed to give rise to the mesoblast, the stroma of the villi, and to the external covering of the villi that continues to be known as trophoblast.

TROPHOBLASTIC LACUNAE
The trophoblastic lacunae are blood spaces created in the early tropho-blast to permit circulation of maternal blood.

UMBILICAL ARTERIES, FETAL
The fetal umbilical arteries, two in number, extend as branches of the internal iliac arteries to the umbilicus. As they emerge from the fetal body, they run through the umbilical cord carrying venous blood to the placenta.

UMBILICAL CORD
The umbilical cord is a long cylindrical cord extending from the fetal umbilicus to the fetal surface of the placenta. The two umbilical arteries and one umbilical vein are bound together within the umbilical cord by Wharton's jelly. The umbilical arteries possess the valvulae Hobokenii and gemmulae Hobokenii.

SYNONYMS: *Funis, Funiculis Umbilicalis* (NA).

UMBILICAL VEIN, FETAL
The fetal umbilical vein emerges from the placenta and carries arterial blood through the umbilical cord to the fetus.

VALVULAE HOBOKENII
The valvulae Hobokenii are protrusions into the lumen of the umbilical arteries where the arteries are twisted or kinked in the umbilical cord.

VASA PREVIA
Vasa previa is an anomaly of umbilical cord insertion in which the umbilical blood vessels traverse the lower uterine segment, presenting in advance of the fetal head. A velamentous insertion of the cord is usually a prerequisite of vasa previa. Fetal mortality in this condition approaches 60 per cent.

VELAMENTOUS INSERTION OF UMBILICAL CORD
Velamentous insertion of the umbilical cord is the condition in which the blood vessels leave the placenta, course between the amnion and chorion, and unite to form the umbilical cord at some distance from the edge of the placenta.

WHARTON'S JELLY
Wharton's jelly is the myxomatous connective tissue constituting the matrix of the umbilical cord and supporting the umbilical vessels.

Embryonic Development of
Genital Organs

EMBRYO

Embryo is a term applied to a human fetus from the time of conception until organogenesis is largely completed (10 gestational weeks). Embryo is an embryologic term and should not be used for purposes of statistical reporting.

BODY STALK

The body stalk is the precursor of the umbilical cord. It is a mesoblastic stalk that connects the developing embryo with the wall of the amniotic sac.

CLOACA

The cloaca is a common entodermal chamber in which urinary, fecal, and reproductive products are passed to be expelled.

CORDS OF PFLUGER

The cords of Pfluger are strands of cells that are in contact with areas of the germinal epithelium of the fetal ovary. Wherever the cords of Pfluger appear, the tunica albuginea is absent.

EXTERNAL GENITALIA

Indifferent Stage

In very young embryos, there is formed in the midline, just cephalic to the proctodeal depression, a vaguely outlined elevation known as the *cloacal* or *genital eminence*. This is soon differentiated into a central prominence, the *genital tubercle*, which will ultimately become differentiated into the penis in the male or into the *clitoris* in the female. Along the caudal surface of the genital tubercle lie the paired *genital folds* extending toward the proctodeum. Between the genital folds is a longitudinal depression into the proximal region of which the urogenital sinus opens. This opening (*urogenital ostium*) is separated from the anal opening when the urorectal fold subdivides the primitive cloaca. Farther laterally, on either side of the genital folds, are paired vaguely outlined elevations known as the *genital swellings*, which become differentiated into the scrotal folds in the male, or into the *labia majora* in the female. In the female, the *genital folds* become the *labia minora*. Although in

322

young female embryos there is for a time a urethral groove homologous with that in the male, the parts of the genital folds extending onto the under surface of the clitoris remain rudimentary and soon regress. Thus the urethral groove in the female is never deepened and closed over to form a urethra in the clitoris corresponding to the penile urethra of the male. In the adult female, there is midventrally in the clitoris only an inconspicuous strand of vascular connective tissue in a position comparable with that occupied by the penile urethra and the corpus cavernosum urethrae in the male. In the female, therefore, there is no secondary projection forward of the urethral orifice, and just the prostatic portion of the male urethra is homologous with the entire urethra in the female. The *minor vestibular glands* should probably be regarded as corresponding to the urethral glands in the male. The seminal vesicles lack any homologues in the female. The curious cryptlike diverticula from the female urethra, called *paraurethral glands*, are ill-developed homologues of the multiple prostatic glandular units of the male. In contrast, the homologues of the bulbourethral glands of the male are relatively more highly developed in the female. They are known as the *major vestibular glands*. Their primordial buds arise during the latter part of the third month.

Anogenital Band

The anogenital band is a cordlike structure that is the first indication of the perineum in the embryo.

INTERNAL REPRODUCTIVE ORGANS

Indifferent Stage

The male ducts are not developed primarily as reproductive ducts, but are appropriated from the regressing mesonephros, some of the mesonephric tubules becoming connected with the developing gonad and the mesonephric duct being used as a discharge passage for the sex cells. The female paramesonephric ducts develop independently alongside the mesonephric ducts and the two duct systems are for a time present together. If the embryo is destined to become a male, the potentially female ducts remain rudimentary and the appropriated mesonephric ducts and tubules undergo further growth and differentiation giving rise to the duct system of the testes. If the embryo develops into a female, the paramesonephric ducts form the fallopian tubes, uterus, and vagina, and the male ducts become rudimentary. The gonads are intimately associated with the nephric system. While the mesonephros is still the dominant excretory organ, the gonads arise as ridgelike thickenings (*gonadal ridges, germinal ridges*) on its ventral border. The *sex cords* are local accumulation of cells that migrate into the mesenchyme forming finger-like structures. If the embryo is to be a male, these cords become increasingly sharply delimited and are eventually differentiated into the seminiferous tubules. If the gonad develops into an ovary, the primordial cell cords tend to break up into cell clusters that become differentiated into primordial ovarian follicles.

Embryonic Fallopian Tube

The embryonic fallopian tube is formed by the part of the para-mesonephric duct between the uterus and the ovary. Near its cephalic end, but not usually at the extreme tip, a more or less funnel-shaped opening develops called the *abdominal ostium.*

Embryonic Hymen

The embryonic hymen is apparent at approximately six to eight weeks of gestation as a solid epithelial plug at the lower end of the fused paramesonephric ducts. If the plug does not become thinned and perforated, an imperforate hymen results.

Embryonic Ovary

The embryonic ovary becomes apparent at approximately the seventh week of gestation. It can be distinguished from the embry-onic testis in that the sex cords are less distinct than in the indifferent or early male gonad, the mesenchyme separating the sex cords is more sparse than in the male, and the outer cellular layer remains active and free of tunica albuginea development.

Embryonic Testis

The embryonic testis becomes apparent at approximately the seventh week of gestation. It can be distinguished from the female gonad by the sex cords. They condense to form the seminiferous tubules, the sex cords become separated by mesenchyme, and the tunica albuginea begins to form between the coelomic epithelium covering the gonads and the sex cords.

Embryonic Uterus

The embryonic uterus is formed by fusion of the paramesonephric ducts. The fusion involves the caudal end of the uterus so that it opens into the vagina in the form of an unpaired neck or *cervix.* The paramesonephric ducts are fused with each other throughout the levels incorporated in the uterus. This results in the formation of what is called a simplex type of uterus. Abnormalities of the uterus result from variations in the extent or manner of fusion of the paramesonephric ducts during early development. Various degrees of partitioning of the fundus of the uterus are among the more frequently encountered abnormalities (uterus subseptus unicollis, uterus septus duplex). In some cases, only the fundal portion of the uterus is involved (uterus bicornis unicollis). In others the partition runs down into the cervical canal (uterus bicornis septus). Com-plete partitioning of the uterus is associated with a double vagina (uterus septus duplex with double vagina). A completely paired uterus with each member of the pair having its own cervix opening into the corresponding member of paired vagina (uterus didelphys with double vagina) is rare.

Embryonic Vagina

The embryonic vagina is formed by the hollowing out of the fused paramesonephric ducts at about the sixth to eighth week of gestation. The lower part of the vagina may fail to acquire a lumen and remain as a solid cord resulting in atresia of the vagina.

MESONEPHRIC DUCT

The mesonephric duct is the duct of the embryo connecting the mesonephros or second excretory organ system. The mesonephric duct is central in the development of the male embryo.

SYNONYMS: *Wolffian Duct, Ductus Mesonephricus* (NA).

PARAMESONEPHRIC DUCT

The paramesonephric duct is an embryonic canal extending along the mesonephros parallel to the mesonephric duct and terminating in the cloaca. The paramesonephric duct is central in the development of female embryos.

SYNONYMS: *Müllerian Duct, Müller's Canal, Müller's Duct, Ductus Paramesonephricus* (NA).

PRIMITIVE GONAD

The primitive gonad is derived from the median aspect of the urogenital ridge and is first distinguishable as a thickening of the coelomic epithelium and the mesenchyme beneath it. The primitive gonad is first detectable at approximately six weeks of gestation.

UROGENITAL RIDGE

The urogenital ridge is a bulging longitudinal mass of cells on each side of the dorsal mesentery.

UROGENITAL SINUS

The urogenital sinus is an elongated embryonic sac. It is derived from the ventral part of the cloaca and is cut off from the rectum by the urorectal fold. The mesonephric ducts empty into the urogenital sinus.

SYNONYM: *Sinus Urogenitalis* (NA).

Section 7: *Obstetrics*

Pregnancy

GENERAL TERMINOLOGY

PREGNANCY

Pregnancy is the state of a female after conception and until termination of the gestation.

SYNONYMS: *Gestation, Cyophoria, Cyesis, Gravidity.*

Abdominal Pregnancy

Abdominal pregnancy is gestation occurring within the peritoneal cavity.

SYNONYM: *Intraperitoneal Pregnancy.*

PRIMARY ABDOMINAL PREGNANCY

Primary abdominal pregnancy is growth of the fetus and placenta within the peritoneal cavity. Fertilization and embryonic growth occur before entrance into the fallopian tube. It is a rare condition.

SECONDARY ABDOMINAL PREGNANCY

Secondary abdominal pregnancy is a pregnancy that develops in the abdominal cavity following tubal abortion or rupture. The fetus may continue to grow until term or become macerated, skeletonized, or mummified.

Ampullar Pregnancy

Ampullar pregnancy is an ectopic pregnancy in the ampullar portion of the fallopian tube. It generally ends in tubal abortion.

Cervical Pregnancy

Cervical pregnancy is gestation that develops when the fertilized ovum becomes implanted in the cervical canal of the uterus.

Combined Heterotopic Pregnancy

Combined heterotopic pregnancy is characterized by the existence of simultaneous intrauterine and extrauterine pregnancies.

SYNONYM: *Compound Pregnancy.*

Cornual Pregnancy

Cornual pregnancy is gestation that has developed in a rudimentary horn of the uterus.

SYNONYM: *Rudimentary Horn Pregnancy.*

Ectopic Pregnancy

Ectopic pregnancy is gestation outside the uterine cavity. It is a broader term than extrauterine pregnancy, because it includes gestations in the interstitial portion of the tube, in a rudimentary horn of the uterus, as well as tubal, abdominal, and ovarian gestations.

SYNONYM: *Heterotopic Pregnancy.*

Extraamniotic Pregnancy

Extraamniotic pregnancy is gestation in which the fetus develops in the uterus but the amnion ruptures early in pregnancy leaving the chorion intact. The shrunken amnion hangs around the insertion of the cord.

SYNONYM: *Graviditas Examnialis.*

Extrachorial Pregnancy

Extrachorial pregnancy is gestation in which the fetus develops in the uterus but outside the chorionic sac. This type of gestation results from rupture and shrinkage of the membranes in the early months of pregnancy.

SYNONYM: *Graviditas Exochorialis.*

Extrauterine Pregnancy

Extrauterine pregnancy is gestation outside the uterine cavity, but it does not include pregnancy in the interstitial portion of the tube.

Interstitial Pregnancy

Interstitial pregnancy is pregnancy in the interstitial portion of the fallopian tube.

SYNONYMS: *Angular Pregnancy, Tubouterine Pregnancy.*

Intraligamentous Pregnancy

Intraligamentous pregnancy is growth of the fetus and placenta between the folds of the broad ligament, after rupture of a tubal pregnancy through the floor of the fallopian tube.

SYNONYMS: *Broad Ligament Pregnancy, Extraperitoneal Pregnancy.*

Intrauterine Pregnancy

Intrauterine pregnancy is a pregnancy within the uterus.

SYNONYM: *Uterine Pregnancy.*

Isthmic Pregnancy

Isthmic pregnancy is a gestation in the narrow portion of the fallopian tube.

Late Pregnancy

Late pregnancy is gestation after the usual childbearing age.

Mesometric Pregnancy

Mesometric pregnancy is gestation within the middle muscular layer of the uterus.

SYNONYM: *Mural Pregnancy.*

Multiple Pregnancy
Multiple pregnancy is the state of being pregnant with two or more fetuses.

Ovarian Pregnancy, Primary
Primary ovarian pregnancy is a rare form of ectopic pregnancy in which impregnation of the ovum by the spermatozoon occurs before the former is extruded from the ovary.

Ovarian Pregnancy, Secondary
Secondary ovarian pregnancy is a rare form of ectopic pregnancy in which the blastocyst implants on the surface of the ovary.

Precocious Pregnancy
Precocious pregnancy is gestation before the usual childbearing age.

Prolonged Pregnancy
Prolonged pregnancy is gestation that has advanced beyond the 42nd completed week (beyond 294 days).

Tubal Pregnancy
Tubal pregnancy is an ectopic pregnancy in a portion of the fallopian tube. It is the most common form of ectopic pregnancy.
SYNONYM: *Salpingocyesis.*

Tuboabdominal Pregnancy
Tuboabdominal pregnancy is growth of the fetus and placenta in the abdominal cavity after rupture of a tubal pregnancy through the roof of the fallopian tube.

Tuboovarian Pregnancy
Tuboovarian pregnancy is growth of the fetus and placenta after implantation in the fimbria ovarica of the fallopian tube. It generally results in a secondary abdominal pregnancy.

Uteroabdominal Pregnancy
Uteroabdominal pregnancy is the growth of the fetus and placenta in the abdominal cavity after rupture of the uterus.

ACCOMMODATION
Accommodation is the process by which the fetus adjusts itself in the uterus.

ANTEPARTUM PERIOD
The antepartum period is the period of gestation from conception to the onset of labor.

CERVICAL MUCUS
Cervical mucus is a secretion of the endocervix during the menstrual cycle and pregnancy. Its composition is altered during the menstrual cycle by the action of estrogen and progesterone. It contains enzymes, mucus, leukocytes, cervical and vaginal cells, and other substances. Dur-

ing pregnancy, it serves as a plug, providing a mechanical and antibacterial barrier to the uterine cavity.

SYNONYMS: *Cervical Secretion, Mucous Plug, Cervical Plug.*

CHAUSSIER'S SIGN

Chaussier's sign is pain in the epigastrium preceding eclampsia.

CHILDBEARING AGE

The childbearing age is a time between puberty and the menopause when conception is most likely to occur.

CHLOASMA

Chloasma is a skin condition of the pregnant woman characterized by the appearance of irregular, variable-sized brownish patches on the face. The condition generally disappears or regresses after pregnancy is terminated.

SYNONYM: *Mask of Pregnancy.*

CREPITUS UTERI

Crepitus uteri is characterized by a crackling sensation felt on palpation of the uterus. It is an indication of air or gas within the uterus.

DECIDUA

The decidua is the endometrium during pregnancy. There are marked hypertrophic and secretory changes. Glands are more prominent with a marked saw-toothed appearance. The epithelium is low, and palestaining, and it actively secretes nutritive substances. The stromal cells are large and polygonal with a wide zone of cytoplasm. The spongy zone is hypertrophic. The basal layer has glands lined with nonsecretory cells.

SYNONYM: *Endometrium of Pregnancy.*

DIASTASIS RECTI

Diastasis recti is separation of the recti muscles due to stretching of the abdominal wall. This condition is sometimes seen during or following pregnancy.

ELDERLY PRIMIGRAVIDA

An elderly primigravida is a woman pregnant for the first time who is more than 30 years of age. The age criterion may vary depending on marital and fertility history, but it is usually at least more than 30 years. It denotes diminished fecundity, high risk for perinatal or maternal complications, and decreased fertility. Such a woman is considered a greater risk than the average woman and should be accorded more intensive care to avoid these problems.

EPULIS OF PREGNANCY

Epulis of pregnancy is a focal, highly vascular swelling of the gums that occurs during pregnancy but regresses spontaneously after birth of the infant.

FIBROMUSCULAR JUNCTION

The fibromuscular junction is the area between the muscular elements of the uterine wall and the fibrous tissue of the cervix. It has considerable functional significance in that it may produce a sphincter-like action, relaxing under estrogen influence and contracting under progesterone action.

GESTATIONAL AGE

Gestational age is the estimated age of the fetus calculated from the first day of the last normal menstrual period. Gestational age is expressed in completed weeks.

GRAVID

Gravid is a general term referring to the pregnant state.

GRAVIDA

Gravida is a woman who is pregnant.

Primigravida

A primigravida is a woman pregnant for the first time.
SYNONYM: *Gravida I.*

Secundigravida

A secundigravida is a woman in her second pregnancy.
SYNONYM: *Gravida II.*

Tertigravida

A tertigravida is a woman in her third pregnancy.
SYNONYM: *Gravida III.*

Quadrigravida

A quadrigravida is a woman in her fourth pregnancy.
SYNONYM: *Gravida IV.*

Quintigravida

A quintigravida is a woman in her fifth pregnancy.
SYNONYM: *Gravida V.*

Sextigravida

A sextigravida is a woman in her sixth pregnancy.
SYNONYM: *Gravida VI.*

Multigravida

A multigravida is a woman who is pregnant and who has been pregnant more than one time.

HALBAN'S SIGN

Halban's sign is the increased growth of the fine hair of the maternal body or face during pregnancy.

HELLIN'S LAW

Hellin's law is a mathematical relationship between the various orders of multiple births. It claims that twins occur once in 89 births, triplets once in 89^2 births, and quadruplets once in 89^3 births.

INTRAPARTUM PERIOD

The intrapartum period is the period of gestation from the onset of labor to the end of the third stage of labor.

LEG CRAMPS

Leg cramps are cramps or contractions of the leg muscles, especially during the night, that occur in many women between the 24th and 34th weeks of gestation.

LIGHTENING

Lightening is the settling or sinking of the fetal vertex or breech downward and forward into the true pelvis. It occurs during the last two or three weeks of pregnancy; in the primigravida, it suggests that the presenting part is not too large for the pelvic inlet.

LOWER UTERINE SEGMENT

The lower uterine segment is the greatly expanded and thinned-out isthmus of the pregnant uterus.

OBSTETRIC INTERNAL OS

The obstetric internal os is the histologic internal os of the gravid uterus.

PARITY

Parity is the state of having given birth to an infant or infants, weighing 500 gm or more, alive or dead. In the absence of known weight, an estimated length of gestation of 20 completed weeks or more, calculated from the first day of the last normal menstrual period, may be used. For the purpose of defining parity, a multiple birth is a single parous experience.

Primipara

A primipara is a woman who has given birth for the first time to an infant or infants, alive or dead, weighing 500 gm or more. In the absence of known weight, an estimated length of gestation of 20 completed weeks or more, calculated from the first day of the last normal menstrual period, may be used.

SYNONYM: *Para I*.

Secundipara

A secundipara is a woman who has given birth for the second time to an infant or infants, alive or dead, weighing 500 gm or more. In the absence of known weight, an estimated length of gestation of 20 completed weeks or more, calculated from the first day of the last normal menstrual period, may be used.

SYNONYM: *Para II*.

Tertipara

A tertipara is a woman who has given birth three times to an infant or infants, alive or dead, weighing 500 gm or more. In the absence of known weight, an estimated length of gestation of 20 completed weeks or more, calculated from the first day of the last normal menstrual period, may be used.

SYNONYM: *Para III.*

Quadripara

A quadripara is a woman who has given birth four times to an infant or infants, alive or dead, weighing 500 gm or more. In the absence of known weight, an estimated length of gestation of 20 completed weeks or more, calculated from the first day of the last normal menstrual period, may be used.

SYNONYM: *Para IV.*

Quintipara

A quintipara is a woman who has given birth five times to an infant or infants, alive or dead, weighing 500 gm or more. In the absence of known weight, an estimated length of gestation of 20 completed weeks or more, calculated from the first day of the last normal menstrual period, may be used.

SYNONYM: *Para V.*

Sextipara

A sextipara is a woman who has given birth six times to an infant or infants, alive or dead, weighing 500 gm or more. In the absence of known weight, an estimated length of gestation of 20 completed weeks or more, calculated from the first day of the last normal menstrual period, may be used.

SYNONYM: *Para VI.*

Multipara

A multipara is a woman who has given birth two or more times to an infant or infants, alive or dead, weighing 500 gm or more. In the absence of known weight, an estimated length of gestation of 20 completed weeks or more, calculated from the first day of the last normal menstrual period, may be used. For the purpose of defining parity, a multiple birth is a single parous experience.

Grand Multipara

Grand multipara is a term applied to a woman who has given birth seven or more times to an infant or infants, alive or dead, weighing 500 gm or more. In the absence of known weight, an estimated length of gestation of 20 completed weeks or more, calculated from the first day of the last normal menstrual period, may be used. For the purpose of defining parity, a multiple birth is a single parous experience.

PARTHENOGENESIS
Parthenogenesis is a form of nonsexual reproduction in which the female reproduces its kind without fertilization of a female germ cell by a male germ cell.

PENDULOUS ABDOMEN
Pendulous abdomen is a relaxed condition of the abdominal wall in which the anterior abdominal wall hangs down over the pubis.

PERIOD OF GESTATION
The period of gestation is the number of completed weeks of pregnancy between the first day of the last normal menstrual period and the date in question, or the date of completion of the pregnancy, irrespective of whether the products of conception include an abortus, fetus, or infant.

PICA
Pica is a craving for unusual substances not normally considered as food.

POSTPARTUM PERIOD
The postpartum period is a general term referring to the period of time following completion of the third stage of labor.
SYNONYM: *Postnatal Period.*

PRENATAL PERIOD
The prenatal period is the period of gestation from conception to the beginning of the birth process.

PSEUDOCYESIS
Pseudocyesis is a false pregnancy. Although conception has not taken place, there are some signs and symptoms of pregnancy.
SYNONYMS: *False Pregnancy, Phantom Pregnancy, Spurious Pregnancy.*

PTYALISM
Ptyalism is excessive salivation occurring during pregnancy.

STRIAE GRAVIDARUM
Striae gravidarum are broad, white, or discolored depressed areas that appear on the skin of the abdomen, breast, buttocks, and occasionally the thighs of a pregnant woman.
SYNONYM: *Lineae Albicantes.*

TRIMESTER, FIRST
The first trimester is the period of pregnancy from the first day of the last normal menstrual period through the completion of 14 weeks (98 days) of gestation.

TRIMESTER, SECOND

The second trimester is the period of pregnancy from the beginning of the 15th through the 28th completed week (99 to 196 days) of gestation.

TRIMESTER, THIRD

The third trimester is the period of pregnancy from the beginning of the 29th through the 42nd completed week (197 to 294 days) of gestation.

UTERINE SACCULATION

Uterine sacculation is a pouch or sac in the uterine wall formed of very thin myometrium and often connected to the gravid uterus by a relatively narrow neck. It is a rare abnormality.

UTERUS, ASYMMETRICAL

An asymmetrical uterus is a disproportionately shaped gravid uterus.

UTERUS, OVOID

An ovoid uterus is an egg-shaped gravid uterus.

SYNONYM: *Oviform Uterus.*

UTERUS, PISKACEK

A Piskacek uterus is a uterus in which implantation of the blastocyst has occurred in one corner, causing asymmetrical enlargement of the corpus. It is a sign of pregnancy.

WALKER'S CHART

Walker's chart is a method of plotting the relative fetal and placental size.

SIGNS AND SYMPTOMS

SIGNS AND SYMPTOMS OF PREGNANCY

The signs and symptoms of pregnancy are classified as subjective and objective indications of pregnancy. The subjective symptoms are noted by the patient; the objective signs are perceived by the physician.

OBJECTIVE SIGNS

The objective signs are noted by the examiner. They differ according to the duration of pregnancy.

Active Fetal Movements

Active fetal movements are motions of the fetus perceived by the mother and felt by the physician through palpation of the abdomen. They may occur as early as the 12th week of gestation and are indicative of fetal life.

Ahlfeld's Sign

Ahlfeld's sign is an irregular circumscribed contraction of the uterus after the third month of pregnancy. It is a presumptive sign of pregnancy.

Auscultatory Sign

The auscultatory sign is the fetal heartbeat heard by the physician. It is a definite sign of pregnancy and a live fetus. The heartbeat normally ranges between 120 and 160 beats per minute.

Ballottement

Ballottement is passive movement ascribed to the fetus. The sign is best elicited with the patient in the lithotomy position. With two fingers in the vagina, the head or breech of the fetus, felt first above the cervix, is given a gentle push. One usually feels the fetus leave and quickly return to the fingers. Ballottement is present from the 16th to the 32nd week of gestation.

SYNONYMS: *Repercussion, Passive Fetal Movements.*

Basal Body Temperature

The basal body temperature is a diagnostic method of determining early pregnancy by continued elevation of body temperature after ovulation. The temperature is taken rectally or orally, on awakening in the morning and before arising. It may indicate pregnancy if the temperature is 37.1 to 37.7 C (98 to 99 F) every day. The temperature should be taken through at least one menstrual cycle prior to pregnancy to establish a base line.

Braun von Fernwald's Sign

Braun von Fernwald's sign is the asymmetric enlargement of the uterus in early pregnancy with a longitudinal furrow separating the two sides.

Braxton Hicks' Sign

Braxton Hicks' sign is painless intermittent contraction of the uterus during pregnancy. Contractions may be perceived by abdominal palpation or felt by the pregnant woman as painless hardening of the uterus. They may occur as early as the tenth week of gestation. These contractions do not cause dilatation of the cervix.

Chadwick's Sign

Chadwick's sign is a bluish discoloration of the vaginal wall and vestibule. It is a presumptive sign of pregnancy and may appear about the 8th to 12th week of pregnancy.

SYNONYMS: *Jacquemier's Sign, Kluge's Sign.*

Goodell's Sign

Goodell's sign is a softening of the cervix and vagina. Softening of the cervix generally occurs at first in the upper and lower portions. Succulence of the vagina and increased leukorrheal discharge are observed. Goodell's sign is determined by bimanual examination.

Gorissenne's Sign

Gorissenne's sign is noted in the early months of pregnancy when the patient's pulse rate is not quickened on rising from a recumbent position.

Hegar's Sign

Hegar's sign is a compressibility and softening of the lower uterine segment. It is elicited by bimanual examination. Hegar's sign is not a positive sign of pregnancy.

Implantation Bleeding

Implantation bleeding is a slight endometrial oozing of blood at the time of blastocyst implantation. It occurs in certain animals and in some women.

Ladin's Sign

Ladin's sign is manifested by an area of softening just above the junction of the cervix and corpus uteri. It is elicited by bimanual examination and is a presumptive sign of pregnancy.

Palpation of Fetal Body

Palpation of the fetal body is perception of the fetal parts through the abdomen and uterus. The fetal parts are designated as small (fetal extremities) and large (vertex or breech). They may be palpated as early as the fourth month of pregnancy.

Piskacek's Sign

Piskacek's sign is manifested by asymmetrical enlargement of the corpus uteri. Early in pregnancy, one lateral half is thicker than the other, or the anterior or posterior wall of the uterus bulges out more than is normal. It is determined by bimanual examination and is a presumptive sign of pregnancy.

Souffle, Fetal

The fetal souffle is a sharp, whistling sound synchronous with the fetal heart. It is due to the rush of blood through the umbilical arteries under circumstances in which they are subject to torsion, tension, or pressure. Fetal souffle is a sign of pregnancy.

SYNONYMS: *Funic Souffle, Umbilical Souffle, Kennedy's Sign.*

Souffle, Uterine

The uterine souffle is a soft, blowing sound synchronous with the maternal heartbeat. It is due to passage of blood through the uterine vessels. Uterine souffle is heard by auscultation through the lower portion of the uterus.

SYNONYM: *Kergaradec's Sign.*

SUBJECTIVE SYMPTOMS

Subjective symptoms are noted by the patient. They differ according to the duration of the pregnancy.

Amenorrhea

Amenorrhea is the absence of menstruation. It may be primary or secondary, and either physiologic or pathologic. It is a subjective, but not a reliable, sign of pregnancy.

SYNONYM: *Menostasis.*

Breast Changes

Breast changes associated with pregnancy are enlargement, fullness, tingling, and soreness. They are not reliable signs of pregnancy.

Irritability of Bladder

Irritability of the bladder is caused by stretching of the base of the bladder due to enlargement and anteversion of the uterus. It is characterized by a frequency and urgency to urinate. Bladder irritability is not a reliable sign of pregnancy.

Nausea and Vomiting

Nausea and vomiting are digestive disturbances that frequently occur in early pregnancy. They are not diagnostic of pregnancy.

Osiander's Sign

Osiander's sign is pulsation of the vagina in early pregnancy.

Quickening

Quickening is the perception of the first active fetal movements by the mother. It is noted generally between the 16th and 18th weeks of gestation.

ESTIMATION OF DURATION

BARTHOLOMEW'S RULE OF FOURTHS

Bartholomew's rule of fourths is a method of determining the duration of pregnancy by measuring the height of the fundus of the uterus above the pubic symphysis. At two months' gestation, the fundus is one-fourth the distance from the pubis to the umbilicus; at three months' gestation, it is one-half the distance; at four months' gestation, it is three-fourths the distance or greater; at five months' gestation, the fundus is at the level of the umbilicus. The fundus then rises one-fourth the way to the ensiform process each month until the ninth month, when it sinks to the level it occupied at eight months.

HAASE'S RULE

Haase's rule is a method of approximating the length of the fetus in centimeters. During the first five months of gestation, the number of the lunar month to which the pregnancy has advanced is squared to give the approximate fetal length. In the second half of pregnancy, the number of the month is multiplied by five.

KNAUS' RULE
Knaus' rule is a rule to determine the approximate date of birth from the date of ovulation. The date of birth is estimated to within five days by counting back three months from the date of ovulation.

MC DONALD'S RULE
McDonald's rule states that the length in centimeters of the contour of the abdomen from the upper margin of the pubic symphysis to the uterine fundus, divided by 3.5, gives the duration of pregnancy in lunar months. This rule can only be applied after the sixth month of gestation.

NÄGELE'S RULE
Nägele's rule is a means of estimating the date of birth by counting back three months from the first day of the last normal menstrual period and adding seven days.

NUMERICAL ESTIMATION
Numerical estimation is a method of calculating the date of birth by counting 266 days from the date of a single fruitful coitus.

PREGNANCY TESTS

BIOLOGIC, IMMUNOLOGIC, AND SEROLOGIC PREGNANCY TESTS
Biologic, immunologic, and serologic pregnancy tests are analyses of blood or urine for the hormones secreted by the products of conception. The tests are as follows: Aschheim-Zondek test, Friedman test, male frog and toad test, ovarian hyperemia test, and immunologic pregnancy test. These tests are based on the fact that the secretion of chorionic gonadotropin by the chorion can be determined by analysis of the urine or blood.

ASCHHEIM-ZONDEK TEST
The Aschheim-Zondek test is a test for the determination of pregnancy. A first morning specimen of urine is injected into four immature white mice. If the woman is pregnant, the ovaries of the mice will become enlarged, hyperemic, and hemorrhagic, and they may also show maturation of the ovarian follicle. It is a reliable test for pregnancy (99 per cent).

FRIEDMAN TEST
The Friedman test is a test for the determination of pregnancy. Ten cubic centimeters of urine from the first morning specimen are injected into the marginal ear vein of a mature, nonpregnant, female rabbit that has been isolated for at least three weeks. The animal is anesthetized 24 hours after the injection. The abdomen is opened and the ovaries are examined in situ for ruptured hemorrhagic follicles. These positive findings are indicative of pregnancy. It is a reliable test (98 per cent). The animal cannot be used again for another four weeks.

IMMUNOLOGIC PREGNANCY TEST

The immunologic pregnancy test is a test for determination of pregnancy in which human chorionic gonadotropin antiserum and an antigen consisting of polystyrene latex particles coated with human chorionic gonadotropin are used. A drop of the antiserum is placed on a dark slide with one drop of urine. The preparation is mixed well, and the slide is rocked gently for 30 seconds. Two drops of the antigen are added and mixed, and the slide is again rocked slowly and gently. The mixture is read for agglutination for no longer than two minutes. The test is negative if agglutination occurs within two minutes and positive if no agglutination occurs within two minutes. It is a reliable test (96 per cent).

MALE FROG AND TOAD TEST

The male frog and toad test is a biologic test for the determination of pregnancy. It is based on the fact that the administration of human chorionic gonadotropin to the *Rana pipiens* frog or the *Bufo americanus* or *Bufo marinus* toads causes spermatozoa to appear in the cloacal fluid. *Bufo marinus* is the most satisfactory animal to use because of less seasonal variation. After the testing of urine from two test animals for absence of spermatozoa, 5 cc of the patient's urine are injected into the dorsal lymph sac of each toad with a 22-gauge needle. At intervals of one hour following injection, the animals are checked for spermatozoa in the cloaca. If both animals are positive at the first check, the test for pregnancy is conclusive and designated "positive." If only one animal is positive, the test is allowed to run four hours. If only one animal is again positive, the test is considered inconclusive and should be repeated.

OVARIAN HYPEREMIA TEST

The ovarian hyperemia test is a biologic test for the determination of pregnancy. Two cubic centimeters of the first urine sample voided in the morning or 1 ml of blood serum is injected intraperitoneally into each of two immature rats, weighing 35 to 75 gm. The animals are sacrificed by chloroform or gas asphyxiation four hours later or at any time up to 24 hours after injection. A reddish injected appearance of the ovaries in comparison to the adjacent coils of the oviduct indicates a positive test for pregnancy. It is rapid, simple, and accurate (98 per cent).

Pelvis

LANDMARKS

BONY PELVIS
The bony pelvis is a ring of bone comprised of the sacrum, coccyx, and the two innominate bones.

ACETABULUM
The acetabulum is a cup-shaped depression on the external surface of the innominate bone into which the head of the femur fits. It is formed medially by the pubis, above by the ilium, laterally and below by the ischium.
SYNONYM: *Acetabulum* (NA).

COCCYX
The coccyx is formed from four rudimentary vertebrae usually ankylosed and articulating with the sacrum above.
SYNONYM: *Os Coccygis* (NA).

ILIAC SPINE, ANTERIOR INFERIOR
The anterior inferior iliac spine is a projection of bone on the anterior surface of the ala of the ilium below the notch adjoining the anterior superior iliac spine. It has no obstetric importance.
SYNONYM: *Spina Iliaca Anterior Inferior* (NA).

ILIAC SPINE, ANTERIOR SUPERIOR
The anterior superior iliac spine is a bony projection at the junction of the iliac crest and anterior border of the ala of the ilium. Its outer border gives attachment to the fascia lata and the tensor fascia lata. Its inner border gives attachment to the iliacus. The extremity affords attachment to the inguinal ligament and origin to the sartorius muscle.
SYNONYM: *Spina Iliaca Anterior Superior* (NA).

ILIAC SPINE, POSTERIOR INFERIOR
The posterior inferior iliac spine is a projection of bone on the inferior surface of the posterior border of the ala of the ilium. It has no particular obstetric importance.
SYNONYM: *Spina Iliaca Posterior Inferior* (NA).

341

ILIAC SPINE, POSTERIOR SUPERIOR

The posterior superior iliac spine is a projection of bone on the superior surface of the posterior border of the ala of the ilium. It serves for the attachment of the oblique portion of the posterior sacroiliac ligament.

SYNONYM: *Spina Iliaca Posterior Superior* (NA).

ILIOPECTINEAL EMINENCE

The iliopectineal eminence is a protuberance on the superior rim of the pelvis, midway between the pubic symphysis and the sacroiliac articulation. It is the point of union of the ilium and pubis.

SYNONYM: *Eminentia Iliopubica* (NA).

ILIUM

The ilium is the superior broad and expanded portion of the innominate bone. It extends upward from the acetabulum.

SYNONYM: *Os Ilium* (NA).

ILIUM, ALA OF

The ala of the ilium is the large expanded portion of the ilium that bounds the greater pelvis laterally.

SYNONYM: *Ala Ossis Ilii* (NA).

ILIUM, CREST OF

The crest of the ilium is the superior surface of the ala of the ilium. It is thinner at the center and ends in the anterior and posterior iliac spines.

SYNONYM: *Crista Iliaca* (NA).

INNOMINATE BONE

The innominate bone is a large, flattened, irregularly shaped bone composed of the ilium, ischium, and pubis. It meets its fellow in the anterior midline to form the sides and anterior wall of the pelvic cavity. The union of the three bones takes place in and around the acetabulum.

SYNONYMS: *Hipbone, Os Coxae* (NA).

ISCHIUM

The ischium is the portion of the innominate bone that forms its lower and back surfaces. It is divided into a body and a ramus.

SYNONYM: *Os Ischii* (NA).

Ischium, Body of

The body of the ischium is the portion of the ischium that constitutes more than two-fifths of the acetabulum. It has an external and internal surface. The external surface forms part of the lunate surface of the acetabulum and a portion of the acetabular fossa. The internal surface is part of the wall of the lesser pelvis and gives origin to some fibers of the obturator internus muscle. A portion of the ischium, formerly known as the superior ramus of the ischium, projects downward and backward from the body. This portion has three surfaces: external, internal, and posterior. The external surface is quadrilateral. It is bounded above by a groove in which the tendon of the obturator externus muscle lodges. Below, it is continuous with the inferior ramus. In front, it is limited by the posterior margin of the obturator foramen. Behind, a prominent margin separates it from the posterior surface. The internal surface of this portion of the ischium forms part of the bony wall of the lesser pelvis. In front, it is limited by the posterior margin of the obturator foramen. Below, it is bounded by a sharp ridge that gives attachment to a falciform prolongation of the sacrotuberous ligament, and more anteriorly, it gives origin to the transverse perineal and ischiocavernosus muscles. The posterior surface of this portion of the ischium forms the tuberosity of the ischium.

SYNONYM: *Corpus Ossis Ischii* (NA).

Ischium, Ramus of

The ramus of the ischium, formerly known as the *inferior ramus,* is the portion of the ischium that ascends from the body of the ischium to join the inferior ramus of the pubis. It has an outer and inner surface and a median border. The latter forms part of the outlet of the pelvis. Colles' fascia is attached to the outer surface, and the inferior fascia of the urogenital diaphragm is attached to its inner surface.

SYNONYM: *Ramus Ossis Ischii* (NA).

Ischium, Spine of

The spine of the ischium is a pointed, triangular eminence that protrudes from the posterior border of the internal surface of the body of the ischium. It gives attachment to the gemellus superior muscle. Its internal surface gives attachment to the coccygeus and levator ani muscles and the pelvic fascia. The sacrospinous ligament is attached to the pointed extremity. The greater sciatic notch is situated above the spine; the lesser sciatic notch is located below. The pudendal nerve and the pudendal vein and artery pass beneath the spine.

SYNONYM: *Spina Ischiadica* (NA).

Ischium, Tuberosity of

The tuberosity of the ischium is a large protuberance on the posterior aspect of the body of the ischium.

SYNONYM: *Tuber Ischiadicum* (NA).

OBTURATOR FORAMEN

The obturator foramen is a large aperture, situated between the ischium and pubis. In the male it is large and oval, its longest diameter slanting obliquely from front to back. In the female, it is smaller and more triangular. It is bounded by a thin, uneven margin, to which a strong membrane is attached, and presents superiorly a deep groove, the *obturator groove,* which runs from the pelvis obliquely mediad and downward. This groove is converted into a canal by a ligamentous band, a specialized part of the obturator membrane, attached to two tubercles: one, the *posterior obturator tubercle*, on the medial border of the ischium, just in front of the acetabular notch; the other, the *anterior obturator tubercle*, on the obturator crest of the superior ramus of the pubis. The obturator vessels and nerve pass out of the pelvis through the canal.

SYNONYMS: *Thyroid Foramen, Foramen Obturatum* (NA).

PUBIC SYMPHYSIS

The pubic symphysis is an articulation between the pubic bones. It is an amphiarthrodial joint formed between the two oval articular surfaces of the bones. The connective tissue supports of this articulation are the superior pubic and arcuate pubic ligaments and the interpubic fibrocartilaginous lamina.

SYNONYMS: *Symphysis Pubis, Pubic Joint, Articulation of the Pubic Bones, Symphysis Pubica* (NA).

PUBIS

The pubis is the anterior part of the innominate bone and is divided into the body, superior ramus and inferior ramus.

SYNONYM: *Os Pubis* (NA).

Pubis, Body of

The body of the pubis is the part of the pubis that forms one-fifth of the acetabulum. Its external surface forms the lunate surface and the acetabular fossa. Its internal surface forms part of the wall of the lesser pelvis. It gives origin to a portion of the obturator internus muscle.

SYNONYM: *Corpus Ossis Pubis* (NA).

Pubis, Inferior Ramus of

The inferior ramus of the pubis is that portion of the pubis which extends laterally and downward from the medial end of the superior ramus of the pubis. It becomes narrower as it descends and joins with the ramus of the ischium below the obturator foramen. It has an external and internal surface, and a medial and a lateral border. The internal surface is smooth and gives origin to the obturator internus muscle and to the constrictor muscle of the urethra. The medial border presents two ridges which extend downward and are continuous with similar ridges on the ramus of the ischium. Colles' fascia is attached to the external surface while the inferior fascia of the urogenital diaphragm is attached to the internal ridge. The lateral border forms part of the obturator foramen and gives attachment to the obturator membrane.

SYNONYMS: *Descending Ramus of Pubis, Ramus Inferior Ossis Pubis* (NA).

Pubis, Superior Ramus of

The superior ramus of the pubis is the portion of the pubis that extends from the body to the median plane, where it articulates with the opposite ramus. The internal surface forms part of the anterior wall of the pelvis. It gives origin to the levator ani and obturator internus muscles, attachment to the pubovesical ligaments, and attachment to a few muscular fibers prolonged from the bladder.

SYNONYMS: *Ascending Ramus of Pubis, Ramus Superior Ossis Pubis* (NA).

RHOMBOID OF MICHAELIS

The rhomboid of Michaelis is the diamond-shaped area over the sacrum outlined by the insertions of the gluteal muscles, the groove at the end of the spine, and the posterior superior spines of the ilia.

SACROILIAC ARTICULATION

The sacroiliac articulation is an amphiarthrodial joint formed between the articular surfaces of the sacrum and the ilium. The articular surface of each bone is covered with a thin plate of cartilage, thicker on the sacrum than on the ilium. These cartilaginous plates are in close contact with each other and to a certain extent are united by irregular patches of softer fibrocartilage, and at their upper and posterior part by fine interosseous fibers. In a considerable part of their extent, especially at advanced ages, they are separated by a space containing synovialike fluid, and the joint presents the characteristics of diarthrosis. The ligaments of the joint are the anterior sacroiliac, posterior sacroiliac, and the interosseous.

SYNONYMS: *Sacroiliac Joint, Sacroiliac Synchondrosis, Articulatio Sacroiliaca* (NA).

SACRUM

The sacrum is a large triangular bone situated in the lower part of the vertebral column and at the upper and back part of the pelvic cavity.

SYNONYM: *Sacrum* (NA).

PASSAGE

PELVIS

The pelvis is a canal that is bony, fibrous, and muscular. The bony portion is divided into the false and true pelvis by the iliopectineal line. The anterior surface of the canal normally measures 4.5 cm in length, and the posterior surface measures 12.5 cm. The upper portion of the canal is directed downward and backward; the lower portion, downward and forward.

SYNONYMS: *Birth Canal, Pelvic Excavation, Pelvis* (NA).

False Pelvis

The false pelvis is the area situated above the iliopectineal line and bounded posteriorly by the lumbar vertebrae, laterally by the iliac fossa, and anteriorly by the anterior abdominal wall.

SYNONYMS: *Greater Pelvis, Pelvis Major* (NA).

True Pelvis

The true pelvis is the area of the pelvis below the iliopectineal line. The true pelvis may be divided into the inlet, outlet, and cavity.

SYNONYMS: *Lesser Pelvis, Pelvis Minor* (NA).

PLANES

Planes are areas or portions of the pelvis. They are not planes in the geometric sense.

Plane of Greatest Pelvic Dimension

The plane of greatest pelvic dimension extends from the middle of the posterior surface of the pubic symphysis to the junction of the second and third sacral vertebrae, and laterally passes through the ischial bones over the middle of the acetabulum.

SYNONYMS: *Second Parallel Pelvic Plane* (Hodge's System), *Wide Plane*.

Plane of Inlet

The plane of inlet is bounded by the upper border of the pubis, anteriorly; the iliopectineal line, laterally; and the sacral promontory, posteriorly. This plane is usually heart-shaped because of the indentation due to the promontory of the sacrum.

SYNONYMS: *First Parallel Pelvic Plane* (Hodge's System), *Superior Strait, Pelvic Brim, Apertura Pelvis Superior* (NA).

Plane of Least Pelvic Dimension

The plane of least pelvic dimension extends from the end of the sacrum to the inferior border of the pubic symphysis. It is bounded posteriorly by the end of the sacrum, laterally by the ischial spines, and anteriorly by the inferior border of the pubic symphysis.

SYNONYMS: *Third Parallel Pelvic Plane* (Hodge's System), *Midplane, Midpelvic plane*.

Plane of Outlet

The plane of outlet is the lower boundary of the bony pelvis. It passes through the pubic arch, the pubic rami, the ischial tuberosities, and the tip of the coccyx. Its anatomic relationship creates two triangles, the anterior and the posterior.

SYNONYMS: *Fourth Parallel Pelvic Plane* (Hodge's System), *Inferior Strait, Apertura Pelvis Inferior* (NA).

AXIS OF PELVIS

The axis of the pelvis is the hypothetical curved line joining the center point of each of the four planes of the pelvis.

SYNONYM: *Axis Pelvis* (NA).

CURVE OF CARUS

The curve of Carus is a segment of the circle that would be inscribed if the center of the pubic symphysis were taken as the central point and the midpoint of the anteroposterior diameter of the inlet were taken as a point on the circumference.

PELVIC INCLINATION

The pelvic inclination is the angle that the inlet of the pelvis forms with the horizon. It is normally 55° to 60° with the patient in an erect position.

SYNONYM: *Inclinatio Pelvis* (NA).

DIAMETERS

DIAMETER

A diameter is the distance between any two arbitrarily selected points.

PLANE OF INLET

Diameter, Anteroposterior

The anteroposterior diameter of the plane of the inlet is the distance from the posterior surface of the pubic symphysis to the promontory of the sacrum. It generally measures 11 cm.

Diameter, Left Oblique

The left oblique diameter of the plane of the inlet is the distance from the left sacroiliac articulation to the right iliopectineal eminence. It generally measures 12.5 cm.

Diameter, Right Oblique

The right oblique diameter of the plane of the inlet is the distance from the right sacroiliac articulation to the left iliopectineal eminence. It generally measures 12.75 cm.

Diameter, Transverse

The transverse diameter of the plane of the inlet is the distance from points midway between the promontory of the sacrum and the superior surface of the pubic symphysis. It generally measures 13.5 cm.

PLANE OF GREATEST PELVIC DIMENSION

Diameter, Anteroposterior

The anteroposterior diameter of the plane of greatest pelvic dimension is the distance from the middle of the pubic symphysis to the junction of the second and third sacral vertebrae. It generally measures 13.5 cm.

Diameter, Transverse

The transverse diameter of the plane of greatest pelvic dimension is the distance between the lateral surfaces of the pelvis. It generally measures 12.5 cm.

PLANE OF LEAST PELVIC DIMENSION

Diameter, Anteroposterior

The anteroposterior diameter of the plane of least pelvic dimension is the distance from the inferior border of the pubic symphysis to the end of the sacrum. It generally measures 11.5 cm.

Diameter, Transverse

The transverse diameter of the plane of least pelvic dimension is the distance between the ischial spines. It generally measures 10.5 cm.

PLANE OF OUTLET

Diameter, Anteroposterior

The anteroposterior diameter of the plane of the outlet is the distance from the inferior border of the pubic symphysis to the end of the coccyx. It generally measures 9.5 cm. The coccyx can be displaced posteriorly about 2 cm; thus this measurement may be increased 2 cm.

Diameter, Transverse

The transverse diameter of the plane of the outlet is the distance between the ischial tuberosities. It generally measures 11 cm.

Triangle, Anterior

The anterior triangle of the plane of the outlet is a triangle with the base at the imaginary line between the ischial tuberosities and the apex at the inferior border of the pubic symphysis. The lateral boundaries of the triangle are formed by the rami of the ischia.

Triangle, Posterior

The posterior triangle of the plane of the outlet is a triangle with the base at the imaginary line between the ischial tuberosities and the apex at the tip of the coccyx. The lateral boundaries of the triangle are formed by the sacrotuberous ligaments.

PELVIMETRY

PELVIMETRY

Pelvimetry is the clinical measurement of the pelvis. Pelvimetry may be either external or internal.

SYNONYM: *Pelvic Mensuration.*

EXTERNAL PELVIMETRY

External pelvimetry is measurement of the external pelvic diameters. These measurements are as follows: external conjugate, interspinous, intercristal, intertrochanteric, transverse of the outlet, and oblique diameters.

Diameter, External Conjugate

The external conjugate diameter is the measurement from the depression below the last lumbar vertebra to the upper border of the pubic symphysis. It generally measures 19 to 20 cm.

SYNONYM: *Baudelocque's Diameter.*

Diameter, Intercristal

The intercristal diameter is the distance between the outermost parts of the iliac crests. It usually measures 28 cm.

Diameter, Interspinous

The interspinous diameter is the distance between the anterior superior iliac spines. It usually measures 25 cm.

Diameter, Intertrochanteric

The intertrochanteric diameter is the distance between the great trochanters of the femurs. It usually measures 29 cm.

Diameter, Oblique

The oblique diameter is the distance from the posterior superior iliac spine on one side to the anterior superior iliac spine on the opposite side. It is generally designated from the posterior point. The left oblique usually measures 22 cm; the right oblique measures 22.5 cm.

SYNONYM: *Deventer's Diameter.*

Diameter, Transverse Outlet

The transverse diameter of the outlet is the distance between the inner aspects of the ischial tuberosities. It usually measures 11 cm. Generally 1.5 to 2 cm is subtracted from the measurement to allow for thickness of skin and subcutaneous fat.

SYNONYM: *Intertuberous Diameter.*

INTERNAL PELVIMETRY

Internal pelvimetry is the measurement of the internal pelvic diameters. It is performed by an internal pelvic examination.

Internal Pelvimetry of Outlet

DIAMETER, ANTEROPOSTERIOR

The anteroposterior diameter is the distance from the inferior border of the pubic symphysis to the tip of the coccyx. It generally measures 9.5 cm, and 2 cm is added for the posterior displacement of the coccyx. The total distance is 11.5 cm. It is measured by inserting two fingers into the vagina with the patient in the lithotomy position. The tip of the coccyx is palpated by the middle finger, and the measurement is made from this point to the inferior border of the pubic symphysis.

DIAMETER, ANTERIOR SAGITTAL

The anterior sagittal diameter is the distance between the midpoint of the transverse diameter of the outlet and the inferior border of the pubic symphysis. It generally measures 6 cm.

DIAMETER, BISPINOUS

The bispinous diameter is the distance between the spines of the ischia. It generally measures 10.5 cm.

DIAMETER, POSTERIOR SAGITTAL

The posterior sagittal diameter is the distance from the midpoint of the transverse diameter of the plane of the outlet to the tip of the sacrum. It is calculated by inserting the index finger into the rectum, palpating the tip of the sacrum, and measuring from the midpoint on the transverse diameter. It generally measures 9 cm.

Internal Pelvimetry of Inlet

DIAMETER, DIAGONAL CONJUGATE
The diagonal conjugate diameter is the distance from the promontory of the sacrum to the inferior border of the pubic symphysis. It generally measures 12.5 cm. It is measured by inserting two fingers into the vagina with the patient in the lithotomy position. The promontory is palpated by the middle finger, and the measurement is made from this point to the inferior border of the pubic symphysis.

DIAMETER, OBSTETRIC CONJUGATE
The obstetric conjugate diameter is the distance from the promontory of the sacrum to a point on the inner surface of the pubic symphysis a few millimeters below its upper margin. It generally measures 11 cm.

DIAMETER, TRUE CONJUGATE
The true conjugate diameter is the distance from the promontory of the sacrum to the superior border of the pubic symphysis. It generally measures 11 cm. It is estimated by subtracting 1 to 2 cm from the diagonal conjugate.

SYNONYMS: *Pubosacral Diameter, Anatomic Conjugate Diameter, Median Conjugate Diameter, Conjugata Vera.*

CEPHALOMETRY, ULTRASONIC
Ultrasonic cephalometry is the use of ultrasonic waves to measure the biparietal diameter of the fetal head in utero.

MENGERT'S INDICES
Mengert's indices are mathematical computations to determine the degree of difficulty to be expected when pelvic midplane and inlet contraction is present, and birth by the vaginal route is anticipated. Mengert's indices are calculated as follows:

$$\text{Midplane: } \frac{\text{anterior-posterior} \times \text{interspinous}}{125} \times 100 = \% \text{ of normal}$$

$$\text{Inlet: } \frac{\text{anterior-posterior} \times \text{transverse}}{145} \times 100 = \% \text{ of normal}$$

RULE OF OUTLET
The rule of outlet is a means of determining the size of the outlet that should enable a normal-sized fetus to successfully pass through the pelvis. It is the sum of the posterior sagittal diameter (internal) and the transverse diameter of the plane of the outlet (external). It must measure at least 15 cm.

STEREOSCOPIC PELVIMETRY

Stereoscopic pelvimetry is roentgenographic measurement of the pelvic diameters by means of two films taken under the same conditions but with the x-ray tube shifted a standard predetermined distance, and subsequent correction of the distortion.

X-RAY PELVIMETRY

X-ray pelvimetry is a method of estimating the size and shape of the pelvis by roentgenographic examination. It also gives a relative estimation of the size of the fetus and its presenting part.

NORMAL AND ABNORMAL PELVES

ANDROID PELVIS

An android pelvis is a female pelvis with major masculine characteristics. It has a wedge-shaped inlet; a narrow retropubic angle; a wide, flat posterior segment; a narrow sacrosciatic notch; a forward sacral inclination; a narrow and wedge-shaped subpubic arch (Gothic); converging side walls; and narrow interspinous and intertuberous diameters. The bones range from medium to heavy.

SYNONYMS: *Funnel Pelvis, Male Pelvis.*

ANTHROPOID PELVIS

An anthropoid pelvis is a pelvis with a long, narrow, oval inlet; a long, narrow, well-rounded anterior segment; a very wide, shallow sacrosciatic notch; a slightly narrow subpubic arch; a long, narrow sacrum of average inclination; and straight side walls.

SYNONYM: *Ape Pelvis.*

ASSIMILATION PELVIS, HIGH

A high assimilation pelvis is a pelvic deformity in which the union of the ilia with the spinal column is higher than normal, occurring at the 24th, 25th, or 26th vertebra. The sacrum has six segments instead of five, and five foramina instead of four.

ASSIMILATION PELVIS, LOW

A low assimilation pelvis is a pelvic deformity in which the union of the ilia with the spinal column is lower than normal, occurring at the 26th, 27th, or 28th vertebra. Six lumbar vertebrae instead of five are present, and the sacrum has three or four foramina.

BEAKED PELVIS

A beaked pelvis is a pelvis with lateral compression of the pelvic bones and with the anterior junction protruding anteriorly.

SYNONYM: *Rostrate Pelvis.*

BLUNDERBUSS PELVIS

A blunderbuss pelvis is a pelvis with divergent side walls. It is often associated with congenital dislocation of the hips or paralysis of the lower extremities.

BRACHYPELLIC PELVIS

A brachypellic pelvis is a pelvis that is flatter than normal and oval; the anteroposterior diameter of the inlet is shorter than the transverse diameter.

CONTRACTED PELVIS

A contracted pelvis is a pelvis that has a contraction of 1 cm or more in any important diameter.

Generally Contracted Pelvis

A generally contracted pelvis is a pelvis that is contracted in all diameters.

CORDATE PELVIS

A cordate pelvis is heart-shaped.

SYNONYM: *Cordiform Pelvis.*

COXALGIC PELVIS

A coxalgic pelvis is a pelvic deformity created by disease of the hip joint in infancy. The deformity generally causes no severe dystocia.

COXARTHROLISTHETIC PELVIS

A coxarthrolisthetic pelvis is a deformed pelvis, with local softening near the acetabulum. The base of one or both acetabula yields to the pressure exerted by the head of the femur and projects into the pelvic cavity, thus causing unilateral or bilateral transverse contraction.

DEVENTER'S PELVIS

Deventer's pelvis is a pelvis that is shortened anteroposteriorly.

DOLICHOPELLIC PELVIS

A dolichopellic pelvis is a long pelvis from back to front, with the anteroposterior diameter of the inlet longer than the transverse diameter of the inlet.

DWARF PELVIS

A dwarf pelvis is a very small pelvis in which the bones are united by cartilage as in the infant.

SYNONYM: *Pelvis Nana.*

Chondrodystrophic Dwarf Pelvis

A chondrodystrophic dwarf pelvis is a pelvis characterized by an extreme anteroposterior flattening. The flattening results from the imperfect development of the portion of the iliac bone entering into the formation of the iliopectineal line. As a result, the sacral articulation is brought nearer to the pubic bone than usual.

Cretin Dwarf Pelvis

A cretin dwarf pelvis is a generally contracted pelvis of imperfectly developed bones. Unlike the true dwarf pelvis, it does not present infantile characteristics.

Hypoplastic Dwarf Pelvis

A hypoplastic dwarf pelvis is a normal pelvis in miniature. It differs significantly from the true dwarf pelvis in that it is completely ossified.

Rachitic Dwarf Pelvis

A rachitic dwarf pelvis is small and deformed due to rickets.

GIANT PELVIS

A giant pelvis is a symmetric but unusually large pelvis.
SYNONYM: *Pelvis Aequabiliter Justo Major.*

GYNECOID PELVIS

A gynecoid pelvis is a normal pelvis with a round to elliptic inlet, a wide and well-rounded forepelvis, a spacious and well-rounded posterior segment, a medium-sized sacrosciatic notch, average sacral curvature and inclination, a wide subpubic arch, and straight side walls with wide intertuberous and interspinous diameters.
SYNONYM: *Normal Pelvis.*

INFANTILE PELVIS

An infantile pelvis is a generally contracted pelvis with a high sacrum, marked inclination of the walls, and an oval inlet.
SYNONYM: *Juvenile Pelvis.*

INVERTED PELVIS

An inverted pelvis is a pelvis with congenital separation at the pubic symphysis.
SYNONYM: *Split Pelvis.*

JUSTOMINOR PELVIS

A justominor pelvis is a symmetrically small female pelvis.
SYNONYMS: *Pelvis Aequabiliter Justo Minor, Pelvis Nimis Parva, Reduced Pelvis, Small Pelvis.*

KYPHORACHITIC PELVIS

A kyphorachitic pelvis is a deformed pelvis. When it is caused by pure rachitic kyphosis, the pelvic changes are slight, because the effect of kyphosis is counterbalanced to a great extent by that of the rachitis. The kyphosis leads to an elongation and the rachitis to a shortening of the true conjugate, while tending, respectively, to narrow and to widen the inferior strait.

KYPHOSCOLIORACHITIC PELVIS

A kyphoscoliorachitic pelvis is a pelvis that does not differ materially from that observed in scoliorachitis, except that the tendency to anteroposterior flattening is counteracted by the action of the kyphotic vertebral column. The oblique deformity of the superior strait is usually quite marked, but this type of pelvis is more favorable from an obstetric standpoint than that resulting from scoliorachitis alone.

KYPHOSCOLIOTIC PELVIS

A kyphoscoliotic pelvis is an evenly contracted rachitic pelvis associated with rachitic kyphoscoliosis.

KYPHOTIC PELVIS

A kyphotic pelvis is a deformed pelvis associated with kyphoscoliosis. The pelvis is contracted transversely, possessing some of the characteristics of an android pelvis. The sacrum is drawn upward and out of the pelvis. The sacrum rotates on a transverse axis, throwing the promontory up and back and the coccyx forward and inward. There is a marked inclination.

LORDOTIC PELVIS

A lordotic pelvis is a pelvis deformed by an anterior lumbar curvature of the vertebral column.

MESATIPELLIC PELVIS

A mesatipellic pelvis is a rounded pelvis with anteroposterior and transverse diameters of the inlet being almost equal.

OBLIQUE PELVIS

An oblique pelvis is a pelvis contracted in one of the oblique diameters of the inlet, with complete ankylosis of the sacroiliac synchondrosis on one side associated with imperfect development of the sacrum and innominate bone on the same side. There is rotation of the sacrum toward the same side and deviation of the pubic symphysis to the opposite side.

SYNONYM: *Nägele's Pelvis.*

OSTEOMALACIC PELVIS

An osteomalacic pelvis is a pelvis deformed as a result of osteomalacia. The pressure of the trunk and head of the femurs, and the traction of the muscles and ligaments on the softened bones crowd the pelvis together. There is downward and forward sinking of the sacrum, beaklike distortion of the horizontal pubic rami, and inward rolling of the iliac crests. The pelvic cavity may be almost obliterated.

SYNONYMS: *Kilian's Pelvis, Halisteretic Pelvis, India Rubber Pelvis, Caoutchouc Pelvis, Malacosteon Pelvis.*

OTTO PELVIS

An Otto pelvis is a pelvis that is narrowed owing to depression of an acetabulum, with protrusion of the femoral head into the pelvis.

PELVIS ANGUSTA

Pelvis angusta is a narrow pelvis with abnormal reduction of the transverse diameter of the inlet.

PELVIS OBTECTA

Pelvis obtecta is a kyphotic pelvis with extension of the vertebral column horizontally across the inlet of the pelvis.

PELVIS SPINOSA
Pelvis spinosa is a pelvis with a very sharp pubic crest resulting from rickets.

SYNONYMS *Hauder's Pelvis, Acanthopelys Pelvis.*

PLATYPELLOID PELVIS
A platypelloid pelvis is a pelvis contracted in the anteroposterior diameter of the inlet. There are two types: simple flat and rachitic flat.
SYNONYM: *Pelvis Plana.*

Rachitic Flat Pelvis
A rachitic flat pelvis is deformed owing to rickets. The bones are smaller and thinner than normal. The ilia flare outward. The pelvic inclination is increased, the pubic arch is broad, the angle that the pubis makes with the inlet is obtuse, and the tuberosities are widely separated. The sacrum is forced downward into the pelvic cavity, and the concavity of the anterior surface is changed and may be convex from side to side, straight from above downward. There may be a second, false, promontory. The outlet is generally enlarged, with its transverse diameter increased.
SYNONYM: *Rickety Pelvis.*

Simple Flat Pelvis
A simple flat pelvis is contracted, generally owing to rachitis. It has a sacrum that sinks downward and forward, causing the outline of the inlet to be broad and reniform. The pelvic cavity is also slightly flattened.

PSEUDOOSTEOMALACIC PELVIS
A pseudoosteomalacic pelvis is a deformed pelvis that resembles the osteomalacic pelvis, but it is not due to osteomalacia.

RENIFORM PELVIS
A reniform pelvis is a modified cordate pelvis with a long, transverse diameter of the inlet, giving the brim its kidney shape.

ROBERT'S PELVIS
Robert's pelvis is a transversely contracted pelvis caused by osteoarthritis. Both sacroiliac joints are affected causing the inlet to assume the form of a narrow wedge. The narrowing of the pelvis usually extends to the outlet.

ROUND PELVIS
A round pelvis is a pelvis with a nearly circular inlet.

SCOLIOTIC PELVIS
A scoliotic pelvis is deformed, usually owing to rachitis, but the deformity is minor. When scoliosis involves the upper portion of the vertebral column, there is usually a corresponding compensatory curvature in the opposite direction lower down, thus giving rise to a double

or S-shaped curve. In such cases, the body weight is transmitted to the sacrum in the usual manner, so that the pelvis is not involved. When the scoliosis is lower down and involves the lumbar region, the sacrum takes part in the compensatory process and accordingly assumes an abnormal position, leading to slight asymmetry of the pelvis.

SPONDYLOLISTHETIC PELVIS

The spondylolisthetic pelvis is a deformed pelvis whose brim is more or less occluded by a forward dislocation of the body of the lower lumbar vertebrae. The pelvic inclination is obliterated, and the lower lumbar spine projects over and into the inlet. The true conjugate diameter is reduced to approximately 5 cm, and the pelvis tends to become funnel-shaped.

SYNONYMS: *Rokitansky's Pelvis, Prague Pelvis.*

CLASSIFICATION OF PELVES

BERMAN CLASSIFICATION OF PELVES

The Berman classification of pelves is a functional working classification based on pelvic size and shape related to the outcome of labor. The pelvis is evaluated in both its anteroposterior and transverse aspects. Each pelvic level is studied individually. The size is determined from the roentgen measurements and the shape from the pelvic architecture.

Pelvic Variations
  Ample or adequate pelves
  Contracted pelves
    Inlet contraction
    Midpelvic contraction
    Outlet contraction
    Upper pelvic contraction
    Lower pelvic contraction
    Complete pelvic contraction

Pelvic Deformities
  Congenital abnormality
  Musculoskeletal disease
  Pelvic trauma

CALDWELL-MOLOY CLASSIFICATION

The Caldwell-Moloy classification is a classification of pelves by division into four basic types: anthropoid, gynecoid, android, and platypelloid.

Intermediate Pelvic Types

Intermediate pelvic types are classified by Caldwell-Moloy using a combined terminology in which the first term refers to the shape of the posterior segment and the second term to the anterior segment. Caldwell-Moloy described ten intermediate types—for example, gynecoid-anthropoid.

SYNONYM: *Mixed Pelvic Types*.

THOMS CLASSIFICATION

The Thoms classification is based on the pelvic index, using the relationship of the anteroposterior and transverse inlet diameters without considering the lower pelvic architecture. The four basic types are brachypellic, mesatipellic, dolichopellic, and platypellic.

Fetus (Passenger)

GENERAL TERMINOLOGY

FETAL HEAD

The fetal head is a structure composed of a solid bony base and compressible vault. The vault is composed of soft, pliable bones held together by fibrous tissue. The points of union of these bones are designated as *sutures*. The bones of the cranial vault are the parietals, occipitals, frontals, and temporals.

ATLOID ARTICULATION

The atloid articulation is the attachment of the base of the fetal skull to the spinal column. The articulation is nearer the posterior than the anterior border of the head. The base of the skull is thus considered as two levers resting on a fulcrum, the spinal column. The longer lever arm is anterior to the articulation. As power during labor is exerted equally on the cranial vault forcing the fetus into the birth canal, the head becomes flexed because of this long-lever action.

CEPHALIC PROMINENCE

The cephalic prominence is the greatest prominence of the fetal head palpated over the brim of the pelvis. In case of flexion, the forehead forms the cephalic prominence. When the head is extended or deflexed, the occiput becomes the cephalic prominence. When the head is partially extended, the two portions of the head stand out equally.

CHONDROCRANIUM

The chondrocranium is a membrane that joins the parietal, occipital, and frontal bones of the fetal head.

CRANIAL VAULT

The cranial vault is the part of the skull composed of the parietal, occipital, frontal, and temporal bones. Certain areas are used as landmarks to determine the position of the fetus in the pelvis.

Bregma

The bregma is the area around the anterior fontanel.

Brow

The brow is the area of the skull just anterior to the anterior fontanel.

SYNONYM: *Sinciput.*

Occiput
The occiput is the area of the skull directly posterior to the lambdoid sutures or posterior fontanel.

Parietal Boss
The parietal boss is a rounded protuberance on the fetal head formed by the parietal bones.

Vertex
The vertex is the area of the skull between the coronal and lambdoid sutures composed of the two parietal bones. The term *vertex* is also used in the descriptive sense when referring to a cephalic presentation of the fetus.

DEVELOPMENTAL AGE
The developmental age is the age of the embryo or fetus calculated from the time of implantation.

SYNONYM: *Fetal Age.*

DIAMETERS OF THE HEAD

Biparietal Diameter
The biparietal diameter is the distance between the two parietal bosses or eminences. It generally measures 9.25 cm.

SYNONYM: *Parietal Diameter.*

Bitemporal Diameter
The bitemporal diameter is the distance between the extremities of the coronal sutures. It generally measures 8 cm.

Cervicobregmatic Diameter
The cervicobregmatic diameter is the distance from the junction of the neck and occipital bone to the center of the anterior fontanel.

Frontomental Diameter
The frontomental diameter is the distance from the forehead to the chin.

Occipitofrontal Diameter
The occipitofrontal diameter is the distance from the posterior fontanel to the root of the nose. It generally measures 11.5 cm in anteroposterior diameter, 9 cm in the transverse diameter and 34 cm in circumference.

SYNONYM: *Anteroposterior Diameter of the Head.*

Occipitomental Diameter
The occipitomental diameter is the distance from the tip of the chin to the most prominent portion of the occiput. It generally measures 13.5 cm in diameter and 39 cm in circumference.

Suboccipitobregmatic Diameter

The suboccipitobregmatic diameter is the distance from the junction of the neck and occipital bone to the anterior fontanel. It generally measures 9.5 cm in the anteroposterior diameter, 9 cm in the transverse diameter, and 29 cm in circumference.

Suboccipitofrontal Diameter

The suboccipitofrontal diameter is the distance from the junction of the neck and occipital bone to the root of the nose. It generally measures 10.5 cm in the anteroposterior diameter, 9 cm in the transverse diameter, and 31 cm in circumference.

FETAL ANOXIA

Fetal anoxia is a condition of oxygen deficiency below the physiologic level due either to failure of tissue to receive or to utilize an adequate amount of oxygen.

SYNONYM: *Fetal Hypoxia.*

FETAL BRADYCARDIA

Fetal bradycardia is a fetal heart rate of less than 100 beats per minute.

FETAL CIRCULATION

Fetal circulation is the circulation of blood through the vessels of the fetus, umbilical cord, and placenta. Fetal venous blood courses through the long umbilical arteries; the oxygenated blood passes through the umbilical vein at a relatively higher pressure.

FETAL DEATH

Fetal death is the cessation of fetal life before termination of the pregnancy.

FETAL DISTRESS

Fetal distress is an adverse or threatening condition resulting from a temporary or permanent stress. The criteria for the identification of fetal distress include bradycardia, tachycardia, cardiac arrhythmia, or passage of meconium by a fetus in a vertex presentation.

FETAL TACHYCARDIA

Fetal tachycardia is a fetal heart rate of 160 beats or more per minute.

FETUS

Fetus is the term applied to the unborn offspring from the date of conception until the termination of the pregnancy.

FONTANEL

A fontanel is a space in the fetal and infant skull at the junction of three or more bones. It is covered only by a thin membrane and skin until ossification.

SYNONYM: *Fonticulus.*

Anterior Fontanel
The anterior fontanel is located in the anterior portion of the skull. It is formed by the junction of the sagittal, frontal, and coronal sutures.

SYNONYMS: *Greater Fontanel, Fonticulus Anterior.*

Lateral Fontanel
The lateral fontanel is a small, triangular space at the side of the fetal skull formed by the intersection of the lambdoid structure and temporal sutures.

SYNONYM: *Temporal Fontanel.*

Mastoid Fontanel
The mastoid fontanel is the membranous area at the junction of the parietal, temporal, and occipital bones.

SYNONYMS: *Posterolateral Fontanel, Fonticulus Mastoideus.*

Posterior Fontanel
The posterior fontanel is formed by the junction of the sagittal suture with the lambdoid sutures.

SYNONYMS: *Lesser Fontanel, Fonticulus Posterior.*

Sagittal Fontanel
The sagittal fontanel is an occasional defect in the sagittal suture that resembles a fontanel.

SYNONYM: *Gerdy's Fontanel.*

Sphenoidal Fontanel
The sphenoidal fontanel is formed by the junction of the parietal, frontal, and temporal bones.

SYNONYMS: *Anterolateral Fontanel, Fonticulus Sphenoidalis.*

LANUGO
Lanugo is fine, soft hair that occasionally appears on the face and chest of the pregnant woman and over the body of the fetus.

SUTURE
A suture is a line of impingement of bones in the fetal and infant skull, particularly before ossification.

Coronal Sutures
The coronal sutures are the sutures between the frontal and the parietal bones.

SYNONYM: *Sutura Coronalis* (NA).

Frontal Suture
The frontal suture is the suture between the frontal bones.

SYNONYMS: *Metopic Suture, Sutura Frontalis* (NA).

Lambdoid Sutures
The lambdoid sutures are the sutures between the parietal and occipital bones.

SYNONYM: *Sutura Lambdoidea* (NA).

Sagittal Suture

The sagittal suture is the suture between the parietal bones.
SYNONYMS: *Longitudinal Suture, Sutura Sagittalis* (NA).

Temporal Suture

The temporal suture is a suture between the temporal and parietal bones.
SYNONYM: *Lateral Suture.*

VAGITUS UTERINUS

Vagitus uterinus is intrauterine fetal crying. It is made possible by rupture of the membranes, which permits the entrance of air into the uterine cavity.

VIABILITY

Viability is a term implying that a fetus is capable of survival.

POINTS OF DIRECTION

POINT OF DIRECTION

A point of direction is an arbitrary point on the presenting part of the fetus by which the topographic relation of the presenting part to the designated point in the maternal pelvis is determined.

DESIGNATED POINTS—FETUS

The designated points of the fetus are specific areas of the presenting part that are used to determine the position of the fetus in the maternal pelvis. They are as follows: occiput, brow, mentum, sacrum, and acromion.

Acromion

The acromion is the outer end of the spine of the scapula, which projects as a broad, flattened process overhanging the glenoid fossa. It articulates with the clavicle and gives attachment to the deltoid muscle and some fibers of the trapezius muscles.

Brow

The brow is the area of the skull just anterior to the anterior fontanel.
SYNONYM: *Sinciput.*

Mentum

The mentum is the lower jaw of the fetal face.
SYNONYM: *Chin.*

Occiput

The occiput is the area of the skull directly posterior to the lambdoid sutures or posterior fontanel.

Sacrum
The sacrum is a large triangular bone situated in the lower part of the vertebral column and at the upper and back part of the pelvic cavity.

SYNONYM: *Sacrum* (NA).

DESIGNATED POINTS—MATERNAL PELVIS
The designated points of the maternal pelvis are created by divisions of the pelvis into four quadrants. They are the right anterior and posterior and the left anterior and posterior quadrants.

PRESENTATIONS AND POSITIONS

PRESENTATION
Presentation is the relationship of the long axis of the fetus to the long axis of the mother. There are two major categories of presentation: longitudinal and transverse.

SYNONYM: *Lie*.

PRESENTING PART
The presenting part is the part of the fetus that is lowest in the maternal pelvis. It is the part that the examining finger palpates on vaginal or rectal examination—for example, vertex, breech, or acromion.

POSITION*
Position is the relationship of a designated point on the presenting part of the fetus to a designated point in the maternal pelvis.

LONGITUDINAL PRESENTATION
In longitudinal presentation, the long axis of the fetus is parallel to the long axis of the mother. This is further differentiated into cephalic and breech presentation. Of all cases, 99.5 per cent are longitudinal.

SYNONYM: *Polar Presentation*.

Cephalic Presentation
In cephalic presentation, the fetal head is the presenting part. The various points of direction are the occiput, mentum, or brow.

VERTEX PRESENTATION
In vertex presentation, the fetal head is the presenting part. The occiput is the point of direction or the designated point on the presenting part.

---

* Position should not be designated as presentation. Each presenting part may so occupy the pelvis that its point of direction should be stated first and then the side of the maternal pelvis in which the point of direction is situated. However, most published works specify the right or left side of the pelvis before the point of direction. This committee would like to recommend that the point of direction be stated first. This would eliminate confusion—for example, ORA = occiput right anterior instead of ROA = right occiput anterior. Also, it should be noted that findings listed as "rectal findings" may also be ascertained vaginally.

POSITIONS

Occiput Left Anterior

Occiput left anterior is the position of the fetus in which the occiput is located in the left anterior quadrant of the maternal pelvis.

RECTAL FINDING: The sagittal suture is located in the right oblique diameter of the pelvis.

ABDOMINAL FINDINGS: The greatest cephalic prominence is in the right side above the pelvic brim, the fetal back is on the left, small parts are on the right and posterior, and the fetal heart is heard loudest in the left lower quadrant of the abdomen.

SYNONYM: *Left Occiput Anterior Position.*

ABBREVIATIONS: OLA, LOA.

Occiput Right Anterior

Occiput right anterior is the position of the fetus in which the occiput is located in the right anterior quadrant of the maternal pelvis.

RECTAL FINDING: The sagittal suture is situated in the left oblique diameter of the pelvis.

ABDOMINAL FINDINGS: The greatest cephalic prominence is on the left, the fetal back is on the right, and the fetal heart is heard loudest in the right lower quadrant of the abdomen.

SYNONYM: *Right Occiput Anterior Position.*

ABBREVIATIONS: ORA, ROA.

Occiput Right Transverse

Occiput right transverse is the position of the fetus in which the occiput is located between the right anterior and posterior quadrants of the maternal pelvis.

RECTAL FINDING: The sagittal suture is situated in the transverse diameter of the pelvis.

ABDOMINAL FINDINGS: The greatest cephalic prominence is on the left side above the pelvic brim, the fetal back is on the right, and the fetal heart is heard loudest in the right lower quadrant of the abdomen.

SYNONYM: *Right Occiput Transverse Position.*

ABBREVIATIONS: ORT, ROT.

Occiput Left Transverse

Occiput left transverse is the position of the fetus in which the occiput is located between the left anterior and posterior quadrants of the maternal pelvis.

RECTAL FINDING: The sagittal suture is situated in the transverse diameter of the pelvis.

ABDOMINAL FINDINGS: The greatest cephalic prominence is on the right side above the pelvic brim, the fetal back is on the left, the small parts on the right, and the fetal heart is heard loudest in the left lower quadrant of the abdomen.

SYNONYM: *Left Occiput Transverse Position.*

ABBREVIATIONS: OLT, LOT.

Occiput Left Posterior

Occiput left posterior is the position of the fetus in which the occiput is located in the left posterior quadrant of the maternal pelvis.

RECTAL FINDING: The sagittal suture is situated in the left oblique diameter of the pelvis.

ABDOMINAL FINDINGS: The greatest cephalic prominence is on the right and anterior, the fetal back is on the left and posterior, and the fetal heart is heard loudest at the posterior aspect of the left lower quadrant of the abdomen.

SYNONYM: *Left Occiput Posterior Position.*

ABBREVIATIONS: OLP, LOP.

Occiput Right Posterior

Occiput right posterior is the position of the fetus in which the occiput is located in the right posterior quadrant of the maternal pelvis.

RECTAL FINDING: The sagittal suture is situated in the right oblique diameter of the pelvis.

ABDOMINAL FINDINGS: The greatest cephalic prominence is on the left and anterior, the fetal back is on the right and posterior, and the fetal heart is heard loudest in the posterior aspect of the right lower quadrant of the abdomen.

SYNONYM: *Right Occiput Posterior Position.*

ABBREVIATIONS: ORP, ROP.

Occiput Anterior

Occiput anterior is the position of the fetus in which the occiput is located directly anterior.

RECTAL FINDINGS: The sagittal suture is situated in the anteroposterior diameter of the maternal pelvis, and the posterior fontanel is located directly behind the pubic symphysis.

ABDOMINAL FINDINGS: The fetal back is directly anterior, and the fetal heart is heard loudest in the lower midline of the abdomen.

SYNONYM: *Anterior Occiput Position.*

ABBREVIATIONS: OA, AO.

Occiput Posterior

Occiput posterior is the position of the fetus in which the occiput is located directly posterior in the hollow of the sacrum.

RECTAL FINDINGS: The sagittal suture is situated in the anteroposterior diameter of the pelvis, and the posterior fontanel is located directly posterior in the hollow of the sacrum.

ABDOMINAL FINDINGS: Cephalic prominence is equal on each side of the abdomen, the small parts are anterior, and the fetal heart is heard loudest in the lower midline of the abdomen.

SYNONYM: *Posterior Occiput Position.*

ABBREVIATIONS: OP, PO.

Face Presentation

Face presentation is a position of the fetus in which the face is the presenting part. The mentum (chin) is the point of direction or the designated point on the face.

Positions

Mentum Right Anterior

Mentum right anterior is the position of the fetus in which the chin is located in the right anterior quadrant of the maternal pelvis.

RECTAL FINDINGS: The chin is located in the right anterior quadrant of the pelvis; other structures of the fetal face palpated in the pelvis are the eyes, nose, and mouth.

ABDOMINAL FINDINGS: The greatest cephalic prominence can be palpated on the left side above the pelvic brim, the fetal back is on the left, and the fetal heart is heard loudest in the right lower quadrant of the abdomen.

SYNONYM: *Right Mentum Anterior Position.*
ABBREVIATIONS: MRA, RMA.

Mentum Right Posterior

Mentum right posterior is a position of the fetus in which the chin is located in the right posterior quadrant of the maternal pelvis.

RECTAL FINDINGS: The chin is located in the right posterior quadrant of the pelvis; other structures of the fetal face palpated in the pelvis are the eyes, nose, and mouth.

ABDOMINAL FINDINGS: The greatest cephalic prominence can be palpated on the left lower quadrant of the abdomen above the pelvic brim, the fetal back is on the left, and the fetal heart is heard loudest in the left lower quadrant of the abdomen.

SYNONYM: *Right Mentum Posterior Position.*
ABBREVIATIONS: MRP, RMP.

Mentum Left Anterior

Mentum left anterior is a position of the fetus in which the chin is located in the left anterior quadrant of the maternal pelvis.

RECTAL FINDINGS: The chin is located in the left anterior quadrant of the maternal pelvis; other structures of the fetal face palpated in the pelvis are the eyes, nose, and mouth.

ABDOMINAL FINDINGS: The greatest cephalic prominence can be palpated on the right side above the pelvic brim, the fetal back is on the right, and the fetal heart is heard loudest in the left lower quadrant of the abdomen.

SYNONYM: *Left Mentum Anterior Position.*
ABBREVIATIONS: MLA, LMA.

Mentum Left Posterior

Mentum left posterior is a position of the fetus in which the chin is located in the left posterior quadrant of the maternal pelvis.

RECTAL FINDINGS: The chin is located in the left posterior quadrant of the pelvis; other structures of the fetal face palpated in the pelvis are the eyes, nose, and mouth.

ABDOMINAL FINDINGS: The greatest cephalic prominence can be palpated on the right lower quadrant above the pelvic brim, the fetal back is on the right, and the fetal heart is heard loudest in the right lower quadrant of the abdomen.

SYNONYM: *Left Mentum Posterior Position.*

ABBREVIATIONS: MLP, LMP.

Mentum Right Transverse

Mentum right transverse is a position of the fetus in which the chin is located in the transverse position midway between the right anterior and posterior quadrants.

RECTAL FINDINGS: The chin is located in the right side of the pelvis; other structures of the fetal face palpated in the pelvis are the eyes, nose, and mouth.

ABDOMINAL FINDINGS: The greatest cephalic prominence is located in the left lower quadrant of the abdomen above the pelvic brim, the fetal back is on the left, and the fetal heart is heard loudest in the right or left lower quadrant of the abdomen.

SYNONYM: *Right Mentum Transverse Position.*

ABBREVIATIONS: MRT, RMT.

Mentum Left Transverse

Mentum left transverse is a position of the fetus in which the chin is located in the transverse position midway between the left anterior and posterior quadrants.

RECTAL FINDINGS: The chin is located on the left side of the pelvis; other structures of the fetal face palpated in the pelvis are the eyes, nose, and mouth.

ABDOMINAL FINDINGS: The greatest cephalic prominence is located in the right lower quadrant of the abdomen above the pelvic brim, the fetal back is on the right, and the fetal heart is heard loudest in either the right or left lower quadrant of the abdomen.

SYNONYM: *Left Mentum Transverse Position.*

ABBREVIATIONS: MLT, LMT.

BROW PRESENTATION

Brow presentation is a position of the fetus in which the brow is the presenting part. The brow is the point of direction or the designated point on the presenting part.

POSITIONS

Brow Right Anterior

Brow right anterior is a position of the fetus in which the brow is located in the right anterior quadrant of the maternal pelvis.

RECTAL FINDINGS: The brow is situated in the right anterior quadrant of the pelvis, the frontal and sagittal sutures are in the left oblique diameter of the pelvis, and the anterior fontanel is situated in the center of the pelvis.

ABDOMINAL FINDINGS: The cephalic prominence is equal on each side of the lower quadrants of the abdomen, the fetal back is on the left and posterior, and the fetal heart is heard loudest in the left lower quadrant of the abdomen.

SYNONYM: *Right Brow Anterior Position.*

ABBREVIATIONS: BRA, RBA.

Brow Right Posterior

Brow right posterior is a position of the fetus in which the brow is located in the right posterior quadrant of the maternal pelvis.

RECTAL FINDINGS: The brow is situated in the right posterior quadrant of the pelvis, frontal and sagittal sutures are in the right oblique diameter of the pelvis, and the anterior fontanel is situated in the center of the pelvis.

ABDOMINAL FINDINGS: The cephalic prominence is equal on each side of the lower quadrants of the abdomen, the fetal back is on the left, and the fetal heart is heard loudest in the left lower quadrant rather posteriorly.

SYNONYM: *Right Brow Posterior Position.*

ABBREVIATIONS: BRP, RBP.

Brow Left Anterior

Brow left anterior is a position of the fetus in which the brow is located in the left anterior quadrant of the pelvis.

RECTAL FINDINGS: The brow is situated in the left anterior quadrant of the pelvis, the frontal and sagittal sutures are situated in the right oblique diameter, and the anterior fontanel is located in the center of the pelvis.

ABDOMINAL FINDINGS: The cephalic prominence is equal on each side of the lower quadrants of the abdomen, the fetal back is on the right and posterior, and the fetal heart is heard loudest in the right lower quadrant of the abdomen.

SYNONYM: *Left Brow Anterior Position.*

ABBREVIATIONS: BLA, LBA.

Brow Left Posterior

Brow left posterior is a position of the fetus in which the brow is located in the left posterior quadrant of the maternal pelvis.

RECTAL FINDINGS: The brow is situated in the left posterior quadrant of the pelvis, the frontal and sagittal sutures are situated in the left oblique diameter, and the anterior fontanel is in the center of the pelvis.

ABDOMINAL FINDINGS: The cephalic prominence is equal on both sides of the lower quadrants of the abdomen, the fetal back is on the right, and the fetal heart is heard loudest in the right lower quadrant of the abdomen.

SYNONYM: *Left Brow Posterior Position.*

ABBREVIATIONS: BLP, LBP.

Brow Right Transverse

Brow right transverse is a position of the fetus in which the brow is located transversely between the right anterior and posterior quadrants of the pelvis.

RECTAL FINDINGS: The brow is situated in the right side of the pelvis, and the frontal and sagittal sutures are situated in the transverse diameter of the pelvis.

ABDOMINAL FINDINGS: The cephalic prominence is equal on each side of the lower quadrants of the abdomen, the fetal back is on the left, and the fetal heart is heard loudest in the left lower quadrant of the abdomen.

SYNONYM: *Right Brow Transverse Position.*

ABBREVIATIONS: BRT, RBT.

Brow Left Transverse

Brow left transverse is a position of the fetus in which the brow is located transversely between the left anterior and posterior quadrants of the pelvis.

RECTAL FINDINGS: The brow is situated in the left side of the pelvis, and the frontal and sagittal sutures are situated in the transverse diameter of the pelvis.

ABDOMINAL FINDINGS: The cephalic prominence is equal on each side of the lower quadrants of the abdomen, the fetal back is on the right, and the fetal heart is heard loudest in the right lower quadrant of the abdomen.

SYNONYM: *Left Brow Transverse Position.*

ABBREVIATIONS: BLT, LBT.

BREECH PRESENTATION

In breech presentation, the fetal breech is the presenting part. The sacrum is the point of direction or the designated point on the presenting part.

Complete Breech Presentation

In complete breech presentation, the buttocks descend first. The legs are flexed on the fetal abdomen, and the feet are alongside the fetal buttocks.

SYNONYMS: *Double Breech Presentation, Full Breech Presentation.*

Frank Breech Presentation

In frank breech presentation, the legs lie extended alongside the fetal body so that the buttocks descend first.

SYNONYMS: *Pelvic Presentation, Single Breech Presentation.*

Incomplete Breech Presentation

Incomplete breech presentation is a breech presentation with one or both feet or knees prolapsed into the vagina.

DOUBLE FOOTLING PRESENTATION: In double footling presentation, both feet have prolapsed into the vagina.

SINGLE FOOTLING PRESENTATION: In single footling presentation, one foot has prolapsed into the vagina.

POSITIONS

Sacrum Right Anterior

Sacrum right anterior is a position of the fetus in which the sacrum is located in the right anterior quadrant of the maternal pelvis.

RECTAL FINDINGS: The fetal sacrum is in the right anterior quadrant, and the gluteal crease is located in the left oblique diameter of the maternal pelvis. The fetal anus and ischial tuberosities can be palpated.

ABDOMINAL FINDINGS: The fetal head can be palpated in the uterine fundus, the presenting part is triangular, the fetal soft parts are on the left side of the abdomen, and the fetal heart is heard loudest in the upper quadrant of the abdomen.

SYNONYM: *Right Sacrum Anterior Position.*

ABBREVIATIONS: SRA, RSA.

Sacrum Right Transverse

Sacrum right transverse is a position of the fetus in which the sacrum is located between the right anterior and posterior quadrants of the maternal pelvis.

RECTAL FINDINGS: The sacrum is palpated on the right, and the gluteal crease is in the transverse diameter of the maternal pelvis. The fetal anus and ischial tuberosities can be palpated.

ABDOMINAL FINDINGS: The fetal head can be palpated in the uterine fundus, the fetal back is on the right, the fetal soft parts are on the left side of the maternal abdomen, and the fetal heart is heard loudest in the right quadrant of the abdomen slightly posterior.

SYNONYM: *Right Sacrum Transverse Position.*

ABBREVIATIONS: SRT, RST.

Sacrum Right Posterior

Sacrum right posterior is a position of the fetus in which the sacrum is located in the right posterior quadrant of the maternal pelvis.

RECTAL FINDINGS: The fetal sacrum can be palpated in the right posterior quadrant of the pelvis, and the gluteal crease is in the right oblique diameter of the maternal pelvis. The fetal anus and ischial tuberosities can be palpated.

ABDOMINAL FINDINGS: The fetal head can be palpated in the uterine fundus, the back is on the right, the fetal soft parts are on the left and anterior side of the maternal abdomen, and the fetal heart is heard loudest in the right upper quadrant of the abdomen slightly posterior.

SYNONYM: *Right Sacrum Posterior Position.*

ABBREVIATIONS: SRP, RSP.

Sacrum Posterior

Sacrum posterior is a position of the fetus in which the sacrum is located directly posterior in the hollow of the maternal sacrum.

RECTAL FINDINGS: The fetal sacrum can be palpated directly posterior, and the gluteal crease is in the anteroposterior diameter of the maternal pelvis. The fetal anus and ischial tuberosities can be palpated.

ABDOMINAL FINDINGS: The fetal head can be palpated in the uterine fundus, the fetal soft parts are directly anterior, and the fetal heart is heard loudest in the upper midline of the abdomen.

SYNONYM: *Posterior Sacrum Position.*

ABBREVIATIONS: SP, PS.

Sacrum Left Posterior

Sacrum left posterior is a position of the fetus in which the sacrum is located in the left posterior quadrant of the maternal pelvis.

RECTAL FINDINGS: The fetal sacrum can be palpated in the left posterior quadrant, and the gluteal crease is located on the left oblique diameter of the maternal pelvis. The fetal anus and ischial tuberosities can be palpated.

ABDOMINAL FINDINGS: The fetal head can be palpated in the uterine fundus, and the presenting part is triangular. The fetal soft parts are in the right side of the abdomen, and the fetal heart is heard loudest in the left upper quadrant of the abdomen slightly posterior.

SYNONYM: *Left Sacrum Posterior Position.*

ABBREVIATIONS: SLP, LSP.

Sacrum Left Transverse

Sacrum left transverse is a position of the fetus in which the sacrum is located between the left anterior and posterior quadrants of the maternal pelvis.

RECTAL FINDINGS: The fetal sacrum can be palpated on the left, and the gluteal crease is in the transverse diameter of the maternal pelvis. The fetal anus and ischial tuberosities can be palpated.

ABDOMINAL FINDINGS: The fetal head can be palpated in the uterine fundus, the fetal back is on the left, the soft parts are

on the right side of the maternal abdomen, and the fetal heart is heard loudest in the upper left quadrant of the abdomen.
SYNONYM: *Left Sacrum Transverse Position.*
ABBREVIATIONS: SLT, LST.

Sacrum Left Anterior

Sacrum left anterior is a position of the fetus in which the fetal sacrum is located in the left anterior quadrant of the maternal pelvis.
RECTAL FINDINGS: The fetal sacrum can be palpated in the left anterior quadrant of the maternal pelvis, and the gluteal crease is in the right oblique diameter of the maternal pelvis. The fetal anus and ischial tuberosities can be palpated.
ABDOMINAL FINDINGS: The fetal head can be palpated in the uterine fundus, the small parts are on the right of and posterior to the maternal abdomen, and the fetal heart is heard loudest in the left upper quadrant of the abdomen.
SYNONYM: *Left Sacrum Anterior Position.*
ABBREVIATIONS: SLA, LSA.

Sacrum Anterior

Sacrum anterior is a position of the fetus in which the fetal sacrum is directly anterior or behind the pubic symphysis.
RECTAL FINDINGS: The fetal sacrum can be palpated directly behind the pubic symphysis, and the gluteal crease is in the anteroposterior diameter. The fetal anus and ischial tuberosities can be palpated.
ABDOMINAL FINDINGS: The fetal head can be palpated in the uterine fundus, the small parts are directly posterior, and the fetal heart is heard loudest in the upper midline of the abdomen.
SYNONYM: *Anterior Sacrum Position.*
ABBREVIATIONS: SA, AS.

TRANSVERSE PRESENTATION

In transverse presentation, the long axis of the fetus is perpendicular to the long axis of the mother.
SYNONYMS: *Torso Presentation, Trunk Presentation.*

Acromion Presentation

In acromion presentation, the long axis of the fetus is perpendicular to the long axis of the mother, and the shoulder is the presenting part. The acromion process of the scapula is the point of direction or the designated point on the presenting part. There are only four positions of the shoulder.
SYNONYM: *Shoulder Presentation.*

POSITIONS

Acromion Left Anterior

Acromion left anterior is a position of the fetus in which the acromion process is located in the left anterior quadrant of the maternal pelvis.

RECTAL FINDINGS: Generally, the presenting part is not engaged in the pelvis, and the acromion process is palpated in the left anterior quadrant of the maternal pelvis. The fetal ribs can be palpated in the anteroposterior diameter of the maternal pelvis.
ABDOMINAL FINDINGS: The fetal head can be palpated on the left side of the maternal abdomen, the fetal back is anterior, and the fetal heart is heard loudest in the left lower quadrant of the maternal abdomen.
SYNONYM: *Left Acromion Anterior Position.*
ABBREVIATIONS: ALA, LAA.

Acromion Left Posterior

Acromion left posterior is a position of the fetus in which the acromion process is located in the left posterior quadrant of the maternal pelvis.
RECTAL FINDINGS: Generally, the presenting part is not engaged in the pelvis, and the acromion process can be palpated in the left posterior quadrant of the maternal pelvis. The fetal ribs can be palpated in the anteroposterior diameter of the pelvis.
ABDOMINAL FINDINGS: The fetal head can be palpated on the left side of the maternal abdomen, the fetal back is posterior, the small parts are anterior and easily palpable through the anterior wall of the uterus and abdomen, and the fetal heart is heard loudest in the left lower quadrant of the abdomen.
SYNONYM: *Left Acromion Posterior Position.*
ABBREVIATIONS: ALP, LAP.

Acromion Right Anterior

Acromion right anterior is a position of the fetus in which the acromion process is located in the right anterior quadrant of the maternal pelvis.
RECTAL FINDINGS: Generally, the presenting part is not engaged in the pelvis and the acromion process is palpated in the right anterior quadrant of the maternal pelvis. The fetal ribs can be palpated in the anteroposterior diameter of the pelvis.
ABDOMINAL FINDINGS: The fetal head can be palpated in the right side of the maternal abdomen, the fetal back is anterior, the fetal small parts are posterior and difficult to palpate, and the fetal heart is heard loudest in the right lower quadrant of the abdomen.
SYNONYM: *Right Acromion Anterior Position.*
ABBREVIATIONS: ARA, RAA.

Acromion Right Posterior

Acromion right posterior is a position of the fetus in which the acromion process is located in the right posterior quadrant of the maternal pelvis.
RECTAL FINDINGS: Generally, the presenting part is not engaged in the pelvis, and the acromion process can be palpated in the right posterior quadrant of the maternal pelvis. The fetal ribs can be palpated in the anteroposterior diameter of the pelvis.

ABDOMINAL FINDINGS: The fetal head can be palpated on the right side of the maternal abdomen, the fetal back is posterior, the fetal soft parts are easily palpated through the anterior wall of the uterus and abdomen, and the fetal heart is heard loudest in the lower right quadrant of the abdomen.

SYNONYM: *Right Acromion Posterior Position.*

ABBREVIATIONS: ARP, RAP.

COMPOUND PRESENTATION

In compound presentation, an extremity prolapses alongside the presenting part so that both enter the pelvic cavity at the same time.

FUNIC PRESENTATION

In funic presentation, the umbilical cord has prolapsed into the maternal vagina. The cord becomes the presenting part.

OBLIQUE PRESENTATION

In oblique presentation, the fetus lies at a marked angle to the long axis of the mother.

PARIETAL PRESENTATION

In parietal presentation, the parietal portion or side of the fetal head presents in the pelvis.

SECTION 7: OBSTETRICS

Labor

GENERAL TERMINOLOGY

LABOR
Labor is the physiologic process by which the uterus expels, or attempts to expel, the fetus and placenta at 20 weeks or more of gestation. Labor is divided into three stages.
SYNONYM: *Parturition.*

First Stage of Labor
The first stage of labor refers to the period from the onset of labor through complete dilatation of the cervix.

Second Stage of Labor
The second stage of labor refers to the period from complete dilatation of the cervix through birth of the fetus.

Third Stage of Labor
The third stage of labor refers to the period from birth of the fetus through expulsion or extraction of the placenta and membranes.

LABOR, ACTIVE
Active labor is regular uterine contraction with progressive dilatation of the cervix and descent of the presenting part.

LABOR, ARRESTED
Arrested labor is labor that has failed to proceed through the normal stages. It may be due to obstructions in the maternal pelvis, uterine inertia, cephalopelvic disproportion, or general systemic diseases.

LABOR, INDUCTION OF
Induction of labor is the deliberate initiation of uterine contractions prior to their spontaneous onset.

LABOR, MISSED
Missed labor is labor that begins at the proper time, but then ceases. Some degree of cervical dilatation may be attained, but the contractions cease and the gestation continues for weeks or months.

LABOR, NORMAL
Normal labor is the progressive dilatation and effacement of the cervix with descent of the presenting part.
SYNONYM: *Eutocia.*

375

LABOR, ONSET OF
The onset of labor is the establishment of regular uterine contractions together with beginning dilatation of the cervix.

LABOR, PRECIPITATE
Precipitate labor is labor that terminates in the expulsion of the fetus in less than three hours.

LABOR, PROLONGED
Prolonged labor is active labor that continues longer than 20 hours.

LABOR, STIMULATION OF
Stimulation of labor is the induced augmentation of uterine contractions after their spontaneous or induced onset.

LABOR, TRIAL OF
A trial of labor is allowing a woman to be in labor long enough to determine if vaginal birth may be anticipated.

DYSTOCIA
Dystocia is abnormal labor resulting from any variation of the normal patterns in the latent or active phases of cervical dilatation, such as prolonged latent phase, protracted active phase, or secondary arrest of cervical dilatation. Other causes are cephalopelvic disproportion, malpresentation, tumor, or resistance of maternal nonbony tissue.
SYNONYM: *Dysfunctional Labor.*

FRIEDMAN CURVE
The Friedman curve is a graph on which duration of labor in hours is plotted against cervical dilatation in centimeters.

MEMBRANES, RUPTURE OF
Rupture of the membranes is a bursting or tearing of the amniotic sac. Rupture of the membranes may be classified as artificial (amniotomy), premature, prolonged, or spontaneous.

Amniotomy
Amniotomy is the surgical rupture of the amniotic sac as a means of inducing or expediting labor.
SYNONYM: *Artificial Rupture of Membranes.*

Premature Rupture of Membranes
Premature rupture of the membranes is rupture of the amniotic sac before the onset of uterine contractions.

Prolonged Rupture of Membranes
Prolonged rupture of the membranes is rupture of the amniotic sac that occurs 24 hours or more prior to the onset of labor.

Spontaneous Rupture of Membranes
Spontaneous rupture of the membranes is rupture of the amniotic sac without manual interference.

PARTURIENT
A parturient is a woman in the process of giving birth to a fetus.

PHYSIOLOGIC RETRACTION RING
The physiologic retraction ring is an area of constriction at the junction of the upper or contracting portion and the lower dilating or passive part of the uterus.

PRODROMAL STAGE OF LABOR
The prodromal stage of labor is the period preceding labor characterized by lightening and increased pressure in the pelvis.

STATION
Station is the location of the presenting part in the birth canal.

Station —3
Station —3 is attained when the presenting part is 3 cm above the biischial spines.

Station —2
Station —2 is attained when the presenting part is 2 cm above the biischial spines.

Station —1
Station —1 is attained when the presenting part is 1 cm above the biischial spines.

Station 0
Station 0 is attained when the presenting part has reached the level of the biischial spines.

Station +1
Station +1 is attained when the presenting part is 1 cm below the biischial spines.

Station +2
Station +2 is attained when the presenting part is 2 cm below the biischial spines.

Station +3
Station +3 is attained when the presenting part is on the perineum.

Station +4 or +5
Station +4 or +5 is attained when the presenting part is about to crown.

POWERS

POWERS OF LABOR
The powers of labor are the contractions of the uterine muscles during the first stage of labor and contraction of the uterine and abdominal muscles during the second stage of labor.

AMNIOTIC PRESSURE
Amniotic pressure is the pressure within the amniotic sac. The pressure is proportional to the tension of the uterine wall and is an accurate measurement of myometrial contraction.

CERVIX, DILATATION OF
Dilatation of the cervix is the enlargement of the cervical opening caused by the upward retraction of the muscle fibers of the cervix during labor. The phases involved are the latent and the active phases.

Latent Phase
The latent phase is the time between the onset of regular uterine contractions and appreciable cervical dilatation. During this phase, the cervix becomes effaced but dilates only slightly.

Active Phase
The active phase extends from the end of the latent phase to the end of the first stage of labor. It may be divided into three periods: acceleration, steady, and deceleration.

ACCELERATION PERIOD
The acceleration period is the time during which the rate of cervical dilatation is continuously changing and increasing.

STEADY PERIOD
The steady period is the time during which the cervix dilates at a regular and steady rate.

DECELERATION PERIOD
The deceleration period is the time during which the rate of cervical dilatation decreases. Complete dilatation is effected during this period and signals the end of the first stage of labor.

CERVIX, EFFACEMENT OF
Effacement of the cervix is accomplished when the cervix is completely retracted, the cervicovaginal angle has disappeared, and only the external cervical os remains. Dilatation now begins or continues.

CONTRACTION, UTERINE
Uterine contraction is a temporary shortening of uterine muscular fibers, which on relaxation return to their original length.

Acme of Contraction
Acme of contraction is the period of maximum uterine contractility.

Diastolic Phase of Contraction
The diastolic phase of contraction is the period of relaxation following the acme of contraction.

Systolic Phase of Contraction
The systolic phase of contraction is the progressive contraction of an area of the uterus. Thirty to 60 seconds is required for the uterus to achieve the acme of contraction. With contractile waves,

the activity is so well coordinated that the peak of the contraction is attained almost simultaneously in all parts of the uterus even though the waves reach them at different times.

FREQUENCY OF CONTRACTIONS

The frequency of contractions is expressed as the number of contractions in ten minutes.

FUNDAL DOMINANCE

Fundal dominance is the dominance of contractility found in the uterine fundus. Contractions in the fundus are stronger than those in the midportion of the uterus.

INTENSITY, INTRAUTERINE

Intrauterine intensity is intrauterine pressure that increases with each uterine contraction.

SYNONYM: *Amplitude*.

INTRAMYOMETRIAL PRESSURE

Intramyometrial pressure is the pressure created within the muscle fibers of the uterus by their contraction.

INVERSION OF GRADIENT

Inversion of the gradient is an abnormal contractile wave that starts in the lower part of the uterus and spreads upward. It may be stronger in the lower segment than in the upper part of the uterus. Contractions with inverted gradients are inefficient for dilating the cervix; in fact, they may cause the cervix to close.

IRRITABILITY, UTERINE

Uterine irritability is the reaction that causes the uterus to respond to external stimulation, resulting in contractions.

LONGITUDINAL SHORTENING OF LOWER UTERINE SEGMENT

Longitudinal shortening of the lower uterine segment is caused by the retraction of longitudinal muscle fibers of that segment before and during labor. It facilitates retraction and dilatation of the cervix.

PACEMAKER, UTERINE

The uterine pacemaker is one of two areas of propagation on the uterine wall in which the contraction waves are initiated. Normal contraction spreads throughout the uterus at the rate of 2 cm per second, invading the whole organ within 15 seconds.

RETRACTION, UTERINE

Uterine retraction is the intermittent permanent shortening of the muscle fibers of the uterus with the inability to return to their original size as long as retraction continues.

SENSIBILITY, UTERINE
Uterine sensibility is the reaction of the uterus during labor, changing from a nonsensitive to a sensitive structure.

TRIPLE DESCENDING GRADIENT
The triple descending gradient is the characteristic normal contractile wave of the uterus during labor. The gradient has three components: propagation of the contraction, duration of the systolic phase of the contraction, and intensity of the contraction.

Propagation of Contraction
Propagation of contraction is a term that denotes the spreading of the contractile muscle wave of the uterus to several parts of the uterus. The activity of the upper parts of the uterus adjacent to the uterine pacemaker is greater than and dominates that of the lower parts.

Duration of Contractions
The duration of contractions is the length of uterine contractions. Contractions usually range from 30 to 90 seconds with an average of one minute.

Intensity of Contraction
The intensity of the contraction is the strength of the contraction.

MECHANICS

MECHANICS OF LABOR
The mechanics of labor are the factors involved in the passage of the fetus through the birth canal.

ASYNCLITISM, ANTERIOR
Anterior asynclitism occurs when the sagittal suture approaches the maternal sacral promontory and the anterior parietal bone is the designated point on the presenting part.
SYNONYMS: *Nägele's Obliquity, Anterior Parietal Position.*

ASYNCLITISM, POSTERIOR
Posterior asynclitism occurs when the sagittal suture approaches the maternal pubic symphysis and the posterior parietal bone is the designated point on the presenting part.
SYNONYMS: *Litzmann's Obliquity, Posterior Parietal Position.*

DESCENT
Descent is the passage of the presenting part into and through the birth canal. It begins at the onset of labor, proceeds during the simultaneous effacement and dilatation of the cervix, and continues during the second stage of labor. Descent is correlated with engagement, inasmuch as engagement cannot take place without descent.

DISENGAGEMENT
Disengagement is the emergence of the presenting part from the vulva during birth.

ENGAGEMENT
Engagement is the mechanism by which the biparietal diameter of the fetal head, in vertex presentation, enters the plane of the inlet. Clinically, the criteria for engagement are met when the presenting part reaches the level of the ischial spines (station zero), covers three-fourths of the pubic symphysis, and covers two-thirds of the anterior surface of the sacrum.

EXTENSION
Extension is the process by which the base of the occiput is brought into direct contact with the inferior margin of the pubic symphysis. The fetal head is directed forward and somewhat upward in the direction of the vulvar ring. This process follows internal rotation of the fetal head.
SYNONYM: *Deflexion.*

FETAL ATTITUDE
Fetal attitude is the relationship of one fetal part to another. The fetus generally is in universal flexion in utero.
SYNONYM: *Habitus.*

FLEXION
Flexion is the normal bending forward of the fetal head in the uterus or birth canal. This is caused by resistance encountered by the descending fetal head either from the margins of the plane of the inlet, the cervix, the walls of the pelvis, or the pelvic floor.

Lateroflexion
Lateroflexion is the bending of the fetal head to one side of the body.

Universal Flexion
Universal flexion is flexion of the fetal parts on the body. The head is flexed with the chin on the chest. The occiput presents into the pelvis.

FLOATING HEAD
A floating head is a fetal head that is not engaged and is freely movable on palpation.

OVERROTATION
Overrotation is the turning of the fetal head, after expulsion, from one side of the mother to the other. It is due to overrotation of the shoulders.

RESTITUTION
Restitution is the return of the fetal head to the normal position in relation to the fetal body, after delivery of the head.

ROTATION
Rotation is the turning of the presenting part of the fetus from one position to another around the pelvic axis.

Rotation, External
External rotation is turning of the presenting part of the fetus after its expulsion.

Rotation, Internal
Internal rotation is turning of the presenting part of the fetus from one position to another in the pelvis as the fetus accommodates to the curve of the lower portion of the birth canal.

SYNCLITISM
Synclitism occurs when the fetal head presents into the pelvis with the sagittal suture midway between the maternal pubic symphysis and sacral promontory.
SYNONYM: *Parallelism.*

THEORY OF ROTATION
The theory of rotation is an explanation of internal rotation of the fetus. According to this theory, the fetus is compressed during labor into a semiflexible cylinder that resists bending differently in various directions. The fetus must accommodate itself to the curve of the solid birth canal in order to be expelled.
SYNONYM: *Sellheim's Theory.*

FIRST STAGE OF LABOR

FIRST STAGE OF LABOR
The first stage of labor refers to the period from the onset of labor through complete dilatation of the cervix.

BLOODY SHOW
Bloody show is the blood-tinged mucous discharge from the vagina that accompanies dilatation of the cervix during the first stage of labor.

CERVIX, DILATATION OF
Dilatation of the cervix is the enlargement of the cervical opening caused by the upward retraction of the muscle fibers of the cervix during labor. The phases involved are the latent and the active phases.

Latent Phase
The latent phase is the time between the onset of regular uterine contractions and appreciable cervical dilatation. During this phase, the cervix becomes effaced but dilates only slightly.

Active Phase

The active phase extends from the end of the latent phase to the end of the first stage of labor. It may be divided into three periods: acceleration, steady, and deceleration.

ACCELERATION PERIOD

The acceleration period is the time during which the rate of cervical dilatation is continuously changing and increasing.

STEADY PERIOD

The steady period is the time during which the cervix dilates at a regular and steady rate.

DECELERATION PERIOD

The deceleration period is the time during which the rate of cervical dilatation decreases. Complete dilatation is effected during this period and signals the end of the first stage of labor.

CERVIX, EFFACEMENT OF

Effacement of the cervix is accomplished when the cervix is completely retracted, the cervicovaginal angle has disappeared, and only the external cervical os remains. Dilatation now begins or continues.

ENGAGEMENT

Engagement is the mechanism by which the biparietal diameter of the fetal head, in vertex presentation, enters the plane of the inlet. Clinically, the criteria for engagement are met when the presenting part reaches the level of the ischial spines (station zero), covers three-fourths of the pubic symphysis, and covers two-thirds of the anterior surface of the sacrum.

LONGITUDINAL SHORTENING OF LOWER UTERINE SEGMENT

Longitudinal shortening of lower uterine segment is caused by the retraction of longitudinal muscle fibers of that segment before and during labor. It facilitates retraction and dilatation of the cervix.

ONSET OF LABOR

The onset of labor is the establishment of regular uterine contractions together with beginning dilatation of the cervix.

SECOND STAGE OF LABOR

SECOND STAGE OF LABOR

The second stage of labor refers to the period from complete dilatation of the cervix through birth of the fetus.

BEARING DOWN

Bearing down is a reflex effort of the mother to coordinate the activity of the abdominal muscles with the uterine contractions.

BIRTH

Birth is the process by which a liveborn infant or a stillborn infant is expelled or extracted from the mother.

CROWNING

Crowning occurs when the fetal head has negotiated the pelvic outlet and the largest diameter of the head is encircled by the vulvar ring. This occurs usually late in the second stage of labor. Clinically, crowning is visualization of the fetal head at the introitus.

DENMAN'S METHOD

Denman's method is spontaneous evolution of the fetus from the transverse presentation. The fetal head rotates posteriorly, and as the breech descends, the shoulder ascends in the pelvis. The back of the fetus is generally posterior.

DISENGAGEMENT

Disengagement is the emergence of the presenting part from the vulva during birth.

DOUGLAS' METHOD

Douglas' method is spontaneous evolution of the fetus from transverse presentation. An arm prolapses, the fetus becomes pointed, and the head is arrested above the inlet and rotates to the pubis. The chest, abdomen, and breech roll down alongside the shoulder, the legs drop out, then the other arm, and finally the head appears.

EPISIOTOMY

An episiotomy is an incision or incisions into the perineum and vagina to enlarge the vaginal opening and to protect the underlying fascia and muscles. It is performed for obstetric purposes. Incision may be made in the median, mediolateral, or lateral direction. The incisions may be bilateral.

Bilateral Episiotomy

A bilateral episiotomy is performed by making incisions into the sides of the perineum at right angles to the median line. This operation is rarely performed because of the resulting tissue damage, excessive bleeding, and the small additional space obtained.

Median Episiotomy

A median episiotomy is an incision made from the fourchette in the midline of the perineum to facilitate delivery.
    SYNONYM: *Central Episiotomy.*

Mediolateral Episiotomy

A mediolateral episiotomy is an incision made from the fourchette into the perineum at approximately 45° from midline to protect perineal structures, particularly the sphincter ani, and to facilitate delivery.

LACERATION, OBSTETRIC

An obstetric laceration is a tearing of the vulvar, vaginal, and occasionally the rectal tissues.

First-degree Obstetric Laceration

A first-degree obstetric laceration is a tear that involves the fourchette, perineal skin, and vaginal mucous membrane without involving any of the muscles.

Second-degree Obstetric Laceration

A second-degree obstetric laceration is a tear that involves, in addition to perineal skin and vaginal mucous membrane, the muscles of the perineal body, but not the sphincter ani.

Third-degree Obstetric Laceration

A third-degree obstetric laceration is a tear that extends completely through the perineal skin, vaginal mucous membrane, perineal body, and sphincter ani.

Fourth-degree Obstetric Laceration

A fourth-degree obstetric laceration is a tear that extends completely through the perineal skin, vaginal mucous membrane, perineal body, sphincter ani, and rectal mucosa.

SYNONYM: *Complete Tear of the Perineum.*

MOLDING

Molding is the change in shape, and to a lesser degree the size, of the fetal head during labor. Such changes are due to forces of labor, the resistance of the bony pelvis, and loose connection and softness of the fetal skull bones.

ROEDERER'S METHOD

Roederer's method is spontaneous evolution of a fetus from transverse presentation without prolapse of the arm. The fetus becomes folded like a V, the shoulder and back advance, and the head presses deep into the chest and abdomen.

THIRD STAGE OF LABOR

THIRD STAGE OF LABOR

The third stage of labor refers to the period from birth of the fetus through expulsion or extraction of the placenta and membranes.

BRANDT-ANDREWS MANEUVER

The Brandt-Andrews maneuver is a method of expressing the placenta from the uterus. It is performed by grasping the cord with the left hand while the right hand is placed on the maternal abdomen, so that the palmar surfaces of the fingers are over the anterior surface of the uterus at the junction of the corpus uteri and the lower uterine segment.

By gently pressing the right hand backward and slightly upward and making gentle traction on the cord with the left hand, the placenta and membranes are easily extracted if separation has occurred.

CALKINS' SIGN

Calkins' sign is the anatomic change of the uterus from a discoid to ovoid shape. It is a sign of separation of the placenta from the uterine wall.

CREDÉ METHOD OF EXPRESSING PLACENTA

The Credé method of expressing the placenta is forceful expulsion of the placenta and membranes by squeezing and pressure on the uterine fundus. It may be traumatic, resulting in tearing or rupture of the uterus and only partial expulsion of the placenta.

DUNCAN MECHANISM

The Duncan mechanism is expulsion of the placenta with the maternal surface appearing at the vulva.

INTRAPLACENTAL PRESSURE

Intraplacental pressure is the pressure of the fetal blood in the placenta and in the umbilical vein.

MANUAL EXPRESSION OF PLACENTA

Manual expression of the placenta is the method of expressing the placenta from the uterus in which the uterus is grasped in the whole hand, with the thumb in front, and is gently, without squeezing, pushed down onto the placenta in the axis of the pelvic inlet. This should only be done when the uterus is firmly contracted and the placenta has separated.

MANUAL REMOVAL OF PLACENTA

Manual removal of the placenta is the method of extracting the placenta from the uterus in which, after grasping the uterus through the abdominal wall with one hand, the other hand is introduced into the vagina and the uterus. As soon as the placenta is reached, its margin should be located and the ulnar border of the hand insinuated between it and the uterine wall. Then, with the back of the hand in contact with the uterus, the placenta should be peeled from its attachment.

PLACENTA

The placenta is the structure providing the principal means of communication between the mother and the fetus. It increases in size until the end of pregnancy, by which time it is a round or oval disc covering about one fifth of the inner surface of the uterus. It is composed of villi containing vessels that carry fetal blood. The villi penetrate the maternal decidua and are bathed in maternal blood. The portion of the decidua basalis superior to Nitabuch's layer forms a thin covering on the maternal surface of the placenta. The fetal surface is composed of chorion to which the amnion is adherent. The placental chorion and the amnion form the amniotic sac. The placenta performs the functions of respiration, nutrition, and excretion, and secretes estrogen, progesterone, and other hormones.

SYNONYMS: *Afterbirth, Placenta* (NA).

SCHULTZ MECHANISM

The Schultz mechanism is expulsion of the placenta with the fetal surface appearing at the vulva.

SEPARATION OF PLACENTA

Separation of the placenta is the detachment of the placenta from the uterine wall.

SPONTANEOUS EXPULSION OF PLACENTA

Spontaneous expulsion of the placenta is the expulsion of the placenta and membranes by the spontaneous contraction of the uterus or of the abdominal muscles.

COMPLICATIONS OF LABOR

DYSTOCIA

Dystocia is abnormal labor resulting from any variation of the normal patterns in the latent or active phases of cervical dilatation such as prolonged latent phase, protracted active phase, or secondary arrest of cervical dilatation. Other causes are cephalopelvic disproportion, malpresentation, tumor, or resistance of maternal nonbony tissue.

SYNONYM: *Dysfunctional Labor.*

Cervical Dystocia

Cervical dystocia is abnormal labor caused by cervical factors such as cervical edema, scarring, displacement, rigidity, tumor, conglutination, or suture.

Contraction Ring Dystocia

Contraction ring dystocia is abnormal labor resulting in the formation of a spastic, contracted muscle zone or ring on the uterus. It is caused by contraction of the circular muscle fibers above or below a depression in the fetal body.

SYNONYM: *Constriction Ring Dystocia.*

Fetal Dystocia

Fetal dystocia is abnormal labor due to an anomaly, abnormal size, or abnormal position of the fetus.

Shoulder Girdle Dystocia

Shoulder girdle dystocia is abnormal labor caused by contracted pelvis, disproportionately large fetal shoulders, short umbilical cord, large fetal chest, locked twins, or a monster. The fetal head is expelled with little or no difficulty, but the shoulders do not immediately follow even upon gentle traction.

ARM, PROLAPSED

A prolapsed arm is the protrusion of a fetal arm through the uterine cervix in advance of the presenting part. One or both arms may protrude through the cervix.

ARREST, DEEP TRANSVERSE

Deep transverse arrest is cessation of labor with the presenting part of the fetal head in the transverse position (occiput left transverse or occiput right transverse) 1 cm below the ischial spines.

ARREST, HIGH TRANSVERSE

High transverse arrest is cessation of labor with the fetal head in the transverse position (occiput left transverse or occiput right transverse) above the ischial spines.

CERVIX, CONGLUTINATION OF

Conglutination of the cervix is failure of cervical dilatation due to a small cervical opening or no cervical opening as a result of fibrous scarring caused by adhesions between the edges of the external os.

CERVIX, PROLAPSE OF ANTERIOR LIP

Prolapse of the anterior lip of the cervix is the impingement of the anterior lip of the cervix between the presenting part and the pubic symphysis. The edematous prolapsed portion of the cervix may obstruct labor.

COLPORRHEXIS

Colporrhexis is a laceration that extends more or less circularly around the vagina near the cervix. It results from overdistention of the birth canal.

CONTRACTIONS, FALSE UTERINE

False uterine contractions are contractions of the uterus that occur preparatory to labor. Dilatation of the cervix does not occur with these contractions, but effacement of the cervix may be enhanced.

CONTRACTION, TETANIC

Tetanic contraction is a state of continuous, tempestuous uterine contraction. It may be caused by intrauterine bleeding, excessive administration of oxytocics, or other sources of uterine irritation.

CONTRACTIONS, TUMULTUOUS

Tumultuous contractions are strong, violent uterine contractions, causing rapid labor and usually endangering the fetus and the maternal soft parts.

CORD, OCCULT PROLAPSE OF

Occult prolapse of the cord is the descent of the umbilical cord alongside the presenting part. It can only be detected by internal examination.

CORD, PROLAPSE OF
Prolapse of the cord is the descent of the umbilical cord through the cervical os in advance of the presenting part.

DISPROPORTION, BORDERLINE PELVIC
Borderline pelvic disproportion is the degree of pelvic contraction that would make the safe passage of the fetus questionable.

DISPROPORTION, CEPHALOPELVIC
Cephalopelvic disproportion is spatial inadequacy of the maternal pelvis in relation to the fetal head. Pelvic contraction, large fetus, or tumorous obstruction of the birth canal may make passage of the fetus difficult or impossible.

DYSTOCIA-DYSTROPHIA SYNDROME
The dystocia-dystrophia syndrome is a syndrome that concerns the improbability of normal vaginal birth of an overmature fetus, the head of which does not engage and the position of which is occiput posterior. Both fetal and maternal dystocia contribute to the failure of normal events. As a rule the mother has conceived for the first time rather late in life, or perhaps has had previous unsuccessful pregnancies. In body habitus, she is heavyset, with girdle obesity; has a masculine type of pelvis, small cervix, and narrow, rigid vagina; and exhibits other signs of dystrophia adiposogenitalis. The pelvic measurements are decreased. Pregnancy is prolonged, and there is disproportion between the fetal head and the maternal pelvis. The fetal head is not engaged when labor begins, the membranes rupture prematurely, and uterine contractions are weak resulting in a protracted first stage of labor.

GIRDLE OF RESISTANCE
The girdle of resistance is composed of the maternal bony pelvis and soft tissues. It opposes the progress of the presenting part during labor.

INERTIA, UTERINE
Uterine inertia is failure of the uterine muscles to contract and retract with normal strength and frequency.
SYNONYM: *Uterine Dysfunction.*

Primary Uterine Inertia
Primary uterine inertia is failure of the uterus to contract and retract normally at the onset of labor. It results in slow dilatation and retraction of the cervix, prolonged labor, and a possible uterine hemorrhage.
SYNONYM: *Hypertonic Uterine Dysfunction.*

Secondary Uterine Inertia
Secondary uterine inertia is failure of the uterus to maintain normal contractions and retractions after labor has been in progress. It results in prolonged labor and a possible uterine hemorrhage.
SYNONYMS: *Hypotonic Uterine Dysfunction, Uterine Atony.*

INVERSION, UTERINE

Uterine inversion is the abnormal turning of the uterus inside out, so that the internal surface of the corpus uteri lies in or outside of the vagina. It may be spontaneous or forced.

Forced Inversion

Forced inversion is uterine inversion created by pulling on the cord, or by forceful manual expression of the placenta when the uterus is atonic.

Spontaneous Inversion

Spontaneous inversion is uterine inversion following spontaneous action of the patient such as bearing down, sudden action of the abdominal muscles, coughing, or increased intraabdominal pressure.

LABOR, ARRESTED

Arrested labor is labor that has failed to proceed through the normal stages. It may be due to obstructions in the maternal pelvis, uterine inertia, cephalopelvic disproportion, or general systemic diseases.

LABOR, MISSED

Missed labor is labor that begins at the proper time, but then ceases. Some degree of cervical dilatation may be attained, but the contractions cease and the gestation continues for weeks or months.

LABOR, PRECIPITATE

Precipitate labor is labor that terminates in the expulsion of the fetus in less than three hours.

POSITION, PERSISTENT OCCIPUT POSTERIOR

The persistent occiput posterior position is a condition in which the fetal occiput remains located in either posterior quadrant of the maternal pelvis. In this position, spontaneous anterior rotation does not occur.

PRESENTATION, ACROMION

In acromion presentation, the long axis of the fetus is perpendicular to the long axis of the mother, and the shoulder is the presenting part. The acromion process of the scapula is the point of direction or the designated point on the presenting part. There are only four positions of the shoulder.

SYNONYM: *Shoulder Presentation.*

PRESENTATION, BREECH

In breech presentation, the fetal breech is the presenting part. The sacrum is the point of direction or the designated point on the presenting part.

PRESENTATION, BROW

Brow presentation is a position of the fetus in which the brow is the presenting part. The brow is the point of direction or the designated point on the presenting part.

PRESENTATION, COMPOUND

In compound presentation, an extremity prolapses alongside the presenting part so that both enter the pelvic cavity at the same time.

PRESENTATION, FACE

Face presentation is a position of the fetus in which the face is the presenting part. The mentum (chin) is the point of direction or the designated point on the face.

PRESENTATION, FUNIC

In funic presentation, the umbilical cord has prolapsed into the maternal vagina. The cord becomes the presenting part.

PRESENTATION, OBLIQUE

In oblique presentation, the fetus lies at a marked angle to the long axis of the mother.

PRESENTATION, PARIETAL

In parietal presentation, the parietal portion or side of the fetal head presents in the pelvis.

RING, PATHOLOGIC RETRACTION

The pathologic retraction ring is a zone of constriction at the junction of the thinned lower uterine segment and the thick, retracted, upper uterine segment. It results from obstructed labor and may be a sign of impending uterine rupture.

SYNONYMS: *Bandl's Ring, Constriction Ring.*

SHOCK, OBSTETRIC

Obstetric shock is sudden maternal collapse during labor or the puerperium. It may be caused by rupture of the uterus, embolism, postpartum hemorrhage, cerebral hemorrhage, vasomotor collapse, inversion of the uterus, anesthesia, prolonged labor, retroperitoneal hemorrhage, acute pulmonary edema, rupture of the uterine or ovarian veins, bacterial shock, pituitary necrosis, ruptured ectopic pregnancy, or perforation of the uterus by trophoblastic tissue.

UTERINE INCOORDINATION, FIRST-DEGREE

First-degree uterine incoordination is deviation from the normal pattern of contraction caused by interference between the actions of the two uterine pacemakers. This incoordination may combine with inverted gradient, hypoactivity, and hypertonicity to give rise to a great variety of abnormal clinical conditions.

UTERINE INCOORDINATON, SECOND-DEGREE

Second-degree uterine incoordination is the independent and asynchronous contraction of the muscle fibers in numerous zones of the uterus.

This results in a variation of amniotic pressure, irregular contractions, and a high frequency of contractions superimposed on a slightly elevated uterine tonus. These local contractions are totally ineffective in advancing the progress of labor.

BREECH BIRTH

BREECH BIRTH
Breech birth is the birth of a fetus presenting by the buttocks or feet.

Spontaneous Breech Birth
Spontaneous breech birth is a breech birth in which the entire fetus is expelled by natural forces of labor without traction or manipulation other than support of the body of the fetus.

Partial Breech Extraction
Partial breech extraction is a breech birth in which the fetus is expelled as far as the umbilicus by natural forces of labor, but the remainder of the body is extracted by the attendant.
SYNONYM: *Assisted Breech Extraction.*

Total Breech Extraction
Total breech extraction is a breech birth in which the entire body of the fetus is extracted by the attendant.

BREECH PRESENTATION
In breech presentation, the fetal breech is the presenting part. The sacrum is the point of direction or the designated point on the presenting part.

Complete Breech Presentation
In complete breech presentation, the buttocks descend first. The legs are flexed on the abdomen, and the feet are alongside the fetal buttocks.
SYNONYMS: *Double Breech Presentation, Full Breech Presentation.*

Frank Breech Presentation
In frank breech presentation, the legs lie extended alongside the fetal body so that the buttocks descend first.
SYNONYMS: *Pelvic Presentation, Single Breech Presentation.*

Incomplete Breech Presentation
Incomplete breech presentation is a breech presentation with one or both feet or knees prolapsed into the vagina.

DOUBLE FOOTLING PRESENTATION
In double footling presentation, both feet have prolapsed into the vagina.

SINGLE FOOTLING PRESENTATION
In single footling presentation, one foot has prolapsed into the vagina.

MANEUVER, BRACHT

The Bracht maneuver is a method of extraction of the aftercoming head. The breech is expelled spontaneously up to the umbilicus. The body and extended legs are held together, with both hands maintaining upward anterior rotation of the fetal body. When anterior rotation is almost complete, the fetal body is held against the maternal pubic symphysis. Sometimes moderate pressure is exerted from above by an assistant.

MANEUVER, KRISTELLER'S

Kristeller's maneuver is an attempt to express the fetus by pressure on the fundus of the uterus toward the axis of the inlet. It is a dangerous procedure and may result in rupture of the uterus.

MANEUVER, LØVSET'S

Løvset's maneuver is a method of extracting the arms in breech birth by clockwise and counterclockwise rotation of the fetus. This maneuver is performed after the fetus has been expelled up to the umbilicus.

MANEUVER, MAURICEAU-SMELLIE-VEIT

The Mauriceau-Smellie-Veit maneuver is a method of extraction of the aftercoming head in breech presentation. After the legs, abdomen, and shoulders are expelled, the infant is straddled over the operator's arm. The middle finger of the operator's hand is inserted into the fetal mouth, and the ring and index fingers are placed on the maxillary bones of the fetal face. The other hand is placed over the fetal shoulders to apply traction. The combined traction of both hands is used to flex and extract the fetal head. An assistant pushes the fetal head into and through the pelvis. It is a dangerous maneuver.

MANEUVER, PINARD

The Pinard maneuver is a method of extraction of an extended leg in breech presentation. The hand is passed into the uterus avoiding the umbilical cord. The index finger or thumb is pressed into the popliteal space of the anterior fetal leg, pressing the thigh against the fetal abdomen. The other fingers are passed over the fetal knee to the ankle, and the leg is rotated medially on the fetal body and brought down into the pelvis and vagina. Deep anesthesia is needed for this procedure.

MANEUVER, PRAGUE

The Prague maneuver is a method of extraction of the aftercoming head when the fetal chin is anterior over the pubic rami. The fetal back, which is posterior, rests on the forearm of the operator, and the operator's hand is placed forklike over the fetal shoulder. The fetal legs are grasped by the other hand of the operator and the fetal body is flexed over the pubic rami.

MANEUVER, VAN HOORN

The Van Hoorn maneuver is a modified Prague maneuver. In this maneuver, an assistant applies gentle pressure on the fetal head, attempting to cause flexion and downward pressure.

MANEUVER, WIGAND-MARTIN

The Wigand-Martin maneuver is a method of extraction of the after-coming head in breech presentation. After the legs, abdomen, and shoulders are expelled, the infant is straddled over the operator's arm. The middle finger of the operator's hand is inserted into the fetal mouth and the ring and index fingers are placed on the maxillary bones of the fetal face. The head is then flexed and brought into the pelvis. The other hand aids flexion of the head by pushing it into the pelvis. It is a relatively safe maneuver.

NUCHAL HITCH POSITION

Nuchal hitch position is a condition in which one or both arms become extended behind the head during breech birth. It is generally due to an undilated cervix, contracted pelvis, or undue manipulation by the operator.

    RELATED TERMS: Single Nuchal Hitch Position, Double Nuchal Hitch Position.

PINARD'S SIGN

Pinard's sign is a sharp pain on pressure over the uterine fundus. After the sixth month of pregnancy, the Pinard sign indicates breech presentation.

VERSION, CEPHALIC

Cephalic version is the conversion of a fetus from a breech presentation into a vertex presentation. It is rarely performed.

VERSION, PODALIC

Podalic version is a method of changing the polarity of the fetus by inserting the operator's hand into the uterus, pushing the fetal head upward, and pulling the fetal extremities into the pelvis. The cervix should be completely or almost completely dilated, the pelvis must be adequate, and anesthesia should be deep and under good control.

    SYNONYM: *Internal Podalic Version.*

INDUCTION OF LABOR

INDUCTION OF LABOR

Induction of labor is the deliberate initiation of uterine contractions prior to their spontaneous onset.

INDUCTION OF LABOR, MEDICAL

Medical induction of labor is induction of labor by the use of an oxytocic.

STIMULATION OF LABOR
Stimulation of labor is the induced augmentation of uterine contractions after their spontaneous or induced onset.

AMNIOTOMY
Amniotomy is the surgical rupture of the amniotic sac as a means of inducing or expediting labor.

SYNONYM: *Artificial Rupture of Membranes.*

OXYTOCICS
Oxytocics are substances that stimulate the uterine musculature to contract. These substances include the principal product of posterior pituitary secretion and synthetic products of similar activity.

OXYTOCIN SENSITIVITY TEST
The oxytocin sensitivity test is a determination of the readiness of the uterus for induction of labor. After a preliminary rest period, the basic uterine activity is recorded by external tocography. Synthetic oxytocin, 0.01 I.U., is given intravenously. This is repeated every minute for ten doses or until the uterus responds with a strong contraction. The test is positive and the uterus is ready for induction only if response occurs with 0.02 I.U. or less. Response to a greater concentration indicates labor is not imminent—that is, not to be expected within 48 hours.

STRIPPING OF THE MEMBRANES
Stripping of the membranes is a method of inducing labor. It involves the digital separation of the fetal membranes from their loose areolar attachment to the lower uterine segment without actually rupturing the membranes.

SECTION 7: OBSTETRICS

Puerperium

GENERAL TERMINOLOGY

PUERPERIUM
The puerperium is the period of 42 days following the birth of the fetus, and expulsion or extraction of the placenta and membranes. During this time, the generative organs ordinarily return to normal.

AFTERPAINS
Afterpains are painful uterine contractions that occur for one to three days postpartum or longer.

INVOLUTION OF THE UTERUS
Involution of the uterus is the return of the puerperal uterus to its normal nonpregnant state.

LACTATION
Lactation is the postpartum production of milk by the breast.

LACTATION CYCLE
The lactation cycle is composed of the period of filling, the period of emptying, and the refractory period.

Period of Filling
The period of filling is the 10 to 30 minutes during which the breast fills with milk.

Period of Emptying
The period of emptying is the period during which the breast is emptied of milk.

Refractory Period
The refractory period is the period after the breast has been emptied. It lasts from two to three hours.

LOCHIA
Lochia is the vaginal discharge during the puerperium. It usually lasts approximately two weeks and is classified as lochia rubra, lochia serosa, and lochia alba.

Lochia Rubra
Lochia rubra is the bloody discharge occurring during the first one to three postpartum days. It consists of blood, shreds of mem-

brane and decidua, and occasionally fetal remnants, vernix caseosa, lanugo, and meconium.

SYNONYM: *Lochia Cruenta.*

Lochia Serosa
Lochia serosa is a thick, maroon vaginal discharge occurring from the fourth to ninth days postpartum. It contains blood, wound exudate, leukocytes, erythrocytes, shreds of decidua in a state of fatty degeneration, mucus from the cervix, and microorganisms.

SYNONYM: *Lochia Sanguinolenta.*

Lochia Alba
Lochia alba is a white, creamy vaginal discharge generally occurring from the 10th to 14th postpartum day. It contains decidual cells; large, mononucleated, irregular round or fusiform cells in the process of degeneration; leukocytes; flat and cylindrical epithelium; fat and debris from the uterus and puerperal wounds; mucus; cholesterin crystals; and many microorganisms.

SYNONYM: *Lochia Purulenta.*

PUERPERA
A puerpera is a woman who has given birth to a fetus during the previous 42 days.

SUPERINVOLUTION OF THE UTERUS
Superinvolution of the uterus is prolonged involution of the puerperal uterus resulting in an extremely small uterus. It only occurs in nursing mothers.

SYNONYM: *Lactation Atrophy.*

COMPLICATIONS OF PUERPERIUM

ABSCESS, BREAST
A breast abscess is a late, usually suppurative sequel to acute mastitis.

ABSCESS, SUBMAMMARY
A submammary abscess is a form of mastitis in which the infection passes directly through the gland to the underlying areolar tissue.

SYNONYMS: *Submammary Mastitis, Retromammary Mastitis.*

AGALACTIA
Agalactia is the absence of lactation.

BREAST ENGORGEMENT
Breast engorgement is a temporary inflammatory condition caused by increased blood flow preceding the formation of milk. It is characterized by fullness, redness, and hardness of the breast.

SYNONYMS: *Caked Breast, Stagnation Mastitis.*

CHIARI-FROMMEL SYNDROME

The Chiari-Frommel syndrome is a condition characterized by persistent postpartum amenorrhea and galactorrhea, and atrophy of the uterus and ovaries probably due to hypothalamic dysfunction. The diagnosis is generally entertained in women who have amenorrhea and lactation for more than a year following delivery or cessation of nursing, and in whom no organic lesion of the central nervous system can be demonstrated by appropriate studies. Gonadotropins and estrogens are markedly diminished. Other endocrine studies are generally normal. Spontaneous recovery may occur after prolonged intervals. Recurrence may be noted after subsequent pregnancies.

SYNONYMS: *Frommel's Disease, Persistent Postpartum Amenorrhea-Galactorrhea Syndrome.*

GALACTOCELE

A galactocele is a true milk-duct cyst due to obstruction of a lactiferous duct.

GALACTORRHEA

Galactorrhea is the constant leakage of milk from the breast.

HERPES GESTATIONIS SYNDROME

The herpes gestationis syndrome is a relatively rare exanthema that occurs as a complication of the latter half of pregnancy or during the early phase of the puerperium. The condition occurs most commonly in women 30 to 35 years old. Symptoms include fever, malaise, dyspnea, burning sensation, neuralgic pains, and an intense pruritus. The cutaneous lesions consist of bullae and vesicles that are present over the chest, abdomen, and extremities. The syndrome may occur with each gestation or during every second or third pregnancy. Exacerbations are likely, even during treatment. Recurrences may occasionally extend into the puerperium as episodes of severe pruritus, prior to the first few menstrual periods. These episodes are called *herpes menstrualis recidivans.* The higher incidence of erythroblastosis fetalis, spontaneous abortions, monstrosities, and stillborn infants among women who seem predisposed to herpes gestationis may be an expression of Rh incompatibility or isosensitization.

SYNONYMS: *Fetal Anomaly Syndrome, Dermatitis Herpetiformis Gestationis Syndrome, Herpes Circinatus Bullosus, Hydroa Gravidarum, Hydroa Herpetiformis, Pemphigus Pruriginosus, Prurigo Gestationis Syndrome, Duhring's Disease, Brocq-Duhring Disease, Dermatitis Herpetiformis, Dermatitis Multiformis, Dermatitis Neurotica, Dermatitis Polymorpha Dolorosa, Dermatitis Pruriginosa, Dermatitis Trophoneurotica, Pemphigus Circinatus, Hydroa Pruriginosa.*

HOMANS' SIGN

Homans' sign is pain at the back of the knee or calf when the ankle is forcibly dorsiflexed. The sign indicates beginning or established thrombophlebitis of the veins of the leg.

LOCHIOCOLPOS
Lochiocolpos is the retention of lochia in the vagina.

LOCHIOMETRA
Lochiometra is the retention of lochia within the uterus.

MASTITIS, ACUTE
Acute mastitis is acute inflammation of the breast, usually associated with a cracked or fissured nipple and occurring in the period of lactation.

MASTITIS, GLANDULAR
Glandular mastitis is an inflammatory disease of the breast that involves the lactiferous tubules.
SYNONYMS: *Galactophoritis, Parenchymatous Mastitis.*

MASTITIS, INTERSTITIAL
Interstitial mastitis is an inflammatory disease of the breast in which bacteria gain access to the connective tissue through a crack or deep fissure. The infection occurs in the fat around the lobes or lobules.
SYNONYMS: *Phlegmonous Mastitis, Lymphangitis Mastitis.*

MASTITIS, PUERPERAL
Puerperal mastitis is an inflammation of the breast that occurs in the puerperium.

METRITIS DISSECANS
Metritis dissecans is a rare sequel to metritis. The endometrium and also portions of the myometrium become necrotic.
SYNONYM: *Gangrene of Uterus.*

METROPHLEBITIS
Metrophlebitis is inflammation of the uterine veins, usually occurring only in the puerperium.

MILK LEG
Milk leg is an extreme edematous swelling of the leg occurring in the puerperium. It is due to thrombosis of the femoral or iliac vein.
SYNONYM: *Phlegmasia Alba Dolens.*

MYOMETRITIS, ACUTE
Acute myometritis is a severe form of infection of the myometrium resulting from a puerperal streptococcal infection. There is marked edema, muscle hypertrophy, and leukocytic infiltration.

NONINVOLUTION OF THE UTERUS
Noninvolution of the uterus is failure of the puerperal uterus to return to a normal nonpregnant state. It is characterized by failure of the physiologic process of obliteration of the large vessels underlying the placental site.

OOPHORITIS
Oophoritis is an inflammation of the ovary, generally associated with pelvic inflammatory disease.

SYNONYM: *Ovaritis.*

PARAMETRITIS
Parametritis is a form of puerperal infection that is extended to the pelvic connective tissue surrounding the uterus. Generally, the apex of infection is from the cervix, lower uterine segment, or vagina. The infection generally subsides after adequate therapy, but it may persist to form a parametrial abscess.

SYNONYM: *Pelvic Cellulitis.*

PELVIC PERITONITIS
Pelvic peritonitis is inflammation of the pelvic peritoneum that may accompany any form of puerperal infection such as parametritis, endometritis, and salpingitis.

PHLEBOTHROMBOSIS
Phlebothrombosis is the formation of a thrombus in a vein in the absence of a pre-existing inflammation. There is a greater danger of pulmonary embolism in this type of thrombosis. The condition may occur in the superficial or deep veins of the legs, or the pelvic veins surrounding the uterus.

SYNONYM: *Blood Thrombosis.*

POLYGALACTIA
Polygalactia is the excessive flow of milk from the breast.

POSTPARTUM CYSTITIS
Postpartum cystitis is infection in the urinary bladder occurring in the puerperium. It is characterized by urgency, dysuria, and a low-grade fever, rarely over 38.3 C (101 F). Diagnosis is made on the demonstration of bacteriuria and pus cells associated with residual urine in the bladder.

POSTPARTUM PSYCHOSES
Postpartum psychoses are characterized by severe degrees of personality disorganization that impair the patient's ability to function responsibly. They are classified as manic-depressive psychosis, puerperal psychosis, schizophrenia, and toxic confusional states.

Manic-Depressive Psychosis
Manic-depressive psychosis is the most common serious psychiatric illness. It usually occurs from a few days to several weeks postpartum. The onset is sudden, with characteristic features of shifts in mood and energy levels.

Puerperal Psychosis

Puerperal psychosis is a special complication of the puerperium. It may be a variant of manic-depressive disease. Its onset most often is within the first 48 hours postpartum. Early symptoms are refusal of food, insomnia, quietness and suspicion, and delusions about the infant. Such patients may be suicidal risks and may do harm to their infants.

Schizophrenia

Schizophrenia is a common psychosis. These patients during pregnancy are rather shy, timid, introverted, and unsociable, and behave eccentrically. The onset of an acute schizophrenic reaction may occur from within a few days to several weeks postpartum.

Toxic Confusional States

Toxic confusional states are acute psychotic reactions precipitated by various factors such as acute sepsis, drug intoxications, metabolic disease crises, and organic brain damage. Disorientation, hallucinations, periods of amentia, restlessness, and insomnia are clinical manifestations. Symptoms appear almost immediately postpartum.

POSTPARTUM PITUITARY NECROSIS SYNDROME

The postpartum pituitary necrosis syndrome is due to postpartum thrombosis of sinuses, and ischemic infarction and necrosis of the pituitary gland, usually as a result of obstetric hemorrhage and shock that occur at term. If both the anterior and posterior lobes are involved and the gonadotropins, thyrotropin, and corticotropin are all absent, the appropriate descriptive term is *panhypopituitarism.* These deficiences indicate secondary atrophy and failure of the adrenal cortices, the thyroid, and the ovaries. Excretion of corticoids in the urine is reduced. The resulting symptoms appear insidiously, and usually after several months. Symptoms of the multiglandular deficiency are variable. Some patients exhibit the characteristics of myxedema. There is pallor, asthenia, apathy, atrophy of the breasts with loss of areolar pigment, inhibition of lactation, loss of pubic and axillary hair, and genital atrophy. Amenorrhea may be temporary or permanent; rarely some women continue to menstruate indefinitely. Lipemia and xanthomatosis are sometimes present. Diabetes mellitus, if present, vanishes. Hypoglycemia is usually found and may be sufficiently severe to produce coma. A flat glucose tolerance curve and extreme sensitivity to insulin may be demonstrated.

SYNONYMS: *Sheehan's Syndrome, Postpartum Panhypopituitary Syndrome.*

POSTPHLEBITIC SYNDROME

The postphlebitic syndrome is characterized by the progressive development of venous insufficiency, caused by thrombosis of the deep venous system of the lower extremities and the pelvis. The syndrome becomes manifest clinically when the thrombosis has extended into the superficial veins of the legs. Clinical features follow a definite sequence and consist of varicosities, edema, induration, stasis dermatitis, pigmentation especially above the medial malleolus, and perhaps ulceration.

SYNONYMS: *Postthrombotic Syndrome, Venous-Ulcer Leg Syndrome.*

PRIMARY THYROID FAILURE

Primary thyroid failure is a rare complication that results from postpartum hemorrhage and shock. It may be related to Sheehan's syndrome.

PUERPERAL BACTEREMIA

Puerperal bacteremia is a form of acute puerperal infection resulting from the entrance of bacteria and their toxins into the bloodstream causing dissolution of the blood, degenerative changes in the organs, and rapid intoxication.

SYNONYM: *Puerperal Septicemia.*

PUERPERAL ENDOMETRITIS

Puerperal endometritis is infection of the endometrium in association with puerperal infection. The endometrium is swollen, hyperemic, and edematous. In the severe type, bacterial toxin causes destructive effects on the endometrium with necrosis and ulceration. Thrombosis of the uterine vessels may result in thrombophlebitis of the uterine and pelvic vessels. Septic emboli may pass to other structures, causing distant abscesses and bloodstream infection.

PUERPERAL HEMATOMAS

Puerperal hematomas are collections of blood in the soft tissues of the pelvis. They may occur above or below the levator ani, beneath the vaginal mucosa, or beneath the skin of the external genitalia.

PUERPERAL INFECTION

Puerperal infection is any infection of the genital tract occurring during the puerperium, or as a complication of abortion. Puerperal infection may be presumed in the presence of a temperature of 38 C (100.4 F) or above on any two successive days, exclusive of the first 24 hours postpartum, granted that other causes of fever are not apparent.

SYNONYM: *Puerperal Sepsis.*

PUERPERAL METRITIS

Puerperal metritis is infection of the uterus during the puerperium.

PUERPERAL MORBIDITY

Puerperal morbidity is a morbid condition occurring during the first ten postpartum days. This condition is often indicated by a temperature of 38 C (100.4 F) on any two of the first ten postpartum days, exclusive of the first 24 hours. The patient's temperature must be taken orally, using a standard technic at least four times a day to establish the diagnosis.

PUERPERAL PYEMIA

Puerperal pyemia is a chronic form of puerperal infection. The essential pathologic process is a metrophlebitis with thrombi from which bacteria, bits of fibrin, and pus are released and carried to distant organs, producing purulent processes.

SYNONYMS: *Puerperal Septicopyemia, Puerperal Metastatic Septicemia.*

PUERPERAL SALPINGITIS

Puerperal salpingitis is a form of puerperal infection produced by extension of a uterine infection into the fallopian tubes. It may extend to the ovaries and may be a cause of secondary sterility.

PUERPERAL VAGINITIS

Puerperal vaginitis is a form of puerperal infection limited to the vagina. Prolonged labor, trauma, and frequent examinations predispose the patient to this condition.

PUERPERAL VULVITIS

Puerperal vulvitis is a form of puerperal infection limited to the vulva. It is caused by trauma and infection during labor. Previous disease, such as bartholinitis, abscess, and fistula, predisposes to vulvitis.

SUPERFICIAL THROMBOPHLEBITIS

Superficial thrombophlebitis is inflammation and thrombosis of the superficial veins of the legs.

THROMBOPHLEBITIS

Thrombophlebitis is the formation of a thrombus after inflammation of the wall of a vein. This condition generally occurs in the leg or pelvic veins during pregnancy or the puerperium. The clot is quite adherent in this type, decreasing the danger of embolism.

Anesthesia and Analgesia

ANALGESIA
Analgesia is the absence of the feeling of pain.

ANESTHESIA
Anesthesia is the loss of feeling or sensation.

Caudal Anesthesia
Caudal anesthesia is anesthesia resulting from a single injection of an anesthetic drug into the caudal canal.

Continuous Caudal Anesthesia
Continuous caudal anesthesia is continuous injection of an anesthetic drug into the caudal canal to provide analgesia in the first stage of labor and anesthesia for the second and third stages of labor.

Endotracheal Anesthesia
Endotracheal anesthesia is inhalation anesthesia administered through an endotracheal tube.
SYNONYM: *Intratracheal Anesthesia.*

Epidural Anesthesia
Epidural anesthesia is the anesthesia resulting from the injection of a local anesthetic drug into the extradural space.

General Anesthesia
General anesthesia is the loss of sensation with loss of consciousness produced by inhalation of an anesthetic agent.

Inhalation Anesthesia
Inhalation anesthesia is general anesthesia achieved by inhaling anesthetic vapors or gases.

Intravenous Anesthesia
Intravenous anesthesia is the injection of an anesthetic solution into the venous circulation.

Local Anesthesia
Local anesthesia is the injection of an anesthetic agent that acts on a limited area.

INFILTRATION ANESTHESIA
Infiltration anesthesia is anesthesia produced by injecting a local anesthetic solution directly into the tissues.

404

PUDENDAL BLOCK ANESTHESIA
Pudendal block anesthesia is the injection of an anesthetic agent into the pudendal nerve and other perineal nerves, either transvaginally or directly into the perineal body.

Paracervical Block Anesthesia
Paracervical block anesthesia is the injection of an anesthetic agent in the area along the base of the broad ligaments and lateral walls of the lower uterine segment to anesthetize the inferior hypogastric plexus and ganglia.

SYNONYM: *Uterosacral Block Anesthesia.*

Parasacral Block Anesthesia
Parasacral block anesthesia is the injection of an anesthetic agent near the anterior sacral foramen.

Paravertebral Block Anesthesia
Paravertebral block anesthesia is the injection of an anesthetic agent in the paravertebral space at the level of the 11th and 12th thoracic and first and second lumbar somatic nerves.

Presacral Block Anesthesia
Presacral block anesthesia is the injection of an anesthetic agent into the posterior sacral foramen.

Rectal Anesthesia
Rectal anesthesia is a form of general anesthesia produced by administration of an anesthetic drug such as ether into the rectum.

Regional Anesthesia
Regional anesthesia is the production of insensibility of a part by interrupting the sensory nerve conductivity of any region of the body.

SYNONYMS: *Block Anesthesia, Conduction Anesthesia.*

Saddle Block Anesthesia
Saddle block anesthesia is injection of an anesthetic agent into the fourth lumbar interspace to anesthetize the perineum and buttocks.

Spinal Anesthesia
Spinal anesthesia is injection of an anesthetic agent into a spinal subarachnoid space.

Twilight Sleep
Twilight sleep is the analgesia and amnesia resulting from the simultaneous administration of morphine and scopolamine.

ABDOMINAL DECOMPRESSION SUIT
An abdominal decompression suit is an apparatus applied to the abdomen and back for relieving pain of labor by reducing the pressure on the abdominal wall by 20 to 50 mm of Hg. This is believed to result

from a reduction of the forces resisting the change of the shape of the uterus from ellipsoid to spheroid.

HYPNOSIS

Hypnosis is an artificially induced state resembling deep sleep or a trancelike state in which the patient is highly susceptible to suggestion and responds readily to the commands of others. The hypnotic trance produces comfortable painless labor.

Obstetric Operations

GENERAL TERMINOLOGY

AMNIOCENTESIS
Amniocentesis is the procedure by which a small amount of amniotic fluid is aspirated from the amniotic sac.
SYNONYM: *Uterocentesis.*

CESAREAN SECTION
Cesarean section is the extraction of the fetus, placenta, and membranes through an incision in the abdominal and uterine walls.

Classical Cesarean Section
Classical cesarean section is the extraction of the fetus, placenta, and membranes through a vertical incision made into the corpus uteri.

Extraperitoneal Cesarean Section
Extraperitoneal cesarean section is the extraction of the fetus, placenta, and membranes through an incision made into the lower uterine segment without entering the peritoneal cavity.
SYNONYM: *Water's Operation.*

Low Cervical Cesarean Section
Low cervical cesarean section is the extraction of the fetus, placenta, and membranes through an incision made into the lower uterine segment, either in a transverse or longitudinal direction.
SYNONYM: *Laparotrachelotomy.*

Postmortem Cesarean Section
Postmortem cesarean section is the extraction of the fetus through an incision in the abdominal and uterine walls immediately following maternal death.

DÜHRSSEN'S INCISIONS
Dührssen's incisions are three symmetrically placed incisions in the cervix for the purpose of enlarging the cervical opening when dilatation is inadequate. The cervix should be completely effaced, and dilated from 4 to 6 cm before operation is considered. Incisions are made at 10, 2, and 6 o'clock positions.

EPISIOTOMY

An episiotomy is an incision or incisions into the perineum and vagina to enlarge the vaginal opening and to protect the underlying fascia and muscles. It is performed for obstetric purposes. Incision may be made in the median, mediolateral, or lateral direction. The incisions may be bilateral.

Bilateral Episiotomy

A bilateral episiotomy is performed by making incisions into the sides of the perineum at right angles to the median line. This operation is rarely performed because of the resulting tissue damage, excessive bleeding, and the small additional space obtained.

Median Episiotomy

A median episiotomy is an incision made from the fourchette in the midline of the perineum to facilitate delivery.

SYNONYM: *Central Episiotomy.*

Mediolateral Episiotomy

A mediolateral episiotomy is an incision made from the fourchette into the perineum at approximately 45° from midline to protect perineal structures, particularly the sphincter ani, and to facilitate delivery.

FORCEPS OPERATION

A forceps operation is an operation for the extraction of the fetal head from the mother by the use of obstetric forceps. Forceps operations are classified in relation to the location or station of the fetal skull and bear no relation to the type of instrument employed. This classification also applies to the vacuum extraction operation. (The term "forceps delivery" should not be employed.)

Low Forceps Operation

A low forceps operation is the application of obstetric forceps to the fetal skull when the scalp is or has been visible at the introitus without separating the labia, the skull has reached the pelvic floor, and the sagittal suture is in the anteroposterior diameter of the outlet of the pelvis.

Midforceps Operation

A midforceps operation is the application of obstetric forceps to the fetal skull when the head is engaged, but the conditions for low forceps have not been met. In the context of this term, any forceps operation requiring artificial rotation, regardless of the station from which extraction is begun, shall be designated a "midforceps operation."

High Forceps Operation

A high forceps operation is the application of obstetric forceps at any time prior to the engagement of the fetal head.

Vacuum Extraction Operation

A vacuum extraction operation is an operation for the extraction of the fetal head from the mother by use of a vacuum extractor applied to the fetal scalp. Vacuum extraction operations are classified in relation to the location or station of the fetal skull (see forceps operation).

HYSTERECTOMY, CESAREAN

Cesarean hysterectomy is an operation in which the fetus is removed through an incision in the abdomen and the uterus followed by either incomplete or complete hysterectomy.

SYNONYM: *Porro's Operation.*

SYMPHYSIOTOMY

A symphysiotomy is the division of the pubic symphysis with a wire saw or knife to increase the size of the bony pelvis.

MANEUVERS

MANEUVER

A maneuver is a planned movement, manipulation, or procedure.

Bracht Maneuver

The Bracht maneuver is a method of extraction of the aftercoming head. The breech is expelled spontaneously up to the umbilicus. The body and extended legs are held together, with both hands maintaining upward anterior rotation of the fetal body. When anterior rotation is almost complete, the fetal body is held against the maternal pubic symphysis. Sometimes moderate pressure is exerted from above by an assistant.

Brandt-Andrews Maneuver

The Brandt-Andrews maneuver is a method of expressing the placenta from the uterus. It is performed by grasping the cord with the left hand while the right hand is placed on the maternal abdomen, so that the palmar surfaces of the fingers are over the anterior surface of the uterus at the junction of the corpus uteri and the lower uterine segment. By gently pressing the right hand backward and slightly upward and making gentle traction on the cord with the left hand, the placenta and membranes are easily extracted if separation has occurred.

Key-in-Lock Maneuver

The key-in-lock maneuver is a method of rotating the fetal head from a posterior or transverse position to an anterior position in the maternal pelvis. Obstetric forceps are applied to fit the pelvic curve and the fetal head is rotated. The forceps are reapplied and the procedure repeated until the fetal head is in an anterior position.

SYNONYM: *DeLee's Operation.*

Kristeller's Maneuver

Kristeller's maneuver is an attempt to express the fetus by pressure on the fundus of the uterus toward the axis of the inlet. It is a dangerous procedure and may result in rupture of the uterus.

Levret Maneuver

The Levret maneuver is the completion of an internal version by pushing the fetus up and rotating it around the long axis of the body. This maneuver is used when the fetus has become wedged at the pelvic brim.

SYNONYMS: *Deutsch Maneuver, Mauriceau-Levret Maneuver.*

Løvset's Maneuver

Løvset's maneuver is a method of extracting the arms in breech birth by clockwise and counterclockwise rotation of the fetus. This maneuver is performed after the fetus has been expelled up to the umbilicus.

Mauriceau-Smellie-Veit Maneuver

The Mauriceau-Smellie-Veit maneuver is a method of extraction of the aftercoming head in breech presentation. After the legs, abdomen, and shoulders are expelled, the infant is straddled over the operator's arm. The middle finger of the operator's hand is inserted into the fetal mouth and the ring and index fingers are placed on the maxillary bones of the fetal face. The other hand is placed over the fetal shoulders to apply traction. The combined traction of both hands is used to flex and extract the fetal head. An assistant pushes the fetal head into and through the pelvis. It is a dangerous maneuver.

Müller-Hillis Maneuver

The Müller-Hillis maneuver is a method of determining whether the fetal head can be engaged in the maternal pelvis. With the patient in the lithotomy position, the examining finger in the rectum locates the tips of the ischial spines and notes the relation of the lowest part of the fetal skull to a line drawn between them. The hand on the outside is placed above the breech and is sunk as deeply as possible toward the maternal spine, the forearm parallel to the long axis of the mother. Pressure is then made on the breech toward the inlet, and the descent of the head is noted with reference to the interspinous line, allowance being made for the thickness of the lower uterine segment, the cervix, or caput succedaneum if present. If the head cannot be impressed to the spines, an assistant places the palm of one hand flatly over the middle of the fetal back to prevent flexion, and the fingers of the other hand, placed palmar surface downward above the head over the pubic symphysis, press the head downward and backward in the axis of the inlet, while the examiner makes pressure on the breech and notes descent with the internal finger.

Pajot Maneuver

The Pajot maneuver is a procedure for extraction of the fetal head from the maternal pelvis by the use of obstetric forceps. The handle of the forceps is pressed upward while the shank of the forceps is depressed downward by the other hand of the operator. This procedure is supposed to create an axis-traction effect, fitting the fetal head to curves of the pelvis.

SYNONYMS: *Saxtorph Maneuver, Osiander's Maneuver.*

Pinard Maneuver

The Pinard maneuver is a method of extraction of an extended leg in breech presentation. The hand is passed into the uterus avoiding the umbilical cord. The index finger or thumb is pressed into the popliteal space of the anterior fetal leg, pressing the thigh against the fetal abdomen. The other fingers are passed over the fetal knee to the ankle, and the leg is rotated medially on the fetal body and brought down into the pelvis and vagina. Deep anesthesia is needed for this procedure.

Prague Maneuver

The Prague maneuver is a method of extraction of the after-coming head when the fetal chin is anterior over the pubic rami. The fetal back, which is posterior, rests on the forearm of the operator, and the operator's hand is placed forklike over the fetal shoulder. The fetal legs are grasped by the other hand of the operator, and the fetal body is flexed over the pubic rami.

Ritgen Maneuver, Modified

The modified Ritgen maneuver is a method of extraction of the fetal head by exerting forward pressure on the fetal chin through the perineum, while exerting downward pressure with the other hand on the occiput. It should be performed between uterine contractions.

Scanzoni Maneuver

The Scanzoni maneuver is rotation of the fetal head 180°, from a posterior to anterior position in the maternal pelvis, by use of forceps.

SYNONYM: *Smellie Maneuver.*

Schatz Maneuver

The Schatz maneuver is a method to convert a face position into an occiput position. It is performed by external manipulation, attempting to flex the fetal body on itself and then forcing the fetal head into the pelvis. It is not highly successful.

Thorn Maneuver

The Thorn maneuver is a method to convert a face position into an occiput position. It is performed by inserting a hand through the cervix and pushing the chin or brow upward and out of the pelvic inlet. Then, in the following order, face, brow, foreskull, and occiput are pushed up forward to flex the head. By so doing, it becomes possible for the external hand to shove the occiput down into the pelvis. It is not usually successful.

Van Hoorn Maneuver

The Van Hoorn maneuver is a modified Prague maneuver. In this maneuver, an assistant applies gentle pressure on the fetal head, attempting to cause flexion and downward pressure.

Wigand-Martin Maneuver

The Wigand-Martin maneuver is a method of extraction of the aftercoming head in breech presentation. After the legs, abdomen, and shoulders are expelled, the infant is straddled over the operator's arm. The middle finger of the operator's hand is inserted into the fetal mouth, and the ring and index fingers are placed on the maxillary bones of the fetal face. The head is then flexed and brought into the pelvis. The other hand aids flexion of the head by pushing it into the pelvis. It is a relatively safe maneuver.

VERSION

Version is the manual conversion of the polarity of the fetus with reference to the mother.

Cephalic Version

Cephalic version is the conversion of a fetus from a breech presentation into a vertex presentation. It is rarely performed.

Combined Version

Combined version is a procedure to change the polarity of the fetus by external and internal manipulation.

Podalic Version

Podalic version is a method of changing the polarity of the fetus by inserting the operator's hand into the uterus, pushing the fetal head upward, and pulling the fetal extremities into the pelvis. The cervix should be completely or almost completely dilated, the pelvis must be adequate, and anesthesia should be deep and under good control.

SYNONYM: *Internal Podalic Version.*

Wigand's External Version

Wigand's external version is version performed for the correction of a transverse presentation by forcing the fetal head into the pelvic inlet. This method is not satisfactory.

DESTRUCTIVE OPERATIONS—FETUS

CLEIDOTOMY

Cleidotomy is division of the clavicle or clavicles to facilitate the extraction of the fetal shoulders.

CRANIOTOMY

Craniotomy is an operation to decrease the size of the fetal head. It is not justified in a living fetus. The fetal head is perforated and its contents are evacuated. This operation is seldom performed today.

DECAPITATION

Decapitation is removal of the fetal head, particularly in neglected transverse presentation, to facilitate birth of a stillborn infant. This operation is rarely performed today.

EMBRYOTOMY

Embryotomy refers to either removal of the fetal viscera through an opening in the thorax or abdomen, or to decapitation.

EVISCERATION

Evisceration is incision into the fetal abdomen or chest and removal of the contents that are unusually enlarged or tumorous and that have prevented passage of the fetus through the birth canal.

SYNONYM: *Exenteration.*

Complications of Pregnancy

ABORTION

ABORTION

Abortion is the expulsion or extraction of all (complete) or any part (incomplete) of the placenta or membranes, without an identifiable fetus or with a liveborn infant or a stillborn infant weighing less than 500 gm. In the absence of known weight, an estimated length of gestation of less than 20 completed weeks (139 days), calculated from the first day of the last normal menstrual period, may be used. Abortion is a term referring to the birth process culminating before the 20th completed week of gestation.

Complete Abortion

Complete abortion is the expulsion of all the products of conception before the 20th completed week of gestation.

Contagious Abortion

Contagious abortion is an abortion produced by *Brucella abortus* (Bang's bacillus). The bacillus is the causative agent of contagious abortion in cattle but also may produce abortion in the human.

Habitual Abortion

Habitual abortion is the occurrence of three or more consecutive spontaneous abortions.

Incomplete Abortion

Incomplete abortion is the expulsion of some, but not all, of the products of conception before the 20th completed week of gestation.

Induced Abortion

Induced abortion is the deliberate interruption of pregnancy by any means before the 20th completed week of gestation. It may be therapeutic or nontherapeutic.

Inevitable Abortion

Inevitable abortion is the state in which bleeding of intrauterine origin occurs before the 20th completed week of gestation with continuous and progressive dilatation of the cervix, without expulsion of the products of conception.

Infected Abortion

Infected abortion is an abortion associated with infection of the genital organs.

Missed Abortion

Missed abortion is an abortion in which the embryo or fetus dies in utero before the 20th completed week of gestation, but the products of conception are retained in utero for eight weeks or more.

Nontherapeutic Abortion

Nontherapeutic abortion is the illegal interruption of pregnancy by any means before the 20th completed week of gestation. *Criminal abortion* and *illegal abortion* are not appropriate medical terms.

Septic Abortion

Septic abortion is an infected abortion in which there is dissemination of microorganisms and their products into the maternal systemic circulation.

Spontaneous Abortion

Spontaneous abortion is the expulsion of the products of conception before the 20th completed week of gestation without deliberate interference.

Therapeutic Abortion

Therapeutic abortion is the interruption of pregnancy before the 20th completed week of gestation for legally acceptable, medically approved indications.

Threatened Abortion

Threatened abortion is a state in which bleeding of intrauterine origin occurs before the 20th completed week of gestation, with or without uterine colic, without expulsion of the products of conception, and without dilatation of the cervix.

ABORTION RATE

The abortion rate is the number of abortions per 1000 terminated pregnancies for a given period.

ABORTUS

Abortus is the term applied to a stillborn infant expelled before attaining a weight of 500 gm. In the absence of known weight, an estimated length of gestation of less than 20 completed weeks (139 days), calculated from the first day of the last normal menstrual period, may be used.

BLIGHTED OVUM

A blighted ovum is a small, relatively hydramniotic sac in which the fetus is completely absent or represented by a small amorphous mass.

SYNONYMS: *Pathologic Ovum, Dropsical Ovum.*

CARNEOUS MOLE

A carneous mole is a shapeless mass of placental secundines. It sometimes occurs in association with abortion.

SYNONYMS: *Fleshy Mole, True Mole, Blood Mole.*

POSTABORTAL SEPSIS
Postabortal sepsis is a severe infection, usually a bloodstream infection, resulting from an abortion.

TARNIER'S SIGN
Tarnier's sign is an indication of impending abortion and is denoted by the straightening of the angle between the corpus uteri and lower uterine segment.

ABRUPTIO PLACENTAE

ABRUPTIO PLACENTAE
Abruptio placentae is the complete or partial detachment of the normally implanted placenta from the uterine wall at 20 weeks or more of gestation. Abruptio placentae may occur in conjunction with placenta previa.

> SYNONYMS: *Premature Separation of the Placenta, Placental Abruption, Accidental Hemorrhage, Ablatio Placentae.*

ABRUPTIO PLACENTAE SYNDROME
The abruptio placentae syndrome is a syndrome characterized by the abnormal separation of a normally implanted placenta, hypofibrinogenemia, hemorrhage, and shock. The incidence varies from 1 in 85 to 1 in 250 deliveries. The onset of symptoms is subacute or abrupt and consists of severe abdominal pain caused by tetanic contractions of the uterus, marked vaginal hemorrhage from incoagulable blood, and beginning shock. Abruptio placentae is the most widely recognized complication of hypofibrinogenemia. Clinical symptoms occur at a level below 150 mg/100 cc of plasma fibrinogen concentration, with a critical level at 90 mg or below. The degree of defibrination is coincident with and apparently directly proportional to the severity of the placental abruption. The placenta often shows either many infarcts or a large retroplacental hematoma. Uterine infiltration of suffused blood sometimes is found, the so-called Couvelaire uterus. The cause of the syndrome may be hypertensive disorders of pregnancy, chronic glomerulonephritis, chronic vascular disease, or trauma. Differential diagnosis should exclude placenta previa, in which the bleeding is painless and tetanic contractions of the uterus and fibrinogen depression are absent; and a ruptured uterus, in which pain is localized at the site of the rupture.

CONCEALED HEMORRHAGE
A concealed hemorrhage is an accumulation of blood within the uterus or amniotic sac associated with abruptio placentae.

PLACENTA PREVIA

PLACENTA PREVIA
Placenta previa is the implantation of any part of the placenta in the lower uterine segment. The term expresses the anatomic relationship

between the placental site and the lower uterine segment. The placenta encroaches on or covers (completely or incompletely) the internal cervical os. Placenta previa is classified as marginal, partial, or total.

Marginal Placenta Previa
Marginal placenta previa is present when some part of the placenta is attached to the lower uterine segment and extends to, but does not cover, any part of the internal cervical os.

Partial Placenta Previa
Partial placenta previa is present when any part of the placenta incompletely covers the internal cervical os.
SYNONYM: *Incomplete Placenta Previa.*

Total Placenta Previa
Total placenta previa is present when any part of the placenta completely covers the internal cervical os.
SYNONYM: *Complete Placenta Previa.*

POSTPARTUM HEMORRHAGES

POSTPARTUM HEMORRHAGE
Postpartum hemorrhage is the loss of 500 cc or more of blood from the reproductive organs after the completion of the third stage of labor. Postpartum hemorrhage is classified as either early or late.

Early Postpartum Hemorrhage
Early postpartum hemorrhage is excessive bleeding that occurs during the first 24 hours after completion of the third stage of labor.

Late Postpartum Hemorrhage
Late postpartum hemorrhage is excessive bleeding that occurs during the puerperium, excluding the first 24 hour period after completion of the third stage of labor.

MC CLINTOCK'S SIGN
McClintock's sign is a maternal pulse rate over 100, recorded an hour or more postpartum, often indicating hemorrhage.

ECTOPIC PREGNANCY

ECTOPIC PREGNANCY
Ectopic pregnancy is gestation outside the uterine cavity. It is a broader term than extrauterine pregnancy, because it includes gestations in the interstitial portion of the tube, in a rudimentary horn of the uterus, as well as tubal, abdominal, and ovarian gestations.
SYNONYM: *Heterotopic Pregnancy.*

ABDOMINAL PREGNANCY

Abdominal pregnancy is gestation occurring within the peritoneal cavity.

SYNONYM: *Intraperitoneal Pregnancy.*

Primary Abdominal Pregnancy

Primary abdominal pregnancy is growth of the fetus and placenta within the peritoneal cavity. Fertilization and embryonic growth occur before entrance into the fallopian tube. It is a rare condition.

Secondary Abdominal Pregnancy

Secondary abdominal pregnancy is a pregnancy that develops in the abdominal cavity following tubal abortion or rupture. The fetus may continue to grow until term or become macerated, skeletonized, or mummified.

AMPULLAR PREGNANCY

Ampullar pregnancy is an ectopic pregnancy in the ampullar portion of the fallopian tube. It generally ends in tubal abortion.

ARIAS-STELLA REACTION

The Arias-Stella reaction is an atypical glandular proliferation of the endometrium associated with ectopic pregnancy. A decidual cast, containing no villi, may be expelled.

BOLT'S SIGN

Bolt's sign is characterized by severe tenderness when the examiner lifts the uterine cervix. It is a sign of ruptured tubal pregnancy.

CERVICAL PREGNANCY

Cervical pregnancy is gestation that develops when the fertilized ovum becomes implanted in the cervical canal of the uterus.

COMBINED HETEROTOPIC PREGNANCY

Combined heterotopic pregnancy is the existence of simultaneous intrauterine and extrauterine pregnancies.

SYNONYM: *Compound Pregnancy.*

CORNUAL PREGNANCY

Cornual pregnancy is gestation that has developed in a rudimentary horn of the uterus.

SYNONYM: *Rudimentary Horn Pregnancy.*

CULLEN'S SIGN

Cullen's sign is a blue discoloration of the periumbilical skin. It suggests intraperitoneal hemorrhage, especially in ruptured ectopic pregnancy.

DANFORTH'S SIGN
Danforth's sign is the occurrence of shoulder pain on inspiration. It is a sign of ruptured tubal pregnancy.

EXTRACAPSULAR RUPTURE
Extracapsular rupture is a complication of tubal pregnancy resulting in bursting of the wall of the fallopian tube. It is caused by hemorrhage, overdistention, necrosis, and penetration by the chorionic villi.

EXTRAUTERINE PREGNANCY
Extrauterine pregnancy is gestation outside the uterine cavity, but it does not include pregnancy in the interstitial portion of the tube.

GOLDEN'S SIGN
Golden's sign is a paleness of the cervix. It is a sign of tubal pregnancy.

HEMATOSALPINX
Hematosalpinx is the distention of a fallopian tube by blood. The condition occurs in incomplete tubal abortion when the fimbriated end of the tube is occluded.

INTERSTITIAL PREGNANCY
Interstitial pregnancy is a pregnancy in the interstitial portion of the fallopian tube.
SYNONYMS: *Tubouterine Pregnancy, Angular Pregnancy.*

INTRACAPSULAR RUPTURE
Intracapsular rupture is a complication of tubal pregnancy resulting in rupture of the amniotic sac and escape of the embryo into the lumen of the fallopian tube.

INTRALIGAMENTOUS PREGNANCY
Intraligamentous pregnancy is growth of the fetus and placenta between the folds of the broad ligament, after rupture of a tubal pregnancy through the floor of the fallopian tube.
SYNONYMS: *Broad Ligament Pregnancy, Extraperitoneal Pregnancy.*

ISTHMIC PREGNANCY
Isthmic pregnancy is a gestation in the narrow portion of the fallopian tube.

MESOMETRIC PREGNANCY
Mesometric pregnancy is gestation within the middle muscular layer of the uterus.
SYNONYM: *Mural Pregnancy.*

OVARIAN PREGNANCY, PRIMARY
Primary ovarian pregnancy is a rare form of ectopic pregnancy in which impregnation of the ovum by the spermatozoon occurs before the former is extruded from the ovary.

OVARIAN PREGNANCY, SECONDARY
Secondary ovarian pregnancy is a rare form of ectopic pregnancy in which the blastocyst implants on the surface of the ovary.

SALMON'S SIGN
Salmon's sign is dilatation of the pupil of one eye in ruptured ectopic pregnancy.

SPIEGELBERG'S CRITERIA FOR OVARIAN PREGNANCY
Spiegelberg's criteria for ovarian pregnancy are conditions that must be met in order to establish a diagnosis of ovarian pregnancy: (1) the fallopian tube on the affected side must be intact. (2) The fetal sac must occupy the position of the ovary. (3) The fetal sac must be connected to the uterus by the ovarian ligament. (4) Definite ovarian tissue must be found in the wall of the fetal sac.

TUBAL PREGNANCY
Tubal pregnancy is an ectopic pregnancy in a portion of the fallopian tube. It is the most common form of ectopic pregnancy.
SYNONYM: *Salpingocyesis.*

Tuboabdominal Pregnancy
Tuboabdominal pregnancy is growth of the fetus and placenta in the abdominal cavity after rupture of a tubal pregnancy through the roof of the fallopian tube.

Tuboovarian Pregnancy
Tuboovarian pregnancy is growth of the fetus and placenta after implantation in the fimbria ovarica of the fallopian tube. It generally results in a secondary abdominal pregnancy.

UTEROABDOMINAL PREGNANCY
Uteroabdominal pregnancy is the growth of the fetus and placenta in the abdominal cavity after rupture of the uterus.

EXTRAMEMBRANOUS PREGNANCIES

EXTRAAMNIOTIC PREGNANCY
Extraamniotic pregnancy is a gestation in which the fetus develops in the uterus but the amnion ruptures early in pregnancy leaving the chorion intact. The shrunken amnion hangs around the insertion of the cord.
SYNONYM: *Graviditas Examnialis.*

EXTRACHORIAL PREGNANCY
Extrachorial pregnancy is a gestation in which the fetus develops in the uterus but outside the chorionic sac. This type of gestation results from rupture and shrinkage of the membranes in the early months of pregnancy.
SYNONYM: *Graviditas Exochorialis.*

DISEASES AND ABNORMALITIES OF THE TROPHOBLAST

BLIGHTED OVUM
A blighted ovum is a small, relatively hydramniotic sac in which the fetus is completely absent or represented by a small amorphous mass.
SYNONYMS: *Pathological Ovum, Dropsical Ovum.*

CARNEOUS MOLE
A carneous mole is a shapeless mass of placental secundines. It sometimes occurs in association with abortion.
SYNONYMS: *Fleshy Mole, True Mole, Blood Mole.*

CHORIOADENOMA DESTRUENS
Chorioadenoma destruens is an invasive tumor that generally follows a hydatidiform mole. One or more villi and associated trophoblast may invade the myometrium, its blood vessels, or both. Although it has invasive power, it has a low degree of malignancy.
SYNONYMS: *Invasive Mole, Penetration Mole.*

CHORIOCARCINOMA
Choriocarcinoma is a malignant trophoblastic neoplasm. It is derived from syncytiotrophoblasts and cytotrophoblasts that form irregular sheets and cords surrounded by lakes of blood. Villi are not formed. The neoplastic cells are highly invasive, and profusely infiltrate the myometrium and blood vessels. Metastases develop relatively early in the course of the illness, and they are frequently found in the lungs, liver, brain, vagina, and various pelvic organs. Choriocarcinoma occurs about once in 40,000 pregnancies. It follows hydatidiform mole in 40 per cent of instances, abortion in 40 per cent, and full-term pregnancy in 20 per cent. Choriocarcinoma occasionally originates in teratoid neoplasms of the ovaries.
SYNONYMS: *Chorioma, Chorionic Epithelioma, Chorioepithelioma, Gestational Chorionepithelioma, Nonteratomatous Chorionepithelioma, Syncytioma Malignum.*

HYDATIDIFORM MOLE
Hydatidiform mole is a pathologic condition of the chorion characterized by cystic degeneration of the villi with hydropic swelling, avascularity, and notable proliferation of the trophoblastic tissue. Microscopically, the cysts show hydropic degeneration of the stroma and proliferation of Langhans' and syncytial cells. Hydatidiform mole is usually benign.
SYNONYMS: *Cystic Mole, Grape Mole, Vesicular Mole.*

STONE MOLE
A stone mole is a carneous mole that has undergone calcareous degeneration.
SYNONYMS: *Uterine Calculus, Wombstone.*

HYPERTENSIVE STATES OF PREGNANCY—
CLASSIFICATION

There are certain vascular derangements that either antedate or arise in pregnancy or the early puerperium that have been designated as the *toxemias of pregnancy, EPH complex, gestosis,* and other terms. These generic terms have grouped together several conditions that have been characterized by hypertension sometimes associated with proteinuria, edema, convulsions, coma, and other signs. Because these terms have been all-inclusive, discrepancies in statistical reporting have occurred. The Committee on Terminology of The American College of Obstetricians and Gynecologists, after careful consideration and consultation with authorities in the field, discourages the use of the term "toxemia" and suggests the following:

Gestational Edema

Gestational edema is the occurrence of a general and excessive accumulation of fluid in the tissues of greater than 1+ pitting edema after 12 hours' rest in bed, or of a weight gain of five pounds or more in one week due to the influence of pregnancy.

Gestational Proteinuria

Gestational proteinuria is the presence of proteinuria, during or under the influence of pregnancy, in the absence of hypertension, edema, renal infection, or known intrinsic renovascular disease.

Gestational Hypertension

Gestational hypertension is the development of hypertension during pregnancy, or within the first 24 hours postpartum, in a previously normotensive woman. No other evidence of preeclampsia or hypertensive vascular disease is present. The blood pressure returns to normotensive levels within ten days following parturition. Some patients with gestational hypertension may in fact have preeclampsia or hypertensive vascular disease, but they do not satisfy the criteria for either of these diagnoses.

Preeclampsia

Preeclampsia is the development of hypertension with proteinuria, edema, or both, due to pregnancy or the influence of a recent pregnancy. It occurs after the 20th week of gestation, but it may develop before this time in the presence of trophoblastic disease. Preeclampsia is predominantly a disorder of primigravidas.

Eclampsia

Eclampsia is the occurrence of one or more convulsions, not attributable to other cerebral conditions such as epilepsy or cerebral hemorrhage, in a patient with preeclampsia.

Superimposed Preeclampsia or Eclampsia

Superimposed preeclampsia or eclampsia is the development of preeclampsia or eclampsia in a patient with chronic hypertensive vascular or renal disease. When the hypertension antedates the pregnancy, as established by previous blood pressure recordings, a rise in the systolic pressure of 30 mm of Hg, or a rise in the diastolic pressure of 15 mm of Hg, and the development of proteinuria, edema, or both are required during pregnancy to establish the diagnosis.

Chronic Hypertensive Disease

Chronic hypertensive disease is the presence of persistent hypertension, of whatever cause, before pregnancy or before the 20th week of gestation, or persistent hypertension beyond the 42nd postpartum day.

Unclassified Hypertensive Disorders

Unclassified hypertensive disorders are those in which information is insufficient for classification. They should compose a minority of the hypertensive disorders in pregnancy.

EDEMA

Edema is a general and excessive accumulation of fluids in the tissues, commonly demonstrated by swelling of the extremities and face.

HYPERTENSION

Hypertension is a rise in the systolic pressure of at least 30 mm of Hg, or a rise in the diastolic pressure of at least 15 mm of Hg, or the presence of a systolic pressure of at least 140 mm of Hg, or a diastolic pressure of at least 90 mm of Hg. Hypertension may also be determined by a *mean arterial pressure* of 105 mm of Hg or more, or by a rise of 20 mm of Hg or more. The levels cited must be manifest on at least two occasions six or more hours apart, and should be based on previously known blood pressure levels.

PROTEINURIA

Proteinuria is the presence of urinary protein in concentrations greater than 0.3 gm per liter in a 24-hour urine collection, or in concentrations greater than 1 gm per liter (1+ to 2+ by standard turbidometric methods) in a random urine collection on two or more occasions at least six hours apart. The specimens must be clean, voided midstream, or obtained by catheterization.

MATERNAL DEATHS—CLASSIFICATION

MATERNAL DEATH

Maternal death is the death of any woman, from any cause, while pregnant or within 42 days of termination of pregnancy, irrespective of the duration and the site of pregnancy.

For world statistical evaluation, it is necessary to divide the 42 days into two periods.

Period I: 1 to 7 days following termination of pregnancy.

Period II: 8 to 42 days following termination of pregnancy.

CLASSIFICATION OF MATERNAL DEATHS

Direct Maternal Death

Direct maternal death is an obstetric death resulting from obstetric complications of the pregnancy state, labor, or puerperium; and from interventions, omissions, incorrect treatment, or a chain of events resulting from any of the above.

Indirect Maternal Death

Indirect maternal death is an obstetric death resulting from previously existing disease, or disease that developed during pregnancy, labor, or the puerperium; it is not directly due to obstetric causes, but aggravated by the physiologic effects of pregnancy.

Nonmaternal Death

Nonmaternal death is an obstetric death resulting from accidental or incidental causes not related to the pregnancy or its management.

MATERNAL MORTALITY COMMITTEE

The maternal mortality committee is a committee established to determine by scientific and confidential analysis all factors involved in maternal deaths in order that avoidable factors in maternal deaths may be reduced or eliminated, and better maternal care may be assured through improvement in teaching and practice.

The functions of the committee include, among others:

1. Full scientific analysis and frank discussion of the causes of all maternal deaths in its jurisdiction, with rigid adherence to ethical and legal principles ensuring anonymity of all parties involved.

2. Determination of the existence and nature of avoidable factors.

3. Objective and impersonal report and dissemination of knowledge gained.

4. Education of all medical and nonmedical personnel connected with obstetrics, and of the lay public in order to accomplish the purposes of the committee.

For worldwide statistical evaluation, maternal mortality should be recorded as preventable, nonpreventable, and unexplained.

Preventable

Preventable maternal deaths are due to inadequate care, inadequate facilities in obstetric units, inadequate facilities in other maternal services before admission to the unit, or adverse conditions in the community—for example, inadequate transportation, lack of confidence in the maternity service, or the patient's failure to seek or accept advice or treatment.

Nonpreventable

Nonpreventable maternal deaths are due to irreversible causes; such as advanced chronic nephritis, severe cardiac diseases, and automobile accidents.

Unexplained

Unexplained maternal deaths are those for which the cause of death is unknown.

MATERNAL DEATH RATE

Maternal death rate is the number of maternal deaths (direct, indirect, or nonmaternal) per 100,000 terminated pregnancies for any specified period. Contributions to the numerator and denominator must be within the same time period.

RUPTURE OF THE GRAVID UTERUS—CLASSIFICATION

GRAVID UTERUS, RUPTURE OF

Rupture of the gravid uterus is disruption of the uterine wall. Rupture of the gravid uterus may occur in the antepartum or intrapartum period.

CLASSIFICATION OF RUPTURE OF THE GRAVID UTERUS

Incidental Rupture

Incidental rupture is an asymptomatic variety of spontaneous rupture of the gravid uterus. Such a rupture may involve all or a small part of a previous scar.

SYNONYMS: *Silent Rupture of Gravid Uterus, Occult Rupture of Gravid Uterus.*

Traumatic Rupture

Traumatic rupture includes ruptured uteri associated with pharmacologic agents (oxytocics), intrauterine manipulations, external pressure (Kristeller maneuver), or instrumental procedures. Traumatic rupture may occur in a scarred or unscarred uterus.

Spontaneous Rupture

Spontaneous rupture occurs in the absence of iatrogenic trauma. Ruptured uteri associated with an unstimulated obstructed labor fall into this category. Spontaneous rupture may occur in a scarred or unscarred uterus.

SCARRED UTERUS

A scarred uterus is a uterus that bears the scar of cesarean section, other hysterotomy, amputation of the cervix, or previous uterine rupture.

UNSCARRED UTERUS

An unscarred uterus is a uterus that does not have a scar.

EMBOLISM

EMBOLISM

An embolism is the obstruction or occlusion of a blood vessel by a transported thrombus, a mass of bacteria, or other foreign matter.

AIR EMBOLISM

An air embolism is an accumulation of air forced into the circulation by a venous or arterial route. It is estimated that from 100 to 150 ml of air is necessary to produce death.

AMNIOTIC FLUID EMBOLISM

An amniotic fluid embolism is the presence of amniotic fluid, lanugo hair, squamous cells, and mucus in the pulmonary vessels and also in the venous system of the uterus. The fluid is forced into the circulation after rupture of the amniotic sac and during forceful uterine contractions.

AMNIOTIC FLUID SYNDROME

The amniotic fluid syndrome is caused by the sudden intravenous infusion of a large volume of amniotic fluid, which causes pulmonary edema and pulmonary embolic phenomena. Clinically, cardiopulmonary distress, obstetric shock, and sometimes sudden death occur. The postulated factors consist of defibrination, massive fibrin embolism, and embolization from the particulate material contained in the amniotic fluid. Laboratory studies usually reveal a depression of fibrinogen, characteristic of defibrination with hemorrhagic phenomena, and evidence of a fibrinogen-fibrin conversion syndrome. The embolic syndrome is the result of a break in the wall of a blood vessel. It occurs during long labors, in traumatic births (forceps operation), in the dead fetus syndrome, in elderly women, and with large fetuses. The syndrome should be differentiated from other causes of sudden death, including massive intraabdominal hemorrhage from a ruptured uterine vein. The course is rapid, and the prognosis is always serious, with survival in doubt.

EMBOLUS

An embolus is a plug composed of a detached thrombus, mass of bacteria, or other foreign substances that occludes a blood vessel.

PULMONARY EMBOLISM

A pulmonary embolism is an occlusion of a portion of the pulmonary arterial circulation by a thrombus that has originated usually from a leg or thigh vein, occasionally from a pelvic vein, and rarely from the inferior vena cava or the right side of the heart. If there is sufficient collateral circulation and adequate venous outflow, the affected area of the lung remains unvascularized and incapable of pulmonary gas diffusion. With insufficient collateral circulation or inadequate venous outflow, the affected lung area becomes edematous, congested, and gangrenous. The latter process is known as infarction and is most often seen in patients with congestive heart failure. The clinical pattern therefore depends on the size of the embolus and the degree of infarction.

SYNONYM: *Blood Clot Embolism.*

BLOOD AND BLOOD DYSCRASIAS

ABO INCOMPATIBILITY

ABO incompatibility is incompatibility of a type O female with naturally occurring anti-A or anti-B circulatory antibodies to the sperm of a type A or type B secretor male, especially if the male is homozygous. It is postulated that his sperm carry or are coated with his antigen, which is neutralized or immobilized by the corresponding antibody in the cervical secretion.

AFIBRINOGENEMIA

Afibrinogenemia is an abnormality in blood-clotting factors. There is no demonstrable fibrinogen in the plasma, and the blood does not coagulate, even after standing for several weeks. Severe bleeding often leads to death in childhood. In heterozygous individuals, there is occasionally a decrease in fibrinogen without clinical symptoms.

MODE OF INHERITANCE: Autosomal recessive.

AGGLUTINATION

Agglutination is a phenomenon in which cells distributed in a fluid are collected into clumps.

AGGLUTININ

Agglutinin is an antibody that aggregates a particular antigen.

Anti-Rh Agglutinin

Anti-Rh agglutinin is an agglutinin not normally present in human plasma, but it may be produced in Rh-negative mothers carrying an Rh-positive fetus or after a transfusion of Rh-positive blood into an Rh-negative patient.

Cold Agglutinin

Cold agglutinin is an agglutinin that reacts only at temperatures below 37 C.

Warm Agglutinin

Warm agglutinin is an incomplete antibody, detectable by the antiglobulin (Coombs') test, that sensitizes and reacts optimally with erythrocytes at body temperature (37 C).

AGGLUTINOGEN

Agglutinogen is any substance that, acting as an antigen, stimulates the production of agglutinin, or is the antigen or suspension of cells containing the antigen used in conducting agglutination tests.

ANAMNESTIC

Anamnestic is, in immunology, a reaction in which antibodies that have previously existed and have disappeared from the blood are redeveloped on the injection of a nonspecific antigen.

ANEMIA

Anemia is a condition in which the red blood cells are deficient in number, the total hemoglobin concentration per unit volume of blood is reduced, or the relative volume of packed red blood cells is less than normal. This varies with age, sex, and other conditions such as pregnancy. Anemia results in decreased concentration of oxygen transporting material.

Acquired Hemolytic Anemia

Acquired hemolytic anemia is a nonhereditary, acute or chronic anemia characterized by an increased rate of destruction of the red blood cells and usually associated with or produced by extracorpuscular factors such as infection, blood loss, burns, chemicals, and autoantibodies.

Acute Posthemorrhagic Anemia

Acute posthemorrhagic anemia is caused by rapid loss of a large amount of blood. Morphologically, the erythrocytes are normochromic and normocytic, and the bone marrow is hyperplastic. The reticulocyte count becomes elevated, and in severe cases there may be nucleated red blood cells and a left shift of white blood cells.

Aplastic Anemia

Aplastic anemia is a normochromic, normocytic anemia often with associated leukopenia and thrombopenia; it is resistant to treatment and frequently fatal.

Congenital Hemolytic Anemia

Congenital hemolytic anemia is an inherited chronic disease characterized by increased hemolysis of red blood cells.

SYNONYMS: *Chronic Familial Icterus, Congenital Hemolytic Icterus, Chronic Acholuric Jaundice, Familial Spherocytosis, Spherocytic Anemia.*

Hypochromic Anemia

Hypochromic anemia is a form of anemia in which the mean corpuscular hemoglobin (MCH) content and the mean corpuscular hemoglobin concentration (MCHC) are less than normal. The cells, therefore, contain less hemoglobin than normal.

Iron Deficiency Anemia

Iron deficiency anemia in its more severe form is a microcytic, hypochromic anemia characterized by small, pale red blood cells, low reticulocyte activity, and depleted iron reserves. Serum iron concentration is below 60 μg/100 ml. Iron deficiency anemia occurs rather frequently during pregnancy.

Megaloblastic Anemia

Megaloblastic anemia is a rare complication of pregnancy caused in part by a defect in the metabolism of nucleic acid. The bone marrow pattern of erythropoiesis changes from normoblastic to megaloblastic. The condition may be accompanied by leukopenia, thrombocytopenia, low hemoglobin, and increased plasma iron concentration.

Pernicious Anemia

Pernicious anemia is a chronic macrocytic anemia, characterized by achlorhydria and certain other gastrointestinal and neurologic disturbances. It occurs most often in Caucasians after the fifth decade of life, but rarely occurs in pregnancy. Pernicious anemia is caused by a lack of vitamin B_{12}.

SYNONYMS: *Addisonian Anemia, Biermer's Anemia.*

Refractory Anemia

Refractory anemia is characterized by hypoplastic bone marrow, decreased numbers of normoblasts, leukopenia, thrombocytopenia, and normal or elevated plasma iron concentration. It is resistant to all hematinics.

Sickle Cell Anemia

Sickle cell anemia is a form of hemolytic anemia that occurs almost exclusively in Negroes. Crystallization of abnormal hemoglobin S in the presence of low oxygen tension and reduced blood pH is responsible for the sickling phenomenon, resulting in the appearance of oat-shaped and sickle-shaped red cells in the blood and increased viscosity of the capillary blood. The onset usually occurs during the first year of life, after normal hemoglobin is replaced with hemoglobin S. The most common clinical signs are arthralgia and abdominal crises. Thrombosis, sterility, disorders in pregnancy, susceptibility to infections, heart diseases, and liver diseases are frequent complications, and there may be sudden death.

MODE OF INHERITANCE: Incomplete dominance.

SYNONYMS: *African Anemia, Drepanocytic Anemia, Hemoglobin S Disease, Homozygous Hemoglobin S Disease, Meniscocytosis, Sicklemia, Herrick's Syndrome.*

ANTIBODY

Antibody is a modified type of serum globulin synthesized by lymphoid tissue in response to an antigenic stimulus.

Anti-Rh (Anti-D, Anti-Rh₀)

Anti-Rh is an antibody formed against the Rh antigen.

Anti-Rh' (Anti-C)

Anti-Rh' is an antibody formed against the Rh' antigen.

Anti-Rh" (Anti-E)

Anti-Rh" is an antibody formed against the Rh" antigen.

Anti-Hr'

Anti-Hr' is an antibody formed against the Hr' antigen.

Anti-Hr″

Anti-Hr″ is an antibody formed against the Hr″ antigen.

Blood Group Antibodies

Blood group antibodies are immunoglobulins produced by an individual after exposure to foreign red cells possessing a blood group antigen lacking in the host.

Complete Antibody

A complete antibody is an Rh antibody capable of directly agglutinating Rh-positive erythrocytes in physiologic saline. The term "complete antibody" implies that the antibody is multivalent—that is, it possesses two or more reactive groups.

Female Antispermatozoal Antibodies

Female antispermatozoal antibodies are presumably developed by the reticuloendothelial system in the female, following the repeated absorption of foreign protein from spermatozoa. Repeated coitus presumably results in the maintenance of a high titer of circulating antibodies, which prevents conception by immobilizing or agglutinating sperm.

Incomplete Antibody

Incomplete antibody is an immune globulin, originally described as a univalent antibody, combining specifically with Rh-positive erythrocytes without causing visible agglutination. In the presence of anti-human globulin (Coombs' serum) or high molecular weight media (albumin), it will cause red cell clumping.

Inhibiting Antibody

Inhibiting antibody is an antibody that possesses the same specificity as one from another source, but interferes with the action of the other, because of dissimilar associated properties in regard to the expected mode of that action.

SYNONYMS: *Blocking Antibody, Glutinin* (obsolete).

Irregular Antibodies

Irregular antibodies is a term intended to designate all blood factor antibodies other than those associated with A, B, O, and Rh_o (D).

Rh′(C)	K ⎫	Kele	S
Rh″(E)	k ⎭		s
Hr′(c)	Fy^a ⎫	Duffy	M
Hr″(e)	Fy^b ⎭		N
rh^{wi} (C^w)	JK^a ⎫	Kidd	P′
f(hr)	JK^b ⎭		L^{ua} ⎫ Lutheran
V(hr^v) hr^v	Le^a ⎫	Lewis	L^{ub} ⎭
	Le^b ⎭		

Neutralizing Antibody

Neutralizing antibody is an antibody that on mixture with a homologous infectious agent reduces or destroys infectivity by partial or complete destruction of the agent.

Sensitizing Antibody

Sensitizing antibody is a term applied to antibodies that are attached to body cells and that sensitize the cells, or render them susceptible to destruction by body defenses.

Specificity of Antibody

Specificity of antibody can be determined from tests of the individual's serum against cells that have been typed for all the known blood group antigens. A suggested set comprises eight known cells.

Titration of Antibodies

Titration of antibodies consists of serial dilution of the serum in an appropriate medium and testing each dilution against red cells containing the antigen.

ANTIGEN

Antigen is a high molecular weight protein or protein-polysaccharide complex that is lacking from the susceptible organism. On gaining access to the tissues of an animal lacking the antigen, the antigen stimulates the formation of a specific antibody and reacts specifically in vivo or in vitro with its homologous antibody—that is, the Rh antibody.

D^u Antigen

D^u antigen is a variant of the Rh_o (D) factor and is of two types, the hereditary type or the gene-interaction type. The individual who is D^u of either the hereditary or gene-interaction type should *donate* blood as Rh-positive. Because he has the D gene, he is capable of immunizing the Rh-negative person. As a recipient, the hereditary type usually carries the Hr' (c) antigen and should receive Rh-negative blood. The gene-interaction type carries the Rh' (C) antigen and should receive blood lacking in the Hr' (c) antigen because the Hr' (c) antigen is second to Rh_o (D) in antigenicity.

ANTI–HUMAN GLOBULIN

Anti-human globulin is made by injecting rabbits with human serum and then bleeding these animals after a suitable interval. After various adsorptions have been carried out, the anti-human globulin is used in detecting antibodies.

BILIRUBIN

Bilirubin is a yellow pigment transported in the blood and excreted in high concentrations in bile. It is sometimes found in urine and occurs in the blood and tissues in jaundice. It is formed from the heme of hemoglobin in the reticuloendothelial cells.

BILIVERDIN
Biliverdin is a green pigment formed from bilirubin by oxidation.

C HEMOGLOBIN DISEASE
C hemoglobin disease is characterized by a mild to moderately severe anemia in Negroes, and it is due to an inherited abnormality of hemoglobin formation and increased red blood cell destruction.

CHRISTMAS DISEASE
Christmas disease is a hemorrhagic diathesis caused by an abnormality of blood clotting factors. It is similar to hemophilia but tends to be milder. The specific defect is a deficiency of plasma thromboplastin component. The diagnosis is suggested by abnormal results from prothrombin consumption tests.

MODE OF INHERITANCE: Sex-linked recessive.

SYNONYMS: *Hemophilia B, Deficiency of PTC factor.*

CLASSICAL HEMOPHILIA
Classical hemophilia is a hereditary hemorrhagic disorder occurring almost exclusively in males and transmitted through females. It is caused by a deficiency of antihemophilic globulin (Factor VIII), which results in a serious clotting defect.

MODE OF INHERITANCE: Sex-linked recessive.

COMPLEMENT
Complement is a lytic substance in normal serum that combines with antigen-antibody complex to promote lysis of intact cells that contain the antigen.

COOMBS' TEST
Coombs' test is used to detect sensitized red cells in erythroblastosis fetalis and to identify antibodies in other syndromes. It is a nonspecific test, in that it reveals the presence of blocking antibodies but does not define them.

CONGLUTINATION
Conglutination is erythrocyte agglutination that is dependent on complement and antibodies.

CRYPTOAGGLUTINOID
Cryptoagglutinoid is an agglutinin that reacts only in the antiglobulin (Coombs') test.

DYSFIBRINOGENEMIA
Dysfibrinogenemia is a qualitative alteration of fibrinogen in the blood.

ELLIPTOCYTOSIS
Elliptocytosis is a disorder characterized by the presence of oval or elliptic red blood cells. It usually is a benign condition, but some affected

persons have a significant hemolytic anemia. The cause is unknown.

MODE OF INHERITANCE: Autosomal dominant (intermediate dominance).

SYNONYMS: *Ovalocytosis, Dresbach's Syndrome.*

ELININ

Elinin is a lipoprotein fraction of red blood cells containing the Rh and A and B factors.

ERYTHROBLASTOSIS FETALIS

Erythroblastosis fetalis is a congenital hemolytic disease caused both by the presence of Rh antibodies in maternal blood and the antigen in fetal red cells. It is the pathologic state produced in the fetus as a result of exposure to maternal antibodies—for example, Rh, Hr, A-B, and those designated in other blood systems.

SYNONYMS: *Erythroblastis Fetalis Syndrome, Erythroblastosis Neonatorum Syndrome, Congenital Hemolytic Disease of Newborn.*

ERYTHROCYTE

An erythrocyte is a non-nucleated, agranular, circulating blood cell that contains hemoglobin for the purpose of accepting, transporting, and delivering oxygen.

ERYTHROPHAGOCYTOSIS

Erythrophagocytosis is the engulfment of erythrocytes by other cells, such as the histiocytes of the reticuloendothelial system.

EXCHANGE TRANSFUSION

An exchange transfusion is essentially a flushing-out process, whereby the circulating blood of the individual is gradually replaced with donor blood. The exchange process is used most commonly to remove Rh-positive red cells from an infant with hemolytic disease and elevated bilirubin concentration.

FIBRIN

Fibrin is an elastic filamentous protein derived from fibrinogen by the action of thrombin in the coagulation of blood.

FIBRINOGEN

Fibrinogen is a globulin of the blood plasma that is converted into fibrin by the action of thrombin in the presence of ionized calcium.

SYNONYM: *Factor I.*

FIBRINOGEN–FIBRIN CONVERSION SYNDROME

The fibrinogen-fibrin conversion syndrome is characterized by a degree of hypofibrinogenemia that causes incoagulable blood. It is a factor in three obstetric complications: abruptio placentae, amniotic fluid syndrome, and prolonged retention of a dead fetus in an Rh-isosensitized mother. The failure of coagulation, which relates to fibrinogen-fibrin conversion, may also occur in Sheehan's syndrome, bilateral renal cortical necrosis, hemolytic blood reactions, and surgical or accidental trauma. Clinically, this syndrome has two pathologic potentialities—embolism and hemorrhage. Decreasing fibrinogen values, determined by serial blood studies, indicate the degree of depletion due to intravascular conversion of fibrinogen to fibrin. Hyperthromboplastinemia, with its defibrinating influence, is one accepted cause. Blood incoagulability occurs when fibrinogenopenia reaches a critical level of 90 mg/100 cc. If the seriously depressed level is reached suddenly, embolic phenomena may predominate, or hemorrhage and embolic manifestations may occur. Shock is a common sequel to either state. Other accompanying abnormalities include decreased Ac-globulin, prothrombin, and platelets. The onset of the syndrome may not depend on placental separation. If decreasing fibrinogen blood values continue to drop downward from 150 mg/100 cc to the critical level, pregnancy should be terminated.

SYNONYMS: *Acquired Afibrinogenemia, Defibrination Syndrome.*

GLUCOSE–6–PHOSPHATE DEHYDROGENASE DEFICIENCY

Glucose-6-phosphate dehydrogenase deficiency is an enzyme defect of red blood cells that may present clinically as a drug-induced *acute hemolytic anemia* (primaquine sensitivity), *favism*, or *congenital nonspherocytic hemolytic anemia*. Many oxidant drugs such as antimalarials, sulfonamides, nitrofurans, and antipyritics cause hemolytic episodes in sensitive individuals. Glucose-6-phosphate dehydrogenase deficiency occurs in Negroes, Mediterranean races, and other ethnic groups. Many genetic variants have been described. It is estimated that about one-third of patients with congenital nonspherocytic hemolytic anemia have glucose-6-phosphate dehydrogenase deficiency.

MODE OF INHERITANCE: Sex-linked gene of partial dominance.

HAGEMAN TRAIT

The Hageman trait is a disorder of blood coagulation with prolonged clotting time of venous blood. It is due to a deficiency of the Hageman Factor. Affected patients are free of significant bleeding difficulties.

MODE OF INHERITANCE: Autosomal recessive.

HEMOPHILIA A

Hemophilia A is a hereditary hemorrhagic disorder, occurring almost exclusively in males and transmitted through females. It is characterized by a deficiency of antihemophilic globulin (Factor VIII).

MODE OF INHERITANCE: Sex-linked recessive.

HETEROIMMUNITY

Heteroimmunity is immunity to cells of a different type than the type that furnishes the immune serum.

HETEROZYGOUS

Heterozygous refers to the presence of different allelic genes for a given character.

HYDROPS

Hydrops is the accumulation of edema fluid in the body of the new-born infant.

HYPOFIBRINOGENEMIA

Hypofibrinogenemia is a serious and important complication of pregnancy. It may be characterized by sudden, uncontrollable hemorrhage due to incoagulability of the blood.

SYNONYM: *Fibrinogenopenia.*

HYPOPROCONVERTINEMIA

Hypoproconvertinemia is a disorder of blood coagulation characterized by an absence of Factor VII, which is required for conversion of pro-thrombin to thrombin.

MODE OF INHERITANCE: Autosomal recessive.

SYNONYM: *Deficiency of Stable Factor.*

ICTERUS INDEX

The icterus index is a measure of the severity or degree of jaundice—that is, of the bilirubin concentration in the plasma.

ICTERUS GRAVIS NEONATORUM

Icterus gravis neonatorum most often results from maternal isoimmunization due to the Rh factor. There is usually a severe anemia present at birth or appearing soon after birth associated with an increase in immature red cells in the circulating blood. The spleen and liver are commonly enlarged, and severe jaundice is frequent.

IMMUNIZATION

Immunization is a process of rendering a subject immune or of becoming immune. Active immunization is inoculation with a specific antigen to promote antibody formation in the body. Immunization is usually specific, and antibodies that are formed ordinarily combine only with the particular antigen causing their production.

ISOAGGLUTINATION

Isoagglutination is agglutination of erythrocytes caused by an agglutinating antibody from another person.

ISOAGGLUTININS

Isoagglutinins are naturally occurring antibodies that react with cells of the same species. This is in contrast to *heteroagglutinins,* which are produced in response to the injection of cells from another species.

SYNONYM: *Isohemolysis.*

JAUNDICE

Jaundice is a syndrome characterized by hyperbilirubinemia and deposition of bile pigment in the skin and other structures, with a resulting yellow appearance of the person.

SYNONYM: *Icterus.*

KERNICTERUS

Kernicterus is characterized by severe neurologic changes and high levels of bilirubin in the blood. There is deep, yellow staining of the basal nuclei, globus pallidus, putamen and caudate nuclei, the cerebellar and bulbar nuclei, and the white and gray substance of the cerebrum with destructive changes. This condition is frequently found in an Rh-positive infant born of an Rh-negative mother who has developed antibodies against the Rh factor, unless exchange transfusion of the infant is performed.

LEUKEMIA

Leukemia is a general proliferative neoplastic disorder of the blood-forming tissues primarily involving the white blood cells.

Acute Leukemia

Acute leukemia is a rapidly fatal form of leukemia characterized by replacement of normal bone marrow by primitive or stem cells of the blood-forming series. Death occurs in untreated cases within a few weeks to six months of the clinical onset of the disease.

Chronic Lymphocytic Leukemia

Chronic lymphocytic leukemia is abnormal proliferation of the lymphocytic elements of the lymph nodes and lymphoid tissues, with infiltration of the bone marrow and replacement of the normal hemopoietic elements.

Chronic Myelocytic Leukemia

Chronic myelocytic leukemia is abnormal proliferation of the granulocytic elements of the blood, usually progressing in a relatively slow manner and responsive to treatment during the major period of the disease.

Monocytic Leukemia

Monocytic leukemia usually has a fairly rapid course marked by excessive proliferation of the monocytic elements of the bone marrow, liver, and spleen.

LEUKOCYTE

A leukocyte is any colorless, ameboid cell mass. The term is applied especially to one of the formed elements of the blood consisting of a colorless granular mass of protoplasm.

PANOCELL

Panocell is a panel of known cells used in testing the serum of the Rh-negative person who has become sensitized, in order to determine the antigen or antigens causing the presence of antibodies.

PARAHEMOPHILIA A SYNDROME

The parahemophilia A syndrome is a congenital disorder in which deficiency of Factor V (proaccelerin) results in hemophiloid hemorrhagic diathesis with epistaxis, susceptibility to bruising, hemorrhage after dental extractions, and menorrhagia.

MODE OF INHERITANCE: Autosomal recessive.

SYNONYMS: *Owren's Syndrome II, Ac-Globulin Deficiency, Factor V Deficiency, Hemophiloid State A, Hypoprothrombinemia, Labile Factor Deficiency, Proaccelerin Deficiency.*

PHENOTYPE

The phenotype is the expression of the hereditary constitution of an organism. It is potentially variable, reflecting the interaction between genotype and nongenetic environment.

POLYCYTHEMIA

Polycythemia is an abnormal increase in the red cell concentration in the blood. More commonly, it is related to hypoxia, the result of congenital cardiac disease or pulmonary disorder.

PROTHROMBIN

Prothrombin is a protein in blood plasma that is the inactive precursor of thrombin.

SYNONYM: *Factor II.*

RH

Rh is an antigenic substance attached to red blood cells that is capable of causing the production of antibodies when introduced intravascularly into an individual whose cells fail to possess Rh—that is, when Rh-positive blood enters the circulation of an Rh-negative person.

RH–HR NOMENCLATURE

The six basic Rh-Hr factors are:

Rh_o (D)	Hr_o (d)
Rh' (C)	Hr' (c)
Rh" (E)	Hr" (e)

Rh-positive persons are those whose erythrocytes show the presence of Rh_o (D) antigen when tested with anti-Rh_o (anti-D) serum.

Rh-negative persons are those whose erythrocytes show the absence of Rh_o (D) antigen when tested with anti-Rh_o (anti-D) serum.

Rh' (C) persons are those whose erythrocytes show the presence of Rh' (C) when tested with anti-Rh' (anti-C) serum.

Rh" (E) persons are those whose erythrocytes show the presence of Rh" (E) when tested with anti-Rh" (anti-E) serum.

Hr_o (d) —No anti-Hr_o (anti-d) serum available.

Hr' (c) persons are those whose erythrocytes show the presence of Hr' (c) when tested with anti-Hr' (anti-c) serum.

Hr" (e) persons are those whose erythrocytes show the presence of Hr" (e) when tested with anti-Hr" (anti-e) serum.

S—C HEMOGLOBIN DISEASE

S–C hemoglobin disease is an inherited type of hemoglobinopathy in which the erythrocytes contain two abnormal hemoglobins, S and C. Clinically, gross hematuria, anemia, retinal hemorrhage, and aseptic necrosis of the femoral head are common features of S–C hemoglobin disease.

SELECTOGEN TEST

The selectogen test is a test using known cells ideally suited for detecting atypical antibodies that are capable of causing transfusion reactions or hemolytic disease of the newborn.

STUART—PROWER FACTOR DEFICIENCY

The Stuart-Prower Factor deficiency (Factor X) is a disorder of blood coagulation characterized by a prolonged prothrombin time. Mucocutaneous hemorrhages, bleeding into tissues, and prolonged bleeding after injury may occur.

MODE OF INHERITANCE: Autosomal recessive.

THALASSEMIAS

Thalassemias are a group of chronic, familial anemias occurring mostly in populations from countries bordering the Mediterranean, and in Negroes. Thalassemias are characterized by the production of an abnormally thin red blood cell. The disorder, transmitted as a dominant characteristic, manifests itself in the homozygous subject as a severe anemia during the first year of life. In the heterozygous subject, the anemia may be low-grade.

RELATED TERMS: *Mediterranean Anemia, Cooley's Anemia, Hereditary Leptocytosis, Thalassemia Major and Minor.*

THROMBIN

Thrombin is an enzyme formed from prothrombin in the blood; it initiates the conversion of fibrinogen to fibrin.

THROMBOCYTOPENIC PURPURA

Thrombocytopenic purpura is characterized by purpuric lesions of the skin, decreased platelet count, prolonged bleeding, impaired clot retraction, decreased prothrombin consumption, and variable numbers of megakaryocytes in the bone marrow.

SYNONYM: *Thrombopenic Purpura.*

Idiopathic Thrombocytopenic Purpura

Idiopathic thrombocytopenic purpura is a form of the disease that in some instances appears to result from the development of platelet agglutinins in the blood.

Secondary Thrombocytopenic Purpura

Secondary thrombocytopenic purpura has a demonstrable cause such as sensitivity to toxic materials in the environment, abruptio placentae, lupus erythematosus, or vitamin deficiency.

VAN DEN BERGH TEST
The van den Bergh test is used to measure bilirubin body fluids.

VON WILLEBRAND'S DISEASE
Von Willebrand's disease is an abnormality of blood-clotting factors, characterized by a prolonged bleeding time and a depression of Factor VIII. The clinical features are recurrent hemorrhages, such as nose bleeds, and prolonged bleeding after trauma.

MODE OF INHERITANCE: Autosomal dominant (intermediate dominance).

SYNONYMS: *Willebrand-Jurgens Thrombopathy, Vascular Hemophilia, Willebrand-Jurgens Syndrome, Minot-von Willebrand Syndrome, von Willebrand's Syndrome, Angiohemophilia, Constitutional Thrombopathy, Hereditary Hemorrhagic Thrombasthenia, Hereditary Pseudohemophilia, Pseudohemophilia.*

DIABETES—CLASSIFICATION

CLASSIFICATION OF DIABETES MELLITUS*
A classification of diabetes mellitus based on abnormalities of carbohydrate metabolism is given below. Progression or regression from one stage to the next may never occur, may proceed slowly over many years, or may be very rapid. This classification does not reflect the presence or absence of vascular disease, for patients with minimal glucose intolerance or even normal tolerance may have angiopathy.

Overt Clinical Diabetes Mellitus
Overt clinical diabetes mellitus is frank diabetes, either of the ketosis-prone or ketosis-resistant type. Fasting hyperglycemia is present. Symptoms of hyperglycemia and glucosuria may be present. A glucose tolerance test is not required for diagnosis.

Latent Diabetes
Latent diabetes is asymptomatic diabetes. The fasting blood glucose level may be elevated, but is usually normal and the postprandial level is frequently elevated. Oral or intravenous glucose tolerance tests performed in the absence of stress give results in the ranges accepted for diabetes.

SYNONYM: *Chemical Diabetes.*

Suspected Diabetes Mellitus
Suspected diabetes mellitus, including stress hyperglycemia, is a temporary carbohydrate intolerance in certain physiologic or pathologic situations. Persons with temporary carbohydrate intolerance should be suspected of having diabetes mellitus, particularly when there is a family history of diabetes. Symptoms due to severe hyper-

---

*This classification has been approved by the Committee on Professional Education of the American Diabetes Association.

glycemia occurring during periods of stress should be regarded as indicating overt diabetes until proved otherwise. Asymptomatic or symptomatic derangement of carbohydrate tolerance should be re-evaluated after total recovery from the stress.

Impaired carbohydrate tolerance in the following situations requires long-term evaluation:

1. The term *gestational diabetes* indicates the presence of abnormal glucose tolerance that reverts to normal values following delivery. In these women, follow-up studies have revealed a high risk of development of diabetes. Diabetes should also be suspected in a woman whose obstetric history includes large babies, unexplained abortion, fetal deaths, neonatal deaths, or polyhydramnios.
2. Obesity with an abnormal glucose tolerance that returns promptly to normal with moderate weight loss.
3. Infections, trauma, vascular accidents, burns, impaired nutrition, and severe emotional disturbances.
4. Treatment with certain pharmacologic agents, such as corticosteroids or thiazides.
5. Endocrinopathies such as acromegaly, Cushing's syndrome, thyrotoxicosis, and pheochromocytoma.

Diabetes must also be suspected in elderly subjects without symptoms and signs of the disease but with a glucose tolerance test that in younger individuals would be considered abnormal.

Prediabetes

Prediabetes is a conceptual term identifying the interval between fertilization of the ovum and the demonstration of impaired glucose tolerance in an individual predisposed to diabetes on genetic grounds. It cannot be diagnosed with certainty in the current state of our knowledge except in the nondiabetic identical twin of a diabetic patient and possibly in the offspring of two diabetic parents.

OTHER ABNORMAL GLUCOSE METABOLISM SYNDROMES

SCREENING TESTS FOR DIABETES MELLITUS:

POSTPRANDIAL BLOOD SUGAR TEST

The postprandial blood sugar test is a procedure for ascertaining the presence of hyperglycemia, utilizing a sample of blood drawn two hours after the completion of a meal containing 100 gm of carbohydrate. True glucose values of venous blood above 130 gm/100 ml indicate diabetes. Venous blood sugar levels are more stable than arterial values, and they are preferred in diagnostic studies of diabetes.

SIMPLIFIED GLUCOSE TOLERANCE TEST

The simplified glucose tolerance test is performed as follows: Glucose (100 gm) is given after an overnight fast. Specimens of urine and blood are obtained two hours after its ingestion. Blood sugar values between

110 and 130 mg/100 ml are inconclusive, but values above 130 mg usually indicate diabetes.

STANDARD GLUCOSE TOLERANCE TEST

The standard glucose tolerance test requires the intake of 300 gm or more of carbohydrate a day for three days prior to the test. A specimen of blood is drawn after an overnight fast and prior to the ingestion of 100 gm of glucose. Specimens are then obtained at intervals of one-half, 1, 2, and 3 hours. Levels indicative of diabetes are as follows:

Fasting	normal or less than 100 mg/100 ml
½ hour	more than 150 mg/100 ml
1 hour	more than 160 mg/100 ml
2 hours	120 mg/100 ml or more
3 hours	normal or more than 120 mg/100 ml

ABBREVIATION: GTT.

CORTISONE–GLUCOSE TOLERANCE TEST

The cortisone-glucose tolerance test aids identification of preclinical diabetes in persons predisposed to diabetes by heredity, obesity, or by other factors and who have responded normally to the standard glucose tolerance test. The intake of carbohydrate should be 300 gm or more a day for three days before the test. A urine specimen and a blood sample are taken after an overnight fast. Cortisone acetate (50 mg) is given 8½ and 2 hours before ingestion of 100 gm of glucose. For patients exceeding 160 pounds, 62.5 gm of cortisone acetate is substituted for each 50 mg dose. True glucose blood levels indicative of preclinical diabetes are as follows:

Fasting	140-200 mg/100 ml
½ or 1 hour	180-200 mg/100 ml
2 hours	more than 140 mg/100 ml

HEART DISEASE—CLASSIFICATION

CLASSIFICATION OF DISEASES OF THE HEART*

A complete diagnosis of heart disease should include one or more titles from each of the principal diagnostic rubrics of this nomenclature: etiologic, anatomic, physiologic, functional, and therapeutic. This classification should be used for all obstetric patients with heart disease.

Etiologic Diagnosis

The etiologic diagnosis may be derived from the patient's history, physical examination, and laboratory data, including the electro-

---

* The material under the heading "Classification of Diseases of the Heart" was excerpted by permission from *Diseases of the Heart and Blood Vessels—Nomenclature and Criteria for Diagnosis*, Little, Brown & Co., Boston, by the New York Heart Association, 1964.

cardiogram, angiocardiogram, and cardiac catheterization. Both structural and functional disturbance should be considered in the determination of the cause of the heart disease. If two or more possible causes of heart disease are present, each should be mentioned.

Anatomic Diagnosis

A correct anatomic diagnosis can be made clinically in the majority of diseases of the heart. Of the various diagnostic methods available, the minimum that should be employed are: history-taking and physical examination, including a determination of blood pressure in multiple extremities, if necessary; electrocardiography; and roentgenography, including fluoroscopy. In some instances the following may be necessary: angiocardiography, phonocardiography, determination of venous pressure and circulation times, catheterization of the right or left heart, or both, and recording of indicator-dilution curves or their equivalents.

Finally, a variety of tests may be required to support a diagnosis suspected on other grounds. These may include complete blood count; serologic test for syphilis; urinalysis and estimation of renal function (blood urea nitrogen and others); determination of the acute phase reactants (erythrocyte sedimentation rate, C-reactive protein), serum enzymes, and serum electrolytes; and performance of pulmonary functional studies. Although ordinarily used for appraisal of function, stress tests (for example, electrocardiographic exercise or hypoxia tests) may yield evidence in support of a specific anatomic diagnosis.

Physiologic Diagnosis

Clinical manifestations of physiologic disturbances in cardiodynamics may be classified thus: disturbance in cardiac rhythm and conduction (for example, arrhythmias, intraventricular block); disturbance in myocardial contractility (for example, heart failure, pulsus alternans); and clinical syndromes (for example, anginal syndrome, Adams-Stokes syndrome). The physiologic diagnosis should include a title from one or more of these categories if the criteria for the disturbance are met. If no disturbance is present, the physiologic diagnosis is normal sinus rhythm.

Functional Classification

The classification of patients according to their cardiac functional capacity gives only part of the information needed to plan the management of the patient's activities. A recommendation or prescription regarding physical activity should be based on information derived from many sources. The functional classification is an estimate of what the patient's heart will allow him to do and should not be influenced by the character of the structural lesions nor by an opinion as to treatment or prognosis.

Class I

Patients with cardic disease but without resulting limitations of physical activity. Ordinary physical activity does not cause undue fatigue, palpitation, dyspnea, or anginal pain.

Class II

Patients with cardiac disease resulting in slight limitation of physical activity. They are comfortable at rest. Ordinary physical activity results in fatigue, palpitation, dyspnea, or anginal pain.

Class III

Patients with cardiac disease resulting in marked limitation of physical activity. They are comfortable at rest. Less than ordinary physical activity causes fatigue, palpitation, dyspnea, or anginal pain.

Class IV

Patients with cardiac disease resulting in inability to carry on any physical activity without discomfort. Symptoms of cardiac insufficiency or of the anginal syndrome may be present even at rest. If any physical activity is undertaken, discomfort is increased.

Therapeutic Classification

The therapeutic classification is intended as a guide to the management of the activities of cardiac patients. It gives a prescription for the amount of physical activity which is advised for those in each functional class. From a practical point of view, it should be translated into terms of daily physical activity, such as walking a certain number of yards, climbing a specified number of stairs, lifting a certain number of pounds, and standing for an unlimited or limited part of the working day.

There is frequently a difference between the amount of activity which a patient can undertake in terms of his functional capacity and that which he should attempt in order to prevent aggravation of his disease. The recommendation of physical activity is based not only upon the amount of effort possible without discomfort but also upon the nature and severity of the cardiac disease.

It should be stressed that in prescribing activity for the cardiac patient an excessively conservative attitude is as harmful to the patient as is an overpermissive attitude.

The therapeutic classification is as follows:

Class A

Patients with cardiac disease whose ordinary physical activity need not be restricted in any way.

Class B

Patients with cardiac disease whose ordinary physical activity need not be restricted, but who should be advised against severe or competitive efforts.

CLASS C

Patients with cardiac disease whose ordinary physical activity should be moderately restricted, and whose more strenuous efforts should be discontinued.

CLASS D

Patients with cardiac disease whose ordinary physical activity should be markedly restricted.

CLASS E

Patients with cardiac disease who should be at complete rest, confined to bed or chair.

RENAL DISEASES

BACTERIURIA

Bacteriuria is the presence of bacteria in the urine. This condition is diagnosed by the discovery of more than 10^5 organisms per milliliter of urine when a clean voided midstream specimen is collected and cultured. SYNONYM: *Bacilluria*.

CYSTITIS

Cystitis is an acute or chronic inflammation of the urinary bladder. It is rarely a primary condition and is usually secondary to an infection of the kidney or urethra. The direct agents causing cystitis are: bacteria, chemical irritants, mechanical irritants, parasites, and fungi.

DIABETIC NEPHROPATHY

Diabetic nephropathy is a disease of the kidney, due to diabetes mellitus, that results in severely compromised renal function.

GLOMERULONEPHRITIS, ACUTE HEMORRHAGIC

Acute hemorrhagic glomerulonephritis is hemorrhage into the glomerulus of the kidney resulting from infection elsewhere in the body. A beta hemolytic streptococcus is the usual infecting organism. Hematuria, proteinuria, oliguria, edema, and hypertension are frequently present. It may proceed through subacute to chronic glomerulonephritis.

GLOMERULONEPHRITIS, CHRONIC

Chronic glomerulonephritis is a disease of the glomerulus of the kidney. The clinical features are divided into persistent proteinuria without other symptoms, chronic glomerulonephritis with significant renal decompensation, and nephrotic syndrome.

Chronic Glomerulonephritis with Renal Decompensation

Chronic glomerulonephritis with renal decompensation is an advanced form of acute or chronic nephritis in which kidney function determined by kidney function tests is below normal. Abortion, increased frequency of perinatal mortality, and abruptio placentae are some of the complications of the disease.

Nephrotic Syndrome
Nephrotic syndrome results from many underlying diseases such as glomerulonephritis, lupus nephritis, diabetic nephropathy, and amyloidosis. Clinically there is edema, massive proteinuria, hypoalbuminemia, and increased blood cholesterol levels.

SYNONYMS: *Epstein's Syndrome, Idiopathic Nephrotic Syndrome.*

Persistent Proteinuria
Persistent proteinuria is the presence of protein in the urine, generally resulting from the previous acute hemorrhagic glomerulonephritis or nephrosis. It may be difficult to ascertain the true predisposing causes.

LACTOSURIA
Lactosuria is the presence of lactose in the urine, the sugar having been absorbed into the bloodstream from the breasts. The lactose is excreted by glomerular filtration and is not reabsorbed by the renal tubules so that all the filtered lactose appears in the urine.

LUPUS NEPHRITIS
Lupus nephritis is a diffuse glomerulonephritis occurring in some patients with systemic lupus erythematosus. It is characterized by hematuria and progressive renal failure, often without hypertension. It is found most frequently in women in the childbearing age.

NECROSIS, ACUTE TUBULAR
Acute tubular necrosis is a lesion resulting from shock, related to either acute blood loss, sudden intravascular hemolysis, severe sepsis, or toxins. It is the major cause of acute renal failure during pregnancy.

NECROSIS, BILATERAL CORTICAL
Bilateral cortical necrosis is a lesion resulting from thrombosis of segments of the renal vascular system. These lesions may be focal, patchy, confluent, or gross. Clinically, the disease follows the course of acute renal failure with oliguria or anuria, uremia, and generally death in 7 to 14 days.

POLYCYSTIC KIDNEY DISEASE
Polycystic kidney disease is a rare familial condition in which the parenchyma of both kidneys is replaced by cysts.

PROTEINURIA, ORTHOSTATIC
Orthostatic proteinuria is the presence of protein in the urine when the patient is in the erect posture. Urine should be tested for protein, the specimen of clean voided urine being collected when the patient is erect and when recumbent.

PYELONEPHRITIS, ACUTE
Acute pyelonephritis is an ascending infection from the bladder involving the ureters, renal pelves, and kidney. Dilatation and atony of the ureter contribute to a partial obstruction in urinary flow.

PYELONEPHRITIS, CHRONIC

Chronic pyelonephritis is a slowly progressing, frequently bilateral infection in the renal pelvis and parenchyma. The condition may have its origin in an acute pyelonephritis in childhood, especially in females, or during pregnancy.

RENAL FAILURE, ACUTE

Acute renal failure is the inability of the kidney to excrete urine. The condition is generally caused by acute tubular necrosis that has followed severe preeclampsia, eclampsia, profuse hemorrhage, septic abortion, and abruptio placentae. The diagnosis is confirmed if oliguria with fixed specific gravity or anuria develops.

RENAL GLYCOSURIA

Renal glycosuria is the excretion of sugar in the urine. It is due to an increased volume of glomerular filtrate, which exceeds the maximal tubule capacity to reabsorb glucose.

RENAL TUBERCULOSIS

Renal tuberculosis is an infection of the kidney, caused by *Mycobacterium tuberculosis*, which usually is blood-borne from a distant focus such as a pulmonary lesion or one in the gastrointestinal tract, lymph nodes, or bone.

FETAL DEATH IN UTERO

FETAL DEATH

Fetal death is the cessation of fetal life before termination of the pregnancy.

DEAD FETUS SYNDROME

The dead fetus syndrome is characterized by the lengthy intrauterine retention of a dead fetus associated with hemorrhage of incoagulable blood. Decreased fibrinogen values between 250 and 150 mg/100 cc of plasma concentration have been observed in this syndrome, although frank hemorrhage seldom occurs until the level reaches 90 mg or less. Few accompanying symptoms may be present before onset of the hemorrhage aside from persistent tachycardia, which is almost a constant feature. The syndrome is not always associated with Rh incompatibility inasmuch as Rh-positive patients with a negative Coombs' test have been observed. Fibrinogen depression usually develops in chronic fashion. Defibrination may become apparent weeks before the onset of labor. Although fibrinogen recovery begins with the emptying of the uterus, low values may continue. The optimum time for interrupting the pregnancy in the dead fetus syndrome depends on the level of fibrinogen recovery after transfusion or the administration of fibrinogen.

KANTER'S SIGN

Kanter's sign is absence of the fetal movements normally produced by pressure on the fetal head. It is a sign of fetal death.

LITHOPEDION

A lithopedion is a calcified fetus in situ.
SYNONYMS: *Lithokelyphos, Osteopedion, Ostembryon.*

MUMMIFICATION OF THE FETUS

Mummification of the fetus is the drying up of the fetus after absorption of the amniotic fluid from the uterus.

MISCELLANEOUS COMPLICATIONS

ABRUPTIO PLACENTAE SYNDROME

Abruptio placentae syndrome is a syndrome characterized by the abnormal separation of a normally implanted placenta, hypofibrinogenemia, hemorrhage, and shock. The incidence varies from 1 in 85 to 1 in 250 deliveries. The onset of symptoms is subacute or abrupt and it consists of severe abdominal pain caused by tetanic contractions of the uterus, marked vaginal hemorrhage from incoagulable blood, and beginning shock. Abruptio placentae is the most widely recognized complication of hypofibrinogenemia. Clinical symptoms occur at a level below 150 mg/100 cc of plasma fibrinogen concentration, with a critical level at 90 mg or below. The degree of defibrination is coincident with and apparently directly proportional to the severity of the placental abruption. The placenta often shows either many infarcts or a large retroplacental hematoma. Uterine infiltration of suffused blood is sometimes found, a so-called Couvelaire uterus. The cause of the syndrome may be hypertensive states of pregnancy, chronic glomerulonephritis, chronic vascular disease, or trauma. Differential diagnosis should exclude placenta previa, in which the bleeding is painless and tetanic contractions of the uterus and fibrinogen depression are absent; and a ruptured uterus, in which pain is localized at the site of the rupture.

AMNION NODOSUM

The amnion nodosum are nodules in the amnion occurring most commonly in that part of the amnion in contact with the chorionic plate. They usually appear near the insertion of the cord as multiple, rounded or oval, opaque elevations that vary from less than 1 to 5 or 6 mm in diameter. Microscopically, they consist of typical stratified squamous epithelium, the upper layers of which are increasingly flattened and pale-staining toward the surface. They may become calcified and are common enough to be found as isolated nodules in about 60 per cent of placentas. The nodules occur in greater concentration in association with oligohydramnios and renal agenesis.
SYNONYMS: *Amniotic Caruncles, Squamous Metaplasia of Amnion.*

ANGIECTID SYNDROME

The angiectid syndrome is characterized by a type of superficial venous lesion that appears during the first trimester of pregnancy. These vascular abnormalities occur on the posterior thigh and calf areas and consist of small, intradermal, raised, sharply circumscribed clumps of blood vessels. The areas are tender, have increased local temperature, and may be painful. They are not related in any way to thrombophlebitis or to the commonplace saphenous varicosities of pregnancy. A distinct etiologic relationship exists between these lesions and the level of female sex hormones, more particularly with variations in the titers of serum estrogen and urinary pregnanediol. Patients with the most painful lesions show the greatest degree of estrogen or pregnanediol deficiency. After a few weeks the lesions sometimes disappear spontaneously, but usually continue longer, often throughout pregnancy and for a few weeks postpartum.

CARDIAC ARREST
Cardiac arrest refers to a sudden, unexpected stoppage of the circulation due to ventricular fibrillation or standstill.

CHORIOANGIOMA
Chorioangioma is a benign tumor of blood vessels usually located on the fetal surface of the placenta, but sometimes occurring within the placenta. Chorioangioma usually has no clinical significance, but approximately one third of these cases are associated with hydramnios.
SYNONYM: *Chorangioma.*

COR PULMONALE
Cor pulmonale is right heart hypertrophy, with or without failure, secondary to disease of the lungs. Cor pulmonale is usually associated with pulmonary artery hypertension.

COUVELAIRE UTERUS
Couvelaire uterus is a uterus in which there is an extravasation of blood into musculature and beneath the uterine serosa. Blood occasionally extends into the broad ligaments and fallopian tubes. The uterus assumes a bluish, purplish, coppery discoloration, with the adnexa showing the same changes. Microscopically, there is fragmentation of the muscle fibers, edema, and extravasation of blood. It is associated with abruptio placentae.
SYNONYM: *Uteroplacental Apoplexy.*

HERPES GESTATIONIS SYNDROME
The herpes gestationis syndrome is a relatively rare exanthema that occurs as a complication of the latter half of pregnancy or during the early phase of the puerperium. The condition occurs most commonly in women 30 to 35 years old. Symptoms include fever, malaise, dyspnea, burning sensation, neuralgic pains, and intense pruritus. The cutaneous lesions consist of bullae and vesicles that are present over the chest, abdomen, and extremities. The syndrome may occur with each gestation or during every second or third pregnancy. Exacerbations are likely, even during treatment. Recurrences may occasionally extend into the puerperium as episodes of severe pruritus, prior to the first few menstrual periods.

These episodes are called *herpes menstrualis recidivans*. The higher incidence of erythroblastosis fetalis, spontaneous abortions, monstrosities, and stillborn infants among women who seem predisposed to herpes gestationis may be an expression of Rh incompatibility or isosensitization.

SYNONYMS: *Duhring's Disease, Brocq-Duhring Disease, Dermatitis Herpetiformis, Dermatitis Multiformis, Dermatitis Neurotica, Dermatitis Polymorpha Dolorosa, Dermatitis Pruriginosa, Dermatitis Trophoneurotica, Herpes Circinatus Bullosus, Hydroa Herpetiformis, Hydroa Pruriginosa, Pemphigus Circinatus, Fetal Anomaly Syndrome, Dermatitis Herpetiformis Gestationis Syndrome, Hydroa Gravidarum, Pemphigus Pruriginosus, Prurigo Gestationis Syndrome.*

HYDRORRHEA GRAVIDARUM

Hydrorrhea gravidarum is a sudden periodic discharge of watery fluid from the vagina during pregnancy. It may simulate spontaneous rupture of the amniotic sac.

HYPEREMESIS GRAVIDARUM

Hyperemesis gravidarum is nausea and vomiting of pregnancy that have progressed to the extent that systemic effects such as acetonuria and substantial weight loss result.

IMPETIGO HERPETIFORMIS

Impetigo herpetiformis is a pyoderma of the vulva and other areas, complicating pregnancy. The eruptions are small, closely aggregated pustules that develop on an inflammatory base. There are severe symptoms and the condition may end in death.

LIVER, ACUTE YELLOW ATROPHY

Acute yellow atrophy of the liver is an extremely rare complication of pregnancy. There are two forms: true yellow atrophy, seen in both pregnant and nonpregnant women, and characterized by massive hepatocellular necrosis; and obstetric yellow atrophy, encountered exclusively in pregnant woman and characterized by fatty infiltration of the hepatic cells without necrosis. This disease is highly fatal.

LYMPHADENOMA

Lymphadenoma is abnormal proliferation, probably neoplastic, of the lymphoid tissues. Transmission of the disease from the mother to the fetus across the placenta has been reported in 10 per cent of cases.

SYNONYMS: *Hodgkin's Disease, Lymphogranulomatosis.*

MATERNAL OBESITY SYNDROME

The maternal obesity syndrome is a syndrome characterized by rapid and excessive gain in weight during pregnancy or after childbirth. Related endocrine factors include the large baby-diabetic syndrome, frank diabetes, a diabetic glucose tolerance curve, and the features of Cushing's syndrome.

MATERNAL SYNDROME

The maternal syndrome is characterized by general pruritus, ankle edema, a sudden marked gain in weight, polyhydramnios, and impending fetal death due to isoimmunization. In addition to the essential features, there may be albuminuria and hypertension. Insofar as can be determined, the fetus remains alive until the onset of the syndrome, which is usually prior to the 36th week of pregnancy. Fetal death varies from 2 to 21 days after the onset of symptoms in the mother. The syndrome does not subside until pregnancy is terminated. The etiologic agent is thought to be the severely affected erythroblastotic fetus or its placenta.

OLIGOHYDRAMNIOS

Oligohydramnios is a deficiency in the amount of amniotic fluid.
SYNONYM: *Oligoamnios.*

PAXSON'S SYNDROME

Paxson's syndrome is a syndrome that may occur as a result of obstetric and gynecologic complications. The features include primary injury to tissue; the presence or absence of shock; suppression of urine with urinary casts and leukocytes; and elevation of blood urea nitrogen, which attains its maximum increase between the fifth and ninth days. The syndrome occurs in three obstetric and gynecologic conditions: placental separation with retroplacental hematoma, ruptured uterus, and hemorrhagic twisted ovarian cyst. It is believed that bloody infiltration into any type of cellular tissue may be responsible for the elaboration of toxic metabolites with resulting renal damage. Thus the presence of this syndrome should be suspected in any severe gynecologic hemorrhagic condition.
SYNONYMS: *Paxson's Crush Syndrome, Obstetric-Gynecologic–Crush Syndrome.*

PLACENTAL HEMANGIOMA SYNDROME

The placental hemangioma syndrome is characterized by placental hemangiomas, polyhydramnios, prematurity, an increased incidence of stillborn infants, and a variety of major congenital abnormalities. Other features consist of antepartum hemorrhage and premature rupture of the membranes. Placental hemangiomas appear to be the primary pathologic feature. These tumors are benign and single or multiple, and they may vary in size. They occur as an elevation on the fetal or maternal surface of the placenta, or occasionally may be attached to the umbilical cord. Large tumors near the cord are most likely to cause symptoms. Polyhydramnios is present in about a third of the cases.

POLYHYDRAMNIOS

Polyhydramnios is an excessive quantity of amniotic fluid (more than 2000 cc). The normal volume of amniotic fluid is about 1000 cc.
SYNONYM: *Hydramnios.*

PORPHYRIA

Porphyria is a group of inherited or, more rarely, acquired disorders of porphyrin metabolism or disturbance of pyrrole biosynthesis.

POSTMATURITY SYNDROME

The postmaturity syndrome is characterized by a prolonged gestation, sometimes an enlarged fetus, diminished placental capacity to supply food and oxygen, and cutaneous and nutritional changes in the newborn infant.

SYNONYMS: *Ballantyne-Runge Syndrome, Ballantyne's Syndrome, Clifford's Syndrome, Runge's Syndrome, Dysmaturity Syndrome, Placental Dysfunction Syndrome, Prolonged Gestation Syndrome, Placental Insufficiency Syndrome.*

POSTRUBELLA SYNDROME

The postrubella syndrome is a syndrome characterized by a high incidence of congenital malformations and defects in the human fetus caused by maternal rubella during the first three months of gestation. The defects and malformations consist of microcephaly, severe mental deficiency, bilateral congenital cataract with blindness, complete or partial deafness, congenital malformation of the heart such as atrial septal defect or patent ductus arteriosus, feeding difficulties, retarded physical development, and many other anomalies.

SYNONYM: *Gregg's Syndrome.*

VARICOSE VEINS

Varicose veins are abnormally lengthened, dilated, and sacculated superficial veins. The long and short saphenous veins and their tributaries are most commonly affected. Forces such as pregnancy, abdominal tumor, ascites, excessive weight, or prolonged weight-bearing tend to increase venous pressure in the lower extremities; the veins may distend to the extent that the valves become incompetent. Further distention and valve incompetence ensue and varicosities result.

YOUNG'S SYNDROME

Young's syndrome is characterized by hyperlactation, rapid weight gain during pregnancy, and the birth of a living child weighing more than 500 gm or termination of pregnancy because of fetal or previous neonatal mortality. In addition, there is a late onset, often after menopause, of diabetes mellitus. A definite hereditary tendency prevails.

SYNONYM: *Somatotrophic Hormone Syndrome.*

SECTION 7: OBSTETRICS

Statistical Reporting

Several of the measures in this section are recommended as ideal calculations, with the full knowledge that the necessary information for the calculation may not generally be available but should be striven for in the future. Similarly, some of the definitions may be at variance with international practice or state or local laws, but these are recommended as improvements over current procedures. Most notable of these variants are the definitions of liveborn infant and stillborn infant.

ABORTION
Abortion is the expulsion or extraction of all (complete) or any part (incomplete) of the placenta or membranes, without an identifiable fetus or with a liveborn infant or a stillborn infant weighing less than 500 gm. In the absence of known weight, an estimated length of gestation of less than 20 completed weeks (139 days), calculated from the first day of the last normal menstrual period, may be used. Abortion is a term referring to the birth process culminating before the 20th completed week of gestation.

ABORTION RATE
The abortion rate is the number of abortions per 1000 terminated pregnancies for a given period.

ABORTUS
Abortus is the term applied to a stillborn infant expelled before attaining a weight of 500 gm. In the absence of known weight, an estimated length of gestation of less than 20 completed weeks (139 days), calculated from the first day of the last normal menstrual period, may be used.

APGAR SCORE
The Apgar score is a system of numerical evaluation that describes the status of the infant at one minute and five minutes after birth. A score of zero indicates a severely jeopardized infant; the higher the score, up to a maximum of 10, the better the condition of the infant. Two cautions: (1) The score should never be given by the one who delivers the infant. It is always too high. (2) The 60 seconds after birth must be timed with a timer that, ideally, rings a bell.

452

Sign	0	1	2
Heart rate	Absent to auscultation	Under 100	Over 100
Respiration	None	Irregular, inadequate	Yelling
Muscle tone	Flaccid	Some tone	Well flexed
Reflexes—sharp slap on feet	None	Grimace	Cry
Color	Pale, blue	Blue hands and feet	Pink all over

BIRTH
Birth is the process by which a liveborn infant or a stillborn infant is expelled or extracted from the mother.

FETAL DEATH
Fetal death is the cessation of fetal life before termination of the pregnancy.

FETUS
Fetus is the term applied to the unborn offspring from the date of conception until the completion of pregnancy.

GESTATIONAL AGE
Gestational age is the estimated age of the fetus calculated from the first day of the last normal menstrual period. Gestational age is expressed in completed weeks.

INFANT
Infant is a pediatric term referring to a liveborn infant from the moment of birth through the completion of the first year of life.

Preterm Infant
A preterm infant is an infant born at any time through the 37th completed week of gestation (259 days).

Term Infant
A term infant is an infant born at any time from the beginning of the 38th week through 41 completed weeks of gestation (260 to 287 days).

Post-Term Infant
A post-term infant is an infant born at any time after the beginning of the 42nd week of gestation (288 days or longer).

INFANT DEATH
Infant death is the death of a liveborn infant at any time from the moment of birth to the end of the first year of life.

INFANT MORTALITY RATE
Infant mortality rate is the number of infant deaths per 1000 liveborn infants for a stated period.

LIVEBORN INFANT
Liveborn infant is a fetus, irrespective of its gestational age, that after complete expulsion or extraction from the mother shows evidence of life —that is, heartbeats or respirations. *Heartbeats* are to be distinguished from several transient cardiac contractions; *respirations* are to be distinguished from fleeting respiratory efforts or gasps. Classification of all liveborn infants will be by gestational age and birth weight.

MATERNAL DEATH
Maternal death is the death of any woman, from any cause, while pregnant or within 42 days of termination of pregnancy, irrespective of the duration and the site of pregnancy.

For world statistical evaluation, it is necessary to divide the 42 days into two periods.

Period I: 1 to 7 days following termination of pregnancy.
Period II: 8 to 42 days following termination of pregnancy.

Direct Maternal Death
Direct maternal death is an obstetric death resulting from obstetric complications of the pregnancy state, labor, or puerperium—from interventions, omissions, incorrect treatment, or a chain of events resulting from any of the above.

Indirect Maternal Death
Indirect maternal death is an obstetric death resulting from previously existing disease, or disease that developed during pregnancy, labor, or the puerperium; it is not directly due to obstetric causes, but aggravated by the physiologic effects of pregnancy.

Nonmaternal Death
Nonmaternal death is an obstetric death resulting from accidental or incidental causes not related to the pregnancy or its management.

MATERNAL DEATH RATE
Maternal death rate is the number of maternal deaths (direct, indirect, or nonmaternal) per 100,000 terminated pregnancies for any specified period. Contributions to the numerator and denominator must be within the same time period.

NEONATAL DEATH
Neonatal death is the death of a liveborn infant within the first 27 days, 23 hours, and 59 minutes of life.

NEONATAL MORTALITY RATE
Neonatal mortality rate is the number of neonatal deaths per 1000 liveborn infants.

NEONATAL PERIOD
The neonatal period is that part of an infant's life from the hour of birth through the first 27 days, 23 hours, and 59 minutes of life. During this period the infant is referred to as a newborn infant.

The neonatal period is divided into three periods: Neonatal Period I is from the hour of birth through 23 hours and 59 minutes; Neonatal Period II is from the beginning of the 24th hour of life through 6 days, 23 hours, and 59 minutes; Neonatal Period III is from the beginning of the seventh day through 27 days, 23 hours, and 59 minutes.

NEWBORN INFANT
Newborn infant refers to a liveborn infant during the first 27 days, 23 hours, and 59 minutes of life.

SYNONYM: *Neonate* (obsolete).

PARITY
Parity is the state of having given birth to an infant or infants, weighing 500 gm or more, alive or dead. In the absence of known weight, an estimated length of gestation of 20 completed weeks or more, calculated from the first day of the last normal menstrual period, may be used. For the purpose of defining parity, a multiple birth is a single parous experience.

PERINATAL DEATH
Perinatal death is an all-inclusive term referring to both stillborn infants and neonatal deaths.

PERINATAL MORTALITY RATE
Perinatal mortality rate is the number of stillborn infants and neonatal deaths per 1000 total births. It is calculated by the following formula:

$$\frac{\text{Perinatal Deaths}}{\text{Liveborn Infants} + \text{Stillborn Infants}} \times 1000$$

Specific perinatal mortality rates may be calculated for any given period, or for any clinical entity such as abruptio placentae and diabetes. The neonatal period (Periods I, II, or III) under consideration should be explicitly stated. Contributions to the numerator and denominator must be within the same category of the variable under consideration— for example, the weight or gestational age of the infants.

EXAMPLE: Diabetics

$$\frac{\text{Neonatal deaths (diabetic mothers)} + \text{stillborn infants (diabetic mothers)}}{\text{Liveborn infants (diabetic mothers)} + \text{stillborn infants (diabetic mothers)}} \times 1000$$

EXAMPLES: Weight

500–999 gm.:

$$\frac{\text{Neonatal deaths (Periods I \& II)} + \text{stillborn infants}}{\text{Liveborn infants} + \text{stillborn infants}} \times 1000$$

1000+ gm.:

$$\frac{\text{Neonatal deaths (Periods I \& II)} + \text{stillborn infants}}{\text{Liveborn infants} + \text{stillborn infants}} \times 1000$$

1500–1900 gm.:

$$\frac{\text{Neonatal deaths (Periods I, II, \& III)} + \text{stillborn infants}}{\text{Liveborn infants} + \text{stillborn infants}} \times 1000$$

PERINATAL MORTALITY RATE (INTERNATIONAL)

For international comparability, the standard perinatal mortality rate includes only stillborn infants of 28 completed weeks (196 days) or more plus deaths occurring in neonatal Periods I and II (or under 7 days). The general formula for determination of perinatal mortality rate is as follows:

$$\frac{\text{Stillborn infants of 28 weeks or more gestation} + \text{Deaths of liveborn infants regardless of period of gestation, under 7 days}}{\text{Stillborn infants of 28 weeks or more gestation} + \text{All liveborn infants regardless of period of gestation.}}$$

PERIOD OF GESTATION

The period of gestation is the number of completed weeks of pregnancy between the first day of the last normal menstrual period and the date in question, or the date of completion of the pregnancy, irrespective of whether the products of conception include an abortus, fetus, or infant.

PREGNANCY

Pregnancy is the state of a female after conception and until termination of the gestation.

SYNONYMS: *Gestation, Cyophoria, Cyesis, Gravidity.*

PREGNANCY TERMINATION

Pregnancy termination is the expulsion or extraction of a dead fetus or other products of conception from the mother, or the birth of a liveborn infant or a stillborn infant.

PREGNANCY TERMINATION—REGISTRATION

Liveborn Infants

All liveborn infants, regardless of birth weight or period of gestation, should be registered in accordance with the regulation or administrative instructions of the particular national, state, or local board of health.

Stillborn Infants

All stillborn infants, regardless of birth weight or period of gestation, should be registered in accordance with the regulation or administrative instructions of the particular national, state, or local board of health.

Other Pregnancy Terminations before the 20th Completed Week of Gestation

Pregnancy terminations before the 20th completed week of gestation, which do not include a liveborn or stillborn infant, should be reported in accordance with the regulation or administrative instructions of the particular national, state, or local board of health.

PRESSURE, MEAN ARTERIAL

The mean arterial pressure is the diastolic pressure in mm Hg plus one-third of the pulse pressure.

STILLBORN INFANT

A stillborn infant is a fetus, irrespective of its gestational age, that after complete expulsion or extraction from the mother shows no evidence of life—that is, heart beats or respirations. *Heart beats* are to be distinguished from several transient cardiac contractions; *respirations* are to be distinguished from fleeting respiratory efforts or gasps. Classification of all stillborn infants will be by gestational age and birth weight.

TOTAL BIRTH RATE

The total birth rate is the number of liveborn and stillborn infants per 1000 population for a given period.

Section 8: *Neonatology*

Infant

GENERAL TERMINOLOGY

INFANT

Infant is a pediatric term referring to a liveborn infant from the moment of birth through the completion of the first year of life.

Preterm Infant

A preterm infant is an infant born at any time through the 37th completed week of gestation (259 days).

Term Infant

A term infant is an infant born at any time from the beginning of the 38th week through 41 completed weeks of gestation (260–287 days).

Post-Term Infant

A post-term infant is an infant born at any time after the beginning of the 42nd week of gestation (288 days or longer).

APGAR SCORE

The Apgar score is a system of numerical evaluation that describes the status of the infant at one minute and five minutes after birth. A score of zero indicates a severely jeopardized infant; the higher the score, up to a maximum of 10, the better the condition of the infant. Two cautions: (1) The score should never be given by the one who delivers the infant. It is always too high. (2) The 60 seconds after birth must be timed with a timer that, ideally, rings a bell.

Sign	0	1	2
Heart rate	Absent to auscultation	Under 100	Over 100
Respiration	None	Irregular, inadequate	Yelling
Muscle tone	Flaccid	Some tone	Well flexed
Reflexes—sharp slap on feet	None	Grimace	Cry
Color	Pale, blue	Blue hands and feet	Pink all over

APNEA
Apnea is a transient cessation of respiration.

BILIRUBIN ENCEPHALOPATHY SYNDROME
Bilirubin encephalopathy syndrome is characterized by damage to the central nervous system from the toxic effects of bilirubin on cerebral tissues. The syndrome follows an attack of icterus gravis neonatorum. A rare recessive gene is thought responsible. Clinical manifestations may include slowing of mental development, an intention tremor, progressive slurring of speech, and perhaps later a disturbance in gait. Among the suspected causes of this syndrome are: incompatibility of the blood of the parents, and diminished capacity of the hepatic cells to metabolize and excrete bilirubin. The syndrome may be differentiated from the neurologic features of kernicterus, a closely related condition, in which deposition of pathologic amounts of biliary pigment is limited essentially to the basal nuclei.

BIRTH PALSY
Birth palsy in the infant is usually due to cerebral hemorrhage occurring during labor or to intrauterine cerebral anoxia.

BRACHIAL BIRTH PALSY
Brachial birth palsy affects the arm of the infant and results from injury during birth. There are three types: whole-arm, upper-arm (Duchenne-Erb), or forearm (Klumpke).

CEPHALHEMATOMA
Cephalhematoma is a collection of blood underneath the periosteum of the fetal skull.
SYNONYMS: *Cephalhematocele, Cephalohematoma, Cephalohematocele.*

ERYTHROBLASTOSIS FETALIS
Erythroblastosis fetalis is a congenital hemolytic disease caused both by the presence of Rh antibodies in maternal blood and the antigen in fetal red cells. It is the pathologic state produced in the fetus as a result of exposure to maternal antibodies—for example, Rh, Hr, A-B, and those designated in other blood systems.
SYNONYMS: *Erythroblastosis Fetalis Syndrome, Erythroblastosis Neonatorum Syndrome, Congenital Hemolytic Disease of Newborn.*

EXSTROPHY OF BLADDER
Exstrophy of the bladder is an anomaly in which the anterior wall of the bladder and the overlying anterior abdominal wall are absent so that the inner surface of the posterior wall of the bladder is everted. The posterior wall protrudes in the region of the lower anterior wall of the abdomen. This anomaly occurs more frequently in the male. Only a few patients have survived well into adult life.

FETAL ASPIRATION SYNDROME

The fetal aspiration syndrome is characterized by aspiration of the amniotic sac contents by the fetus. It may occur at term, but it is often associated with post-term infants. This neonatal distress syndrome ensues when the demands of the fetus for food and oxygen outgrow placental capacity. Aside from malnutrition, there is yellow staining of skin and nails and aspiration of meconium and keratinized squamous cells into distal bronchi. Symptoms are not pathognomonic. Pulmonary findings, often complicated by focal hemorrhage or pneumonia, include hyperresonance, loud breath sounds, and coarse rales. Roentgenographic findings of this syndrome are fairly characteristic with coarse and irregular streaks of interstitial markings and areas of focal irregularities of aeration. By contrast, the roentgenographic pattern in hyaline membrane disease shows a fine, diffuse miliary or stippled increase in density. As a rule, pulmonary features show evidence of clearing within 24 hours. The condition is much less frequent and hazardous than hyaline membrane disease.

FONTANEL

A fontanel is a space in the fetal and infant skull at the junction of three or more bones. It is covered only by a thin membrane and skin until ossification.

SYNONYM: *Fonticulus.*

Anterior Fontanel

The anterior fontanel is located in the anterior portion of the skull. It is formed by the junction of the sagittal, frontal, and coronal sutures.

SYNONYMS: *Greater Fontanel, Fonticulus Anterior.*

Lateral Fontanel

The lateral fontanel is a small, triangular space at the side of the fetal skull formed by the intersection of the lambdoid suture and temporal sutures.

SYNONYM: *Temporal Fontanel.*

Mastoid Fontanel

The mastoid fontanel is the membranous area at the junction of the parietal, temporal, and occipital bones.

SYNONYMS: *Posterolateral Fontanel, Fonticulus Mastoideus.*

Posterior Fontanel

The posterior fontanel is formed by the junction of the sagittal suture with lambdoid sutures.

SYNONYMS: *Lesser Fontanel, Fonticulus Posterior.*

Sagittal Fontanel

The sagittal fontanel is an occasional defect in the sagittal suture that resembles a fontanel.

SYNONYM: *Gerdy's Fontanel.*

Sphenoidal Fontanel

The sphenoidal fontanel is formed by the junction of the parietal, frontal, and temporal bones.

SYNONYMS: *Anterolateral Fontanel, Fonticulus Sphenoidalis.*

GALACTOSEMIA

Galactosemia is a disorder of galactose metabolism caused by a deficiency of galactose-1-phosphate-uridyl transferase or galactokinase. The latter is a relatively benign condition characterized clinically by cataracts. Individuals with the transferase defect manifest hypoglycemia, vomiting and diarrhea, jaundice, hepatomegaly, splenomegaly, cataract formation, and aminoaciduria shortly after milk feedings are begun in the newborn period. Failure to thrive and mental retardation are common. Death occurs in undiagnosed patients when the enzyme deficiency is severe.

MODE OF INHERITANCE: Autosomal recessive.

HYALINE MEMBRANE

A hyaline membrane is a homogenous membrane of eosinophilic material lining the alveoli, alveolar ducts of the lungs, and respiratory bronchioles.

HYALINE MEMBRANE DISEASE

Hyaline membrane disease is a syndrome of newborn infants characterized by a progressive and frequently fatal respiratory disorder, the result of a hyaline type of membrane in the lungs. It occurs most commonly in preterm infants, especially those delivered by cesarean section, and also in large infants whose mothers are diabetic. Hyaline membrane disease also occurs in post-term infants more often than in those of normal gestational age.

HYDROPS

Hydrops is the accumulation of edema fluid in the body of the newborn infant.

ICTERUS GRAVIS NEONATORUM

Icterus gravis neonatorum most often results from maternal isoimmunization due to the Rh factor. There is usually a severe anemia present at birth or appearing soon after birth associated with an increase in immature red cells in the circulating blood. The spleen and liver are commonly enlarged, and severe jaundice is frequent.

INFANT ASPHYXIA

Infant asphyxia is a state of insufficient oxygen-carbon dioxide exchange, generally resulting in respiratory failure.

INFANT DEATH

Infant death is the death of a liveborn infant at any time from the moment of birth to the end of the first year of life.

INFANT MORTALITY RATE

The infant mortality rate is the number of infant deaths per 1000 liveborn infants for a stated period.

KERNICTERUS

Kernicterus is characterized by severe neurologic changes and high levels of bilirubin in the blood. There is deep yellow staining of the basal nuclei, globus pallidus, putamen and caudate nuclei, the cerebellar and bulbar nuclei, and the white and gray substance of the cerebrum with destructive changes. This condition is frequently found in an Rh-positive infant born of an Rh-negative mother who has developed antibodies against the Rh factor, unless exchange transfusion of the infant is performed.

LONGITUDINAL DUCT OF EPOOPHORON

The longitudinal duct of the epoophoron is the remains of the lower part of the mesonephric duct, which may persist as a fibrous cord at the side of the upper half of the vagina.

SYNONYMS: *Gartner's Canal, Malpighian Canal, Ductus Epoophori Longitudinalis* (NA).

MALE CIRCUMCISION

Male circumcision is the operative removal of the prepuce of the penis.

MECONIUM

Meconium is a greenish black, semifluid substance that collects in the intestines of the fetus. It is composed of cellular debris, bile, lanugo, mucopolysaccharides, digestive enzymes, and vernix caseosa.

NEONATAL DEATH

Neonatal death is the death of a liveborn infant within the first 27 days, 23 hours, and 59 minutes of life.

NEONATAL MORTALITY RATE

The neonatal mortality rate is the number of neonatal deaths per 1000 liveborn infants.

NEONATAL MASTITIS

Neonatal mastitis is inflammation of the breast in the newborn.

NEWBORN INFANT

Newborn infant refers to a liveborn infant during the first 27 days, 23 hours, and 59 minutes of life.

SYNONYM: *Neonate* (obsolete).

OMPHALITIS

Omphalitis is inflammation of the umbilicus and surrounding area.

OMPHALOCELE
Omphalocele is a congenital herniation at the umbilicus.
SYNONYM: *Umbilical Hernia.*

OMPHALOPHLEBITIS
Omphalophlebitis is an inflammation of the umbilical veins.

OMPHALORRHAGIA
Omphalorrhagia is bleeding from the umbilicus.

OMPHALOTRIPSY
Omphalotripsy is crushing of the umbilical cord.

OPHTHALMIA NEONATORUM
Ophthalmia neonatorum is acute purulent conjunctivitis of the newborn infant. It is usually due to gonorrheal discharge from the maternal birth canal.

PEMPHIGUS NEONATORUM
Pemphigus neonatorum is an infectious condition of impetigo that occurs in the newborn and is characterized by the appearance of blebs or bullae around the umbilicus, buttocks, and vulva.
SYNONYMS: *Ritter's Disease, Impetigo Neonatorum, Bullous Impetigo of Infants.*

PERINATAL DEATH
Perinatal death is an all-inclusive term referring to both stillborn infants and neonatal deaths.

PERINATAL MORTALITY RATE
Perinatal mortality rate is the number of stillborn infants and neonatal deaths per 1000 total births. It is calculated by the following formula:

$$\frac{\text{Perinatal Deaths}}{\text{Liveborn Infants } + \text{ Stillborn Infants}} \times 1000$$

Specific perinatal mortality rates may be calculated for any given period, or for any clinical entity such as abruptio placentae and diabetes. The neonatal period (Periods I, II, or III) under consideration should be explicitly stated. Contributions to the numerator and denominator must be within the same category of the variable under consideration—for example, the weight or gestational age of the infants.
EXAMPLE: Diabetics

$$\frac{\text{Neonatal deaths (diabetic mothers) } + \text{ stillborn infants (diabetic mothers)}}{\text{Liveborn infants (diabetic mothers) } + \text{ stillborn infants (diabetic mothers)}} \times 1000$$

EXAMPLES: Weight

500–999 gm:

$$\frac{\text{Neonatal deaths (Periods I \& II) + stillborn infants}}{\text{Liveborn infants + stillborn infants}} \times 1000$$

1000+ gm:

$$\frac{\text{Neonatal deaths (Periods I \& II) + stillborn infants}}{\text{Liveborn infants + stillborn infants}} \times 1000$$

1500–1900 gm:

$$\frac{\text{Neonatal deaths (Periods I, II, \& III) + stillborn infants.}}{\text{Liveborn infants + stillborn infants}} \times 1000$$

PHENYLKETONURIA

Phenylketonuria is a hereditary disorder characterized by the excretion of phenylpyruvic acid in the urine. Most untreated patients have seizures, eczema, and mental retardation. The specific defect is a lack of the liver enzyme phenylalanine hydroxylase, which is responsible for the conversion of phenylalanine to tyrosine.

MODE OF INHERITANCE: Autosomal recessive.

SYNONYMS: *Imbecilitas Phenylpyruvica, Phenylpyruvic Oligophrenia, Phenyluria, Fölling's Disease.*

ABBREVIATION: PKU.

POSTMATURITY SYNDROME

The postmaturity syndrome is characterized by a prolonged gestation period, sometimes an enlarged fetus, diminished placental capacity to supply food and oxygen, and cutaneous and nutritional changes in the newborn infant.

SYNONYMS: *Ballantyne-Runge Syndrome, Ballantyne's Syndrome, Clifford's Syndrome, Runge's Syndrome, Dysmaturity Syndrome, Placental Dysfunction Syndrome, Prolonged Gestation Syndrome, Placental Insufficiency Syndrome.*

SUTURE

A suture is a line of impingement of bones in the fetal and infant skull, particularly before ossification.

Coronal Sutures

The coronal sutures are the sutures between the frontal and the parietal bones.

SYNONYM: *Sutura Coronalis* (NA).

Frontal Suture

The frontal suture is the suture between the frontal bones.

SYNONYMS: *Metopic Suture, Sutura Frontalis* (NA).

Lambdoid Sutures

The lambdoid sutures are the sutures between the parietal and occipital bones.

SYNONYM: *Sutura Lambdoidea* (NA).

Sagittal Suture

The sagittal suture is the suture between the parietal bones.

SYNONYMS: *Longitudinal Suture, Sutura Sagittalis* (NA).

Temporal Suture

The temporal suture is a suture between the temporal and parietal bones.

SYNONYM: *Lateral Suture.*

THRUSH

Thrush is an infection of the infant's mouth with *Candida albicans.*

UMBILICUS

The umbilicus is the depression in the anterior abdominal wall at the point where the umbilical cord entered the fetal body.

SYNONYMS: *Navel, Omphalos.*

VERNIX CASEOSA

Vernix caseosa is a cheesy deposit on the skin of the newborn derived from the stratum corneum, sebaceous secretions, and remnants of epithelium.

NORMAL TWINS

TWIN

A twin is one of two individuals developing simultaneously within the uterus.

Compacted Twins

Compacted twins are twins whose presenting parts engage simultaneously, thereby preventing the progress of labor.

Dizygotic Twins

Dizygotic twins result from fertilization of two female germ cells coming from simultaneously developed follicles. Such individuals have a different genetic constitution and may be of the same or different sex.

SYNONYMS: *Binovular Twins, Dichorial Twins, Dichorionic Twins, Dissimilar Twins, False Twins, Fraternal Twins, Heterologous Twins, Hetero-ovular Twins, Two-egg Twins, Unlike Twins.*

Impacted Twins

Impacted twins are twins in which the pressure of any part of one twin onto the surface of the second twin produces incomplete simultaneous engagement of both.

Interlocked Twins

Interlocked twins are twins in which the inferior surface of the chin of the first twin locks with that of the second twin, with one head above and the other below the pelvic inlet.

Monoamniotic Twins

Monoamniotic twins are twins developing with a single amniotic cavity. They come from a single ovum and are always of the same sex and genetic constitution.

Monochorionic Twins

Monochorionic twins are twins developing within a single chorionic sac. They may have separate (diamniotic) or common (monoamniotic) sacs and although they are usually monozygotic they may be dizygotic.

Monozygotic Twins

Monozygotic twins are twins resulting from fertilization of a single female germ cell. The developing zygote splits into halves at an early cleavage phase, each half giving rise to a complete individual. Such twins are always of the same sex and genetic constitution.

SYNONYMS: *Enzygotic Twins, Identical Twins, Monochorial Twins, Mono-ovular Twins, Similar Twins, True Twins, Uniovular Twins.*

Polyovular Twins

Polyovular twins are twins that result from the simultaneous fertilization of two or more female germ cells.

SUPERFECUNDATION

Superfecundation is the impregnation of two or more ova, liberated at the same ovulation, by successive acts of coitus.

SUPERFETATION

Superfetation is the presence of two fetuses of different ages, not twins, in the uterus. It is due to the impregnation of two ova liberated at successive periods of ovulation.

SYNONYM: *Hypercyesia.*

TRIPLET

A triplet is one of three individuals developing simultaneously within the uterus.

ABNORMAL TWINS

ACARDIAC TWIN

An acardiac twin is a malformed monozygous twin without a heart (acardia) or with a very imperfect one (hemicardia), obtaining its circulation by vascular anastomoses with the circulation of the normal twin. Such twins may be divided into acardiac paracephalous (rudimentary head), acardiac acephalous (no head and most often no arms, thoracic or upper abdominal viscera) and acardiac amorphous (no viscera or organized parts).

CEPHALOTHORACOPAGUS TWINS

Cephalothoracopagus twins are conjoined twins in which two fetuses of equal size are fused front to front over much of the trunk region. They have a single neck and head; the face is ordinarily single; the cerebrum irregularly duplicated; the cerebellum, brain stem, and spinal cord completely duplicated.

CONJOINED TWINS

Conjoined twins are twins attached to each other. They vary widely from those in which two well-developed individuals have only a minor superficial connection, to those in which only a small part of the body is duplicated, or in which amorphous masses of tissue are attached to an otherwise normal individual.

SYNONYM: *Siamese Twins.*

Conjoined Equal Twins

Conjoined equal twins are conjoined twins in which both members are approximately of the same size, and fairly normal except for the area of fusion.

SYNONYM: *Symmetric Conjoined Twins.*

Conjoined Unequal Twins

Conjoined unequal twins are conjoined twins in which one fairly normal member serves as the host (autosite) for the other small incompletely developed member (parasite).

SYNONYM: *Asymmetric Conjoined Twins.*

CRANIODIDYMUS TWINS

Craniodidymus twins are conjoined twins with two heads and partial or complete duplication of the spine. The body is usually single with two arms and two legs.

CRANIOPAGUS TWINS

Craniopagus twins are twins with partially fused skulls; the union may be frontal, occipital, or parietal.

SYNONYM: *Cephalopagus.*

DERADELPHUS TWINS

Deradelphus twins are a variety of cephalothoracopagus twins in which there is a single face with two ears and a single, normally formed cerebrum.

DICEPHALUS DIPUS TWINS

Dicephalus dipus twins consist of three types: (1) Dicephalus dipus dibrachius twins are conjoined twins with two heads, two arms, two legs, and partial duplication of the spine. There are varying degrees of duplication of the median shoulder; (2) Dicephalus dipus tribrachius twins are conjoined twins united at the pelvis. They have a partially duplicated spine, two heads, two legs, two arms, and a median third arm or arm rudiment; (3) Dicephalus dipus tetrabrachius twins are conjoined twins united at the pelvis. They have a partially duplicated spine, two heads, four arms, and two legs.

DICEPHALUS DIPYGUS TWINS
Dicephalus dipygus twins are conjoined twins with two heads, fused bodies, and a variable reduction in the number of upper and lower extremities.

DIPYGUS TWINS
Dipygus twins are conjoined twins in which the upper part of the body is single and the lower part irregularly duplicated.

EPIGNATHUS
Epignathus is a teratoma arising from the palate in the region of Rathke's pouch, distending the buccal cavity and often protruding through the mouth. Because these rare tumors contain recognizable fetal structures, they are sometimes considered a parasitic twin.

FETUS ANIDEUS
Fetus anideus is a shapeless simple rounded mass of tissue with slight indications of fetal parts.

FETUS IN FETU
Fetus in fetu is a double fetus in which the small imperfectly formed parasite is contained within the autosite.

FETUS PAPYRACEUS
Fetus papyraceus is a fetus that dies early in pregnancy and becomes paper-thin because of compression by the living twin.
SYNONYM: *Fetus Compressus.*

FETUS SANGUINOLENTUS
Fetus sanguinolentus is a dead fetus that has become dark-colored and macerated.

HETEROPAGUS TWINS
Heteropagus twins are unequal and asymmetric conjoined twins with one component smaller than, and dependent on, the other. The parasite may consist of arms, or head and arms, legs and a portion of pelvis, or arms and legs. It is usually attached to the epigastrium of the autosite, less commonly to the back.

ISCHIOPAGUS TWINS
Ischiopagus twins are twins fused in the ischial region.

JANICEPS TWINS
Janiceps twins are anteriorly fused twins with four arms, four legs, and a single head having faces front and back.

MONOCEPHALUS TWINS

Monocephalus twins are conjoined twins with a single head. The head may exhibit varying degrees of duplication, although the rest of the body is normal, or the entire body may be duplicated except the head.

MONOCEPHALUS DIPROSOPUS TWINS

Monocephalus diprosopus twins are conjoined twins with duplication of the face either complete or with one eye of each face fused with a common median orbit.

MONOCEPHALUS TETRAPUS DIBRACHIUS TWINS

Monocephalus tetrapus dibrachius twins are conjoined twins with a single head and trunk, two arms, partial or complete duplication of the pelvis, and four legs, the pair belonging to one member often being fused in a sirenomelous limb.

MONOCEPHALUS TRIPUS DIBRACHIUS TWINS

Monocephalus tripus dibrachius twins are conjoined twins with a single head and trunk, two arms, partial duplication of the pelvis, and a third median leg (variably developed).

OMPHALOANGIOPAGUS TWINS

Omphaloangiopagus twins are separate twins in which one twin has derived its blood supply from the vessels of the placenta or umbilical cord of the normal twin.

OMPHALOPAGUS TWINS

Omphalopagus twins are conjoined twins united at the umbilicus.
SYNONYM: *Monomphalus Twins.*

PYGOAMORPHUS TWINS

Pygoamorphus twins are conjoined twins in which the parasite is attached to the buttocks of the autosite. It is reduced to a formless mass or embryoma.

PYGODIDYMUS TWINS

Pygodidymus twins are conjoined twins fused in the cephalothoracic region but with doubled buttocks.

PYGOMELUS TWINS

Pygomelus twins are unequal conjoined twins in which the parasite is represented by a fleshy mass or a more fully developed limb attached to the sacral or coccygeal region of the autosite.

PYGOPAGUS TWINS

Pygopagus twins are twins joined back to back in the sacral region. External genitalia, bladder, and other organs of the pelvis are usually separate.

SYNCEPHALUS TWINS

Syncephalus twins are conjoined twins with four arms and four legs, but a single head. There is a single face and four ears, two on the back of the head. The cerebrum may be single or partially duplicated.

THORACOMELUS TWINS

Thoracomelus twins are unequal conjoined twins in which a single arm or leg, representing one fetus, is attached to the thorax of the other.

THORACOPAGUS TWINS

Thoracopagus twins are conjoined twins with fusion in or near the sternal area. The heart and liver may be separate or only partially duplicated.

THORACOPARACEPHALUS TWINS

Thoracoparacephalus twins are conjoined twins in which a parasite with a rudimentary head is attached to the thorax of the autosite.

THORADELPHUS TWINS

Thoradelphus twins are conjoined twins with one head, two arms, and four legs, the bodies being joined above the navel.

Genetics and Genetic Syndromes

ABDOMINAL MUSCLE DEFICIENCY SYNDROME
The abdominal muscle deficiency syndrome consists of partial or complete absence of abdominal musculature; hydroureter, hydronephrosis, and megabladder; undescended testes in males; and malrotation of the intestine. Deficiency or absence of the abdominal muscles includes the lateral groups, the transversus, and the obliques. The recti are often present. Symptoms more often pertain to the genitourinary tract or to one of the other many congenital abnormalities. These include pigeon breast deformity, spina bifida with myelomeningocele, hydrocephalus, congenital bladder-neck obstruction, bilateral hydroureter, urachus, and perhaps talipes. The clinical course is often complicated by episodes of infections that require antibiotics and possible surgery. Many of these patients have a low intelligence quotient and require chronic institutional care.

MODE OF INHERITANCE: Unknown.

SYNONYMS: *Prune Belly Syndrome, Triad Syndrome, Orbinsky's Syndrome.*

ABSENCE OF CENTRAL INCISORS
Absence of the central incisors is an abnormality of the teeth.

MODE OF INHERITANCE: Sex-linked.

ACANTHOCYTOSIS
Acanthocytosis is a disorder characterized by malformed, crenated erythrocytes, atypical retinitis pigmentosa, progressive ataxic neuropathy, and steatorrhea. The intestinal absorption of lipids is defective, and serum beta lipoprotein is absent.

MODE OF INHERITANCE: Probably autosomal recessive.

SYNONYMS: *Abetalipoproteinemia, Acanthrocytosis, Bassen-Kornzweig Syndrome.*

ACATALASIA
Acatalasia is an absence of catalase in the blood and other tissues. There are two main types: *Takahara's disease* (oral gangrene) and *Swiss variant* (asymptomatic). Affected individuals are liable to ulcerating lesions of the mouth, necrosis of the jaw, and loosening and loss of teeth. The disease is more common in the Far East. The specific defect is deficiency of catalase, the enzyme responsible for conversion of hydrogen peroxide into water and oxygen, in the erythrocytes and tissues.

Protection from hydrogen peroxide-producing hemolytic streptococci is reduced.

MODE OF INHERITANCE: Autosomal recessive.

ACHONDROPLASIA

Achondroplasia is a disorder of cartilage that begins prenatally, causing dwarfism. The chief features are the combination of a rather normal-sized trunk with short extremities. The proximal portions of the extremities are shorter than the distal parts, and the limbs are often curved. The head is usually large, with prominent forehead and flattening of the bridge of the nose. Lumbar lordosis is accented, and the gait is waddling. Intelligence is usually normal.

MODE OF INHERITANCE: Autosomal dominant in most cases.

SYNONYMS: *Chondrodystrophy, Kaufmann's Disease, Parrot-Kaufmann Syndrome, Achondrodysplasia, Chondrodysplasia, Chondrodystrophia Fetalis, Chondrogenesis Imperfecta, Fetal Achondroplasia, Osteochondrodystrophia Fetalis, Osteosclerosis Congenita, Parrot's Disease.*

ACROCEPHALOSYNDACTYLY

Acrocephalosyndactyly is a type of hereditary craniosynostosis characterized by acrocephaly, midface hypoplasia, exophthalmos, hypertelorism, ophthalmoplegia; syndactyly, broad distal thumb and toe; and mental deficiency.

MODE OF INHERITANCE: Autosomal dominant.

SYNONYMS: *Typical Apert's Syndrome, Acrocraniodysphalangia, Acrocephaly with Syndactyly, Acrodysplasia, Syndactylic Oxycephaly Syndrome, Apert's Syndrome.*

AFIBRINOGENEMIA

Afibrinogenemia is an abnormality in blood-clotting factors. There is no demonstrable fibrinogen in the plasma, and the blood does not coagulate, even after standing for several weeks. Severe bleeding often leads to death in childhood. In heterozygous individuals, there is occasionally a decrease in fibrinogen without clinical symptoms.

MODE OF INHERITANCE: Autosomal recessive.

AGAMMAGLOBULINEMIA

Agammaglobulinemia is a deficiency of immunoglobulins (γ G).

SYNONYMS: *Antibody Deficiency Syndrome, Hypogammaglobulinemia.*

Bruton's X-Linked Agammaglobulinemia

Bruton's X-linked agammaglobulinemia is characterized by a failure to develop antibodies following antigenic stimulation, and absence of gammaglobulin in the plasma. There is a great deficiency of plasma cells in the liver and lymph nodes. Susceptibility to bacterial infections is increased. The thymus is usually normal. Nearly all affected individuals are males.

MODE OF INHERITANCE: Sex-linked recessive.

SYNONYMS: *Congenital Agammaglobulinemia, Bruton's Disease.*

Congenital Aplasia of Thymus

Congenital aplasia of the thymus is characterized by congenital hypoparathyroidism, neonatal tetany, increased susceptibility to virus and fungus infections, and growth failure. Anomalies of the mouth, neck, and great vessels are present, as well as thymus aplasia.

MODE OF INHERITANCE: Autosomal recessive.

SYNONYM: *Di George's Syndrome.*

Swiss Type Agammaglobulinemia

Swiss type agammaglobulinemia is the absence of all primordial lymphoid tissue and the deficiency of all immunoglobulins: IgG, IgM, and IgA. It is characterized by persistent infection from early infancy due to bacterial, viral, or fungal pathogens, and also by thymic dysplasia, chronic diarrhea, wasting, runting, absence of tonsils, and failure to reject skin grafts.

MODE OF INHERITANCE: Autosomal recessive.

SYNONYMS: *Alymphocytosis, Thymic Alymphoplasia, Hereditary Thymic Dysplasia.*

Dysgammaglobulinemia

Dysgammaglobulinemia is a consistent deficiency of one or two of the three major immunoglobulins (IgG, IgM, IgA). It is characterized by recurrent pyogenic infections with normal or slightly reduced total gammaglobulins.

MODE OF INHERITANCE: Not clear.

ALBINISM

Albinism is a hereditary disorder of tyrosine metabolism resulting in the decrease or absence of melanin. The clinical features are absence of pigmentation, photophobia, nystagmus, and deaf mutism. There are several types of albinism: (1) complete; (2) incomplete—melanin present in the iris; (3) partial (piebald)—absence in scattered isolated areas of the melanin of skin and hair; (4) white forelock; (5) ocular—absence of melanin in retinal pigment epithelium only. The specific defect is the lack of tyrosinase, which is responsible for the formation of melanin from tyrosine.

MODE OF INHERITANCE: The complete and incomplete types are autosomal recessive. The partial and white forelock are autosomal dominant. The ocular is sex-linked recessive.

ALBRIGHT'S HEREDITARY OSTEODYSTROPHY

Albright's hereditary osteodystrophy is an example of lack of end-organ response to normal hormone production (parathyroid hormone). The clinical features are rounded face, short fourth metacarpal bones, obesity, hypocalcemia, soft tissue calcifications, mental retardation, short stature, and resistance to the effect of parathyroid hormone.

MODE OF INHERITANCE: Possibly X-linked dominant.

SYNONYM: *Pseudo-pseudohypoparathyroidism.*

ALKAPTONURIA

Alkaptonuria is a disorder of the metabolism of the amino acids phenylalanine and tyrosine. The clinical features are darkening of the urine caused by the presence of homogentisic acid, ochronosis, and arthritis. The specific defect is a deficiency of homogentisic acid oxidase.

MODE OF INHERITANCE: Autosomal recessive.

ALPORT'S SYNDROME

Alport's syndrome is characterized by hematuria that is usually present shortly after birth, deafness, and nephropathy. During the second decade, deafness that is usually mild becomes evident, and renal failure with hypertension may occur. Complications may include cataract, spherophakia, defective metabolism of amino acids, hypertensive states of pregnancy, and abortions (which occur in high incidence).

MODE OF INHERITANCE: Probably autosomal dominant. Expressivity is more pronounced in males.

SYNONYMS: *Dickinson's Syndrome, Congenital Hereditary Hematuria, Hematuric Familial Nephropathy, Hereditary Familial Congenital Hemorrhagic Nephritis, Hereditary Hematuria-Nephropathy-Deafness Syndrome, Hereditary Nephritis with Deafness.*

AMAUROTIC FAMILIAL IDIOCY

Amaurotic familial idiocy consists of several related forms of disorders of lipid metabolism resulting in accumulation of gangliosides in cells. There are two forms, infantile and juvenile. The infantile form is characterized by progressive loss of muscle strength, progressive blindness, mental deterioration to a state of complete idiocy, and the cherry-red spot in the macula. It occurs most often in Ashkenazi Jews and is usually fatal. In the juvenile form, there is a later onset and the disease progresses slowly. It does not occur predominantly among Jews.

MODE OF INHERITANCE: Autosomal recessive.

SYNONYMS: *Bielschowsky-Jansky Disease* (juvenile form), *Tay-Sachs Disease* (infantile form), *Ganglioside Lipidosis* (juvenile form), *Stock-Spielmeyer-Vogt Syndrome* (juvenile form).

AMELOGENESIS IMPERFECTA

Amelogenesis imperfecta is an abnormality of the teeth. There are two forms: the hypomaturation type and the hypoplastic type. In the hypomaturation type, the enamel is opaque, white, soft, and easily abraded, but it appears to be of normal thickness in unerupted teeth. In the hypoplastic type, the enamel is very hard but is abnormally thin so that the teeth appear small. The surface of the teeth is rough.

MODE OF INHERITANCE: The hypomaturation type is sex-linked recessive. The hypoplastic type is sex-linked dominant.

ANALBUMINEMIA

Analbuminemia is a disorder in which there is a decreased rate of albumin synthesis. There is slight peripheral edema, and the serum cholesterol is often elevated.

MODE OF INHERITANCE: Probably autosomal recessive.

SYNONYM: *Benhold's Disease.*

ANALPHALIPOPROTEINEMIA

Analphalipoproteinemia is the absence of alphalipoprotein. The clinical features are large, orange tonsils, hepatomegaly, splenomegaly, and enlarged lymph nodes. There is cholesterol ester storage in the reticuloendothelial tissues.

MODE OF INHERITANCE: Autosomal recessive.

SYNONYMS: *Tangier Disease, Fredrickson's Disease.*

ANENCEPHALY

Anencephaly is an embryologic axial central nervous system malformation, frequently associated with spina bifida. There is a congested hemorrhagic mass lying on top of the head, the cranial vault is absent, ganglion cells of the retina are absent, and there are other abnormalities. The sex ratio is one male to two females. The incidence of anencephaly varies with geographic distribution, social class (lower classes are more susceptible), season of the year, and parity (higher in first-born children).

ANHYDROTIC ECTODERMAL DYSPLASIA

Anhydrotic ectodermal dysplasia is characterized by aplasia or hypoplasia of sweat, mucous, and sebaceous glands, pilar structures, and tooth buds. The clinical features are high temperature, lack of perspiration, peg-shaped teeth, and alopecia.

MODE OF INHERITANCE: X-linked.

SYNONYM: *Congenital Anhydrotic Ectodermal Defect.*

ANKYLOBLEPHARON

Ankyloblepharon is a congenital fusion of the eyelids along their margins. It may be associated with microphthalmos or anophthalmos.

CAUSAL FACTORS: Probably genetically determined.

ANKYLOSING SPONDYLITIS

Ankylosing spondylitis consists of hardening of the joints of the spinal column and sacroiliac region with rigidity of the spine.

MODE OF INHERITANCE: Autosomal dominant with reduced penetrance in females.

SYNONYMS: *Bekhterev-Strümpell-Marie Syndrome, Bekhterev's Disease, Marie's Disease, Marie-Strümpell Disease, Pierre Marie's Disease, Ankylosing Polyarthritis, Atrophic Ligamentous Spondylitis, Atrophic Spondylitis, Bamboo Spine, Fibrositis Ankylopoietica Dorsi, Infectious Spondylitis, Juvenile-Adolescent Spondylitis, Ossifying Ligamentous Spondylitis, Pelvospondylitis Ossificans, Poker Back, Rheumatismal Ossifying Pelvospondylitis, Rheumatoid Spon-*

dylitis, Rhizomelic Spondylosis, Spondylarthritis An-
kylopoietica, Spondylitis Ankyloarthrica, Spondylitis
Adolescens, Spondylitis Atrophica Ligamentosa, Spondy-
litis Deformans, Spondylitis Ossificans Ligamentosa,
Syndesmitis Ossificans.

ANONYCHIA
Anonychia is congenital absence of the fingernails and toenails.

ANOPHTHALMOS
Anophthalmos is absence of the eyes. It is usually associated with abnormalities of the brain and may occur in the trisomy D (13-15) syndrome.

ANOSMIA
Anosmia is total absence of the sense of smell. There is agenesis of the olfactory lobes.

MODE OF INHERITANCE: Autosomal dominant.

APICAL DYSTROPHY
Apical dystrophy is congenital absence of the terminal portions of the second to fifth fingers.

MODE OF INHERITANCE: Autosomal dominant.

ARGININOSUCCINIC ACIDURIA
Argininosuccinic aciduria is a disorder of amino acid metabolism. The clinical features are severe mental retardation, general seizures, ataxia, short and brittle hair, cranial nerve palsies, liver disease, low blood argininosuccinic acid concentration, excretion of large amounts of argininosuccinic acid in the urine, and normal blood urea. The specific defect is probably an argininosuccinase deficiency in the brain and skin and blood cells.

MODE OF INHERITANCE: Autosomal recessive.

ARTHROGRYPOSIS MULTIPLEX CONGENITA
Arthrogryposis multiplex congenita is a syndrome of congenital contraction of joints. It is characterized by stiffness of one or more joints, with hypoplasia of the attached muscles, dislocation of the hip, and defects of the palate and vertebrae.

MODE OF INHERITANCE: Unknown.

SYNONYMS: *Guérin-Stern Syndrome, Otto's Syndrome, Rocher-Sheldon Syndrome, Rossi's Syndrome, Amyoplasia Congenita, Arthromyodysplasia Congenita, Congenital Amyoplasia, Congenital Arthromyodysplasic Syndrome, Congenital Contractures of the Extremities, Congenital Multiple Articular Rigidity, Multiple Congenital Contractures, Myodysplasia Fibrosa Multiplex, Myodysplasia Fetalis Deformans, Myodystrophia Congenita, Myodystrophia Fetalis Deformans, Neuroarthromyodysplasia, Pterygium Multiplex, Pterygium Universalis, Pterygoarthromyodysplasia Congenita.*

ASPHYXIATING THORACIC DYSTROPHY

Asphyxiating thoracic dystrophy is a skeletal dysplasia characterized by a small and immobile thorax, short ribs, poor air exchange, and repeated respiratory infections.

MODE OF INHERITANCE: Autosomal recessive.

SYNONYM: *Jeune's Syndrome.*

ATAXIA–TELANGIECTASIA

Ataxia-telangiectasia is a neurologic disorder characterized by cerebellar ataxia, familial oculocutaneous telangiectasia, hypogammaglobulinemia (IgA), susceptibility to respiratory and otic infections and to malignant neoplasia, small thymus, gonadal dysgenesis, mental retardation, and short stature. Death usually occurs in the second decade.

MODE OF INHERITANCE: Autosomal recessive.

SYNONYMS: *Louis-Bar's Syndrome, Boder-Sedgwick Syndrome, Ataxia Telangiectasica, Cephalo-oculocutaneous Telangiectasis.*

ATRESIA OF AUDITORY MEATUS

Atresia of the auditory meatus is the developmental failure of the earhole to open, usually with rudimentary auditory ossicles.

MODE OF INHERITANCE: Autosomal dominant.

ATRESIA OF EXTERNAL AUDITORY CANAL

Atresia of the external auditory canal is a condition arising from a failure of development of the first branchial groove with an ectopic development of mesoderm between the outer ectoderm lining and the inner endoderm. It is characterized by some degree of deformed pinna, or the pinna may be absent. Ossicles in the middle ear are maldeveloped with severe conductive deafness. The condition is usually unilateral.

ATRIAL SEPTAL DEFECT

Atrial septal defect is a congenital abnormality of the heart characterized by a defect of the septum separating the atria of the heart.

MODE OF INHERITANCE: Possibly polygenic.

BASAL CELL NEVUS SYNDROME

Basal cell nevus syndrome is characterized by multiple nevoid basal cell epitheliomas, jaw cysts, and bifid ribs. Scoliosis, agenesis of the corpus callosum milia, and broad nasal root may be part of the symptom complex. Sarcomatous degeneration of the tissues surrounding the jaw cysts is noted occasionally.

MODE OF INHERITANCE: Autosomal dominant.

SYNONYMS: *Gorlin's Syndrome, Gorlin-Goltz Syndrome, Nevoid Basal-Cell Carcinoma Syndrome.*

BENIGN FRUCTOSURIA

Benign fructosuria is a rare disorder of carbohydrate metabolism in which there is partial or complete failure to convert fructose to fructose-1-phosphate.

MODE OF INHERITANCE: Autosomal recessive.

BIEMOND'S ATAXIA

Biemond's ataxia is a disorder characterized by cerebellar ataxia, brachydactyly, and nystagmus. Some patients are mentally deficient.

MODE OF INHERITANCE: Autosomal dominant.

BLOOM'S SYNDROME

Bloom's syndrome is a form of dwarfism associated with malformations. The clinical features are telangiectatic erythema, molar hypoplasia, cutaneous photosensitivity, low birth weight after full-term gestation, and a predilection to malignant neoplasia. Chromosomal breakage appears in vitro.

MODE OF INHERITANCE: Autosomal recessive.

SYNONYMS: *Facial Telangiectases in Dwarfs, Bloom-Torre-Machacek Syndrome.*

BRACHYDACTYLY

There are five types of isolated brachydactyly.

Type A Brachydactyly

In type A brachydactyly, shortening is confined mainly to the middle phalanges.

MODE OF INHERITANCE: Autosomal dominant.

Type B Brachydactyly

In type B brachydactyly, middle phalanges are short, and the terminal phalanges are rudimentary or absent. Both fingers and toes are affected, and syndactylism may be present.

MODE OF INHERITANCE: Autosomal dominant.

Type C Brachydactyly

In type C brachydactyly, the characteristic deformities are shortening of the middle and proximal phalanges of the second and third fingers, and hypersegmentation of the proximal phalanx.

MODE OF INHERITANCE: Autosomal dominant.

Type D Brachydactyly

In type D brachydactyly, the terminal phalanges of the thumbs and big toes are short and broad.

MODE OF INHERITANCE: Autosomal dominant.

SYNONYM: *Stub Thumbs.*

Type E Brachydactyly

In type E brachydactyly, the metacarpals and metatarsals are short.

MODE OF INHERITANCE: Autosomal dominant.

SYNONYM: *Brachymetapody.*

CARPENTER'S SYNDROME

Carpenter's syndrome is a syndrome of inherited craniosynostosis. The clinical features are peculiar facies, craniosynostosis, midfacial hypoplasia, polydactyly, brachysyndactyly, obesity, mental retardation, short stature, and hypogenitalism.

MODE OF INHERITANCE: Autosomal recessive.

SYNONYM: *Acrocephalopolysyndactyly.*

CARTILAGE–HAIR HYPOPLASIA

Cartilage-hair hypoplasia is a bone and connective tissue dysplasia characterized by fine sparse hair, bowing of legs, wide irregular metaphyses, intestinal malabsorption, and short stature.

MODE OF INHERITANCE: Autosomal recessive.

CAT CRY SYNDROME

The cat cry syndrome is a congenital abnormality characterized by deletion of part of the short arm of a Group B chromosome (chromosome 5) (5p-). The syndrome is so named because of fancied resemblance of the infant's cry to the mewing of a cat. Mental retardation, characteristic facial appearance, abnormal dermal patterns, microcephaly, and dwarfism characterize this syndrome. The majority of patients are females.

SYNONYMS: *Cri Du Chat Syndrome, B₁ Deletion Syndrome.*

CAT EYE SYNDROME

The cat eye syndrome is a syndrome associated with an extra chromosome that is about half the size of those of the group 21-22. The clinical features are ocular hypertelorism, antimongoloid palpebral fissures, vertical coloboma of iris, preauricular fistula, and anal atresia. Some patients are mentally retarded.

CYTOGENETICS: Very small extra acrocentric chromosome.

SYNONYM: *Schmid-Fraccaro Syndrome.*

CEREBROHEPATORENAL SYNDROME

The cerebrohepatorenal syndrome is a rare, fatal, muscular disorder with associated multiple malformations. This syndrome is characterized by hypotonia, short stature, hepatomegaly, high forehead, flat facies, and death in early infancy.

MODE OF INHERITANCE: Probably autosomal recessive.

CHEDIAK–HIGASHI SYNDROME

The Chediak-Higashi syndrome is a form of oculocutaneous albinism associated with abnormal white blood cells. The clinical features include photophobia, decreased lacrimation, hyperhidrosis, and pigmentary disturbances consisting of partial albinism and excessive pigmentation of areas exposed to sunlight. Anemia, leukopenia, thrombocytopenia, lymphadenopathy, splenomegaly, and hepatomegaly are rather constant findings. Döhle inclusion bodies are found in the polymorphonuclear leukocytes. Inclusions that stain bright red are found in the myeloid cells of the bone marrow and in peripheral lymphocytes.

MODE OF INHERITANCE: Autosomal recessive.

SYNONYMS: *Anomalous Leukocytic Inclusions with Constitutional Stigmata, Béguez César-Steinbrinck-Chediak-Higashi Syndrome, Chediak's Anomaly, Chediak's Disease, Chediak-
Steinbrinck Anomaly.*

CHONDROHYPOPLASIA

Chondrohypoplasia is a mild form of achondroplasia. The proximal
bones such as the humerus and femur are strikingly short, and the pelvis
is reduced in all dimensions.

MODE OF INHERITANCE: Autosomal intermediate dominance.

SYNONYM: *Achondroplasia Tarda.*

CHRISTMAS DISEASE

Christmas disease is a hemorrhagic diathesis caused by an abnormality
of blood-clotting factors. It is similar to hemophilia but tends to be milder.
The specific defect is a deficiency of plasma thromboplastin component.
The diagnosis is suggested by abnormal results from prothrombin consumption tests.

MODE OF INHERITANCE: Sex-linked recessive.

SYNONYMS: *Hemophilia B, Deficiency of PTC Factor.*

CHRONIC BENIGN NEUTROPENIA

Chronic benign neutropenia is a disorder characterized by a decreased
white blood count with a striking diminution of neutrophils, hypergammaglobulinemia, and recurrent infection. There is a maturation arrest in
the bone marrow at the myelocyte or metamyelocyte stage.

MODE OF INHERITANCE: Autosomal dominant.

CITRULLINEMIA

Citrullinemia is a disorder of amino acid metabolism characterized by
mental retardation, increased citrulline in plasma and urine, and hyper-
ammonemia. The formation of argininosuccinic acid from citrulline probably is blocked.

MODE OF INHERITANCE: Unknown.

CLASSICAL HEMOPHILIA

Classical hemophilia is a hereditary hemorrhagic disorder, occurring
almost exclusively in males and transmitted through females. It is caused
by a deficiency of antihemophilic globulin (Factor VIII), which results
in a serious clotting defect.

MODE OF INHERITANCE: Sex-linked recessive.

CLEIDOCRANIAL DYSOSTOSIS

Cleidocranial dysostosis is a syndrome characterized by absence or
maldevelopment of clavicles, delayed ossification of the skull bones,
frontal bossing, and late eruption of the teeth.

MODE OF INHERITANCE: Autosomal dominant.

SYNONYMS: *Scheuthauer-Marie-Sainton Syndrome, Hultkrantz's Syndrome, Marie-Sainton Disease, Scheuthauer-Marie Syndrome, Dysostosis Cleidocranialis, Dysostosis Cleidocraniodigitalis, Dysostosis Cleiodocraniopelvina, Dysostosis Generalisata, Hereditary Cleidocranial Dysostosis, Mutational Dysostosis.*

COCKAYNE SYNDROME

The Cockayne syndrome is a syndrome of premature senility and associated malformations. The clinical features are dwarfism, diminished hair, senile appearance, photosensitivity, retinal degeneration, impaired hearing, and mental retardation.

MODE OF INHERITANCE: Autosomal recessive.

SYNONYMS: *Progeria-like Syndrome, Trisomy 10.*

COLOBOMA OF EYELID

Coloboma of the eyelid is a congenital notch of the eyelid. It may be an isolated defect or associated with other defects in the eye or elsewhere in the body. Ocular defects include dermoids, corneal opacities, and coloboma of the iris.

COMPLETE MONOCHROMATIC COLOR BLINDNESS

Complete monochromatic color blindness is characterized by photophobia, total color blindness, nystagmus, and diminished vision.

MODE OF INHERITANCE: X-linked.

CONGENITAL AGANGLIONIC MEGACOLON

Congenital aganglionic megacolon is characterized clinically by abdominal distention and increasingly severe constipation due to dysfunction of the distal colon. Abnormal peristaltic activity is caused by the absence of parasympathetic ganglion cells in the intramural plexus of the involved segment, which usually extends from the anus to the rectosigmoid. Sometimes there is involvement of the small and large bowel and megaloureter.

MODE OF INHERITANCE: Autosomal recessive.

SYNONYM: *Hirschsprung's Disease.*

CONGENITAL AMPUTATION

Congenital amputation is an abnormality characterized by the absence of one or more extremities or a portion thereof.

MODE OF INHERITANCE: Variable. It may be recessive, incomplete dominant, or dominant.

CONGENITAL DYSKERATOSIS SYNDROME

The congenital dyskeratosis syndrome is a disease characterized by cutaneous pigmentation, dystrophy of the nails, leukoplakia of the oral mucosa, continuous lacrimation due to atresia of the lacrimal ducts, often thrombocytopenia, anemia, and in most cases testicular atrophy.

MODE OF INHERITANCE: Sex-linked recessive, or possibly autosomal recessive.

SYNONYMS: *Zinsser-Engman-Cole Syndrome, Cole's Syndrome, Cole-Rauschkolb-Tommey Syndrome, Engman's Syndrome, Zinsser's Syndrome, Dyskeratosis Congenita.*

CONGENITAL ERYTHROPOIETIC PORPHYRIA

Congenital erythropoietic porphyria is an inborn error of porphyrin metabolism characterized by pink-red fluorescing urine, undue cutaneous sensitivity to light, red pigmented bones and teeth, hemolytic anemia, hypertrichosis, and splenomegaly. An enzymatic defect in the formation of porphyrin results in an excess of uroporphyrin I and coproporphyrin I in the urine and erythrocytes.

MODE OF INHERITANCE: Probably autosomal recessive.

SYNONYMS: *Congenital Photosensitive Porphyria, Günther's Disease, Hematoporphyria Congenita, Günther's Syndrome.*

CONGENITAL POIKILODERMA

Congenital poikiloderma is a rare hereditary condition characterized by erythema and edema of the skin followed by telangiectases, pigmentation, and atrophy. Sometimes there is alteration of hair growth and other abnormalities.

MODE OF INHERITANCE: Autosomal recessive.

SYNONYMS: *Rothmund-Thomson Syndrome, Bloch-Stauffer Dyshormonal Dermatosis, Rothmund's Dystrophy, Congenital Cutaneous Dystrophy, Congenital Poikiloderma-Juvenile Cataract Syndrome, Poikiloderma Congenitale, Telangiectasis-Pigmentation-Cataract Syndrome, Rothmund's Syndrome.*

CORNELIA DE LANGE SYNDROME

The Cornelia de Lange syndrome is a syndrome of obscure cause associated with the following abnormalities: low birth weight after full-term pregnancy; retarded osseous maturation; mental retardation; initial hypertonicity; microbrachycephaly; micrognathia; small nose with inverted nostrils; synophrys and long, curly eyelashes; ocular abnormalities; hirsutism; cutis marmorata; hypoplastic nipples and umbilicus; micromelia or phocomelia; syndactyly, oligodactyly, or clinodactyly; simian creases; and flexion contracture of the elbow. Most of those affected have diminished sucking and swallowing ability. Frequent vomiting results in aspiration pneumonia.

MODE OF INHERITANCE: Not clear.

SYNONYMS: *Brachman-de Lange Syndrome, Lange's Syndrome, Amsterdam Dwarf, Amsterdam Type, Status Degenerativus Amstelodamensis, Typus Degenerativus Amstelodamensis.*

CORONARY XANTHOMATOSIS

Coronary xanthomatosis is a disorder of the heart characterized by yellow deposits or nodules in the heart valves and the coronary arteries, resulting in angina pectoris.

MODE OF INHERITANCE: Autosomal dominant.

CRANIOFACIAL DYSOSTOSIS

Craniofacial dysostosis is a type of congenital craniostosis characterized by acrocephaly, maxillary hypoplasia, short upper and protruding lower lips, exophthalmos, hypertelorism, and a beak-shaped nose.

MODE OF INHERITANCE: Autosomal dominant.

SYNONYMS: *Crouzon's Disease, Dysostosis Craniofacialis, Dysostosis Craniofacialis Hereditaria, Dysostosis Cranio-orbitofacialis.*

CRANIOMETAPHYSEAL DYSPLASIA

Craniometaphyseal dysplasia is a rare skeletal disorder characterized by thickened skull bones, cranial nerve compression, flat nasal bridge, genu valgum, and metaphyseal flaring of the long bones.

MODE OF INHERITANCE: Autosomal recessive.

SYNONYMS: *Pyle's Disease, Bakwin-Krida Syndrome, Pyle-Cohen Disease, Familial Metaphyseal Dysplasia.*

CYSTATHIONINURIA

Cystathioninuria is a disorder of amino acid metabolism characterized by developmental retardation, severe mental deficiency, pituitary deficiency or excess, and increased cystathionine in the urine, plasma, cerebrospinal fluid, and tissues.

MODE OF INHERITANCE: Unknown.

CYSTIC FIBROSIS

Cystic fibrosis of the pancreas is a congenital disorder characterized by clinical evidence of celiac syndrome resulting from pancreatic exocrine deficiency and severe respiratory disease. There is decreased or absent secretion in the mucous glands of the salivary glands, intestine, pancreas, gallbladder, and other organs.

MODE OF INHERITANCE: Autosomal recessive.

DENTINOGENESIS IMPERFECTA

Dentinogenesis imperfecta is an abnormality in which the teeth have a peculiar opalescent, blue to brown color, and their crowns wear down readily. The primary defect is mesodermal, and both deciduous teeth and permanent teeth are affected.

MODE OF INHERITANCE: Autosomal dominant.

SYNONYMS: *Hereditary Opalescent Dentin, Capdepont's Syndrome, Capdepont-Hodge Syndrome, Fargin-Fayelle Syndrome, Stainton's Syndrome, Stainton-Capdepont Syndrome, Dentigenesis Hypoplastica Hereditaria, Hereditary Dark Teeth.*

DOMINANT TYPE METAPHYSEAL DYSOSTOSIS

Dominant type metaphyseal dysostosis is a disorder of bone and connective tissue which resembles achondroplasia. The clinical features are short stature, bowlegs, and extension deformities of the fingers.

MODE OF INHERITANCE: Autosomal dominant.

DOWN'S SYNDROME

Down's syndrome is a congenital abnormality characterized by the presence of an extra chromosome 21. The syndrome is caused by nondisjunction of chromosome 21 during parental gametogenesis and is usually associated with increased maternal age. The clinical features are hypotonia, epicanthic folds, Brushfield spots, a broad flat nose, mental retardation, protruding tongue, high-arched palate, anomalies of the dermal ridge pattern with a simian crease, often cardiac anomalies, and a predilection for acute leukemia.

CYTOGENETICS: Trisomy 21, 47 chromosomes (47 G+); 15/21 translocation, 46 chromosomes; 21/21 translocation, 46 chromosomes; 21/22 translocation, 46 chromosomes.

CARRIERS: Translocation of chromosome 21, 45 chromosomes. Partial trisomy 21 (mosaicism).

SYNONYMS: *Maternal Age Dependent Syndrome, Trisomy 21, Langdon Down Anomaly, Mongolism, Trisomy G, Trisomy 22.*

DUCHENNE'S MUSCULAR DYSTROPHY

Duchenne's muscular dystrophy is the most common form of muscular dystrophy in childhood. Certain muscle groups are enlarged (pseudohypertrophy); atrophic changes are noted in others. The involvement is usually symmetric. Creatine phosphokinase is usually increased in patients with the disease and in asymptomatic carriers. The onset is between 2 and 6 years of age, with rapidly progressive muscular weakness and disability. Death may occur by 15 years.

MODE OF INHERITANCE: Sex-linked recessive or autosomal recessive.

SYNONYMS: *Pseudohypertrophic Muscular Dystrophy, Childhood Muscular Dystrophy, Duchenne-Griesinger Disease, Progressive Muscular Atrophy of Childhood, Pseudohypertrophic Muscular Paralysis.*

DYSCHONDROSTEOSIS

Dyschondrosteosis is an inherited osteochondrodystrophy. In this disorder, the forearms and the lower legs are primarily involved; the proximal parts of the extremities tend to be normal. Madelung's deformity is usually present.

MODE OF INHERITANCE: Autosomal dominant.

SYNONYMS: *Leri-Weill Syndrome, Leri's Syndrome, Polytopic Enchondral Dysostosis.*

EHLERS–DANLOS SYNDROME

The Ehlers-Danlos syndrome is an abnormality of the collagen bundles in which the wickerwork is abnormally loose. This congenital dystrophic anomaly is characterized by hyperelasticity of the skin, hyperlaxity of the joints, subcutaneous tumors, and fragility of the skin and its blood vessels with faulty healing leading to papyraceous scar formation. The skin is excessively elastic, especially over the metacarpal, phalangeal, and large joints, and exceptionally thin and fragile over the entire body. Frequent injuries result in the formation of small pseudotumors composed of blood elements. There is an extreme laxity of the joints, most marked in the fingers and thumbs. Associated abnormalities may include dental defects, clubfeet, and rarely, cardiac anomalies. The condition has been reported in association with other disorders, such as lipomatosis, lymphangiectatic tumors, fibromas, tetralogy of Fallot, syringomyelia, muscular atrophy, and polycystic disease of the kidneys. Associated functional hypopituitarism and acromegaly have also been observed. The features of the syndrome that are first manifested in childhood persist throughout life, but the hyperelasticity of the skin and hyperlaxity of joints tend to decrease in the course of years.

MODE OF INHERITANCE: Autosomal dominant (intermediate dominance).

SYNONYMS: *Danlos' Syndrome, Cutis Hyperelastica Dermatorrhexis, Meekrin-Ehlers-Danlos Syndrome, Cutis Hyperelastica, Dermatorrhexis with Dermatochalasis and Arthrochalasis, Cutis Elastica, Elastic Skin, Fibrodysplasia Elastica, Fibrodysplasia Elastica Generalisata.*

ELLIPTOCYTOSIS

Elliptocytosis is a disorder characterized by the presence of oval or elliptic red blood cells. It usually is a benign condition, but some affected persons have a significant hemolytic anemia. The cause is unknown.

MODE OF INHERITANCE: Autosomal dominant (intermediate dominance).

SYNONYMS: *Ovalocytosis, Dresbach's Syndrome.*

ELLIS–VAN CREVELD SYNDROME

The Ellis-van Creveld syndrome is characterized by dwarfism, chondrodysplasia, ectodermal dysplasia, polydactyly, and congenital heart disease. The anomalies are varied. The long bones of the extremities from the trunk to the distal phalanges are short and thick, resembling the classic picture of achondroplasia. The proximal segments of the limbs tend to be more reduced in length than the distal portions. There may be supernumerary digits on the hands and sometimes on the feet. Other malformations such as talipes equinovarus and epispadias have been reported. In many instances, congenital heart lesions such as patent interventricular septum are present. Defects are seen in the nails, hair, and teeth, but the sweat glands and the skin are normal. There appear to be no mental abnormalities.

MODE OF INHERITANCE: Autosomal recessive.

SYNONYMS: *Chondroectodermal Dysplasia Syndrome, Ellis-van Creveld Disease.*

EPIDERMOLYSIS BULLOSA

Epidermolysis bullosa is a rare, often inherited, skin disturbance in which slight trauma leads to the development of bullae. It is most common on the extremities, but it may occur in any area subject to pressure or trauma. It is of variable severity, and the two principal categories are the simplex and dystrophic types. Either variety may be present at birth, may develop within a few days, or may not be evident for several months.

MODE OF INHERITANCE: Simple form, autosomal dominant; dystrophic form, autosomal recessive.

SYNONYMS: *Fox's Disease, Goldscheider's Disease, Köbner's Disease, Weber-Cockayne Syndrome, Acantholysis Bullosa, Acanthosis Bullosa, Bullous Recurrent Eruption, Dermatitis Bullosa Hereditaria, Dystrophia Bullosa Congenita, Epidermolysis Bullosa Hereditaria, Epidermolysis Dystrophica, Epidermolysis Hereditaria Tarda, Keratolysis Bullosa Hereditaria.*

ERYTHRYOPOIETIC PROTOPORPHYRIA

Erythropoietic protoporphyria is a relatively mild disorder of prophyrin metabolism characterized by itching, erythema, and edema following exposure to ultraviolet light. There is an increase in protoporphyrin and coproporphyrin in red blood cells and in the stool.

MODE OF INHERITANCE: Autosomal dominant.

FABRY'S DISEASE

Fabry's disease is a rare sex-linked lipidosis with onset in childhood or early adulthood. Symptoms usually begin with recurring attacks of fever, limb pain, abdominal pain, proteinuria or hematuria, and angiomatous skin lesions involving the lower trunk and thighs. Later, ankle edema appears and renal function worsens. Intracellular lipid deposits are formed in the autonomic nervous system. There is dystrophy of the corneal epithelium. Ceramide trihexoxidase has been found deficient in some affected individuals.

MODE OF INHERITANCE: X-linked.

SYNONYMS: *Fabry-Anderson Syndrome, Ruiter-Pompen Syndrome, Ruiter-Pompen-Wyers Syndrome, Sweeley-Klionsky Disease, ACD, Angiokeratoma Corporis Diffusum Universale, Angioma Corporis Diffusum Universale, Cardiovasorenal Syndrome, Diffuse Angiokeratosis, Glycolipid Lipidosis, Hereditary Dystropic Lipoidosis, Thesaurismosis Lipoidica, Thesaurismosis Hereditaria, Fabry's Syndrome.*

FACIOSCAPULOHUMERAL MUSCULAR DYSTROPHY

Facioscapulohumeral muscular dystrophy is a type of genetically determined primary myopathy. The onset is usually in the teens and is characterized by slowly progressive weakness of facial and shoulder muscles. Long remissions are common.

MODE OF INHERITANCE: Autosomal dominant.

SYNONYMS: *Landouzy-Déjerine Dystrophy, Facioscapulohumeral Progressive Muscular Dystrophy.*

FAMILIAL BLEPHAROPHIMOSIS

Familial blepharophimosis is a congenital shortening of the palpebral aperture, both horizontally and vertically. It is very rare as an isolated defect and usually occurs in association with epicanthus, inverted inner canthial fold, and ptosis, or with dwarfism or mongolism.

MODE OF INHERITANCE: Autosomal dominant.

FAMILIAL CYSTINURIA

Familial cystinuria is a metabolic disorder involving the renal transport of cystine, lysine, arginine, and ornithine, with recurrent cystine calculus formation. A specific transport system is missing in both kidney and intestine.

MODE OF INHERITANCE: There are two forms of the disease: autosomal recessive with the heterozygotes showing no urinary abnormalities, and autosomal recessive with the heterozygotes showing a moderate increase of cystine and lysine but no increase in arginine in the urine.

FAMILIAL GOITROUS HYPOTHYROIDISM

Familial goitrous hypothyroidism is a metabolic disorder due to an abnormality in the biosynthesis of thyroid hormone. Five separate forms have been described, four representing blocks in the synthesis of thyroid hormone and one caused by an abnormal iodoprotein in the peripheral blood. Affected individuals have goiters caused by increased activity and compensatory growth of the gland. Some people with an enzyme deficiency may develop a goiter without frank hypothyroidism.

FAMILIAL HYPOPHOSPHATEMIA

Familial hypophosphatemia is a disorder characterized by rickets resistant to large doses of vitamin D. Serum calcium levels are nearly always normal, but phosphorus is always low. Intestinal absorption of calcium is low, and there is suppressed renal tubular reabsorption of phosphorus. The cause of the disorder is not well understood.

MODE OF INHERITANCE: Sex-linked dominant with nearly complete penetrance.

SYNONYM: *Vitamin D–Resistant Rickets.*

FAMILIAL MICROCEPHALY

Familial microcephaly is a rare developmental lesion characterized by arrest of brain growth and an abnormally small head. It is accompanied by severe mental retardation.

MODE OF INHERITANCE: Autosomal recessive.

FAMILIAL PERIODIC PARALYSIS

Familial periodic paralysis is a disorder characterized by episodic muscular weakness or paralysis without loss of consciousness or sensory modalities. There are at least three types of disease: *hypokalemic periodic paralysis, hyperkalemic periodic paralysis (adynamia episodica hereditaria)*, and *normokalemic periodic paralysis*. The pathogenesis is not clear.

MODE OF INHERITANCE: Autosomal dominant, sometimes without complete penetrance. Males are more often affected than females.

SYNONYMS: *Westphal's Syndrome, Cavaré-Romberg Syndrome, Cavaré-Westphal Syndrome, Westphal's Neurosis, Familial Paroxysmal Paralysis, Intermittent Myoplegia, Paroxysmal Paralysis, Periodic Paralysis, Cavaré-Romberg-Westphal Syndrome.*

FANCONI'S ANEMIA

Fanconi's anemia is a familial disorder consisting of pancytopenia, bone marrow aplasia, and multiple congenital abnormalities, associated with a wide spectrum of symptoms, such as general purpura present at birth or shortly thereafter, brown patchy pigmentation, dwarfism, microcephaly, hypogonadism, cryptorchism, hypospadias, strabismus, microphthalmia, ptosis, epicanthal folds, nystagmus, deafness, ear deformity, syndactyly, Sprengel's deformity, bone defects of the radial sides of the forearm and hand, obesity, exaggerated tendon reflexes, mental retardation, cleft palate, and splenic atrophy. The hematologic symptoms include severe anemia, thrombocytopenia, and granulocytopenia.

MODE OF INHERITANCE: Autosomal recessive.

SYNONYMS: *Fanconi's Panmyelopathy, Fanconi's Refractory Anemia, Aplastic Anemia with Congenital Anomalies, Aplastic Infantile Funicular Myelosis, Congenital Pancytopenia, Congenital Aplastic Anemia, Familial Aplastic Anemia with Multiple Congenital Defects, Familial Constitutional Panmyelopathy.*

FARBER'S DISEASE

Farber's disease is a rare form of lipidosis, with onset in early life. Hoarse cry, subcutaneous nodules, arthropathy, irritability, nutritional failure, granulomatous lesions of the skin and viscera, central nervous system involvement, and an accumulation of ceramide and ganglioside intracellularly characterize this condition.

MODE OF INHERITANCE: Autosomal recessive.

SYNONYMS: *Disseminated Lipogranulomatosis, Farber's Syndrome, Farber-Uzman Syndrome, Lipogranulomatosis.*

FIBRODYSPLASIA OSSIFICANS MULTIPLEX PROGRESSIVA

Fibrodysplasia ossificans multiplex progressiva is a rare familial disorder in which the connective tissue of skeletal muscle, tendons, ligaments, and fasciae calcifies and ossifies. Other congenital anomalies such as polydactyly, microdactyly, absent teeth, and spina bifida may be present.

MODE OF INHERITANCE: Autosomal dominant.

SYNONYMS: *Myositis Ossificans Progressiva, Münchmeyer's Syndrome, Exostosis Luxurians, Fibrocellulitis Progressiva Ossificans, Fibrositis Ossificans, Hyperplasia Fascialis Ossificans, Hyperplasia Fascialis Progressiva, Myo-ossificatio Progressiva Multiplex, Myopathia Osteoplastica, Myositis Ossificans Multiplex Progressiva, Osteoma Multiplex Intermusculare, Polyossificatio Congenita Progressiva.*

FOCAL DERMAL HYPOPLASIA SYNDROME

Focal dermal hypoplasia syndrome is a congenital syndrome of atrophy and linear pigmentation of the skin with occasional papillomatoses, keratosis, and focal aplasia distributed chiefly on the trunk and limbs; multiple papillomatosis of the labial, oral, and anal mucosa and leukokeratosis of the oral mucosa; occasional alopecia of the scalp; thin dystrophic nails; hypoplasia of the dental enamel with microdontia and notching of the teeth; thin helix of the ear; coloboma of the iris and choroid with strabismus and microphthalmia; adactyly, syndactyly, or polydactyly; dysplasia of the clavicle; scoliosis; spina bifida; and frequent mental retardation. The syndrome almost always occurs in females.

MODE OF INHERITANCE: Autosomal dominant, sex-influenced.

SYNONYM: *Goltz-Gorlin Syndrome.*

FORNEY'S SYNDROME

Forney's syndrome is a rare familial form of congenital heart disease, skeletal defects, and deafness. The syndrome is characterized by freckling on the face and shoulders, fusion of the carpal and tarsal bones, deafness due to stapes defect, mitral insufficiency, and short stature.

MODE OF INHERITANCE: Probably autosomal dominant.

FRASER'S SYNDROME

Fraser's syndrome is a rare familial syndrome associated with craniofacial and gonadal anomalies, fusion of the eyelids, and abnormal auricles.

MODE OF INHERITANCE: Probably autosomal recessive.

FREEMAN–SHELDON SYNDROME

The Freeman-Sheldon syndrome is a rare muscular disorder characterized by a masklike "whistling face," hypoplastic ala nasi, and club feet.

MODE OF INHERITANCE: Probably autosomal dominant.

SYNONYM: *Whistling Face Syndrome, Craniocarpotarsal Dystrophy.*

GALACTOSEMIA

Galactosemia is a disorder of galactose metabolism caused by a deficiency of galactose-1-phosphate-uridyl transferase or galactokinase. The latter is a relatively benign condition characterized clinically by cataracts. Individuals with the transferase defect manifest hypoglycemia, vomiting and diarrhea, jaundice, hepatomegaly, splenomegaly, cataract formation, and aminoaciduria shortly after milk feedings are begun in the newborn period. Failure to thrive and mental retardation are common. Death occurs in undiagnosed patients when the enzyme deficiency is severe.

MODE OF INHERITANCE: Autosomal recessive.

GARDNER'S SYNDROME

Gardner's syndrome is characterized by cystic skin lesions, fibrous tissue tumors, and polyposes of the colon and sometimes stomach and small intestine. The colonic polyps frequently undergo malignant change.

MODE OF INHERITANCE: Autosomal dominant.

SYNONYMS: *Gardner-Bosch Syndrome, Hereditary Adenomatosis, Hereditary Polyposis and Osteomatosis, Intestinal Polyposis III.*

GAUCHER'S DISEASE

Gaucher's disease is a disorder of lipid metabolism characterized by the accumulation of glucocerebrosides in the reticuloendothelial cells. There are several different clinical patterns, but nearly all patients have hepatosplenomegaly, Gaucher cells in the bone marrow, and high serum acid phosphatase. The acute infantile type has cerebral involvement, and the course is rapidly progressive with early death. The chronic adult type without cerebral involvement is more common and may become evident at any age.

MODE OF INHERITANCE: Probably autosomal recessive, but some pedigrees are consistent with a dominant mode of inheritance, distinct predilection among Jews for the noncerebral chronic form.

SYNONYMS: *Gaucher-Schlagenhaufer Syndrome, Cerebroside Lipidosis, Familial Splenic Anemia.*

GENERAL GANGLIOSIDOSIS

General gangliosidosis is a rare familial lipidosis that resembles Hurler's disease. The onset is in early infancy. It is characterized by odd facies, visceromegaly, skeletal changes, central nervous system dysfunction, and death within 1 to 3 years. Foam cells can be found in the viscera, ganglioside (GM1) accumulates in the brain, and mucopolysaccharides are present in the viscera.

MODE OF INHERITANCE: Autosomal recessive.

SYNONYMS: *Norman-Landing Disease, Familial Neurovisceral Lipidosis, Pseudo-Hurler's Disease.*

GILBERT–LEREBOULLET SYNDROME

The Gilbert-Lereboullet syndrome is a benign familial disorder occurring in the absence of overt hemolysis and characterized by low-grade chronic hyperbilirubinemia with considerable daily fluctuations of the bilirubin level. Icterus may be detected shortly after birth or later in life. Asthenia, fatigue, anxiety, nausea, and abdominal pain occur in most cases, and may be precipitated by exercise, alcohol, or infection.

MODE OF INHERITANCE: Not clear, occurs predominantly in males.

SYNONYMS: *Gilbert's Disease, Meulengracht's Icterus, Cholemia Familiaris Simplex, Chronic Intermittent Juvenile Jaundice, Congenital Familial Cholemia, Constitutional Hepatic Dysfunction, Constitutional Hyperbilirubinemia, Familial Cholemia, Familial Nonhemolytic Jaundice, Hereditary Nonhemolytic Bilirubinemia, Hereditary Nonhemolytic Jaundice, Icterus Intermittens Juvenilis, Idiopathic Hyperbilirubinemia, Physiologic Cholemia.*

GLUCOSE–6–PHOSPHATE DEHYDROGENASE DEFICIENCY

Glucose-6-phosphate dehydrogenase deficiency is an enzyme defect of red blood cells that may present clinically as a drug-induced *acute hemolytic anemia* (primaquine sensitivity), *favism,* or *congenital nonspherocytic hemolytic anemia.* Many oxidant drugs such as antimalarials, sulfonamides, nitrofurans, and antipyritics cause hemolytic episodes in sensitive individuals. Glucose-6-phosphate dehydrogenase deficiency occurs in Negroes, Mediterranean races, and other ethnic groups. Many genetic variants have been described. It is estimated that about one-third of patients with congenital nonspherocytic hemolytic anemia have glucose-6-phosphate dehydrogenase deficiency.

MODE OF INHERITANCE: Sex-linked gene of partial dominance.

GLYCINEMIA WITH KETOSIS

Glycinemia with ketosis is a disorder of amino acid metabolism characterized by severe acidosis, ketonuria, mental and physical retardation, periodic thrombocytopenia and neutropenia, and an increased accumulation of glycine in the blood and urine. The specific defect is in the conversion of propionate to methylmalonate.

MODE OF INHERITANCE: Autosomal recessive.

GLYCOGEN STORAGE DISEASES

There are six types of glycogen storage diseases: hepatorenal glycogenosis, general glycogenosis, glycogenosis III, amylopectinosis, glycogenosis V, and glycogenosis VI.

Hepatorenal Glycogenosis

Hepatorenal glycogenosis is one of the glycogen storage diseases causing glycogen accumulation in the liver. It occurs in childhood and is characterized by stunted growth, hepatomegaly, yellowish skin, attacks of hypoglycemia, and possible glycogen infiltration of the renal tubules. The specific defect is a lack of glucose-6-phosphatase responsible for the conversion of glucose-6-phosphate into glucose and phosphate.

MODE OF INHERITANCE: Autosomal recessive.

SYNONYMS: *Von Gierke's Syndrome, Von Gierke-Van Creveld Syndrome, Glycogenosis I, Hepatonephromegalia Glycogenica, Liver Glycogen Disease.*

General Glycogenosis

In general glycogenosis, there are massive glycogen deposits in the cardiac muscle causing cardiac enlargement. Glycogen is also stored in the skeletal muscles. The specific defect is deficient activity of lysosomal alpha-1, 4-glucosidase. Clinical symptoms are related to impaired cardiac function and manifest themselves in the neonatal period. Death usually occurs within the first year of life.

MODE OF INHERITANCE: Autosomal recessive.

SYNONYMS: *Pompe's Disease, Cardiomegalia Glycogenica Diffusa, Congenital Rhabdomyoma of the Heart, Glycogen Heart Disease, Glycogenosis-Cardiac Syndrome, Rhabdomyomatosis Diffusa Cordis, Glycogenosis II.*

Glycogenosis III

In glycogenosis III, abnormal glycogen accumulates in the liver and muscles. The clinical manifestations are similar to those of type I but milder. Muscular weakness is usually present. The specific defect is deficiency of one or both of the two debranching enzymes (amylo-1, 4→1,4-transglucosidase and amylo-1,6-glucosidase).

MODE OF INHERITANCE: Autosomal recessive.

SYNONYMS: *Cori's Disease, Forbes' Disease, Debrancher Deficiency Limit Dextrinosis, Limit Dextrinosis, Glycogenosis of Liver and Muscle.*

Amylopectinosis

In amylopectinosis, an abnormal structured glycogen accumulates in the liver, kidney, spleen, muscle, and nervous tissue. Clinically, there is growth retardation, hepatosplenomegaly, cirrhosis, and ascites. The specific defect is a deficiency of the branching enzyme (amylo-1, 4→1,6-transglucosidase).

MODE OF INHERITANCE: Possibly autosomal recessive.

SYNONYMS: *Brancher Deficiency Amylopectinosis, Andersen's Disease, Glycogenosis IV.*

Glycogenosis V

In glycogenosis V, glycogen accumulation is limited to striated muscle. Clinical features are pain, stiffness, and extreme weakness of the muscles after exertion, marked tachycardia, and absence of hyperlacticacidemia after exercise. The specific defect is a deficiency of muscle phosphorylase.

SYNONYMS: *McArdle's Disease, McArdle-Schmid-Pearson Syndrome, Glycolysis Myopathy Syndrome, Glycometabolic Myopathy Syndrome, Myophosphorylase Deficiency Glycogenosis.*

Glycogenosis VI

In glycogenosis VI, glycogen accumulates in the liver. Clinical manifestations are mild and similar to those of type I. The specific defect is deficient liver phosphorylase enzyme.

MODE OF INHERITANCE: Sex-linked recessive.

SYNONYMS: *Hers' Disease, Hepatophosphorylase Deficiency Glycogenosis.*

GOLDENHAR'S SYNDROME

Goldenhar's syndrome is a rare familial malformation characterized predominantly by facial defects such as malformed ears, preauricular tags, and epibulbar dermoid or epidermoid malar hypoplasia.

MODE OF INHERITANCE: Unknown.

SYNONYMS: *Mandibulofacial Dysostosis with Epibulbar Dermoids, Oculoauricular Dysplasia, Oculoauriculovertebral Dysplasia.*

GREEN–RED COLOR BLINDNESS

Green-red color blindness is partial color blindness to red (protan disturbances) and green (deutan disturbances).

MODE OF INHERITANCE: X-linked recessive with partial manifestation in the heterozygotes.

SYNONYM: *Daltonism.*

HAGEMAN TRAIT

The Hageman trait is a disorder of blood coagulation with prolonged clotting time of venous blood. It is due to a deficiency of the Hageman Factor. Affected patients are free of significant bleeding difficulties.

MODE OF INHERITANCE: Autosomal recessive.

HALLERMANN–STREIF SYNDROME

The Hallermann-Streif syndrome is a syndrome consisting of birdlike facies, congenital cataract, microphthalmia, micrognathia, and hypotrichosis. The head has an abnormal shape, usually brachycephalic or scaphocephalic. The frontal and parietal bones may be enlarged, and the fontanels remain open. The cranial vault appears enlarged in proportion to the small face. Micrognathia is associated with thin lips and high-arched palate. The dental abnormalities may include absence of teeth, persistence of deciduous teeth, malocclusion with open bite, and premature caries. The ears are frequently set low. Nystagmus, strabismus, and other ocular abnormalities may be associated. No definite genetic correlation has been established.

MODE OF INHERITANCE: Probably autosomal dominant.

SYNONYMS: *François' Dyscephaly, Hallermann's Syndrome, Hallermann-Streif-François Syndrome, Ullrich and Fremerey-Dohna Syndrome, Dyscephalia Mandibulo-oculofacialis, Dyscephaly with Congenital Cataract and Hypotrichosis, Mandibulofacial Dysmorphia, Mandibulo-oculofacial Dysmorphism, Oculomandibulodyscephaly with Hypotrichosis.*

HARTNUP DISEASE

Hartnup disease is a disorder in which there is defective transport of tryptophan across the walls of the proximal tubules and across the intestinal walls, especially in the jejunum. Hartnup disease is characterized by constant gross aminoaciduria, attacks of a pellagra-like rash, episodes of cerebellar ataxia, an excess of indole metabolites in the gut, and psychiatric changes.

MODE OF INHERITANCE: Autosomal recessive.

SYNONYMS: *Hart's Syndrome, H Disease, Pellagra-Cerebellar Ataxia-Renal Aminoaciduria Syndrome.*

HEMERALOPIA

Hemeralopia is day blindness, the inability to see clearly in bright light. It is usually associated with color blindness.

MODE OF INHERITANCE: Autosomal recessive, sometimes sex-linked recessive.

HEMOCHROMATOSIS

Hemochromatosis is a disorder of iron metabolism resulting in increased absorption of iron from the intestine and subsequent deposition (as hemosiderin) in various organs. It is characterized by increased iron resorption, a high serum iron level, melanoderma, hepatomegaly, splenomegaly, diabetes mellitus, hypogenitalism, cardiac insufficiency, and hemosiderinuria.

MODE OF INHERITANCE: Autosomal intermediate dominance, sex-linked to males.

SYNONYMS: *Bronze Diabetes, Recklinghausen-Applebaum Disease, Pigmentary Cirrhosis.*

HEMOPHILIA A

Hemophilia A is a hereditary hemorrhagic disorder occurring almost exclusively in males and transmitted through females. It is characterized by a deficiency of antihemophilic globulin (Factor VIII).

MODE OF INHERITANCE: Sex-linked recessive.

HEPARINEMIA

Heparinemia is an oversecretion of heparin from the liver into the blood, with resultant bleeding.

MODE OF INHERITANCE: Autosomal recessive.

HEPATIC PORPHYRIA

Hepatic porphyria includes acute intermittent porphyria and porphyria cutanea tarda hereditaria.

Acute Intermittent Porphyria

Acute intermittent porphyria is characterized by acute attacks of abdominal pain and nervous manifestations including peripheral neuropathy, bulbar symptoms, psychosis, and autonomic disturbances. δ–Aminolevulinic acid and porphobilinogen are increased in the urine during attacks. Fecal coproporphyrin and protoporphyrin are normal.

MODE OF INHERITANCE: Autosomal dominant.

SYNONYM: *Swedish Form Porphyria.*

Porphyria Cutanea Tarda Hereditaria

Porphyria cutanea tarda hereditaria is characterized by cutaneous lesions, acute visceral and neurologic attacks, and continuous excretion of increased amounts of coproporphyrin and protoporphyrin in the feces.

MODE OF INHERITANCE: Autosomal dominant.

HEPATOLENTICULAR DEGENERATION

Hepatolenticular degeneration is a defect of copper metabolism resulting in an increased deposition of copper in the brain, liver, kidney, and cornea. The disease is characterized by cirrhosis of the liver, abnormal renal tubular function, a Kayser-Fleisher ring in the cornea, neurologic symptoms, ceruloplasmin deficiency, and low serum copper in most patients.

MODE OF INHERITANCE: Autosomal recessive.

SYNONYMS: *Wilson's Disease, Kinnier Wilson's Disease, Westphal-Strümpell Syndrome, Cerebral Pseudosclerosis, Hepato-cerebral Degeneration, Neurohepatic Degeneration, Progressive Lenticular Degeneration.*

HEREDITARY ANGIONEUROTIC EDEMA

Hereditary angioneurotic edema is characterized by acute noninflammatory swelling primarily involving skin, subcutaneous tissue, larynx, and gastrointestinal mucosa. It is due to a deficiency of the normal serum inhibitor of C'1 esterase. During an attack, levels of C'2 and C'4 complement components are reduced.

MODE OF INHERITANCE: Autosomal dominant.

SYNONYMS: *Bannister's Disease, Milton's Disease, Milton's Urticaria, Quincke's Disease, Acute Circumscribed Edema, Acute Essential Edema, Cutaneous Angioneurosis, Edema Cutis Circumscriptum, Giant Urticaria, Urticaria Gigantea, Urticaria Edematosa, Wandering Edema, Quincke's Edema.*

HEREDITARY CARDIOVASCULAR DYSPLASIA

Hereditary cardiovascular dysplasia is characterized by an enlarged heart, fibrosis of the myocardium, hypoplasia of the aorta, hypertrophy of the interventricular septum, and a bizarre arrangement of muscle fibers. The condition is associated with dyspnea and syncope.

MODE OF INHERITANCE: Autosomal dominant.

HEREDITARY FRUCTOSE INTOLERANCE

Hereditary fructose intolerance is a disorder caused by deficiency of fructose-1-phosphoaldolase and either deficiency or inhibition of fructose-1, 6-diphosphoaldolase. The condition is characterized by severe hypoglycemia and vomiting shortly after prolonged ingestion of fructose, failure to thrive, jaundice, hepatomegaly, albuminuria, and aminoaciduria. Cirrhosis and mental retardation may develop in untreated patients.

MODE OF INHERITANCE: Autosomal recessive.

HEREDITARY HEMORRHAGIC TELANGIECTASIA

Hereditary hemorrhagic telangiectasia is characterized by widespread telangiectases and angiomas on the fingertips, face, and mucous membranes of the nasopharynx and gastrointestinal tract. Bleeding is a major problem.

MODE OF INHERITANCE: Autosomal intermediate dominance.

SYNONYMS: *Rendu-Osler-Weber Disease, Osler's Disease (2), Osler's Syndrome, Babington's Disease, Goldstein's Hematemesis, Goldstein's Heredofamilial Angiomatosis, Rendu-Osler Syndrome, Angioma Hemorrhagicum Hereditaria, Familial Hemorrhagic Telangiectasia, Generalized Angiomatosis, Hereditary Epistaxis, Hereditary Familial Angiomatosis, Heredofamilial Angiomatosis, Multiple Hereditary Telangiectases with Recurrent Hemorrhage, Telangiectasia Hereditaria Hemorrhagica.*

HEREDITARY OPTIC ATROPHY

Hereditary optic atrophy is characterized by degeneration of the retina and papillomuscular bundle with loss of vision. Associated neurologic disturbances may be present.

MODE OF INHERITANCE: Uncertain, usually sex-linked recessive.

SYNONYMS: *Leber's Syndrome, Leber's Disease, Leber's Atrophy.*

HIDROTIC ECTODERMAL DYSPLASIAS

There are several varieties of hidrotic ectodermal dysplasia: Marshall type (autosomal dominant), Robinson type (autosomal dominant), Feinmesser type (probably autosomal recessive), pili torti and deafness (probably autosomal recessive), enamel hypoplasia and curly hair (autosomal dominant), Clouston type (autosomal dominant), and the Basan type (autosomal dominant). The clinical features are peg-shaped teeth, enamel hypoplasia, hypoplastic or dystrophic nails, smooth palms and soles, and deafness.

MODE OF INHERITANCE: Autosomal dominant or autosomal recessive.

HISTIDINEMIA

Histidinemia is a disorder of amino acid metabolism resulting in the accumulation of large amounts of histidine in the blood and urine. There may be no clinical manifestations, or there may be speech, mental, or developmental retardation. There is a deficiency of histidase, which is responsible for the conversion of histidine to urocanic acid.

MODE OF INHERITANCE: Autosomal recessive.

HOLT–ORAM SYNDROME

The Holt-Oram syndrome is characterized by congenital heart disease (septal defects), narrow shoulders, and defects of the proximal upper extremities, especially the thumb and radius.

MODE OF INHERITANCE: Autosomal dominant.

SYNONYMS: *Atriodigital Dysplasia, Atrioextremital Dysplasia, Upper Limb Cardiovascular Syndrome.*

HOMOCYSTINURIA

Homocystinuria is an inborn error of metabolism in which homocystine is excreted in the urine in large quantities. The condition is characterized by dilatation of the aorta and pulmonary artery, intravascular thrombosis, malar flush, subluxation of the lens, cataracts, osteoporosis, and mental retardation. The specific defect is a cystathionine synthetase deficiency.

MODE OF INHERITANCE: Autosomal recessive.

HUNTINGTON'S CHOREA

Huntington's chorea is a degenerative disease characterized by choreic movements and progressive mental deterioration. The age of onset is variable.

MODE OF INHERITANCE: Autosomal dominant.

SYNONYMS: *Lund-Huntington Chorea, Chorea Chronica Progressiva Hereditaria, Chorea Progressiva Hereditaria, Degenerative Chorea, Hereditary Chorea, Microcellular Striatal Syndrome.*

HYPERPROLINEMIA

Hyperprolinemia is a disorder of amino acid metabolism characterized by elevated plasma proline and by an aminoaciduria of proline, hydroxyproline, and glycine. It apparently can be caused by a deficiency of proline oxidase or pyrroline-5-carboxylate dehydrogenase.

MODE OF INHERITANCE: Unknown.

HYPOGONADOTROPIC HYPOGONADISM WITH ANOSMIA

Hypogonadotropic hypogonadism with anosmia is a disease in which affected males show anosmia and hypogonadism secondary to low gonadotropin production. Carrier females have partial or complete anosmia. The anosmia is due to agenesis of the olfactory lobes.

MODE OF INHERITANCE: Probably sex-linked dominant.

SYNONYMS: *Kallmann Syndrome, Dysplasia Olfactogenitalis.*

HYPOPHOSPHATASIA

Hypophosphatasia is an inborn error of metabolism due to an absence or decrease in alkaline phosphatase activity. The clinical features vary widely, but spontaneous shedding of teeth and skeletal abnormalities resembling rickets are common. Affected individuals excrete increased amounts of phosphorylethanolamine in their urine.

MODE OF INHERITANCE: Autosomal recessive.

SYNONYM: *Rathbun Syndrome.*

HYPOPROCONVERTINEMIA

Hypoproconvertinemia is a disorder of blood coagulation characterized by an absence of Factor VII, which is required for conversion of pro-thrombin to thrombin.

MODE OF INHERITANCE: Autosomal recessive.

SYNONYM: *Deficiency of Stable Factor.*

ICHTHYOSIS VULGARIS

Ichthyosis vulgaris occurs in autosomal dominant and sex-linked forms. The sex-linked form usually appears during the first three months of life, and the skin changes resemble the "collodion baby." Thick, large, grayish scales appear that are most common on the neck, abdomen, legs, and popliteal fossae. Deep corneal opacities are visible on slit-lamp examination. Autosomal ichthyosis vulgaris is the more common form and is seldom seen before the age of three months. It is characterized by a family history of atopy, keratosis pilaris, and increased markings on the palms and soles.

MODE OF INHERITANCE: Sex-linked recessive; autosomal dominant.

IDIOPATHIC FAMILIAL HYPERLIPEMIA

Idiopathic familial hyperlipemia is a rare disorder of lipid metabolism characterized by a striking increase in plasma lipids. The most common type is induced by high fat content in the diet; another type is carbo-hydrate-induced. Some patients have bouts of fever, acute abdominal pain, hepatosplenomegaly, and eruption xanthomas with hyperlipemia.

MODE OF INHERITANCE: Not definitely known, but males are princi-pally affected.

SYNONYMS: *Burger-Grütz Syndrome, Essential Familial Hyperlipemia, Familial Hyperchylomicronemia, Familial Hyperlipopro-teinemia 1, Fat-Induced Hyperlipemia, Hepatosplenomeg-alic Lipoidosis, Hypercholesterinemic Xanthomatosis, Idiopathic Lipoidosis, Retention Hyperlipemia.*

IMIDAZOLE AMINOACIDURIA

Imidazole aminoaciduria is a disorder of amino acid metabolism, char-acterized by cerebral degeneration and blindness. Large amounts of anserine, carnosine, and histidine are excreted in the urine.

MODE OF INHERITANCE: Unknown.

SYNONYMS: *Imidazole Syndrome, Bessman-Baldwin Syndrome.*

INCONTINENTIA PIGMENTI

Incontinentia pigmenti is a congenital disorder characterized by bizarre skin lesions and multiple defects of ectodermal and mesodermal origin. It is found mainly in females. Affected persons have pigmented macules that assume unusual patterns such as whorls, streaks, lines, patches, and spidery forms. Skeletal malformations, seizures, retardation, strabismus, corneal opacities, dental defects, and patchy alopecia are also found.

MODE OF INHERITANCE: Autosomal dominant, sex-influenced.

SYNONYMS: *Bloch-Sulzberger Syndrome, Bloch-Siemens Syndrome, Bloch-Sulzberger Incontinentia Pigmenti, Bloch-Sulzberger Melanoblastosis, Siemens-Bloch Pigmented Dermatosis, Melanoblastosis Cutis Linearis Sive Systematisata, Melanosis Corii Degenerativa, Nevus Pigmentosus Systematicus.*

INFANTILE LETHAL AGRANULOCYTOSIS

Infantile lethal agranulocytosis is characterized by the total absence or marked reduction of neutrophils in young infants who have severe pyogenic infections. It is fatal; the basic defect is not known.

MODE OF INHERITANCE: Autosomal recessive.

KARTAGENER'S SYNDROME

Kartagener's syndrome is a triad that consists of dextrocardia, sinusitis, and bronchiectasis.

MODE OF INHERITANCE: Probably recessive with incomplete penetrance.

SYNONYM: *Sinusitis-Bronchiectasis-Situs Inversus Syndrome.*

KLEIN–WAARDENBURG SYNDROME

The Klein-Waardenburg syndrome is characterized by developmental anomalies of the eyelids, eyebrows, or nose root; pigmentary anomalies of the iris and head hair; and congenital deafness. Although the most serious defect in this syndrome is congenital deafness, it is seldom accepted or mentioned by the patient. Dystopia canthorum is the most conspicuous feature. This displaced palpebral angle is readily apparent, especially in childhood. Other frequently observed anomalies consist of lateral displacement of the medial canthi and lacrimal points; a hyperplastic, broad, high nasal root; hyperplasia of the medial portions of the eyebrows; partial or total heterochromia iridis; and partial, unilateral circumscribed albinism of the frontal head hair (white forelock). There may be blepharophimosis rather than ptosis, hypoplasia of the carunale and of the plica semilunaris, displacement of the puncta, especially the lower, laterally toward the cornea, and a widened interpupillary distance. Occasionally, other anomalies may be present, such as limitation of ocular movements, underdevelopment of the orbit, thickening of the tarsus, epicanthus, and such general defects as brachycephaly.

MODE OF INHERITANCE: Autosomal dominant with variable manifestations.

SYNONYMS: *Klein's Syndrome, van der Hoeve-Halbertsma-Waardenburg Syndrome, van der Hoeve-Waardenburg-Gualdi*

Syndrome, Waardenburg's Syndrome, Dystopia Canthia
Medialis Lateroversa, Embryonic Fixation Syndrome, Pto-
sis-Epicanthus Syndrome.

KLINEFELTER'S SYNDROME

Klinefelter's syndrome, which occurs in the male, is characterized by
small testes of firm consistency, spermatogenic failure with normal or
impaired Leydig cell function, gynecomastia, and high urinary follicle-
stimulating hormone levels. In its true form, this syndrome is a type of
gonadal dysgenesis and is associated with a chromosomal aberration.
Most of these persons are sex chromatin-positive and on chromosomal
analysis have 47 chromosomes with an XXY karyotype. Other patterns
of chromosomal aberration may be present such as XXXXY, XXYY,
XXXY, and a variety of mosaic patterns. Some patients with the clinical
manifestations of this condition are sex chromatin-negative with an XY
karyotype; they are sometimes referred to as "sex chromatin-negative
Klinefelter" patients. It is not known at present whether these also have
a genetic defect or if the disorder results from a postnatal testicular lesion.

SYNONYMS: *Klinefelter-Reifenstein-Albright Syndrome, Gynecomastia-
Aspermatogenesis Syndrome, XXY Sex Chromosome Constitution, Seminiferous Tubule Dysgenesis.*

KLIPPEL–FEIL SYNDROME

The Klippel-Feil syndrome is characterized by multiple hemivertebrae,
a decreased number of cervical vertebrae, spina bifida, platybasia, scoliosis, torticollis, Sprengel's deformity, short neck, and a low hairline.

MODE OF INHERITANCE: Not clear, but probably dominant with reduced penetrance and variable expression.

SYNONYMS: *Brevicollis, Congenital Webbed-Neck Syndrome, Congenital Synostosis of Cervicothoracic Vertebrae, Congenital
Osseous-Torticollis Syndrome.*

LARSEN'S SYNDROME

Larsen's syndrome is a syndrome of flattened facies, with prominent
forehead, depressed nasal bridge, and wide-spaced eyes; bilateral dislocation of the elbows, hips, and knees; talipes equinovalgus or equinovarus; cylindrical fingers that do not taper normally; occasionally cleft
palate or other palate abnormalities; and occasionally an associated
failure of spinal segmentation.

MODE OF INHERITANCE: Probably autosomal recessive.

LAURENCE–MOON–BIEDL SYNDROME

The Laurence-Moon-Biedl syndrome is an autosomal recessive congenital disorder of childhood characterized by obesity, retinal degeneration, genital hypoplasia, polydactylism, and mental retardation. The
complete syndrome is seldom observed in the same individual, but the
characteristics are often scattered among the siblings of one family or
generation. Members of these families have an increased number of abor-

tions and early deaths. In addition to the cardinal features, acrocephaly, syndactyly, dwarfism, atresia ani, deafness, mongolian facies, and dental anomalies may be present. The ophthalmic abnormalities are numerous. Retinal degeneration with varying degrees of pigmentary changes is the chief ocular defect. Microphthalmos, cataracts, macular atrophy, convergent strabismus, hemeralopia, and nystagmus may be present. If the patient reaches adulthood, there may be an absence of body hair and other physical signs of anterior pituitary deficiency. Underdevelopment of the breasts and amenorrhea are present in the female; pseudogynecomastia, impotence, aleydigism, and azoospermia are present in the male.

SYNONYMS: *Laurence-Moon Syndrome, Biedl-Bardet Syndrome, Laurence-Moon-Bardet-Biedl Syndrome.*

LEIGH'S ENCEPHALOMYELOPATHY

Leigh's encephalomyelopathy is a progressive encephalopathy of early childhood characterized by a failure to thrive, progressive mental retardation, seizures, respiratory difficulty, symmetric necrosis of the basal ganglia and brainstem, acidosis, hyperlactacidemia, pyruvemia, and death. The specific defect is a deficiency of pyruvic acid carboxylase, an enzyme that converts pyruvic acid to oxaloacetic acid.

MODE OF INHERITANCE: Autosomal recessive.

SYNONYMS: *Pyruvic Acid Carboxylase Deficiency, Infantile Subacute Necrotizing Encephalomyelopathy.*

LEPRECHAUNISM

Leprechaunism is a congenital disorder manifested by extreme growth retardation and emaciation. The clinical features are large, low-set ears, negroid facies, large hands and feet, enlarged phallus, and hirsutism.

MODE OF INHERITANCE: Autosomal recessive.

SYNONYM: *Donohue's Syndrome.*

LERI'S PLEONOSTEOSIS

Leri's pleonosteosis is characterized by a broad thumb in the valgus position, flexion deformity of the fingers, and mongoloid slanting of the palpebral fissures.

MODE OF INHERITANCE: Autosomal dominant.

SYNONYM: *Pleonosteosis Familiaris.*

LESCH–NYHAN SYNDROME

The Lesch-Nyhan syndrome is a disorder of purine metabolism characterized by mental retardation, choreoathetoid movements, muscle spasticity, self-mutilation, and the overproduction of uric acid. The specific defect is a hypoxanthine-guanine phosphoribosyltransferase deficiency.

MODE OF INHERITANCE: X-linked, female carriers have two populations of cells.

LIMB–GIRDLE MUSCULAR DYSTROPHY

Limb-girdle muscular dystrophy is a type of genetically determined primary myopathy with onset at about the age of puberty. Weakness ordinarily involves the pelvic girdle and less frequently the shoulder girdle. The disease is less severe and less rapidly progressive than the Duchenne type, but eventually causes disablement and death.

MODE OF INHERITANCE: Autosomal recessive.

LIPODYSTROPHY OF BERARDINELLI

Lipodystrophy of Berardinelli is characterized by complete loss of adipose tissue. The clinical features are increased height, hepatomegaly, hirsutism, phallic hypertrophy, muscular hypertrophy, insulin-resistant hyperglycemia, hyperlipemia, and anatomic functional disturbances of the central nervous system.

MODE OF INHERITANCE: Autosomal recessive.

SYNONYMS: *Lipodystrophia Totalis, Seip's Syndrome, Total Lipodystrophy and Acromegaloid Gigantism.*

LOWE'S SYNDROME

Lowe's syndrome is a rare, familial renal tubular dysfunction syndrome. The clinical features are glaucoma, aminoaciduria, organic aciduria, decreased renal ammonia production, cataracts, mental retardation, rickets, and hypotonia.

MODE OF INHERITANCE: Sex-linked, partially dominant. Female carriers may have lenticular opacities.

SYNONYMS: *Oculocerebrorenal Dystrophy, Lowe-Terry-MacLachlan Syndrome.*

MAFFUCCI'S SYNDROME

Maffucci's syndrome is a rare form of skeletal malformation characterized by enchondromas and cavernous hemangiomas.

MODE OF INHERITANCE: Unknown.

SYNONYMS: *Dyschondroplasia with Hemangiomas, Chondrodystrophy and Vascular Hamartoma, Kast's Syndrome, Maffucci-Kast Syndrome, Chondrodysplasia-Angiomatosis Syndrome, Chondrodysplasia-Hemangioma Syndrome, Cutaneous Dyschondroplasia-Dyschromia Syndrome, Dyschondrodysplasia-Angiomatosis Syndrome.*

MALE TURNER'S SYNDROME

The male Turner's syndrome is a syndrome of congenital malformations. These malformations resemble those found in females with Turner's syndrome. The clinical features are webbed neck, hypertelorism, pectus excavatum, pulmonic stenosis, cryptorchidism, and short stature. There usually is no chromosomal abnormality associated with this syndrome.

MODE OF INHERITANCE: Unknown.

SYNONYMS: *Noonan's Syndrome, Pseudo-Turner's Syndrome.*

MAPLE SYRUP URINE DISEASE

Maple syrup urine disease is a disorder of amino acid metabolism. This disease occurs in newborn infants and is characterized by failure to thrive, vomiting, muscular hypertonicity, mental retardation, and a maple syrup-like odor of the urine. The specific defects include failure of oxidative decarboxylation of alpha keto derivatives of certain amino acids, such as leucine, isoleucine, and valine.

MODE OF INHERITANCE: Probably autosomal recessive.

SYNONYMS: *Branched Chain Ketoaciduria, Maple Sugar Urine Disease.*

MARCHESANI'S SYNDROME

Marchesani's syndrome is characterized by short stature, brachydactyly, and spherophakia with associated myopia and glaucoma. The dwarfism is frequently accompanied by short neck, low forehead, short extremities, and stubby, thickened hands, fingers, and toes. Body build tends to be stocky with broad chest and heavy musculature. In addition to the characteristic ocular defects, there may be iridodonesis, subluxation, and blindness.

MODE OF INHERITANCE: Autosomal recessive.

SYNONYMS: *Weil-Marchesani Syndrome, Weill-Marchesani Syndrome, Brachymorphism and Ectopia Lentis, Dysmorphodystrophia Mesodermalis Congenita, Inverted Marfan's Syndrome, Spherophakia-Brachymorphia Syndrome.*

MARFAN'S SYNDROME

Marfan's syndrome is a mesodermal dystrophy. The clinical features are tall stature, arachnodactyly, flaccid muscles, ectopia lentis, hyperextensible joints, cardiac hypertrophy, and aortic medionecrosis or aneurysm. There is an increased excretion of hydroxyprolin in the urine. There is metachromasia in cultured fibroblasts due to a striking increase in hyaluronic acid content.

MODE OF INHERITANCE: Autosomal dominant.

SYNONYMS: *Marfan's Abiotrophy, Marfan-Achard Syndrome, Acrochondrohyperplasia, Arachnodactyly, Congenital Mesodermal Dystrophy, Dolichostenomelia, Hyperchondroplasia, Spider Fingers.*

MARINESCO–SJÖGREN SYNDROME

The Marinesco-Sjögren syndrome is a rare neurologic disorder characterized by cerebellar ataxia, hypotonia, cataracts, sparse hair, mental retardation, and short stature.

MODE OF INHERITANCE: Autosomal recessive.

SYNONYMS: *Marinesco-Garland Syndrome, Torsten Sjögren's Syndrome, Cataract-Oligophrenia Syndrome.*

MENKES' SYNDROME

Menkes' syndrome is a rare neurologic disorder characterized by progressive cerebral deterioration, seizures, brittle stubby hair, short stature, and mental retardation.

MODE OF INHERITANCE: Sex-linked recessive.

METATROPIC DWARFISM

Metatropic dwarfism is a rare form of dwarfism characterized by severe kyphoscoliosis, flattened vertebrae, short extremities, and metaphyseal flare.

MODE OF INHERITANCE: Autosomal recessive.

METHYLMALONIC ACIDEMIA

Methylmalonic acidemia is a disorder of amino acid metabolism caused by a deficiency of the specific isomerase that converts methylmalonic acid to succinic acid. The clinical features are failure to thrive, metabolic acidosis, episodes of vomiting, hypoglycemia and ketosis, and increased methylmalonic acid in the plasma and urine.

MODE OF INHERITANCE: Autosomal recessive.

MICROPHTHALMOS

Microphthalmos is a failure of the globe of the eye to develop to its normal size. It varies in degree and may involve one or both eyes. It is often accompanied by other conditions such as coloboma, cataracts, and aniridia.

MODE OF INHERITANCE: Usually autosomal recessive but may be dominant.

MICROPOLYGYRIA

Micropolygyria is a malformation of the cerebral cortex characterized by broad irregular gyri, with the gray matter extending deep into the brain substance. The clinical features are mental deficiency, epilepsy, and cerebral diplegia and hemiplegia.

MIETEN'S SYNDROME

Mieten's syndrome is a rare congenital malformation characterized by corneal opacities, narrow nose, flexion contracture of the elbow, mental retardation, and dwarfism.

MODE OF INHERITANCE: Probably autosomal recessive.

MOHR'S SYNDROME

Mohr's syndrome is a rare congenital malformation characterized by polydactyly, syndactyly, and brachydactyly, high-arched palate, cleft tongue, supernumerary sutures in the skull, and conductive hearing loss.

MODE OF INHERITANCE: Probably autosomal recessive.

MUCOPOLYSACCHARIDOSIS

Mucopolysaccharidosis is a disorder of mucopolysaccharide metabolism. There are six syndromes associated with this disease: Hurler's syndrome, Hunter's syndrome, Sanfilippo's syndrome, Morquio's disease, Scheie's syndrome, and Maroteaux-Lamy syndrome.

Hurler's Syndrome

Hurler's syndrome is a systemic mucopolysaccharidosis marked by progressive physical and mental deterioration leading to death before the age of ten years. The onset follows a few months of normal growth. The early symptoms include lumbar gibbus, stiff joints, and rhinitis. Dwarfism, hepatosplenomegaly due to deposits of mucopolysaccharides in the liver and spleen, gargoyloid facies, noisy breathing, and respiratory infection appear later. Mental retardation becomes evident during the second year of life. The cornea is usually clear at birth, but shortly thereafter it becomes cloudy with an accumulation of gray punctate opacities in the substantia propria, often masking coexisting retinal degeneration. Mucopolysaccharide deposits in the coronary arteries and heart valves may lead to congestive heart failure. Hydrocephalus with a large head and prominent scalp veins, hypertelorism, flat nasal bridge, snub nose, wide nostrils, large lips, and prominent tongue give the face a peculiar, coarse appearance. Contractures; clawhand; furrowed, thick skin; lanugo; short neck; absence of sexual maturation in spite of apparently normal genitalia; small or peg-shaped teeth; malocclusion; broad stubby fingers; vertebral and skeletal abnormalities including kyphosis, genu valgum, coxa valga, pes planus, pes equinovarus, and funnel chest; congenital heart defects; nasal congestion; and several other defects may be present.

MODE OF INHERITANCE: Autosomal recessive.

SYNONYM: *Mucopolysaccharidosis I.*

ABBREVIATION: MPS type I.

Hunter's Syndrome

Hunter's syndrome is similar to Hurler's syndrome in many respects, except that gibbus and corneal clouding are absent and the symptoms are generally milder, although corneal opacities may appear later in life. Retinitis pigmentosa, nodular skin lesions, hypertrichosis, papilledema, optic atrophy, progressive deafness, and pulmonary hypertension may be present. Death, usually from congestive heart failure, occurs during the third or fourth decade.

MODE OF INHERITANCE: Sex-linked.

SYNONYM: *Mucopolysaccharidosis II.*

ABBREVIATION: MPS type II.

Sanfilippo's Syndrome

Sanfilippo's syndrome is a systemic form of mucopolysaccharidosis characterized by severe progressive mental retardation associated with mild forms of dwarfism, stiff joints, skeletal defects, and hepatosplenomegaly. Excessive amounts of heparitin sulfate are found in the urine, and mild corneal opacities may be seen.

MODE OF INHERITANCE: Autosomal recessive.

SYNONYMS: *Heparitinuria, Mucopolysaccharidosis III.*

ABBREVIATION: MPS type III.

Morquio's Disease

Morquio's disease is a systemic mucopolysaccharidosis marked by early dwarfism followed, at the time the infant begins to walk, by vertebra plana, fusion of the cervical vertebrae, platybasia, enlarged wrists, disproportionately long arms, genu valgum, flat feet, waddling gait, flaccid muscles, barrel chest, pigeon breast, short neck, prominent abdomen, and peculiar facies characterized by a wide mouth, protruding maxilla, and short nose. The teeth are usually widely spaced and have thin and flaky enamel. All patients excrete large amounts of keratosulfate in the urine, and some excrete chondroitin sulfate A in the urine. The eponym *Morquio-Ullrich syndrome* has been used to designate the disease in which, in addition to the skeletal changes, there is corneal opacity; Morquio's disease applies to the variant without corneal changes.

MODE OF INHERITANCE: Autosomal dominant.

SYNONYMS: *Brailsford-Morquio Syndrome, Morquio's Syndrome, Atypical Chondrodystrophy, Chondrodystrophia Tarda, Chondroosteodystrophy, Dysostosis Enchondralis Metaepiphysaria, Eccentro-osteochondrodysplasia, Familial Osseous Dystrophy, Hereditary Osteochondrodystrophy, Hereditary Polytopic Enchondral Dysostosis, Infantile Hereditary Chondrodysplasia, Keratosulfaturia, Mucopolysaccharidosis IV, Osteochondrodystrophia Deformans.*

ABBREVIATION: MPS type IV.

Scheie's Syndrome

Scheie's syndrome is a systemic mucopolysaccharidosis marked by stiff joints, mild bone deformities, clawhand, hirsutism, retinitis pigmentosa, corneal opacities, and broad-mouthed facies. Carpal tunnel syndrome and aortic coarctation occur frequently. Clouding of the cornea, although present at birth in a discrete form, may not become evident until adolescence. Excessive amounts of chondroitin sulfate B are excreted in the urine.

MODE OF INHERITANCE: Autosomal recessive.

SYNONYMS: *Forme Fruste of Hurler's Syndrome, Late Hurler's Syndrome, Mucopolysaccharidosis V.*

ABBREVIATION: MPS type V.

Maroteaux-Lamy Syndrome

The Maroteaux-Lamy syndrome is a systemic mucopolysaccharidosis characterized by dwarfism of the trunk and extremities, genu valgum, lumbar kyphosis, anterior sternal protrusion, stiff joints, hepatosplenomegaly, corneal opacities, varying degrees of deafness due to recurrent otitis media, and peculiar facies with thick lips and enlarged nose. Roentgenography shows defects of the metaphyses and epiphyses, retarded growth of the carpal and tarsal bones, flattening of the vertebrae, and a wedgelike deformity of the lumbar and thoracic vertebrae. Both polymorphonuclear inclusions and lymphocytic inclusions are found in the blood, and excessive amounts of chondroitin sulfate B are excreted in the urine.

MODE OF INHERITANCE: Autosomal recessive.

SYNONYMS: *Mucopolysaccharidosis VI, Mucopolysaccharidosis B, Mucopolysaccharidosis Chondroitin Sulfate B, Polydystrophic Dwarfism.*

ABBREVIATION: MPS type VI.

MULTIPLE EPIPHYSIAL DYSPLASIA

Multiple epiphysial dysplasia is a bone and connective tissue dysplasia characterized by shortened fingers, metaphysial flaring, limitation of the joints, osteoarthritis of the hip, and short stature.

MODE OF INHERITANCE: Autosomal dominant.

MULTIPLE EXOSTOSES

Multiple exostoses are bony growths that are usually bilateral and develop on parts of the skeleton that were previously cartilaginous. They may cause growth retardation and deformity, and interfere with joint motion.

MODE OF INHERITANCE: Autosomal dominant.

SYNONYM: *Osteochondroma.*

MYOTONIA CONGENITA

Myotonia congenita is a rare hereditary disease of muscles characterized by myotonia (delayed relaxation) of voluntary muscles, hypertrophy of limb and trunk muscles, and a herculean appearance. The specific defect is probably a true cholinesterase deficiency at the neuromuscular end plate.

MODE OF INHERITANCE: Autosomal dominant.

SYNONYMS: *Thomsen's Disease, Ataxia Muscularis, Congenital Muscular Dystrophy, Hereditary Myotonia, Paramyotonia Congenita.*

MYOTONIC DYSTROPHY OF STEINERT

Myotonic dystrophy of Steinert is a form of hereditary muscular dystrophy characterized by myotonia with muscle atrophy, hypogonadism, and cataract formation.

MODE OF INHERITANCE: Autosomal dominant.

SYNONYMS: *Curschmann-Batten-Steinert Syndrome, Batten's Disease, Batten-Steinert Syndrome, Curschmann-Steinert Syndrome, Steinert's Disease, Atrophic Myotonia, Dystrophia Myotonica, Myotonia Atrophica.*

NAIL–PATELLA SYNDROME

The nail-patella syndrome is characterized by dystrophy of the nails, absence or hypoplasia of the patellae, abnormality of the elbows interfering with supination and pronation, and other bone dysplasias.

MODE OF INHERITANCE: Autosomal dominant. This is linkage to ABO locus.

SYNONYMS: *Turner-Kieser Syndrome, Arthroonychodysplasia.*

NEPHROGENIC DIABETES INSIPIDUS

Nephrogenic diabetes insipidus is a disorder in which the renal tubules fail to respond to antidiuretic hormone. The clinical features are polyuria, polydipsia, persistently hypotonic urine, dehydration, and growth failure.

MODE OF INHERITANCE: Sex-linked dominant.

SYNONYM: *Vasopressin Resistant Diabetes Insipidus.*

NEUROFIBROMATOSIS

Neurofibromatosis is a slowly progressive disorder characterized by café-au-lait patches, sessile or pedunculated tumors of the skin, neurofibromas along cranial spinal nerves, osteitis fibrosa cystica, and multiple central nervous system lesions that are predominantly nodular.

MODE OF INHERITANCE: Probably autosomal dominant with incomplete dominance.

SYNONYMS: *Recklinghausen's Disease I, von Recklinghausen's Disease, Multiple Neurofibromatosis, Neurinofibrolipomatosis, Neurinomatosis Centralis et Peripherica, Neurinomatosis Universalis.*

NIEMANN–PICK DISEASE

Niemann-Pick disease is a disorder of lipid metabolism resulting in accumulation of sphingomyelin and cholesterol in cells. If the onset is early in life, the disease is characterized by hepatomegaly, splenomegaly, neurologic degeneration, and a cherry-red spot on the macula. Foam cells full of lipids are present in many tissues. Death occurs by five or six years of life. Other less severe forms of the disorder have been described in juveniles and adults.

MODE OF INHERITANCE: Probably autosomal recessive.

SYNONYMS: *Sphingomyelin Lipidosis, Niemann's Disease, Essential Lipoid Histiocytosis, Lipid Histiocytosis, Phosphatidolipoidosis, Phosphatidosis, Sphingomyelinosis.*

OCULODENTODIGITAL SYNDROME

The oculodentodigital syndrome is a rare syndrome in which craniofacial malformations are associated with digital defects. The clinical features are camptodactyly of the fifth fingers, narrow nose, microphthalmos, glaucoma, and enamel hypoplasia.

MODE OF INHERITANCE: Probably autosomal recessive.

SYNONYMS: *Meyer-Schwickerath and Weyers Syndrome, Gillespie's Syndrome, Microphthalmos Syndrome, Oculodentodigital Dysplasia.*

ABBREVIATIONS: ODD syndrome.

OPHTHALMOPLEGIA EXTERNA WITH MYOPIA

Ophthalmoplegia externa with myopia is characterized by bilateral ptosis, complete or partial ophthalmoplegia, myopia, and progressive degeneration of the choroid and retina. Other congenital abnormalities may be present such as spina bifida and absent patellar and Achilles tendon reflexes.

MODE OF INHERITANCE: Sex-linked recessive with partial manifestation in the heterozygous state.

OROFACIODIGITAL SYNDROME

The orofaciodigital syndrome is a rare, possibly lethal, congenital malformation. The clinical features are hypoplasia of the ala nasi and hypertrophic frenuli producing pseudoclefts of the upper lip, tongue, palate, and jaws, and digital asymmetry. Mental retardation is usually present.

MODE OF INHERITANCE: Autosomal dominant, possibly lethal in males.

SYNONYMS: *Papillon-Léage and Psaume Syndrome, Dysplasia Linguofacialis, Orodigitofacial Dysostosis, Orodigitofacial Syndrome.*

ABBREVIATION: OFD syndrome.

OROTIC ACIDURIA

Orotic aciduria is a disorder of pyrimidine metabolism characterized by physical and mental retardation, and anemia that responds to uridine administration. A pyrimidine nucleotide deficiency secondary to reduced activity of both orotidylic pyrophorylase and orotidylic decarboxylase causes the disorder.

MODE OF INHERITANCE: Autosomal recessive.

OSTEOGENESIS IMPERFECTA

Osteogenesis imperfecta is an inherited condition in which the bones are abnormally brittle, and subject to fractures. In *osteogenesis imperfecta congenita,* the fractures occur in intrauterine life and the child is born with deformities. In *osteogenesis imperfecta tarda,* the fractures occur when the child begins to walk. The condition is usually attended by blue coloration of the sclera of the eyes (*Lobstein's disease* or *syndrome*) and sometimes also by otosclerotic deafness (*van der Hoeve's syndrome*).

MODE OF INHERITANCE: Autosomal dominant with wide range of expressivity.

SYNONYMS: *Fragilitas Ossium, Osteopsathyrosis, Brittle Bones, Hypoplasia of the Mesenchyme.*

OSTEOPETROSIS

Osteopetrosis is a rare disorder characterized by brittle and hard bones. Onset begins in utero, and the brittleness predisposes to fractures. General growth is retarded, and deformities frequently develop. There is progressive optic atrophy, progressive deafness, secondary pancytopenia, and hepatosplenomegaly. Mentality is normal.

MODE OF INHERITANCE: Autosomal recessive.

SYNONYMS: *Albers-Schönberg Syndrome, Chalk Bones, Disseminated Condensing Osteopathy, Ivory Bones, Marble Bones, Marble Disease, Osteopetrosis Familiaris, Osteopetrosis Tarda, Osteosclerosis Congenita Diffusa, Osteosclerosis Fragilitas Generalisata, Albers-Schönberg Disease.*

OTOPALATODIGITAL SYNDROME

The otopalatodigital syndrome is a broad-thumb syndrome with associated defects. Broad distal digits, cleft of the soft palate, microstomia, conductive hearing loss, and short stature characterize this syndrome. It may be associated with mental retardation.

MODE OF INHERITANCE: Probably sex-linked.

SYNONYM: *Taybi's Syndrome.*

OTOSCLEROSIS

Otosclerosis is the development of spongy bone in the capsule of the labyrinth, leading to middle-ear deafness.

MODE OF INHERITANCE: Autosomal dominant with reduced penetrance.

OXALOSIS

Oxalosis is a rare disease characterized by widespread deposition of calcium oxalate crystals in the kidneys, bones, arterial media, and myocardium due to excessive formation of oxalate from glycine. Urinary excretion of oxalate is increased, and multiple calculi form in childhood. Patients die of renal insufficiency in late childhood.

MODE OF INHERITANCE: Autosomal recessive. Some may show dominant inheritance.

SYNONYM: *Primary Hyperoxaluria.*

PARAHEMOPHILIA A SYNDROME

The parahemophilia A syndrome is a congenital disorder in which deficiency of Factor V (proaccelerin) results in hemophiloid hemorrhagic diathesis with epistaxis, susceptibility to bruising, hemorrhage after dental extractions, and menorrhagia.

MODE OF INHERITANCE: Autosomal recessive.

SYNONYMS: *Owren's Syndrome II, Ac-Globulin Deficiency, Factor V Deficiency, Hemophiloid State A, Hypoprothrombinemia, Labile Factor Deficiency, Proaccelerin Deficiency.*

PENTA–X SYNDROME

The penta-X syndrome is a variety of the poly-X syndrome associated with congenital malformations. The clinical features are mongoloid slanting of the palpebral fissures, small hands, clinodactyly of the fifth finger, patent ductus arteriosus, mental deficiency, and short stature. Patients are phenotypic females.

CYTOGENETICS: 49 chromosomes with XXXXX. Buccal smear shows four Barr bodies.

PENTOSURIA

Pentosuria is a defect of carbohydrate metabolism resulting in excretion of 5-carbon sugars in the urine. The most important of these sugars, from a clinical standpoint, is xylose. The condition is often misdiagnosed as diabetes mellitus. The specific defect is a block in the glucuronic acid oxidation pathway.

MODE OF INHERITANCE: Autosomal recessive.

PEUTZ–JEGHERS SYNDROME

The Peutz-Jeghers syndrome is a rare inherited condition characterized by intestinal polyps, especially in the jejunum, and pigmentation of the buccal mucosa. The clinical features are recurrent intussusception, gastrointestinal bleeding and anemia due to polyposis, and areas of mucocutaneous, spotty pigmentation. Females tend to develop ovarian tumors. Malignant degeneration of intestinal polyps is rare.

MODE OF INHERITANCE: Autosomal dominant.

SYNONYMS: *Peutz Syndrome, Intestinal Polyposis-Cutaneous Pigmentation Syndrome, Melanoplakia and Small Intestinal Polyposis, Lentigino-Polypose Digestive Syndrome, Intestinal Polyposis II, Hutchinson-Weber-Peutz Syndrome, Jegher's Syndrome, Peutz-Touraine Syndrome.*

PHENYLKETONURIA

Phenylketonuria is a hereditary disorder characterized by the excretion of phenylpyruvic acid in the urine. Most untreated patients have seizures, eczema, and mental retardation. The specific defect is a lack of the liver enzyme phenylalanine hydroxylase, which is responsible for the conversion of phenylalanine to tyrosine.

MODE OF INHERITANCE: Autosomal recessive.

SYNONYMS: *Imbecilitas Phenylpyruvica, Phenylpyruvic Oligophrenia, Phenyluria, Fölling's Disease.*

ABBREVIATION: PKU.

PHOCOMELIA

Phocomelia refers to a great reduction in size of the proximal portions of the limbs.

PIERRE ROBIN SYNDROME

The Pierre Robin syndrome is a congenital hypoplasia of the mandible. The clinical features are micrognathia, microglossia, glossoptosis, and high-arched cleft palate. The retracted position of the tongue obstructs the pharynx, causing asphyxia.

MODE OF INHERITANCE: Not clear.

SYNONYMS: *Robin's Syndrome, Micrognathia-Glossoptosis Syndrome.*

PIGMENTED LIPID HISTIOCYTOSIS

Pigmented lipid histiocytosis is a rare sex-linked lipidosis of childhood characterized by persistent and often fatal infections that are not cured by antibiotics. The clinical features include infections of the skin, lymph nodes, middle ear, and intestinal tract. Lymphadenopathy, hepatosplenomegaly, and pulmonary consolidation develop, together with hypergammaglobulinemia. The basic defect is an inability of polymorphonuclear leukocytes and monocytes to kill ingested bacteria.

MODE OF INHERITANCE: X-linked recessive.

SYNONYM: *Chronic Granulomatous Disease of Childhood.*

POLAND'S SYNDROME

Poland's syndrome is a rare muscular disorder associated with other malformations. The clinical features are unilateral absence of the pectoralis minor muscle, unilateral hypoplasia or absence of the nipple, and unilateral syndactyly of the hand.

MODE OF INHERITANCE: Unknown.

POLYDACTYLY

Polydactyly is the presence of extra digits or portions of digits.

MODE OF INHERITANCE: Usually autosomal dominant.

POLY–X SYNDROME

The poly-X syndrome is a congenital abnormality characterized by the presence of four X chromosomes and a total of 48 chromosomes. The clinical features are mental retardation and sterility.

CYTOGENETICS: Mosaicism may possibly occur. A penta-X syndrome may also occur having XXXXX chromosomes with four sex chromatin bodies.

SYNONYM: *XXXX Sex Chromosome Constitution.*

POPLITEAL WEB SYNDROME

The popliteal web syndrome is a rare hereditary syndrome characterized by a popliteal web, lower lip pits, cleft palate, and digital and genital anomalies.

MODE OF INHERITANCE: Autosomal dominant, sometimes autosomal recessive.

PRADER–WILLI SYNDROME

The Prader-Willi syndrome is a syndrome combining mental retardation, short stature, muscular hypotonia, small hands and feet, obesity, cryptorchism, and hypogonadism, with or without diabetes mellitus. Associated abnormalities may include ocular hypertelorism, epicanthus, and strabismus; low-set ears and overlapping helix; high-arched palate, micrognathia, microdontia, dental caries, and defective dental enamel; acromicria; mesobrachyphalangia, clinodactyly, partial syndactyly of the toes, and fourfingerline. The cause is unknown. Laboratory findings usually fail to reveal a constant pattern of abnormalities. Most cases have been reported in males, but abnormalities of the genitalia may increase the likelihood of recognition in the male. Diabetes mellitus associated with this syndrome is known as *Royer's Syndrome.*

MODE OF INHERITANCE: Not clear.

SYNONYMS: *Prader-Labhart-Willi-Fanconi Syndrome, Hypogenital Dystrophy with Diabetic Tendency, Hypotonia-Hypomentia-Hypogonadism-Obesity Syndrome.*

ABBREVIATION: HHHO syndrome.

PRIMARY GOUT

Primary gout is a disorder of purine metabolism resulting in a raised level of serum uric acid. It is characterized by the formation of tophi composed of monosodium urate, hyperuricemia, recurrent attacks of arthritis, and renal lithiasis.

MODE OF INHERITANCE: It may be autosomal dominant, or multifactorially controlled; it is sex-influenced (male/female ratio is 6 to 7).

PROGRESSIVE ARTHROOPHTHALMOPATHY OF STICKLER

Progressive arthroophthalmopathy of Stickler is a rare form of joint dysplasia characterized by limitation of joints, progressive myopia, retinal detachment, and sensory and neural deafness.

MODE OF INHERITANCE: Autosomal dominant.

PSEUDOXANTHOMA ELASTICUM

Pseudoxanthoma elasticum is a rare disease of elastic tissue marked by small papules, individual, confluent, or massed into plaques; thickening of the skin where the lesions exist; and exaggeration of the normal creases and folds of the skin. Angioid streaks may be found in the retina. Systemic vascular disease eventually develops, especially in the brain and gastrointestinal tract.

MODE OF INHERITANCE: Probably autosomal recessive with partial sex limitation to the female. It may also be partially sex-linked.

SYNONYMS: *Elastoma, Elastosis Atrophicans, Nevus Elasticus, Darier's Syndrome (2).*

PYKNODYSOSTOSIS OF STANESCO

Pyknodysostosis of Stanesco is a form of osteopetrosis. It is characterized by osteosclerosis, relatively short upper arms, brachycephaly with thin cranium, facial bone hypoplasia, and short stature.

MODE OF INHERITANCE: Autosomal dominant.

RADIAL APLASIA–THROMBOCYTOPENIA SYNDROME

The radial aplasia-thrombocytopenia syndrome is a hereditary disorder of platelets. The syndrome is characterized by thrombocytopenia with megakaryocytopenia, radial aplasia, and cardiac defects in some cases.

MODE OF INHERITANCE: Autosomal recessive.

RENAL TUBULAR ACIDOSIS

Renal tubular acidosis is a defect in renal acid-base balance without glomerular insufficiency, and general tubular dysfunction. Most patients cannot acidify urine below pH 6.0 and have persistent hyperchloremia. The tubular defect usually represents an inability to establish a maximum hydrogen ion gradient in the distal nephron. Some patients have associated nephrocalcinosis.

MODE OF INHERITANCE: Probably autosomal dominant; expression may be variable.

RETINITIS PIGMENTOSA

Retinitis pigmentosa is frequently a hereditary disease marked by progressive retinal sclerosis with pigmentation and atrophy. It is attended by contraction of the field of vision and hemeralopia. There are stellate deposits of pigment in the retina, and the retinal vessels become obliterated.

MODE OF INHERITANCE: Variable.

RETINOBLASTOMA

Retinoblastoma is a congenital malignant tumor arising from the nuclear layers of the retina. It may involve one or both eyes.

MODE OF INHERITANCE: Autosomal dominant with somewhat reduced penetrance.

RIEGER'S SYNDROME

Rieger's syndrome is a congenital disorder transmitted as a dominant trait. Principal features include corneal opacities, hypoplastic stroma of the iris, iridotrabecular adhesions, and posterior embryotoxon. Specific ocular findings usually consist of microcornea or megalocornea, cornea plana, aniridia, various pupillary defects, coloboma, ectopia or opacities of the crystalline lens, glaucoma, strabismus, and ametropia. Associated abnormalities may include dental defects, dysgnathia, hypertelorism, agenesis of the facial bones, hydrocephalus, cerebellar hypoplasia, and mental retardation. Rieger's syndrome refers to ocular disorders associated with nonocular abnormalities; ocular disorders without other defects are referred to as *Rieger's anomaly* or *Rieger's malformation*.

MODE OF INHERITANCE: Autosomal dominant.

SYNONYMS: *Dysgenesis Mesodermalis Corneae et Iridis, Dysgenesis Mesostromalis Anterior, Dysplasia Marginalis Posterior, Embryotoxon Corneae Posterius, Mesodermal Dysgenesis of the Anterior Ocular Segment, Posterior Marginal Dysplasia.*

RILEY'S SYNDROME

Riley's syndrome is a rare disorder characterized by macrocephaly, pseudopapilledema, and cutaneous hemangiomas.

MODE OF INHERITANCE: Probably autosomal dominant.

RUBINSTEIN–TAYBI SYNDROME

The Rubinstein-Taybi syndrome is a combination of congenital disorders consisting of short, broad terminal phalanges of the thumbs and great toes (brachydactylia); short stature; mental retardation; motor retardation; facial deformities, including high-arched palate and straight or beaked nose; eye abnormalities, including various combinations of antimongoloid slant, epicanthus, strabismus, cataract, refractive error, high-arched eyebrows, and long lashes; skeletal maturation and head circumference that are below average for the age; and cryptorchism. There is also susceptibility to respiratory infections. Occasionally associated are other skeletal abnormalities, especially of the sternum, ribs, fingers, vertebrae, and toes; deformity of the external ears; congenital defects of the heart; lax ligaments; hypotonia; abnormalities of the urinary tract; simian crease; capillary hemangioma; and abnormal electroencephalographic findings. The possibility of polygenic or multifactorial inheritance has been raised.

MODE OF INHERITANCE: Unknown.

SAWITSKY'S DISEASE

Sawitsky's disease is a rare familial lipidosis characterized by asymptomatic hepatosplenomegaly, anemia, and unidentified glycolipid deposition in reticuloendothelial cells.

MODE OF INHERITANCE: Autosomal recessive.

SYNONYM: *Chronic Reticuloendothelial Cell Storage Disease.*

SCHWARTZ' SYNDROME

Schwartz' syndrome is a familial congenital syndrome characterized by myotonia, shortness of stature, and hip dysplasia, associated with blepharophimosis or blepharospasm, peculiar rigid facies, pectus carinatum, small muscle mass, and rigidity of joints. Muscle biopsy reveals fibrosis and fatty infiltration, glycogen accumulation, and, according to more recent studies, activities of phosphorylase, amylo-1,6-glucosidase, and lysosomal acid α-glucosidase in the muscles.

MODE OF INHERITANCE: Probably autosomal recessive.

SYNONYM: *Schwartz-Jampel Syndrome.*

SECKEL'S SYNDROME

Seckel's syndrome is a hereditary dwarfism associated with facial hypoplasia, prominent nose, microcephaly, multiple skeletal and minor joint abnormalities, and mental retardation.

MODE OF INHERITANCE: Autosomal recessive.

SYNONYMS: *Virchow-Seckel Dwarfism, Ateliosis, Bird-Headed Dwarfism, Intrauterine Growth Retardation, Low Birth Weight Dwarfism, Nanocephalic Dwarfism, Primordial Dwarfism.*

SICKLE CELL ANEMIA

Sickle cell anemia is a form of hemolytic anemia that occurs almost exclusively in Negroes. Crystallization of abnormal hemoglobin S in the presence of low oxygen tension and reduced blood pH is responsible for the sickling phenomenon, resulting in the appearance of oat-shaped and sickel-shaped red cells in the blood and increased viscosity of the capillary blood. The onset usually occurs during the first year of life, after normal hemoglobin is replaced with hemoglobin S. The most common clinical signs are arthralgia and abdominal crises. Thrombosis, sterility, disorders in pregnancy, susceptibility to infections, heart diseases, and liver diseases are frequent complications, and there may be sudden death.

MODE OF INHERITANCE: Incomplete dominance.

SYNONYMS: *African Anemia, Drepanocytic Anemia, Hemoglobin S Disease, Homozygous Hemoglobin S Disease, Meniscocytosis, Sicklemia, Herrick's Syndrome.*

SILVER'S SYNDROME

Silver's syndrome is a syndrome of skeletal asymmetry, low birth weight, and dwarfism associated with triangular hypoplastic facies, downturning mouth, and clinodactyly of the fifth finger.

MODE OF INHERITANCE: Unknown.

SJÖGREN–LARSSON SYNDROME

The Sjögren-Larsson syndrome is a rare neurologic disorder characterized by spasticity of the lower extremities, mental retardation, short stature, and ichthyosis.

MODE OF INHERITANCE: Autosomal recessive.

SMITH–LEMLI–OPITZ SYNDROME

The Smith-Lemli-Opitz syndrome is a rare congenital malformation. The clinical features are syndactyly of the second and third toes, hypospadias, cryptorchism, anteverted nostrils or ptosis of the eyelids, micrognathia, mental deficiency, and failure to thrive.

MODE OF INHERITANCE: Probably autosomal recessive.

SPONDYLOEPIPHYSIAL DYSPLASIA

Spondyloepiphysial dysplasia is a syndrome that resembles achondroplasia. However, affected individuals are normal at birth and then develop short stature, lumbar lordosis, and signs of epiphysial dysplasia after several years of life.

MODE OF INHERITANCE: X-linked recessive or autosomal dominant.

STUART–PROWER FACTOR DEFICIENCY

The Stuart–Prower Factor deficiency (Factor X) is a disorder of blood coagulation characterized by a prolonged prothrombin time. Mucocutaneous hemorrhages, bleeding into tissues, and prolonged bleeding after injury may occur.

MODE OF INHERITANCE: Autosomal recessive.

STURGE–WEBER SYNDROME

The Sturge-Weber syndrome is characterized by venous angiomas of the leptomeninges; ipsilateral telangiectasia or port-wine nevus of the trigeminal region, including the upper third of the face, eyes, mouth, and nasal mucosa; contralateral hemiplegia; and choroidal angioma with late glaucoma. Vascular changes are usually associated with intracranial calcifications, mental retardation, epileptic seizures, crossed hemiparesis, hydrophthalmia, and hemianopsia. *Jahnke's syndrome* is a variant that is not associated with glaucoma; *Schirmer's syndrome* is associated with early glaucoma (hydrophthalmia); *Lawford's syndrome* is accompanied by glaucoma but without increase in the volume of the globe; and angioma of the choroid without glaucoma occurs in *Milles' syndrome*.

MODE OF INHERITANCE: Not clear.

SYNONYMS: *Kalischer's Syndrome, Krabbe's Syndrome, Parkes Weber's Syndrome, Parkes Weber and Dimitri Syndrome, Sturge's Disease, Sturge's Syndrome, Sturge-Weber-Dimitri Syn-*

drome, Weber-Dimitri Syndrome, Angioma Capillare et Venosum Calcificans, Angiomatosis Meningo-oculofacialis, Congenital Ectodermosis, Congenital Neuroectodermal Dysplasia, Cutaneocerebral Angioma, Encephalofacial Neuroangiomatosis, Encephalotrigeminal Angiomatosis, Meningo-oculofacial Angiomatosis, Neuroangiomatosis Encephalofacialis, Neurocutaneous Syndrome, Neuroectodermal Hamartoma, Neuro-oculocutaneous Angiomatosis, Nevoid Amentia, Trigeminoencephaloangiomatosis, Sturge-Weber-Krabbe Disease, Sturge-Kalischer-Weber Syndrome, Krabbe's Disease, Sturge-Parkes Weber-Dimitri Syndrome, Lannois-Bernoud Syndrome, Meningofacial Angiomatosis, Encephalofacial Angiomatosis, Encephalotrigeminal Vascular Syndrome.

SYMPHALANGISM
Symphalangism is bony or fibrous union of the phalanges.
MODE OF INHERITANCE: Autosomal dominant.

SYNDACTYLY
Syndactyly is a common congenital anomaly of the fingers or toes that may consist of webbing of the skin only or fusion of the bones. It most commonly involves the third and fourth fingers and the second and third toes.
MODE OF INHERITANCE: Variable.

TESTICULAR FEMINIZATION SYNDROME
The testicular feminization syndrome is a genetic type of male pseudo-hermaphroditism that occurs in phenotypic females with well-developed breasts and other female sex characteristics but with a paucity of pubic and axillary hair. These patients are generally first seen by the physician because of primary amenorrhea. On pelvic examination, it is noted that pubic hair is sparse or absent, the external genitalia are otherwise usually normal, but the vagina ends in a blind pouch. The uterus and fallopian tubes are absent or rudimentary; the internal ducts are usually predominantly male. The bilateral testes are usually cryptorchid but may descend and in some cases are found as the sole content of inguinal hernias. The gonadal tissue is histologically similar to that of undescended testes. Tubular adenomas are often seen and occasionally malignant tumors are present. Studies indicate that the testes produce both estrogen and androgen. It appears, however, that in these patients there is a genetic target-organ unresponsiveness to androgen, thus accounting for the lack of development of the male genitalia and the lack of pubic and axillary hair. This condition appears to be transmitted by a sex-limited recessive or a sex-limited dominant gene.
SYNONYMS: *Syndrome of Feminizing Testes, Male Pseudohermaphroditism, Syndrome of Hairless Women, Goldberg-Maxwell Syndrome, Androgynoidism.*

THALASSEMIAS

Thalassemias are a group of chronic, familial anemias occurring mostly in populations from countries bordering the Mediterranean, and in Negroes. Thalassemias are characterized by the production of an abnormally thin red blood cell. The disorder, transmitted as a dominant characteristic, manifests itself in the homozygous subject as a severe anemia during the first year of life. In the heterozygous subject, the anemia may be low-grade.

RELATED TERMS: *Mediterranean Anemia, Cooley's Anemia, Hereditary Leptocytosis, Thalassemia Major and Minor.*

THROMBOCYTOPENIC PURPURA WITH HISTIOCYTOSIS OF THE SPLEEN

Thrombocytopenic purpura with histiocytosis of the spleen is a rare familial lipidosis associated with purpura. The clinical features are similar to idiopathic thrombocytopenic purpura. The onset is in middle childhood. Foam cells of the spleen and marrow accumulate phospholipid.

MODE OF INHERITANCE: Autosomal recessive.

TRANSFERRIN DEFICIENCY

Transferrin deficiency is a very rare syndrome characterized by an absence of the plasma protein transferrin, which has a role in iron transport. Affected individuals have anemia, hepatosplenomegaly, cirrhosis, and siderosis.

MODE OF INHERITANCE: Possibly autosomal recessive.

TREACHER COLLINS SYNDROME

The Treacher Collins syndrome is characterized by laterally sloping palpebral fissures, hypoplasia of the facial bones, macrostomia, high palate, abnormal position and malocclusion of the teeth, and malformations of the ear. The auricle is usually low-set. Atresia of the external auditory meatus may be present.

MODE OF INHERITANCE: Dominant mutant gene with variable manifestation.

SYNONYMS: *Incomplete Mandibulofacial Dysostosis, Incomplete Mandibulofacial Syndrome, Eyelid-Malar-Mandible Syndrome.*

TRISOMY D SYNDROME

Trisomy D syndrome is a congenital abnormality characterized by the presence of an extra chromosome in the D group (13-15). The clinical features are mental retardation, severe central nervous system defects, apparent deafness, microphthalmos or anophthalmos, ear malformation, cardiac defects, cleft lip and palate, polydactyly, characteristic dermal pattern, capillary hemangioma, scalp defects, apneic spells, and death in early infancy.

MODE OF INHERITANCE: Sex-linked recessive.

SYNONYMS: *Bartholin-Patau Syndrome, Patau's Syndrome, Trisomy 13-15.*

TRISOMY E SYNDROME

Individuals with trisomy E syndrome have a total chromosome count of 47, the extra chromosome being a number 18. The clinical findings include low-set and malformed ears, micrognathia with high-arched palate, overlapping fingers, pronounced failure to thrive, central nervous system defects, and cardiac defects. Most patients die within a few months.

MODE OF INHERITANCE: Sex-linked.

SYNONYM: *Trisomy 18.*

TRYPSINOGEN DEFICIENCY

Trypsinogen deficiency is a disorder due to inability to synthesize pancreatic trypsinogen. The clinical features are severe malnutrition, growth failure, and hypoproteinemic edema.

MODE OF INHERITANCE: Unclear.

TUBEROUS SCLEROSIS

Tuberous sclerosis is a hereditary syndrome characterized by mental deficiency, epilepsy, and adenoma sebaceum. The symptoms may be present at birth, but more frequently they appear during early childhood. Most patients die before reaching the age of 20. Pathologically, there are many smooth potato-like masses on the cerebral cortex, cerebral ventricles, and other parts of the brain, and intracranial calcifications are frequently observed. The ocular complications may include glaucoma, whitish gray tumors of the conjunctiva, cloudy vitreous, corneal opacity, mushroom-like tumors, plaques and hemorrhage of the retina and choroid, and papilledema. Simian hands, short and incurving little fingers, ear deformities, hypernephroma, rhabdomyoma of the heart, spina bifida, thickened calvarium, exostoses of the frontal bones, accessory thumbs, and honeycomb lung may be associated.

MODE OF INHERITANCE: Autosomal dominant.

SYNONYMS: *Bourneville's Syndrome, Bourneville's Disease, Bourneville-Brissaud Disease, Bourneville-Pringle Syndrome, Pringle's Disease, Adenoma Sebaceum Disseminatum, Epiploia, Nevus Multiplex, Neurinomatosis Centralis, Neurospongio-blastosis Diffusa, Phakomatosis, Sclerosis Tuberosa, Spongioblastosis Centralis Circumscripta.*

TURNER'S SYNDROME

Turner's syndrome is a genetic abnormality occurring in phenotypic females characterized by dwarfism, sexual infantilism, webbing of the neck, and cubitus valgus. These persons have rudimentary gonads consisting of streaks of connective tissue devoid of germ cells. Most of these persons are sex chromatin-negative, and have 45 chromosomes with an XO karyotype. In some instances, a few follicles or epithelioid tissue may be present in the streak gonad. Many variations of the syndrome have been described and are grouped under the general term of *gonadal dysgenesis.* A large variety of other associated somatic stigmata has been noted, including an underdeveloped mandible; a high arched palate; a broad shieldlike chest with widely spaced, immature nipples; large, dark, elevated moles on the face and neck; low-set ears; a low posterior hairline, and many others. When none of the somatic stigmata are present, the condition may be referred to as *pure gonadal dysgenesis*. If a testis is present on one side and a streak gonad on the other with both wolffian and müllerian gonadal accessories, the term *male Turner's syndrome* is used to describe phenotypic males with short stature, webbed neck, and hypoplastic testes. Many types of chromosomal aberrations have been found in patients with gonadal dysgenesis, including a variety of mosaic patterns such as XO/XX, XO/XXX, XO/XX/XXX, and XO/XY, and structural defects of the X and Y chromosomes. Hormonal assays in Turner's syndrome and its variants show markedly elevated urinary gonadotropins, very low estrogen levels, and normal or moderately diminished 17-ketosteroid levels.

SYNONYMS: *Turner-Albright Syndrome, Turner-Varny Syndrome, Gonadal Dysgenesis, Ovarian-Short Stature Syndrome, Gonadal Agenesis, Genital Dwarfism Syndrome, Pterygonuchal Infantilism Syndrome, Ovarian Agenesis, Ovarian Dwarfism, Ovarian Aplasia, Congenitally Absent Ovaries Syndrome, Rudimentary Ovary Syndrome, Morgagni-Turner Syndrome, Morgagni-Turner-Albright Syndrome, Shereshevskii-Turner Syndrome, Primary Ovarian Insufficiency, Pseudonuchal Infantilism, XO Sex Chromosome Constitution, XO Syndrome.*

TYROSINOSIS

Tyrosinosis is a disorder of amino acid metabolism in which tyrosine metabolites are excreted in the urine. There usually are no serious symptoms or signs, although some patients have progressive liver disease. The specific defect is a deficiency of *p*-hydroxyphenylpyruvic acid oxidase.

MODE OF INHERITANCE: Autosomal recessive.

VON HIPPEL–LINDAU SYNDROME

The von Hippel-Lindau syndrome is characterized by angiomas of the retina, hemangioblastoma of the cerebellum, and by tumors or cysts of the abdominal organs, chiefly the kidneys and pancreas.

MODE OF INHERITANCE: Autosomal dominant.

SYNONYMS: *Lindau's Syndrome, Lindau's Disease, Viscerocystic-retinoangiomatosis Syndrome, Lindau-von Hippel Syndrome, Hippel-Lindau Syndrome, Hippel's Disease, Hippel-Czermak Syndrome, Lindau's Tumor, Angiomatosis Retinae, Angiomatosis Retinae Cystica, Angiomatosis Retinocerebellosa, Angioreticuloma Cerebelli, Hereditary Hemangiomatosis of the Central Nervous System, Retinal Angiomatosis.*

VON WILLEBRAND'S DISEASE

Von Willebrand's disease is an abnormality of blood-clotting factors characterized by a prolonged bleeding time and a depression of Factor

VIII. The clinical features are recurrent hemorrhages, such as nose bleeds, and prolonged bleeding after trauma.

MODE OF INHERITANCE: Autosomal dominant (intermediate dominance).

SYNONYMS: *Willebrand-Jurgens Thrombopathy, Vascular Hemophilia, Willebrand-Jurgens Syndrome, Minot-von Willebrand Syndrome, von Willebrand's Syndrome, Angiohemophilia, Constitutional Thrombopathy, Hereditary Hemorrhagic Thrombasthenia, Hereditary Pseudohemophilia, Pseudohemophilia.*

WILDERVANCK SYNDROME

The Wildervanck syndrome is a hereditary familial syndrome characterized by deaf-mutism, Klippel-Feil syndrome, abducens paralysis, retractio bulbi, defective implantation of the hair and teeth, and facial hypoplasia. Subconjunctival neoplasms, status dysraphicus, and facial and cranial asymmetry may occur.

MODE OF INHERITANCE: Uncertain, limited almost completely to females.

SYNONYMS: *Franceschetti-Klein-Wildervanck Syndrome, Wildervanck-Waardenburg-Franceschetti-Klein Syndrome, Cervico-oculoacusticus Syndrome, Cervico-oculofacial Dysmorphia, Cervico-oculofacial Syndrome.*

WISKOTT–ALDRICH SYNDROME

The Wiskott-Aldrich syndrome is a sex-linked recessive disease characterized by eczema, thrombocytopenia, proneness to infection, bloody diarrhea, and early death.

MODE OF INHERITANCE: Sex-linked recessive.

SYNONYMS: *Aldrich's Syndrome, Wiskott-Aldrich-Huntley Syndrome, Eczema-Thrombocytopenia Syndrome.*

XERODERMA PIGMENTOSUM

Xeroderma pigmentosum is a rare hereditary skin disease characterized by dermal sensitivity to sunlight and ultraviolet light, and the development of skin cancer. The specific defect is in the enzyme system that repairs deoxyribonucleic acid.

MODE OF INHERITANCE: Autosomal recessive.

SYNONYMS: *Malignant Freckles, Angioma Pigmentosum et Atrophicum, Lentigo Maligna, Lioderma Essentialis cum Melanosis et Telangiectasia, Melanosis Lenticularis Progressiva, Pigmented Epitheliomatosis, Kaposi's Dermatosis.*

XXX SEX CHROMOSOME CONSTITUTION

The XXX sex chromosome constitution is a congenital abnormality of phenotypic females that is associated with few, if any, somatic abnormalities. However, the incidence of mental retardation is higher in affected individuals than in the general population. Most have normal fertility.

SYNONYMS: *Triple-X Female, Poly-X Female, Superfemale.*

XXXXY SYNDROME

The XXXXY syndrome is a chromosomal imbalance syndrome. Inner epicanthic fold or upslanting of the palpebral fissures, limitation of the elbow, hypogenitalism, mental retardation, and short stature characterize this syndrome. Patients are usually phenotypic males.

CYTOGENETICS: 49 chromosomes (XXXXY). Buccal smears show three Barr bodies.

XYY SYNDROME

The XYY syndrome is a congenital abnormality characterized by XYY sex chromosomes and a total of 47 chromosomes. The clinical features include tallness, increased plasma testosterone levels, verbal/performance IQ discrepancy, and a decreased total ridge count. Aggressive behavior may be present, and skeletal deformities are occasionally found.

Section 9: *Glossary of Congenital Anomalies*

Anencephalus

ACRANIA

Acrania is partial or complete absence of the cranium or skull.

AMYELENCEPHALY

Amyelencephaly is the absence of both the brain and spinal cord.

ANENCEPHALY

Anencephaly is the absence of the brain. Sometimes basal ganglia and cerebellum are present.

SYNONYM: *Anencephalia.*

HEMIANENCEPHALY

Hemianencephaly is the absence of the brain on one side.

HEMICEPHALY

Hemicephaly is the congenital absence of the cerebrum. Usually the cerebellum and basal ganglia are present in rudimentary form.

SYNONYM: *Partial Anencephaly.*

Spina Bifida

FISSURE OF SPINE
Fissure of spine is a spina bifida or a cleft spine.

HOLORACHISCHISIS
Holorachischisis is the absence of vertebral arches along the entire spine.

SYNONYM: *Complete Spina Bifida.*

HYDROMENINGOCELE (SPINAL)
Hydromeningocele is a protrusion of the spinal cord meninges through a bony wall defect.

HYDROMYELOCELE
Hydromyelocele is the protrusion of the spinal cord substance through a spina bifida.

MENINGOCELE
Meningocele is a herniation of the membranes of the brain or spinal cord through a defect in the skull or spinal column.

MIDBRAIN DISPLACEMENT
Midbrain displacement is a displacement of the mesencephalon into the cervical canal with a portion of cerebellum and medulla projecting down the foramen magnum.

SYNONYMS: *Cerebellomedullary Malformation Syndrome, Congenital Foramen Magnum Hernia, Arnold-Chiari Syndrome.*

MYELOCELE
Myelocele is a protrusion of the spinal cord through a spina bifida.

MYELOCYSTOCELE
Myelocystocele is a spina bifida that contains spinal cord substance.

MYELOMENINGOCELE
Myelomeningocele is a protrusion of the spinal cord and meninges through a spina bifida.

SYNONYM: *Myelocystomeningocele.*

RACHISCHISIS
Rachischisis is a congenital opening or fissure of the spinal column and spinal cord.

SPINA BIFIDA

Spina bifida is a defect in the vertebral arches of the spine leaving a gap through which meninges, brain, or spinal cord may protrude.

SPINA BIFIDA (APERTA) WITH HYDROCEPHALUS

Spina bifida (aperta) with hydrocephalus is a spina bifida that has a protruding meningocele or myelocele and associated hydrocephalus.

SPINA BIFIDA (APERTA) WITHOUT HYDROCEPHALUS

Spina bifida (aperta) without hydrocephalus is an obvious palpable defect in the vertebral arches of the spine leaving a gap through which meninges or cord may protrude.

SPINA BIFIDA CYSTICA

Spina bifida cystica is a spina bifida with a fluid-filled sac.

SPINA BIFIDA MANIFESTA

Spina bifida manifesta is a spina bifida that can be seen and felt.

SPINAL HERNIA

Spinal hernia is a protrusion of the spinal cord and meninges through a defect in the vertebra.

SPONDYLOSCHISIS

Spondyloschisis is a fissure of a vertebral arch.

SYRINGOMENINGOCELE

Syringomeningocele is protrusion of fluid-filled meninges through a spina bifida with a communication to the spinal canal.

SYRINGOMYELOCELE

Syringomyelocele is a protrusion of the spinal cord and membranes through an opening in the spinal column.

Hydrocephalus

APERTURA LATERALIS VENTRICULI QUARTI, ATRESIA OF
Atresia of the apertura lateralis ventriculi quarti is an atresia of the lateral aperture of the fourth ventricle.
SYNONYM: *Atresia of the Foramen of Luschka.*

APERTURA MEDIANA VENTRICULI QUARTI, ATRESIA OF
Atresia of the apertura mediana ventriculi quarti is an atresia of the median portion of the fourth ventricle.
SYNONYM: *Atresia of the Foramen of Magendie.*

AQUEDUCTUS CEREBRI, ATRESIA OF
Atresia of the aqueductus cerebri is an absence or closure of the aqueduct of the cerebrum from the third to the fourth ventricle through the mesencephalon.
SYNONYM: *Atresia of the Aqueductus of Sylvius.*

AQUEDUCTUS CEREBRI, SEPTUM OF
Septum of aqueductus cerebri is a partition or division of the aqueduct so that there are two or more channels, usually resulting in obstructive hydrocephalus because the channels are small.
SYNONYM: *Forking of the Aqueductus Cerebri.*

AQUEDUCTUS CEREBRI, STENOSIS OF
Stenosis of aqueductus cerebri is a narrowing of the channel or aqueduct from the third to the fourth ventricle through the mesencephalon.
SYNONYM: *Stenosis of the Aqueductus of Sylvius.*

HYDRANENCEPHALY
Hydranencephaly is almost or complete absence of the cerebral hemispheres, which are only represented by thin glial membranes. The space is filled by cerebrospinal fluid and is readily transilluminated.
SYNONYM: *Internal Hydrocephalus.*

HYDROCEPHALUS, CONGENITAL
Congenital hydrocephalus is the accumulation of excessive amounts of cerebrospinal fluid within the ventricles of the brain.

Nervous System

AGYRIA
Agyria is the absence of convolutions over the cerebral hemispheres associated with thickening of cortical gray mantle.

SYNONYM: *Lissencephalia.*

AMYELIA
Amyelia is absence of the spinal cord.

ATELOMYELIA
Atelomyelia is an imperfect development of the spinal cord.

BRACHIAL PLEXUS, DISPLACEMENT OF
Displacement of brachial plexus is an abnormal placement of the brachial plexus.

CAUDA EQUINA, CONGENITAL DEFECTIVE DEVELOPMENT OF
Congenital defective development of the cauda equina is a malformation of the cauda equina.

CEPHALOCELE, ORBITAL
Orbital cephalocele is a protrusion of brain substance through a defect in the bones surrounding the eye.

CEREBELLUM, ABSENCE OF, AGENESIS OF, APLASIA OF, OR HYPOPLASIA OF

CEREBRAL HERNIA, CONGENITAL
Congenital cerebral hernia is a protrusion of brain substance through a skull defect.

SYNONYM: *Congenital Brain Hernia.*

CEREBRAL HERNIA, ENDAURAL
Endaural cerebral hernia is a protrusion of cerebral meninges and brain into the ear canal.

CEREBRAL MENINGES, CONGENITAL ADHESIONS OF
Congenital adhesions of cerebral meninges are adherent meninges of the brain.

CORPUS CALLOSUM, ABSENCE OF, AGENESIS OF, APLASIA OF, OR HYPOPLASIA OF

DERENCEPHALOCELE
Derencephalocele is the protrusion of a small brain in the cervical spinal canal associated with an open skull.

DIASTEMATOMYELIA
Diastematomyelia is a double or split spinal column, usually separated by bone cartilage or fibrous tissue.

DYSAUTONOMIA, FAMILIAL
Familial dysautonomia is a congenital syndrome with nervous system disturbances, particularly autonomic.
SYNONYM: *Riley-Day Syndrome.*

DYSPLASIA, ENCEPHALOOPHTHALMIC
Encephaloophthalmic dysplasia consists of cerebral and retinal malformations with multiple eye defects and mental retardation.
SYNONYM: *Krause's Syndrome.*

DYSRAPHIA
Dysraphia is an incomplete closure of the neural tube.

ECTOPIA, FACIAL NERVE
Facial nerve ectopia is an inferior displacement of the facial nerve so that it lies between the oval and round windows.

ENCEPHALOCELE
Encephalocele is a protrusion of part of the brain through a congenital opening in the skull.

ENCEPHALODYSPLASIA
Encephalodysplasia is a congenital brain deformity.

ENCEPHALOMENINGOCELE
Encephalomeningocele is a protrusion of brain covered with meninges through a gap in the skull.

ENCEPHALOMYELOCELE
Encephalomyelocele is a herniation of brain and spinal cord or meninges through a defect in the occipital region of the spine.

HOLOPROSENCEPHALY
Holoprosencephaly is a single forebrain resulting from its failure to divide into hemispheres.

HYDROENCEPHALOCELE
Hydroencephalocele is a protrusion of a sac of brain substance, containing cerebrospinal fluid, through a cleft in the skull.

HYDROENCEPHALOMENINGOCELE
Hydroencephalomeningocele is the protrusion of a sac containing brain meninges and cerebrospinal fluid through a defect in the skull.

HYDROMENINGOCELE, CRANIAL
Cranial hydromeningocele is a protrusion of a meningeal sac containing cerebrospinal fluid through a defect in the skull.

HYDROMICROCEPHALY
Hydromicrocephaly is an increased amount of cerebrospinal fluid associated with microcephaly.

HYDRORACHIS EXTERNA
Hydrorachis externa is an increased amount of spinal fluid between cord and membranes.

HYDRORACHIS INTERNA
Hydrorachis interna is an increased amount of spinal fluid in the central canal or in cavities in the cord.

HYDROSYRINGOMYELIA
Hydrosyringomyelia is the presence of abnormal spaces in the spinal cord associated with distention of the spinal canal by fluid.

HYPERPLASIA, FACIAL NERVE

JAW-WINKING SYNDROME
Jaw-winking syndrome is characterized by an increase in width of eyelids during chewing.
SYNONYMS: *Jaw-winking Phenomenon, Marcus Gunn Syndrome.*

JAW-WINKING SYNDROME, REVERSE
Reverse jaw-winking syndrome is characterized by the closure of the eyelids when the mouth is opened widely.
SYNONYM: *Marin Amat Syndrome.*

MACROCEPHALY WITH HEMANGIOMATA AND PSEUDOPAPILLEDEMA SYNDROME
Macrocephaly with hemangiomata and pseudopapilledema syndrome is a syndrome with multiple cutaneous hemangiomata, pseudopapilledema, and macrocephaly without hydrocephalus.
SYNONYM: *Riley-Smith Syndrome.*

MACROGYRIA
Macrogyria is the presence of abnormally large cerebral convolutions.

MEGALENCEPHALY
Megalencephaly is an abnormal largeness of the brain.

MENINGOCELE, CEREBRAL
Cerebral meningocele is a protrusion of the meninges of the brain through a skull defect.

MENINGOENCEPHALOCELE
Meningoencephalocele is a protrusion of brain and meninges through a skull defect.

MICRENCEPHALY
Micrencephaly is an abnormally small brain.
SYNONYMS: *Microencephalon, Microencephaly.*

MICROCEPHALY
Microcephaly is an abnormally small head.
SYNONYM: *Microcephalism.*

MICROGYRIA
Microgyria is the presence of abnormally small brain convolutions.

MYELATELIA
Myelatelia is imperfect development of the spinal cord.
SYNONYM: *Hypoplasia of the Spinal Cord.*

MYELOSCHISIS
Myeloschisis is a failure of closure of the neural folds, resulting in a cleft spinal cord.

NERVE, AGENESIS OF

OCULAR ORBIT, ABSENCE OF ROOF OF
Absence of roof of ocular orbit is agenesis of the roof of the orbit of the eye.

OPTIC ATROPHY–ATAXIA SYNDROME
Optic atrophy-ataxia syndrome is a combination of pyramidal lesions, ataxia, optic nerve atrophy, mental deficiency, and other defects.
SYNONYM: *Behr's Syndrome.*

OPTIC NERVE, HYPOPLASIA OF

PACHYGYRIA
Pachygyria is the presence of unusually thick convolutions of the cerebral cortex.

PORENCEPHALY
Porencephaly is the presence of cavities within the brain.

PORENCEPHALY, FALSE
False porencephaly is the presence of multiple cystic cavities anywhere in the cerebral hemispheres but not communicating with the meningeal space or ventricles.

PSEUDOOPHTHALMOPLEGIA SYNDROME
Pseudoophthalmoplegia syndrome is the loss of control of the voluntary muscles of the eye but with retention of vestibulogenic eye deviation, due to a lesion in the basal ganglia or tectum.
SYNONYM: *Roth-Bielschowsky Disease.*

SCHIZENCEPHALY
Schizencephaly is the presence of abnormal clefts in the brain substance.

SCHIZOGYRIA
Schizogyria is a deformity of the cerebral convolutions by breaks in continuity.

SEPTUM PELLUCIDUM AGENESIS SYNDROME
Septum pellucidum agenesis syndrome is failure of development of the septum pellucidum with lacunar skull, hydrocephalus, spina bifida, and status dysraphicus.
SYNONYM: *Durand-Zunin Syndrome.*

SINUS PERICRANII
Sinus pericranii is a vascular scalp tumor communicating directly with an intracranial sinus through a skull defect.

SPINAL MENINGES, CONGENITAL ADHESIONS OF
Congenital adhesions of the spinal meninges are spinal meninges continuous with adjacent tissues.

SPINAL MENINGES, CONGENITAL ANOMALY OF
Congenital anomaly of the spinal meninges is a malformation of the spinal meninges.

SPINOCEREBELLAR ATAXIA–RETINITIS PIGMENTOSA SYNDROME
Spinocerebellar ataxia-retinitis pigmentosa syndrome is retinitis pigmentosa, deafness, spinocerebellar ataxia, and often mental retardation.
SYNONYM: *Graefe-Sjögren Syndrome.*

SYNENCEPHALOCELE
Synencephalocele is a protrusion of brain substance through a cranial defect with reduction prevented by adhesions.

ULEGYRIA
Ulegyria is the presence of narrow and scarred cerebral gyri.

SECTION 9: GLOSSARY OF CONGENITAL ANOMALIES

Eye

ABLEPHARON

Ablepharon is the absence of an eyelid.

ANEURYSM, CONGENITAL RETINAL

Congenital retinal aneurysm is an arterial dilatation in the retina.

ANIRIDIA

Aniridia is the partial or complete absence of the iris. It is usually bilateral.

SYNONYM: *Irideremia.*

ANISOCORIA, CONGENITAL

Congenital anisocoria is a congenital inequality in the size of both pupils and without associated structural abnormality of the iris or malfunction of the eye.

ANKYLOBLEPHARON FILIFORME ADNATUM

Ankyloblepharon filiforme adnatum is a condition in which there are filamentous adhesions between the upper and lower eyelids.

ANKYLOBLEPHARON, TOTAL

Total ankyloblepharon is adhesion of the eyelids to each other.

ANOPHTHALMOS

Anophthalmos is the congenital absence of one or both eyes.

APHAKIA, CONGENITAL

Congenital aphakia is the absence of the lens.

BLEPHAROCHALASIS

Blepharochalasis is an extra skin fold almost at the margin of the upper lid.

BLEPHAROCLISIS

Blepharoclisis is adhesion of the lid margins.

BLEPHAROCOLOBOMA

Blepharocoloboma is a defect, or a fissure, of an eyelid.

534

BLEPHAROPHIMOSIS
Blepharophimosis is an inability to fully open the eye.
SYNONYM: *Blepharostenosis.*

BLEPHAROPTOSIS, CONGENITAL
Congenital blepharoptosis is a drooping upper eyelid.
SYNONYM: *Blepharoptosia.*

CATARACTA MEMBRANACEA CONGENITA
Cataracta membranacea congenita is an opacification of the lens or its capsule resembling a membrane.

CATARACT, CONGENITAL
Congenital cataract is a hereditary condition characterized by loss of transparency of the lens of the eye or its capsule.
SYNONYM: *Embryonal Cataract.*

CATARACT, FROSTED
Frosted cataract is characterized by white scintillating opacities resembling frost or ice crystals and appearing in the embryonic nucleus.
SYNONYM: *Vogt's Cataract.*

CHOROID, COLOBOMA OF
Coloboma of the choroid is a defect of the choroid and retina. The exposed sclera appears as a white patch and is usually situated below the optic disc.

CHOROID, CONGENITAL CRESCENT OF
Congenital crescent of the choroid is a pigmented half-moon-shaped area, usually along the inferior margin of the disc.
SYNONYM: *Fuch's Coloboma.*

CHOROIDEREMIA
Choroideremia is progressive degeneration and atrophy of the pigment epithelium and choroid.
SYNONYM: *Tapetochoroidal Dystrophy.*

CILIA, ABSENCE OF, OR AGENESIS OF

CILIARY BODY, COLOBOMA OF
Coloboma of the ciliary body is a defect involving the corpus ciliare, the tunica vasculosa between the choroid and the iris.

COLOBOMA
Coloboma is a mutilation, defect, or fissure of any part of the eye.

CONJUNCTIVAL MELANOSIS, CONGENITAL
Congenital conjunctival melanosis is a condition characterized by pigment deposits in the conjunctiva.
SYNONYM: *Eye Melanosis.*

CONUS
Conus is a variation from the normal circular outline of the optic discs.

CORECTOPIA
Corectopia is an abnormal position of the pupil.
SYNONYM: *Ectopia of the Pupil.*

CORNEA, ABSENCE OF

CORNEA, CONGENITAL MACULAR OPACITIES OF
Congenital macular opacities of the cornea are a progressive corneal degeneration characterized by corneal opacities.

CORNEA, CRYSTALLINE DYSTROPHY OF
Crystalline dystrophy of the cornea is the presence of opacities in the anterior stromal layer of the cornea.
SYNONYM: *Schnyder's Corneal Dystrophy.*

CORNEAL EROSIONS, HEREDITARY
Hereditary corneal erosions are the presence of hereditary corneal epithelial dystrophy with corneal erosions.
SYNONYM: *Franceschetti's Dystrophy.*

CORNEAL MELANOSIS, CONGENITAL
Congenital corneal melanosis is the presence of pigment cells, which are usually large and branching, in the substantia propria or in the epithelium near the limbus.

CORNEAL OPACITY, CONGENITAL
Congenital corneal opacity is a nontransparent cornea.

CORNEA, OVAL
Oval cornea is a vertically oval or egg-shaped cornea caused by pre-natal infection or a growth defect.

CORNEA PLANA CONGENITA FAMILIARES
Cornea plana congenita familiares is a flattened cornea.

CORNEA, POLYMORPHOUS ENDOTHELIAL DEGENERATION OF
Polymorphous endothelial degeneration of the cornea is a degenera-tion of the corneal endothelium with vesicles, opacities, and nodules.

CORNEA, SPECKLED DYSTROPHY OF
Speckled dystrophy of the cornea is the presence of scattered opacities in the corneal stroma.
SYNONYM: *Francois' Speckled Dystrophy of Cornea.*

CRYPTOPHTHALMOS
Cryptophthalmos is characterized by failure of eyelid formation so that the skin is continuous from forehead to cheeks. Eyelashes and eyebrows are absent.

DACRYOCYSTIC DUCT, CONGENITAL OBSTRUCTION OF
Congenital obstruction of dacryocystic duct is a blockage of the lacrimal duct resulting from failure to discharge the epithelial plug.

DACRYOSTENOSIS, CONGENITAL
Congenital dacryostenosis is a narrowing or stricture of a lacrimal duct.

DEGENERATION, TAPETORETINAL
Tapetoretinal degeneration is degeneration of the pigment layer of the retina.

DERMOID CYST, ORBITAL
Orbital dermoid cyst is a dermoid cyst occurring in the eye socket.

DERMOID CYST, PERIORBITAL
Periorbital dermoid cyst is a dermoid cyst occurring in the periosteum of the orbit of the eye.

DYSCORIA
Dyscoria is an anomalously shaped pupil.

DYSTOPIA CANTHORUM
Dystopia canthorum is displacement or malposition of the canthus and lacrimal puncta with other associated conditions.

EMBRYOTOXON
Embryotoxon is a band of corneal opacity in the newborn.

EMBRYOTOXON, POSTERIOR
Posterior embryotoxon is a band of opacity on the posterior surface of the cornea.
SYNONYMS: *Posterior Marginal Dysplasia of Cornea, Axenfeld's Syndrome.*

EPIBLEPHARON
Epiblepharon is an extra skin fold almost at the margin of the lower lid.

EPICANTHUS
Epicanthus is a vertical fold of skin alongside the bridge of the nose, extending over and partially hiding the canthus.
SYNONYM: *Plica Palpebronasalis.*

EYE, ANASTOMOTIC VASCULAR ANOMALIES OF
Anastomotic vascular anomalies of the eye may be anastomoses of the cilioretinal arteries, opticociliary arteries, or the choroidovaginal veins.

EYE, APLASIA OF, DYSPLASIA OF, OR HYPOPLASIA OF

EYE, CONGENITAL CYSTIC
Congenital cystic eye is the arrest of development before invagination of an optical vesicle, leaving a large thin-walled cyst.

EYELID, COLOBOMA OF
Coloboma of the eyelid is a vertical fissure of the eyelid.
SYNONYM: *Palpebral Coloboma.*

EYELID, CONGENITAL ECTROPION OF
Congenital ectropion of the eyelid is the turning outward of the margin of the eyelid.

EYE, MACULAR DEFECTS OF
Macular defects of the eye are various congenital abnormalities in the macular area.

EYE MUSCLES, ACCESSORY

EYE REMNANTS, PERSISTENT FETAL VASCULAR
Persistent fetal vascular eye remnants are the presence of an embryonic type of eye vasculature in an infant.

EYE, RUDIMENTARY
Rudimentary eye is an underdeveloped eye.

EYE, SUPERNUMERARY CARUNCLE OF
Supernumerary caruncle of the eye is an extra caruncula lacrimalis of the eye.

FOLD, RETINAL
Retinal fold is a plica or margin formed by the folding of part of the retina.
SYNONYM: *Ablatio Falciformis Congenita.*

GLAUCOMA, CONGENITAL
Congenital glaucoma is characterized by enlargement of the eyeball, thinning and bulging of the cornea, a large and fixed pupil, and a very deep anterior chamber. The disorder is usually bilateral and is seen in infants and children. In this rare condition, the outflow of aqueous is obstructed by a congenital defect in the region of the angle of the anterior chamber, or by a rudimentary or absent canal of Schlemm, with consequent increase of intraocular tension. If the disease progresses, the disc becomes excavated and blindness ensues.
SYNONYMS: *Buphthalmos, Hydrophthalmos, Keratoglobus.*

HYALOID ARTERY, PERSISTENT
Persistent hyaloid artery is failure of atrophy of the hyaloid artery between the lens and the optic disc.

SYNONYM: *Persistent Cloquet's Canal.*

HYALOID CYSTS, PREPAPILLARY
Prepapillary hyaloid cysts are cysts on the disc resulting from incomplete atrophy of the hyaloid vessels.

IRIDECTROPIUM
Iridectropium is eversion of part of the iris.

IRIDOCELE
Iridocele is protrusion of part of the iris through a defect in the cornea.

IRIS, COLOBOMA OF
Coloboma of the iris is a congenital cleft of the iris, often associated with coloboma of the choroid.

SYNONYMS: *Iridoschisis, Iridocoloboma, Coloboma Iridis.*

KERATOCONUS, CONGENITAL
Congenital keratoconus is a conical protrusion of the center of the cornea.

LACRIMAL APPARATUS, ABSENCE OF, OR AGENESIS OF

LACRIMAL CANAL, ACCESSORY

LACRIMAL CANALICULA, SUPERNUMERARY

LACRIMAL CANALICULUS, INCOMPLETE OR ABSENT

LACRIMAL DUCT CLOSURE, CONGENITAL
Congenital lacrimal duct closure is the blockage of one or both tear ducts.

LACRIMAL DUCT, IMPATENCY OF
Impatency of the lacrimal duct is failure of canalization of the nasolacrimal duct, usually at the inferior ostium.

LACRIMAL GLAND, ABERRANT
Aberrant lacrimal gland is a misplaced lacrimal gland.

LACRIMAL GLAND, ECTOPIA OF
Ectopia of the lacrimal gland is an abnormal position of a lacrimal gland.

LACRIMAL PUNCTA, SUPERNUMERARY
Supernumerary lacrimal puncta are additional openings of the lacrimal canal.

LACRIMAL PUNCTUM, ABSENCE OF

LACRIMAL PUNCTUM, INFERIOR, ATRESIA OF
Atresia of the inferior lacrimal punctum is absence of a canal in the inferior lacrimal punctum.

LACRIMONASAL DUCT, SUPERNUMERARY
Supernumerary lacrimonasal duct is an extra passage from the lacrimal sac to the nasal meatus.

LENS, COLOBOMA OF
Coloboma of the lens is a defect in the lens of the eye in which the periphery is incomplete or indented.
SYNONYM: *Coloboma Lentis.*

LENS, PERSISTENT VASCULAR SHEATH
Persistent vascular sheath of the lens is the presence of a posterior portion of the vascular sheath of the lens, and the presence of the hyaloid system.
SYNONYM: *Persistent Primary Hyperplastic Vitreous.*

LENTICONUS, ANTERIOR
Anterior lenticonus is a cone-shaped protrusion of the lens, anteriorly.

LENTICONUS, POSTERIOR
Posterior lenticonus is a cone-shaped protrusion of the lens, posteriorly.

LENTIGLOBUS
Lentiglobus is a spheroid protrusion of the posterior lens surface.

MACROCORNEA
Macrocornea is a large or protruding cornea, with glaucoma as the only abnormality. The size of the cornea is 13 to 18 mm in diameter.
SYNONYM: *Megalocornea.*

MACULA, HETEROTOPIA OF
Heterotopia of macula is the abnormal location of the macula.

MEGALOCORNEA
Megalocornea is an unusually large cornea.

MEGALOPAPILLA
Megalopapilla is an unusually large optic disc.

MEGALOPHTHALMOS
Megalophthalmos is an eye of abnormally large size.

MELANOCYTOSIS, OCULODERMAL
Oculodermal melanocytosis is pigmentation of the facial skin and the eye following first and second trigeminal nerve distribution.
SYNONYMS: *Oculocutaneous Pigmentation, Nevus of Ota.*

MELANOSIS, CONGENITAL SCLERAL
Congenital scleral melanosis is the pigmentation of superficial layers of the sclerotic coat of the eye.
SYNONYM: *Schmidt-Rimpler Syndrome.*

MELANOSIS OCULI
Melanosis oculi is an increase of or excessive pigmentation in part of the eye.

MELANOSIS, RETINAL
Retinal melanosis is migration into the retinal substance and hyperplasia of retinal epithelial cells with developmental failure of subjacent rods and cones.
SYNONYMS: *Bear-track Pigmentation of Retina, Grouped Pigmentation of Retina.*

MEMBRANA CAPSULARIS LENTIS POSTERIOR
Membrana capsularis lentis posterior is a persistent nutritive capsule over the posterior surface of the crystalline lens.

MEMBRANA EPIPAPILLARIS
Membrana epipapillaris is an abnormal fibrous membrane over the optic disc.

MICROBLEPHARON
Microblepharon is an abnormally small eyelid.

MICROCORNEA
Microcornea is an abnormally thin and flat cornea.

MICROPHAKIA
Microphakia is a small spherical lens.
SYNONYMS: *Spherophakia, Microlentia.*

MICROPHTHALMOS
Microphthalmos is an abnormally small eyeball.
SYNONYM: *Microphthalmia.*

NYSTAGMUS, CONGENITAL
Congenital nystagmus is the presence of regular or rhythmic oscillations of the eyeballs. This may be horizontal, vertical, or rotary.

OCULAR MUSCLE, ABSENT

OPACITY, CONGENITAL VITREOUS
Congenital vitreous opacity is nontransparency of the vitreous body.

OPTIC DISC, CONGENITAL PIGMENTATION OF
Congenital pigmentation of the optic disc is the presence of pigment epithelium in or near the optic disc.

OPTIC DISC, GLIOSIS OF
Gliosis of the optic disc is an area of persistent neuroglia covering part or all of the optic disc.

OPTIC DISC, PITS OF
Pits of the optic disc are variable sized excavations of the optic nerve head.

OPTIC DISC, SITUS INVERSUS OF
Situs inversus of optic disc is apparent reversal of the optic disc due to passage of vessels toward the nasal instead of the temporal side.

OPTIC NERVE, APLASIA OF

OPTIC NERVE ENTRY, COLOBOMA OF
Coloboma of the optic nerve entry is a defect in the optic disc, and is usually associated with other eye defects.

OPTIC NERVE FIBERS, ABERRANT
Aberrant optic nerve fibers are small patches of misplaced nerve fibers that can occur nearly anywhere in the wall of the optic vesicle and stalk.

OPTIC NERVE FIBERS, OPAQUE
Opaque optic nerve fibers are characterized by the presence of medullations of optic nerve fibers extending onto the disc and adjacent retina so that they can be seen ophthalmoscopically.
   SYNONYMS: *Medullated Optic Nerve Fibers, Myelinated Optic Nerve Fibers, Papilla Leporina.*

OPTIC NERVE, PIGMENTATION OF
Pigmentation of the optic nerve is discoloration of the optic nerve.

OPTIC PAPILLA, CONGENITAL PSEUDONEURITIS OF
Congenital pseudoneuritis of the optic papilla is a piling of optic nerve fibers on the disc resulting in obliteration of the physiologic cup and some of the disc margin. It must be differentiated from a true neuritis of the optic papilla.
   SYNONYM: *Spurious Optic Neuritis.*

OPTIC PAPILLA, PIGMENTED
Pigmented optic papilla is an abnormal deposition of pigment in the discus nervi optici.

POLYCORIA
Polycoria is the presence of two or more pupils in one eye.

PUPIL, ATRESIA OF
Atresia of pupil is a pupil without an opening.

PUPILLARY MEMBRANE, PERSISTENT
Persistent pupillary membrane is retention of the thin vascular membrane that forms the anterior portion of the lens capsule during fetal life. It occludes the fetal pupil until about the seventh month of fetal life, when it normally disappears.

RETINA, COLOBOMA OF
Coloboma of retina is a defect in the retina.
SYNONYMS: *Coloboma Retinae, Coloboma Maculae.*

RETINA, CONGENITAL PIGMENTATION OF
Congenital pigmentation of the retina is the presence of local patches of pigment in the inner layer of the optic cup.

RETINAL DYSPLASIA SYNDROME
Retinal dysplasia syndrome consists of bilateral retinal dysplasia in the shape of rosettes with microphthalmia and cerebral agenesis .
SYNONYM: *Reese's Syndrome.*

RETINITIS PUNCTATA ALBESCENS
Retinitis punctata albescens is defective vision in bright light with fine white spots in the retina.
SYNONYMS: *Fundus Albipunctatus cum Hemeralopia, Lauber's Disease.*

RETINOSCHISIS, CONGENITAL
Congenital retinoschisis is a splitting of the retinal layers, or a detachment of the retina.

SCLERA, COLOBOMA OF
Coloboma of the sclera is a defect in the sclera or fibrous membrane that forms the outer envelope of the eye.

SCLEROTICS, BLUE
Blue sclerotics is an abnormal translucency of the sclera, enabling the color of the uvea to be seen.

VEILS, PREPAPILLARY
Prepapillary veils are mesodermal remnants of the hyaloid system.
SYNONYM: *Glial Remnants.*

VEILS, VITREOUS
Vitreous veils are preretinal or papillary veils resulting from an occluded and persistent hyaloid artery surrounded by glial tissue.
SYNONYM: *Bergmeister's Papilla.*

SECTION 9: GLOSSARY OF CONGENITAL ANOMALIES

Ear, Face, and Neck

ANOTIA
Anotia is congenital absence of an ear.
SYNONYM: *Congenital Absence of Ear.*

ANTIHELIX, PROMINENT
Prominent antihelix is an ear with disproportionate prominence of the antihelix.
SYNONYM: *Wildermuth's Ear.*

ANULUS TYMPANICUS, MALFORMATION OF
Malformation of anulus tympanicus is a congenital anomaly of the bony ring at the inner end of the external auditory meatus.

APPENDAGE, PREAURICULAR
Preauricular appendage is a supernumerary auricle or tab of skin in front of the ear.

APPENDAGES, AURICULAR
Auricular appendages are growths of the external ear. They are usually round and may contain cartilage.
SYNONYM: *Nevi Auriculares.*

AUDITORY TUBE, ABSENCE OF

AUDITORY TUBE, DIVERTICULA OF
Diverticula of auditory tube are pouchings from the lumen of the eustachian tube.

AUDITORY TUBE, WEBS OF
Webs of the auditory tube are strands of tissue across the pharyngeal end of the eustachian tube associated with an abnormal lumen patency.

AURICLE, CERVICAL
Cervical auricle is a "little ear" or depression in the side of the neck at the site of a branchial groove.

AURICLE, CONGENITAL FISTULA OF
Congenital fistula of the auricle is a tract or sinus in front of the ear at the site of a branchial cleft.
SYNONYMS: *Aural Fistula, Auricular Fistula.*

544

AURICULAR HILLOCKS, PERSISTENT
Persistent auricular hillocks are irregular pedunculated masses of connective tissue covered with skin anterior to the tragus.

BRANCHIAL SINUS, INTERNAL
Internal branchial sinus is a persistent pharyngeal pouch representing the site of a gill cleft.

BRANCHIAL SINUS, EXTERNAL
External branchial sinus is a persistent branchial groove, a depression in the neck at the site of a potential gill cleft.

CERVICO–OCULOACOUSTIC SYNDROME
Cervico-oculoacoustic syndrome is a syndrome characterized by congenital deafness, paralysis of the external eye muscles, low hairline, and a short, stiff neck.

CLEFT, BRANCHIAL
Branchial cleft is persistence of a rudimentary branchial groove.

CHIN, CONGENITAL ABSENCE OF
Congenital absence of the chin is agenesis of the chin.

CRYPTOTIA
Cryptotia is burial of the superior portion of the auricle in the scalp.

CYCLOTIA
Cyclotia is fusion of the earlobes in an infant; it is associated with absence of the mandible and a very small mouth.

CYST, BRANCHIAL
Branchial cyst is a cyst in the neck resulting from persistence of a branchial cleft.

DIVERTICULUM, CERVICAL
Cervical diverticulum is an incomplete fistula leading inward from the skin of the neck (branchial groove) or outward from the pharynx (pharyngeal pouch).

EAR, ACCESSORY TRAGUS OF
Accessory tragus of the ear is a supernumerary or extra tragus.

EAR AURICLE, CONGENITAL ABSENCE OF

EAR, BAT
Bat ear is a pointed ear with a large auricle.

EAR, CAT
Cat ear is inversion of the upper part of the auricle causing it to be cup-shaped, resembling a cat's ear.

EAR DAMAGE, THALIDOMIDE
Thalidomide ear damage is a group of ear deformities due to maternal use of thalidomide in early pregnancy.

EAR, DERMOID CYSTS OF
Dermoid cysts of the ear are cysts containing epithelium, glands, and other cutaneous elements.

EAR, FISTULAS OF
Fistulas of the ear are blind sinus tracts, usually located above the tragus.
SYNONYM: *Fistula Auris Congenita.*

EAR, FUSED CRURA OF HELIX AND ANTIHELIX OF
Fused crura of the helix and antihelix of the ear are abnormal unions of the helix and antihelix.
SYNONYM: *Mozart Ear.*

EARLOBE, CLEFT
Cleft earlobe is the failure of the tragus and antitragus to fuse.

EARLOBE, CONGENITAL ABSENCE OF
Congenital absence of the earlobe is failure of the earlobe to develop.

EAR, LOP
Lop ear is an auricle that hangs down loosely.

EAR LOBULE, SUPERNUMERARY
Supernumerary ear lobule is an extra lobe or lobes.

EAR OSSICLES, FUSION OF
Fusion of the ear ossicles is union of malleus, incus, and stapes.

EAR, POINTED
Pointed ear is an ear with a pointed tip or auricle.
SYNONYM: *Satyr Ear.*

EAR, SUPERNUMERARY
Supernumerary ear is an extra ear or ears.

EXTERNAL AUDITORY CANAL, ABSENCE OF

EXTERNAL AUDITORY CANAL, ATRESIA OF

EXTERNAL AUDITORY CANAL, STRICTURE OF
Stricture of the external auditory canal is narrowing of the outer portion of the ear canal.

EXTERNAL AUDITORY MEATUS, ATRESIA OF
Atresia of the external auditory meatus is blockage of the outer meatus by bone or fibrous tissue.

FACE, ASYMMETRY OF
Asymmetry of face is unequal development of the sides of the face.

FIRST–ARCH SYNDROME
First-arch syndrome is a group of malformations involving derivatives of the first branchial arch.

FISTULA, BRANCHIAL
Branchial fistula is the presence of an open communication between the skin of the neck and the pharynx due to persistence of an opening between a pharyngeal pouch and a branchial groove.
SYNONYMS: *Branchial Cleft Fistula, Branchiogenous Fistula.*

FISTULA, CERVICOAURAL
Cervicoaural fistula is a sinus tract or depression in the side of the neck that may communicate with the pharynx and that is at the site of a branchial groove.

FISTULA, PREAURICULAR
Preauricular fistula is a tract situated in front of the helix and above the tragus, resulting from incomplete fusion of the first and second branchial arches.
SYNONYMS: *Fistula Auris Congenita, Preauricular Sinus.*

HYDROCELE, CERVICAL
Cervical hydrocele is a cyst formed in a persistent branchial fissure.
SYNONYM: *Hydrocele Colli.*

INCUS AND STAPES, NONUNION OF
Nonunion of the incus and stapes is failure of the incus and stapes to unite.

INCUS, CONGENITAL ABSENCE OF

INNER EAR, ABSENCE OF

INNER EAR, AGENESIS OF
Agenesis of the inner ear is the failure of complete inner ear development. There are four types: Michel, Mondini-Alexander, Bing-Siebenmann, and Schiebe.

JUGULAR BULB, HERNIATION OF
Herniation of the jugular bulb is a protrusion of the bulb of the jugular vein through an opening in the floor of the middle ear.

MACROCHEILIA
Macrocheilia are abnormally large lips.
SYNONYM: *Congenital Hypertrophy of the Lips.*

MACROSTOMIA
Macrostomia is a congenitally large mouth.

MACROTIA
Macrotia is an abnormally large pinna of the ear.

MELOSCHISIS
Meloschisis is the failure of fusion that results in a congenital cleft of the cheek.

MELOTIA
Melotia is a displaced auricle.

MEMBRANOUS LABYRINTH, CONGENITAL ANOMALY OF
Congenital anomaly of the membranous labyrinth is an abnormal development of the membranous labyrinth.

MICROCHEILIA
Microcheilia are abnormally small lips.

MICROTIA
Microtia is an unusually small pinna of the ear.

MIDDLE EAR, CONGENITAL ANOMALY OF
Congenital anomaly of the middle ear is abnormal middle ear development.

MIDDLE EAR, SALIVARY GLAND TISSUE IN
Salivary gland tissue in the middle ear is the presence of areas of salivary gland cells in the middle ear.

NECK, WEBBED
Webbed neck is a short, thick fold of skin on either side, usually both sides, of the neck.
SYNONYMS: *Patagium Colli, Pterygium Colli, Pterygium Syndrome.*

ORGAN OF CORTI, ABSENCE OF

ORGAN OF CORTI, CONGENITAL ANOMALY OF
Congenital anomaly of the organ of Corti is abnormal development of the organum spirale.

OSSEOUS MEATUS, ATRESIA OF
Atresia of the osseous meatus is blockage of the bony opening of the outer ear.

OSSEOUS MEATUS, STRICTURE OF
Stricture of the osseous meatus is a narrowing of the osseous meatus.

POLYOTIA
Polyotia is the presence of a supernumerary auricle, or parts of one.

ROUND WINDOW, CONGENITAL ABSENCE OF
Congenital absence of the round window is agenesis of the round window of the ear.

SINUS, PRECERVICAL
Precervical sinus is a depression in the side of the neck at the site of a branchial cleft.

STAPEDIUS MUSCLE, CONGENITAL ABSENCE OF
Congenital absence of the stapedius muscle is absence of the stapedius muscle at birth.

STAPEDIUS TENDON, CONGENITAL OSSIFICATION OF
Congenital ossification of the stapedius tendon is bony hardening of the stapedius tendon.

STAPES FOOTPLATE, CONGENITAL FIXATION OF
Congenital fixation of the stapes footplate is an abnormal adherence of the footplate of the stapes.

SYNOTIA
Synotia is lack of lateral shift of ears so that they remain horizontally below the mandible.

TUBERCULUM AURICULAE
Tuberculum auriculae is a small projection at upper end of the posterior part of the helix as found in some simians.
SYNONYMS: *Darwinian Tubercle, Darwinian Point.*

TYMPANIC CAVITY, ABSENCE OF

VESTIGE, BRANCHIAL
Branchial vestige is a rudimentary structure at the site of a branchial cleft or gill cleft.

SECTION 9: GLOSSARY OF CONGENITAL ANOMALIES

Heart

ANOMALOUS ORIGIN OF LEFT CORONARY ARTERY FROM PULMONARY ARTERY
Anomalous origin of the left coronary artery from the pulmonary artery is the origination of the left coronary artery from the pulmonary artery instead of the aorta, so that only the right coronary artery arises from the aorta.
SYNONYM: *Bland-Garland White Syndrome.*

AORTA AND PULMONARY ARTERY, COMPLETE TRANSPOSITION OF
Complete transposition of the aorta and pulmonary artery is the result of the ridges of the truncus growing straight down so that the pulmonary artery communicates with the left ventricle and the aorta with the right ventricle.
SYNONYM: *Transposition of Great Vessels.*

AORTA, DOUBLE STENOSIS OF
Double stenosis of the aorta is a narrowed ventricular outflow tract and valvular stenosis.

AORTA, TRANSPOSITION OF
Transposition of the aorta is an aorta displaced to the right and communicating with the right ventricle.

AORTIC ARCH, COMPLETE INTERRUPTION OF
Complete interruption of the aortic arch is failure of continuity of the aortic arch.

AORTIC ATRESIA
Aortic atresia is a nonpatent aorta.

AORTIC STENOSIS, CONGENITAL VALVULAR
Congenital valvular aortic stenosis is an obstruction of the aorta due to small or narrowed semilunar or aortic valves.

AORTIC STENOSIS, MUSCULAR OUTFLOW–TRACT TYPE OF
Muscular outflow-tract type of aortic stenosis is a narrowing of the right ventricular outflow tract due to hypertrophy of cardiac musculature.
SYNONYM: *Idiopathic Hypertrophic Subaortic Stenosis.*

550

AORTIC STENOSIS, SUBVALVULAR
Subvalvular aortic stenosis is any narrowing of the outflow tract proximal to the semilunar valves.

AORTIC STENOSIS, SUPRAVALVULAR
Supravalvular aortic stenosis is a narrowing of the aorta distal to the semilunar valves.

ARTERIAL TRUNK, TRANSPOSITION OF
Transposition of the arterial trunk is reversal of the position of the thoracic aorta so that it originates on the right of the vertebral column.

ATRIAL BANDS, ANOMALOUS
Anomalous atrial bands are strips of tissue, bands, or adhesions in the atria.
SYNONYM: *Chiari's Network.*

ATRIOVENTRICULAR CANAL, COMMON
Common atrioventricular canal is persistence of the common canal joining the primitive atrium and ventricle and is due to failure of development of the endocardial cushions.
SYNONYM: *Atrioventricularis Communis.*

ATRIOVENTRICULAR CANAL, DEFECT OF
Defect of the atrioventricular canal is failure of development of the atrioventricular canal.

ATRIOVENTRICULAR CANAL, PERSISTENT
Persistent atrioventricular canal is the presence of the common canal connecting the atrium and ventricle. Arrest in development of endocardial cushions causes the gap between the interatrial and interventricular septa to fail to close.

BIVENTRICULAR PULMONARY ARTERY SYNDROME
Biventricular pulmonary artery syndrome is characterized by transposed aorta, high ventricular septal defect, hypertrophy of the right ventricle, and a large pulmonary artery that partially overrides the ventricular septum while arising primarily from the right ventricle.
SYNONYM: *Taussig-Bing Syndrome.*

BULBUS CORDIS PERSISTENT IN LEFT VENTRICLE
Bulbus cordis persistent in the left ventricle is the presence of the bulbus cordis, which is a primitive embryonic structure, between the pumping ventricle and the ventral aorta.

CARDIAC CONDUCTION DEFECT, CONGENITAL FAMILIAL
Congenital familial cardiac conduction defect is characterized by intraventricular and atrioventricular node conduction defects.

CARDIAC VALVE, ABNORMAL POSITION OF
Abnormal position of the cardiac valve is a congenital downward displacement of the tricuspid valve into the right ventricle.

CARDIAC VALVE, DOUBLE ORIFICE OF
Double orifice of the cardiac valve is the presence of two openings in a cardiac valve.

CARDIAC VALVE, INCOMPLETE DIFFERENTIATION OF
Incomplete differentiation of the cardiac valve is incomplete development of the cardiac valve.

CARDIAC VALVE, MYXOMATOSIS OF
Myxomatosis of the cardiac valve is the presence of myxomas or fibromyxomas on the pulmonary or aortic valves of neonates, probably due to persistence of embryonic tissues.

CARDIOMEGALY, CONGENITAL
Congenital cardiomegaly is an enlarged heart.
SYNONYM: *Congenital Cardiac Dilatation.*

COR BILOCULARE
Cor biloculare is a heart with a common atrium, common ventricle, and common atrioventricular valve.
SYNONYM: *Two-Chambered Heart.*

CORONARY ARTERIOVENOUS FISTULA, CONGENITAL
Congenital coronary arteriovenous fistula is a direct communication or fistula between a coronary artery and either the pulmonary artery, coronary vein, or a cardiac chamber.

CORONARY ARTERY ANEURYSM, CONGENITAL
Congenital coronary artery aneurysm is a congenital dilatation of a coronary artery.

COR PSEUDOTRILOCULARE BIATRIATUM
Cor pseudotriloculare biatriatum is tricuspid atresia with rudimentary right ventricle and passage of blood from the dilated right atrium to the left atrium. The result functionally is a three-chambered heart.

COR TRIATRIATUM
Cor triatriatum is a heart with three atria.
SYNONYM: *Accessory Atrium.*

COR TRILOCULARE
Cor triloculare is a heart with two atria and one ventricle or one having two ventricles and one atrium.

COR TRILOCULARE BIATRIATUM
Cor triloculare biatriatum is a three-chambered heart resulting from absence of the interventricular septum.
SYNONYM: *Common Ventricle.*

CUSPS OR LEAFLETS, ABNORMAL NUMBER OF
An abnormal number of cusps or leaflets is any departure from the normal number of cusps.

DEXTROCARDIA
Dextrocardia is displacement of the heart to the right side, either as a mirror-image transposition, or a simple displacement.

Isolated Dextrocardia
Isolated dextrocardia is dextrocardia without situs inversus of other organs.

Mirror-Image Dextrocardia
Mirror-image dextrocardia is abnormal development of the heart so that all of its components are normal but in a reversed relationship as if seen in a mirror.

Simple Displacement Dextrocardia
Simple displacement dextrocardia is a condition in which the heart is simply pushed to the right.

DISEASE, BLUE
Blue disease is any congenital heart disease with cyanosis.
SYNONYM: *Morbus Caeruleus.*

ECTOPIA CORDIS
Ectopia cordis is a congenital misplacement of the heart resulting in protrusion of most of the heart through an abdominal wall defect.
SYNONYM: *Displaced Heart.*

ENDOCARDIAL CUSHION DEFECT
Endocardial cushion defect is failure of development of the endocardial thickenings of the common canal connecting the atrium with the ventricle.

FIBROELASTOSIS CORDIS
Fibroelastosis cordis is an endocardium that has been replaced by a thick fibroelastic coat or fibrin-like fibers. It is associated with ventricular hypertrophy and fibrosis of the myocardium. The aortic valve leaflets are often damaged.
SYNONYMS: *Endocardial Fibroelastosis, Primary Endocardial Sclerosis, Congenital Endocarditis, Endomyocardial Fibrosis, Endomyocardial Sclerosis, Fetal Endocarditis, Weinberg-Himelfarb Syndrome.*

FORAMEN OVALE, PATENT
Patent foramen ovale is an opening between the atria that remains open.
> SYNONYMS: *Anatomically Patent Foramen Ovale, Functionally Patent Foramen Ovale, Incompetent Valve of Foramen Ovale, Nonclosure of Foramen Ovale, Persistent Foramen Ovale, Probe Patent Foramen Ovale.*

FORAMEN OVALE, PREMATURELY CLOSED
Prematurely closed foramen ovale is closure of the foramen ovale before birth, resulting in failure of the blood to shunt from the right to the left atrium.

GREAT VESSELS, CORRECTED TRANSPOSITION OF
Corrected transposition of the great vessels is the reversal of the position of the great vessels but with inversion of the ventricles or atria, resulting in normal circulation.

HEART ANEURYSM, CONGENITAL
Congenital heart aneurysm is a dilatation and thinning of the wall of the heart.

HEART, ANOMALOUS BANDS OF
Anomalous bands of the heart is the presence of abnormal bands or adhesions within the heart.

HEART BLOCK, CONGENITAL
Congenital heart block is atrioventricular conduction impairment or arrest.

HEART, CONGENITAL IDIOPATHIC HYPERTROPHY OF
Congenital idiopathic hypertrophy of the heart is dilatation and hypertrophy of the heart with myocardial degeneration and fibrosis.
> SYNONYM: *Kugel-Stoloff Syndrome.*

HEART, HYPOPLASIA OF
Hypoplasia of heart is an incompletely or defectively developed heart.

HEART, UNILOCULAR
Unilocular heart is a single-chambered heart.

HEART VALVE, ANOMALIES OF
Anomalies of the heart valve include atresia, insufficiency, stenosis, stricture, double orifice, fenestration of the cusps, fusion of the cusps, and supernumerary cusp.

HYPOPLASTIC LEFT HEART SYNDROME
Hypoplastic left heart syndrome is a group of malformations including hypoplasia of the left ventricle and/or aortic and mitral valve atresia.

LEVOCARDIA
Levocardia is a heart that is normally placed on the left side but with situs inversus of other organs.
SYNONYM: *Sinistrocardia.*

LEVOCARDIA, ISOLATED
Isolated levocardia is a heart with mirror-image transposition of the chambers of the heart without displacement of abdominal viscera.

MICROCARDIA
Microcardia is an abnormally small heart.

MITRAL INSUFFICIENCY, CONGENITAL
Congenital mitral insufficiency is an inadequate mitral valve.

MITRAL VALVE, ATRESIA OF
Atresia of the mitral valve is nonpatency of the mitral valve.

MITRAL VALVE, CLEFT LEAFLET OF
Cleft leaflet of the mitral valve is a mitral valve having a bifid leaflet.

MITRAL VALVE, DUPLICATION OF
Duplication of the mitral valve is the presence of two mitral valves.

MITRAL VALVE, STENOSIS OF
Stenosis of the mitral valve is a narrowing of the mitral valve.
SYNONYM: *Duroziez's Disease.*

OSTIUM ARTERIOSUM PRIMUM, PERSISTENT
Persistent ostium arteriosum primum is an opening or perforation that develops in the septum primum dividing the atria.
SYNONYMS: *Interatrial Foramen Primum, Foramen Ovale I.*

OSTIUM ARTERIOSUM SECUNDUM, PERSISTENT
Persistent ostium arteriosum secundum is an opening between the atria resulting from incomplete development of the septum secundum.
SYNONYMS: *Interatrial Foramen Secundum, Foramen Ovale II.*

PENTALOGY SYNDROME
Pentalogy syndrome is a syndrome characterized by ventricular septal defect, pulmonic stenosis, dextraposition of the aorta, right ventricular hypertrophy, and an atrioseptal defect.
SYNONYM: *Fallot's Pentalogy.*

PERICARDIUM, ABSENCE OF

RIGHT VENTRICLE, HYPOPLASIA OF
Hypoplasia of the right ventricle is inadequate development of the myocardium of the right ventricle, which may be paper-thin, like parchment.
SYNONYM: *Uhl's Anomaly.*

SEPTAL DEFECT, AORTIC

Aortic septal defect is a communication between the aorta and the pulmonary artery just above the valves.

SYNONYMS: *Aorticopulmonary Window, Partial Truncus Arteriosus, Absent Aortic Septum.*

SEPTAL DEFECT, INTERATRIAL

Interatrial septal defect is any persistent opening in the partition between the left and right atria.

SYNONYMS: *Interauricular Septal Defect, Common Atrium, Cor Triloculare Biventriculare, Atrioseptal Defect.*

SEPTAL DEFECT, INTERATRIAL, WITH MITRAL STENOSIS AND ENLARGED RIGHT ATRIUM

SYNONYM: *Lutembacher's Syndrome.*

SEPTAL DEFECT, VENTRICULAR

Ventricular septal defect is a defect or absence of the septum between the ventricles.

SYNONYMS: *Interventricular Septal Defect, Roger's Disease.*

SEPTAL DEFECT, VENTRICULAR, WITH HYPERTROPHIED RIGHT VENTRICLE

Ventricular septal defect with hypertrophied right ventricle is a ventricular septal defect with overriding aorta, and hypertrophy of the right ventricle.

SYNONYM: *Eisenmenger Complex.*

SINUS VENOSUS, REMNANTS OF VALVES OF

Remnants of the valves of the sinus venosus is persistence of portions of the valves of the sinus venosus.

STENOSIS, SUBAORTIC

Subaortic stenosis is a narrowed ventricular outflow ring of fibrous tissue just below the aortic valve.

TETRALOGY SYNDROME

Tetralogy syndrome is a syndrome characterized by ventricular septal defect, pulmonic stenosis or atresia, dextraposition (overriding) of aorta, and hypertrophy of the right ventricle.

SYNONYM: *Fallot's Tetralogy.*

TRICUSPID VALVE, ATRESIA OF

TRICUSPID VALVE, BICUSPID

Bicuspid tricuspid valve is a valve between the right atrium and the right ventricle that has only two cusps.

TRICUSPID VALVE, CLEFT LEAFLET OF

Cleft leaflet of the tricuspid valve is a tricuspid valve with a bifid leaflet.

TRICUSPID VALVE, DOWNWARD DISPLACEMENT OF

Downward displacement of the tricuspid valve is displacement down into the right ventricle of the tricuspid valve.

SYNONYMS: *Ebstein's Anomaly, Ebstein's Malformation.*

TRICUSPID VALVE, QUADRICUSPID

Quadricuspid tricuspid valve is a valve between the right atrium and the right ventricle that has four cusps.

TRILOGY SYNDROME

Trilogy syndrome is a syndrome characterized by pulmonic stenosis, atrial septal defect, and hypertrophy of right ventricle.

SYNONYM: *Fallot's Trilogy.*

TRUNCUS ARTERIOSUS COMMUNIS

Truncus arteriosus communis is persistence of the truncus due to failure in the development of the septum between the aorta and pulmonary artery.

SYNONYM: *Common Truncus.*

TRUNCUS ARTERIOSUS, PERSISTENT

Persistent truncus arteriosus is the result of failure of the bulbus aortae to divide longitudinally to form the aorta and pulmonary artery.

VENTRICLE, RIGHT DOUBLE-OUTLET

Right double-outlet ventricle is a malformation in which the aorta and the pulmonary artery arise from the right ventricle.

Circulatory System

ANEURYSM, ARTERIOVENOUS (PERIPHERAL)

ANEURYSM, CONGENITAL PERIPHERAL

AORTA, ABSENCE OF, APLASIA OF, ATRESIA OF, OR HYPOPLASIA OF

AORTA, COARCTATION OF
Coarctation of the aorta is atresia or stenosis of the thoracic aorta just beyond the origin of the left subclavian artery.

AORTA, CONGENITAL ANEURYSM OF
Congenital aneurysm of the aorta is a dilatation and thinning of a section of the aorta.

AORTA, CONGENITAL DILATATION OF
Congenital dilatation of the aorta is congenital enlargement of the aorta.

AORTA, DEXTROPOSITION OF
Dextroposition of the aorta is displacement of the aorta to the right and communication between the aorta and the right ventricle.

AORTA, OVERRIDING OF
Overriding of the aorta is a shift in the aortic orifice so that it is over (overrides) the defect in the septal opening; it thus receives blood from both the left and right openings. It is due to absence of the membranous portion of the septum of the ventricle with a resultant shift in position of the aorta.

AORTA, POSTDUCTAL COARCTATION OF
Postductal coarctation of the aorta is a stenosis of the aorta beyond the ductus arteriosus; it is called the adult type of coarctation.

AORTA, PREDUCTAL COARCTATION OF
Preductal coarctation of the aorta is a stenosis of the aorta before the origin of the ductus arteriosus; it is called the fetal or infantile type of coarctation.

AORTIC ANEURYSM, CONGENITAL RUPTURED
Congenital ruptured aortic aneurysm is the rupture of an aortic aneurysm before birth is completed.

AORTIC ARCH, DOUBLE
Double aortic arch results from persistence of the right fourth aortic arch, so that there is a right aortic arch as well as a left aortic arch.

AORTIC ARCH, PERSISTENT CONVOLUTIONS OF
Persistent convolutions of the aortic arch is the presence of embryonic configurations of the aortic arch.

AORTIC ARCH, PERSISTENT RIGHT
Persistent right aortic arch is the presence and development of the fourth right aortic arch as a functioning aorta in communication with the descending aorta.

ARTERIOVENOUS FISTULA, CONGENITAL PULMONARY
Congenital pulmonary arteriovenous fistula is any communication between artery and vein in the lung other than through the normal capillary bed.

ARTERIOVENOUS FISTULA, CONGENITAL
Congenital arteriovenous fistula is a communication between artery and vein with massive bypassing of normal circulatory routes. It usually occurs in thorax, liver, or brain.
SYNONYM: *Massive Systemic Arteriovenous Fistula.*

ARTERY, CONGENITAL STRICTURE OF

ARTERY OR VEIN, ABSENCE OF OR ATRESIA OF

ASCENDING AORTA, STENOSIS OF
Stenosis of the ascending aorta is a stricture of the ascending aorta.

BRAIN, ARTERIOVENOUS ANEURYSM OF

BRAIN, ARTERIOVENOUS MALFORMATIONS OF
Arteriovenous malformations of the brain are variable collections of blood vessels—arterial, venous, or aneurysmal. They may be in a mass within the brain or distributed over the surface of the cortex.

BRAIN, CONGENITAL ANEURYSM OF

BRAIN, VASCULAR ANOMALIES OF

CARDINAL VEIN, PERSISTENT LEFT POSTERIOR
Persistent left posterior cardinal vein does not unite with the left anterior cardinal vein but persists and empties into the sinus venosus.

COMMUNICATION, PULMONARY VEIN–CARDINAL VEIN
Pulmonary vein-cardinal vein communication is persistence of some communication between pulmonary veins and some vessels arising from the anterior cardinal veins.

DUCTUS ARTERIOSUS, DOUBLE
Double ductus arteriosus is due to persistence of the sixth aortic arch on the right side, as well as on the left.

DUCTUS ARTERIOSUS, PATENT
Patent ductus arteriosus is the result of the nonclosure of the fetal vessel connecting the left pulmonary artery to the descending aorta.
SYNONYMS: *Patent Ductus Botalli, Nonclosure of Ductus Arteriosus, Persistent Ductus Arteriosus.*

DUCTUS ARTERIOSUS, RIGHT–SIDED
Right-sided ductus arteriosus is persistence of the sixth right aortic arch rather than the left.

FISTULA, SINUS AORTAE
Sinus aortae fistula is a defective development of an aortic sinus with aneurysm formation and rupture into the right or left ventricle or left atrium.
SYNONYMS: *Sinus of Valsalva Fistula, Ruptured Aneurysm of Sinus of Valsalva.*

HYPOPLASIA, AORTIC ARCH (TUBULAR)
Aortic arch (tubular) hypoplasia is a stenosis of the ascending aortic arch due to maldevelopment.

LEVOATRIOCARDINAL VEIN
Levoatriocardinal vein is the presence of a left common cardinal vein draining (venous) blood from left side of the body into the left atrium with resultant moderate cyanosis.

PATENT DUCTUS ARTERIOSUS–REVERSED FLOW SYNDROME
Patent ductus arteriosus-reversed flow syndrome is the shunting of blood from the pulmonary artery to the aorta.

PHARYNX, VASCULAR RING OF
Vascular ring of the pharynx is a complex of anomalous arteries surrounding the trachea and esophagus.

PHLEBECTASIA, CONGENITAL
Congenital phlebectasia is a widespread reddish, reticulated mottling of the skin associated with red telangiectasia. Flat blue angiomata are often present.
SYNONYMS: *Van Lohuizen's Disease, Cutis Marmorata Telangiectatica.*

PORTAL VEIN, ABSENCE OF

PORTAL VEIN, ANOMALOUS TERMINATION OF
Anomalous termination of the portal vein is termination of the portal vein in a location other than in the liver.

PSEUDOTRUNCUS ARTERIOSUS
Pseudotruncus arteriosus is an anomaly with pulmonary valve atresia, and no main pulmonary artery. The blood supply to lungs is through a patent ductus or through bronchial arteries from the aorta.

RIGHT PULMONARY VEIN, ANOMALOUS TERMINATION OF
Anomalous termination of the right pulmonary vein is termination of the right pulmonary vein directly into the right atrium.

SEQUESTRATION, PULMONARY ARTERY
Pulmonary artery sequestration is separation of the pulmonary artery from the bronchial tree.

SUPERIOR LEFT VENA CAVA, PERSISTENCE OF
Persistence of the superior left vena cava results from the failure of the innominate vein to develop so that the left common cardinal vein persists as a left superior vena cava.

TUNNEL, AORTIC–LEFT VENTRICULAR
Aortic-left ventricular tunnel is an aneurysmal communication from the aortic root, above the valves into the left ventricle, through the upper part of the septum of the ventricle.

UMBILICAL ARTERY, SINGLE
Single umbilical artery is the presence of a single artery in the amniotic cord. It is often associated with other anomalies.

VARIX, CONGENITAL
Congenital varix is a congenitally enlarged vein, artery, or lymphatic vessel.

VENOUS DRAINAGE, ANOMALOUS PULMONARY
Anomalous pulmonary venous drainage is drainage of the pulmonary vein into the vena cava or into the left innominate vein with associated septal defects.
SYNONYM: *Taussig-Snellen-Albers Syndrome.*

VENOUS RETURN, TOTAL ANOMALOUS PULMONARY
Total anomalous pulmonary venous return is an anomalous emptying into the right atrium or its tributaries of all four pulmonary veins.

Respiratory System

ARHINIA

Arhinia is absence of the nose.

ARYTENOID CARTILAGE, DISPLACEMENT OF, DEFORMITY OF, OR ABSENCE OF

ATRESIA, CHOANAL

Choanal atresia is failure of communication of the nose with the pharynx, a blockage of posterior nares.

SYNONYM: *Congenital Closure of the Nose.*

BRONCHUS, ABSENCE OF, OR AGENESIS OF

BRONCHUS, BLIND

Blind bronchus is a bronchus that does not end in bronchioles and alveolar tissue.

BRONCHUS, DIVERTICULUM OF

Diverticulum of the bronchus is an outpouching of the wall of a bronchus.

BRONCHUS, TRACHEAL

Tracheal bronchus is an ectopic or anomalous bronchus extending to the upper lobe of right lung from the trachea.

COLUMELLA NASI, ABSENCE OF

COLUMELLA NASI, CONGENITAL SHORTENING OF

CRICOID CARTILAGE, ABSENCE OF, DEFORMITY OF, OR ANOMALY OF

CYST, BRONCHIOGENIC

Bronchiogenic cyst is a pulmonary cyst that is usually centrally located, single, and arising from a major bronchus.

EPIGLOTTIS, ATRESIA OF, OR ABSENCE OF

EPIGLOTTIS, FISSURE OF

FISTULA, LARYNGOTRACHEAL

Laryngotracheal fistula is an abnormal communication between larynx and trachea.

FISTULA, TRACHEAL
Tracheal fistula is any abnormal communication of the trachea with the skin surface, esophagus, or larynx.

GLOSSOPTOSIS
Glossoptosis is the downward displacement or recession of the tongue, which may cause laryngeal obstruction.

GLOTTIS, ATRESIA OF

LARYNGOCELE
Laryngocele is an air sac communicating with the lumen of the larynx. It is usually visible on the neck.

LARYNX, ABSENCE OF, AGENESIS OF, OR ATRESIA OF

LARYNX AND TRACHEA, ABNORMAL UNION OF
Abnormal union of the larynx and trachea is an abnormally close junction or fusion of the larynx and trachea.

LARYNX, CHONDROMALACIA OF
Chondromalacia of the larynx is the presence of soft laryngeal cartilage. SYNONYM: *Laryngomalacia.*

LARYNX, CONGENITAL FISSURE OF
Congenital fissure of the larynx is an abnormal opening into larynx.

LARYNX, CONGENITAL STENOSIS OF

LARYNX, DOUBLE
Double larynx is the presence of two larynxes with a single pharynx.

LARYNX, WEB OF
Web of the larynx is a membranous septum across the larynx. It may be perforate or imperforate.

LUNG, ABERRANT LOBE OF
Aberrant lobe of the lung is a misplaced lobe of lung.

LUNG, ABSENCE OF, AGENESIS OF, OR APLASIA OF

LUNG, ABSENCE OF LOBE OR FISSURES OF

LUNG, ACCESSORY LOBE OF
Accessory lobe of the lung is a supernumerary lobe of a lung that is part of the lung proper.

LUNG, ANOMALOUS FISSURE FORMATION OF
Anomalous fissure formation of the lung is an anomaly of the development of the lung fissures.

LUNG, AZYGOUS LOBE OF
Azygous lobe of the lung is an extra lobe, which may be found at either lung apex.

LUNG, BILOBED RIGHT
Bilobed right lung is the absence of one of the lobes of the normally trilobed right lung.

LUNG, CONGENITAL CYSTIC
Congenital cystic lung is one comprised of multiple small cysts.

LUNG, CONGENITAL CYSTS OF

LUNG, CYSTIC ADENOMATOID
Cystic adenomatoid lung is the presence of multiple microscopic cysts with a great overgrowth of bronchi.

LUNG, CYST OF PERIPHERY OF
Cyst of the periphery of the lung is a cyst with irregular plates of cartilage in the walls; it resembles dilated bronchi.
SYNONYM: *Solitary Cyst of the Lung.*

LUNG, EXTRAPULMONIC ACCESSORY LOBE OF
Extrapulmonic accessory lobe of the lung is a supernumerary lobe separate from the lung proper.

LUNG, HETEROTOPIC BRAIN TISSUE IN
Heterotopic brain tissue in the lung is the presence of small amounts of brain tissue in the lungs of anencephalic monsters.

LUNG, HONEYCOMB
Honeycomb lung is characterized by the presence of many thin-walled cysts in the lung.

LUNG HYPOPLASIA, PRIMARY
Primary lung hypoplasia is the failure of normal development of lung tissue in an otherwise normal infant.

LUNG HYPOPLASIA, SECONDARY
Secondary lung hypoplasia is the failure of lung development resulting from a condition that has reduced the capacity of the thoracic cage.

LUNG, POLYCYSTIC DISEASE OF
Polycystic disease of the lung is characterized by the presence of multiple small cysts in the lung.

LUNG, RUDIMENTARY
Rudimentary lung is an imperfectly developed lung.

LUNG, SEQUESTERED LOBE OF
Sequestered lobe of the lung is a mass of lung tissue not communicating with the bronchial tree.

LUNG, VARIATIONS OF LOBULATIONS OF
Variations of lobulations of the lung are deviations from the normal lobulation of the lungs.

LYMPHANGIECTASIS, PULMONARY
Pulmonary lymphangiectasis is characterized by an increase in number and size of the pulmonary lymphatic channels.

MEDIASTINUM, CONGENITAL CYST OF

NARES, ATRESIA OR STENOSIS OF

NASAL SEPTUM, CONGENITAL DEVIATION OF

NASAL SEPTUM, LATERAL DISPLACEMENT OF
Lateral displacement of the nasal septum is displacement of the lower border of the septum into one nasal canal.

NASOPHARYNX, ATRESIA OF

NOSE, ACCESSORY

NOSE, CLEFT
Cleft nose is a broad groove in the midline, dividing the nose more or less symmetrically.
SYNONYM: *Double Nose.*

NOSE, CONGENITAL NOTCHING OF
Congenital notching of the nose is indentation of tip of the nose due to maldevelopment of the frontonasal process.

NOSE, HALF
Half nose is the absence of half of the external nose due to maldevelopment of the frontonasal process.

NOSE, TUBULAR PROBOSCIS OF
Tubular proboscis of the nose is protrusion of the nose due to failure of migration downward of the frontonasal process.

PARANASAL SINUS, CONGENITAL DEFORMITY OF

PARANASAL SINUS, PERFORATION OF

PERICARDIAL SAC, ABNORMAL COMMUNICATION OF PLEURAL SAC WITH

PLEURAL FOLDS, ANOMALY OF

SEPTAL CARTILAGE, ABSENCE OF

SEQUESTRATION, CONGENITAL BRONCHOPULMONARY
   Congenital bronchopulmonary sequestration is the loss of the connection between the bronchial tree and a mass of lung tissue. A separate bronchus and separate circulation are present.
   SYNONYMS: *Intralobar Bronchopulmonary Sequestration, Pulmonary Sequestration.*

THYROID CARTILAGE, CONGENITAL ABSENCE OF, OR DEFORMITY OF

THYROID CARTILAGE, CONGENITAL CLEFT OF
   Congenital cleft of the thyroid cartilage is a partial or complete opening in the midline anteriorly of the cartilago thyroidea.

TRACHEA, ABSENCE OF, AGENESIS OF, OR ATRESIA OF

TRACHEA, CARTILAGINOUS OCCLUSION OF
   Cartilaginous occlusion of the trachea is blockage of the trachea below the vocal cords by a mass of cartilage.

TRACHEA, CONGENITAL DILATATION OF

TRACHEA, CONGENITAL STENOSIS OF

TRACHEOCELE, CONGENITAL
   Congenital tracheocele is a pouching or protrusion outward of the mucous membrane through the tracheal wall.

VOCAL CORDS, CONGENITAL PAPILLOMAS OF
   Congenital papillomas of the vocal cords are papillomas occurring on the vocal cords.

Cleft Palate and Cleft Lip

CLEFT, FACIAL
Facial cleft is the failure of closure of the cheek from the side of the nose to the medial canthus of the eye.

CLEFT LIP, CLEFT PALATE WITH

CLEFT MAXILLA, CENTRAL
Central cleft maxilla is a failure of development of the frontonasal process, and occurs only in association with cebocephalus.

CLEFT PALATE, COMPLETE

CLEFT PALATE, FLAT FACE, AND MULTIPLE DISLOCATION SYNDROME
SYNONYM: *Larsen's Syndrome.*

CLEFT PALATE, INCOMPLETE

LIP, CLEFT
Cleft lip is a fissure in the upper lip. It may be unilateral or bilateral.
SYNONYMS: *Congenital Fissure of Lip, Split Lip, Harelip, Labium Leporinum, Cheiloschisis, Cheilognathus.*

LIP, COMMISSURAL PITS OF
Commissural pits of the lip are fistulas located at commissures of lips.

PALATE, FISSURE OF

PALATE, FISTULAS OF
Fistulas of the palate are the result of failure of fusion at the junction of the soft palate and anterior pillar of the fauces; they are usually bilateral.

PALATOSCHISIS
Palatoschisis is cleft palate.

UVULA, SPLIT
Split uvula is a cleft of the soft palate or uvula palatina.
SYNONYMS: *Bifid Uvula, Cleft Uvula, Staphyloschisis.*

Upper Alimentary Tract

AGLOSSIA–ADACTYLIA SYNDROME
Aglossia-adactylia syndrome consists of lingual hypoplasia and failure of development of the digits.

AGLOSSIA, CONGENITAL

ANKYLOGLOSSIA
Ankyloglossia is an abnormally short frenulum linguae.
SYNONYM: *Tongue-tie.*

ANKYLOGLOSSIA SUPERIOR SYNDROME
Ankyloglossia superior syndrome consists of adherence of the tongue to the hard palate with microglossia, dental defects, and digital hypoplasia or aplasia.

ATELOSTOMIA
Atelostomia is imperfect development of the mouth and parts.

ATRESIA, PREPYLORIC
Prepyloric atresia is an obstruction by a membrane at the outlet of the stomach above the pylorus.

CARDIOSPASM
Cardiospasm is a spasm of the sphincter at the cardiac end of stomach.

CHEILOGNATHOGLOSSOSCHISIS
Cheilognathoglossoschisis is a syndrome of cleft in the tongue, in the middle of the lower lip, and in the mandible.

CONTRACTION RING, ESOPHAGEAL
Esophageal contraction ring is a circular zone of muscle in spasm causing stenosis of the esophagus.
SYNONYM: *Schatzki's Ring.*

DIVERTICULUM, ESOPHAGEAL
Esophageal diverticulum is a pouching of the esophageal wall.
SYNONYM: *Esophageal Pouch.*

ESOPHAGUS, ABSENCE OF, ATRESIA OF, IMPERFORATE, CONGENITAL STENOSIS OF, OR CONGENITAL STRICTURE OF

ESOPHAGUS, DILATATION OF
SYNONYM: *Esophagectasia.*

ESOPHAGUS, DISPLACEMENT OF

ESOPHAGUS, DUPLICATION OF

ESOPHAGUS, GIANT
SYNONYMS: *Congenital Megaloesophagus, Congenital Megaesophagus.*

ESOPHAGUS, SHORT
Short esophagus is an abnormally short esophagus usually associated with, or the result of, an esophageal hiatus hernia.

ESOPHAGUS, WEBBED
Webbed esophagus is an esophagus with bands or strands of tissue across the lumen.

FISTULA, BRONCHOESOPHAGEAL
Bronchoesophageal fistula is a communication between the esophagus and a bronchus.

FISTULA, GASTROCOLIC
Gastrocolic fistula is a direct connection between the stomach and colon.

FISTULA, SALIVARY GLAND

FISTULA, SUBLINGUAL
Sublingual fistula is an abnormal communication of a sublingual salivary gland with the skin surface.

FISTULA, TRACHEOESOPHAGEAL
Tracheoesophageal fistula is a communication between the trachea and esophagus.

GASTRIC MUCOSA, DISPLACEMENT OF
Displacement of the gastric mucosa is the presence of gastric mucosa in unusual or abnormal places. It usually appears as a cyst behind the pleura.

GULLET, ATRESIA OF

HOLOGASTROSCHISIS
Hologastroschisis is an abdomen with an opening extending its whole length.

LARYNGEAL NERVE DUOSYNDROME
Laryngeal nerve duosyndrome is the combination of unilateral facial weakness with contralateral vocal cord weakness due to pressure in utero on laryngeal nerve or its blood supply.
SYNONYM: *Chopple's Syndrome.*

LINGUA PLICATA
Lingua plicata is a tongue with papillae in clumps separated by small fissures and resembling the skin of the scrotum.
SYNONYM: *Congenital Scrotal Tongue.*

LIP, DOUBLE
Double lip is a sagging of the inner villous portion of the mucous membrane of the lip (pars villosa) below the smooth outer zone of the lip (pars glabra), giving the appearance of a double lip.

LIP PITS, LOWER
Lower lip pits are small fistulas or sinuses on the midportion of lower lip.
SYNONYMS: *Midlip Pits, Lip Fistulas.*

LIPS, ECTOPIC SEBACEOUS GLANDS OF
Ectopic sebaceous glands of the lips are hypertrophic sebaceous glands of the lips and mouth.
SYNONYMS: *Pseudocolloid of Lips, Fordyce's Disease* (mouth).

MACROGLOSSIA
Macroglossia is an abnormally large tongue.
SYNONYM: *Megaloglossia.*

MEGAESOPHAGUS–BRONCHIECTASIS SYNDROME
Megaesophagus-bronchiectasis syndrome is enlarged esophagus with tracheoesophageal fistula, skeletal deformities, and bronchiectasis.
SYNONYM: *Turpin's Syndrome.*

MEGALOGASTRIA
Megalogastria is an abnormally large stomach.

MICROGASTRIA
Microgastria is a small stomach.

MICROGLOSSIA
Microglossia is a small tongue.

MOUNDS, LIP
Lip mounds are puckerings or protrusions of tissue on the midportion of the lower lips.

PALATE, HIGH–ARCHED

PAROTID GLANDS, ABSENCE OF

PHARYNX, DIVERTICULUM OF
Diverticulum of the pharynx is a pouching of the wall of the pharynx.
SYNONYM: *Pharyngoesophageal Diverticulum.*

PHARYNX, IMPERFORATE

PHARYNX, POLYP OF

POUCH, PHARYNGEAL
A pharyngeal pouch is a bulging outward of the pharyngeal entoderm between the branchial arches.

PYLORUS, SPASM OF
Spasm of the pylorus is a narrowing of the lumen due to excessive contractions of the pyloric sphincter without an increase in volume of the pyloric sphincter muscles.

RANULA
Ranula is a retention cyst of the submaxillary or sublingual gland.

SALIVARY DUCT, ATRESIA OF, OR DUPLICATE OF

SALIVARY GLAND, ABSENCE OF, OR ACCESSORY

STENOSIS, HYPERTROPHIC PYLORIC
Hypertrophic pyloric stenosis is stenosis due to hypertrophy of the circular and longitudinal muscles of the pyloric sphincter.

STENOSIS, PYLORIC
Pyloric stenosis is hypertrophy chiefly of the circular layer of muscle in the pyloric sphincter.
SYNONYM: *Congenital Pyloric Constriction.*

STOMACH, DISPLACEMENT OF
Displacement of the stomach is any abnormal position of the stomach, usually resulting from failure of normal rotation of the stomach to the left, or from herniation through the diaphragm.

STOMACH, DUPLICATION OF
Duplication of the stomach is usually manifested by a small, closed cavity or cyst lined with gastric mucosa.

STOMACH, HOURGLASS CONTRACTION OF

STOMACH, TRANSPOSITION OF
Transposition of the stomach is failure or reversal of rotation so that the cardiac end of the stomach lies to the right of midline and the pyloric end to the left.

SUBMAXILLARY GLANDS, ABSENCE OF

SYNCHILIA
Synchilia is partial or complete adhesion of the lips, that is, atresia of the mouth.

THORACIC CYSTS, GASTRIC

Gastric thoracic cysts are intrathoracic cysts parallel to or attached to the esophagus and usually originating from the esophagus.

TONGUE, ABSENCE OF

TONGUE, CONGENITAL ADHESIONS OF

TONGUE, CONGENITAL HYPERTROPHY OF

TONGUE, DOUBLE

Double tongue is a tongue that is split at the end for a variable distance.
SYNONYMS: *Schistoglossia, Bifid Tongue, Cleft Tongue, Forked Tongue.*

TONGUE, DOWNWARD DISPLACEMENT OF

TONGUE, FISSURED

Fissured tongue is a tongue with grooves or fissures parallel to or at right angles to the midline groove of tongue.
SYNONYM: *Lingua Fissurata.*

TONGUE, HYPOPLASIA OF

TONGUE, TRIFID

Trifid tongue is a tongue divided longitudinally into three parts.

UPPER ALIMENTARY TRACT, ABSENCE OF

UPPER ALIMENTARY TRACT, HYPOPLASIA OF

UPPER ALIMENTARY TRACT, MALPOSITION OF

UVULA, ABSENCE OF

Digestive System

ADHESIONS, ANOMALOUS OMENTAL

ADHESIONS, PERITONEAL
   Peritoneal adhesions are fibrous bands, or areas of peritoneal surface, that have fused.

AGENESIS, ANORECTAL
   Anorectal agenesis is absence of the anus and part of rectum.

ALIMENTARY TRACT, ABSENCE OF

ANUS, ABSENCE OF

ANUS, ATRESIA OF
   Atresia of the anus is an occluded anus, one without a canal.

ANUS, COVERED
   Covered anus is a normally situated anal canal leading into a sub-cutaneous tunnel running forward in the midline, opening on the under-surface of the perineum, scrotum, or penis.

ANUS, DUPLICATION OF
   Duplication of the anus is the presence of two anal orifices.

ANUS, ECTOPIC
   An ectopic anus is one that is not in its normal position but may be situated anywhere in the midline between the normal position and the vagina or scrotum.

ANUS, HYPOPLASIA OF

ANUS, IMPERFORATE
   Imperforate anus is one in which the anal canal does not communicate with the exterior.
   SYNONYM: *Occlusion of Anus.*

ANUS, STRICTURE OF
   Stricture of the anus is a narrowing of the anal canal.

APPENDIX, DUPLICATION OF
   Duplication of the appendix is the presence of more than one appendix.

573

APPENDIX, TRANSPOSITION OF
Transposition of the appendix results from failure of rotation of the bowel so that the appendix is in the left side of the abdomen.

BAR, ANAL
Anal bar is a median anteroposterior bridge of soft tissue dividing the anus into two separate openings.

BILE DUCT, ATRESIA OF
Atresia of the bile duct is a bile duct without a lumen.

BILE DUCT, DUPLICATION OF
Duplication of the bile duct is the presence of two bile ducts, partial or complete.

BILE DUCT, HYPOPLASTIC
Hypoplastic bile duct is failure of normal development of the bile duct.

BILE DUCT, MALPOSITION OF
Malposition of the bile duct is failure of the bile duct to develop in the normal anatomic relationships.

BILE DUCT OR PASSAGE, OBSTRUCTION OF
Obstruction of the bile duct or passage is blockage of the bile duct.

BILE DUCT, STRICTURE OF
Stricture of the bile duct is a narrowed lumen of a bile duct.

BOWEL, INCOMPLETE ROTATION OF
Incomplete rotation of the bowel is failure of the bowel to complete its normal turning or migration from the midline to the right side of the abdomen.

CECUM, ATRESIA OF
Atresia of the cecum is a cecum without a lumen.

CECUM, DUPLICATION OF
Duplication of the cecum is the presence of two cecums.

CECUM, INCOMPLETE ROTATION OF
Incomplete rotation of the cecum is failure of the cecum to migrate to the right side of the abdomen.

CECUM, MOBILE
Mobile cecum is a cecum that is loose due to failure of the mesocolon of the ascending colon to fuse with the adjacent peritoneum.

CLOACA, EXSTROPHY OF
Exstrophy of the cloaca is the presence of two bladder areas, each having its own ureter. Between these vesical areas lies intestinal mucosa. Below this is an imperforate anus.

CLOACA, PERSISTENT
Persistent cloaca is a single orifice for the passage of feces and urine due to inadequate separation of the urethra from the rectum, resulting in common canal.

CLOACA, RECTOVESICAL FISTULA OF
Rectovesical fistula of the cloaca is a communication between the rectum and bladder in a patient with a cloaca.

CLOACAL DIVISION, FAILURE OF
Failure of cloacal division is the nonabsorption of the wedge-shaped septum separating the urogenital sinus from rectum.

CLOACAL SEPTUM, PERSISTENT
Persistent cloacal septum is the persistence of the urorectal septum, a wedge of mesenchyme.

COLON, ADHESIONS OF
Adhesions of the colon are thin, vascular, veil-like, congenital adhesions covering the anterior of the colon from the hepatic flexure to the cecum.
SYNONYMS: *Jackson's Membrane, Jackson's Veil.*

COLON, ATRESIA OF
Atresia of the colon is a large bowel without a lumen.

COLON, DIVERTICULUM OF
Diverticulum of the colon is a pouching of the wall of the colon.
SYNONYM: *Congenital Diverticulitis of Colon.*

COLON, MALROTATION OF
Malrotation of the colon is failure of the cecal end of the colon to migrate to the right side of the abdomen.

COLON, STENOSIS OF
Stenosis of the colon is a narrowing of the large bowel.

COLON, TRANSPOSITION OF
Transposition of the colon is a colon that is on the wrong side due to failure of normal rotational development.

COMMON DUCT, STRICTURE OF
Stricture of the common duct is a narrowing of the common duct.

COMMON MESENTERY, PERSISTENT
Persistent common mesentery is the persistence of the two layers of splanchnic mesoderm (peritoneum) that support the intestines and are attached dorsally and ventrally to the body wall, thus dividing the peritoneal cavity into two parts.
SYNONYMS: *Universal Mesentery, Primary Mesentery, Primitive Mesentery.*

CYSTIC DUCT, ANOMALIES OF
Anomalies of the cystic duct are quite frequent abnormalities of cystic duct formation and implantation into the common hepatic duct.

DIMPLE, ANAL
Anal dimple is the depression in skin over anal canal if the canal is imperforate.

DIVERTICULUM ILEI
Diverticulum ilei is a blind pouch of the ileum representing the remains of the omphalomesenteric duct.
SYNONYM: *Meckel's Diverticulum.*

DOLICHOCOLON
Dolichocolon is an abnormally long colon.

DUODENUM, AGENESIS OF
Agenesis of the duodenum is failure of development of the duodenum.

DUODENUM, ATRESIA OF
Atresia of the duodenum is a duodenum without a lumen.

DUODENUM, STENOSIS OF
Stenosis of the duodenum is a narrowing of the duodenum.

FISSURE, ANAL
An anal fissure is a crack or ulceration along the anal margin.

FISTULA, ANAL
An anal fistula is an abnormal position of the anal opening or openings.

FISTULA, CYSTIC DUCT
Cystic duct fistula is an abnormal communication between the cystic duct and skin surface.

FISTULA, FECAL
Fecal fistula is an abnormal communication between the intestines and the skin surface or another viscus.

FISTULA, RECTOPERINEAL
A rectoperineal fistula is an abnormal tract or communication between the rectum and perineum.

GALLBLADDER, ABSENCE OF

GALLBLADDER, BILOBED
A bilobed gallbladder is a gallbladder with two lobes or sacculations.

GALLBLADDER, DIVERTICULUM OF
Diverticulum of the gallbladder is an outpouching of the wall of the gallbladder.

GALLBLADDER, DUPLICATION OF
Duplication of the gallbladder is the presence of two gallbladders. SYNONYM: *Double Gallbladder*.

GALLBLADDER, ECTOPIC
Ectopic gallbladder is a gallbladder not in its normal location.

GALLBLADDER, FLOATING
Floating gallbladder is one that is abnormally mobile, a wandering gallbladder.

GALLBLADDER, HOURGLASS CONTRACTION OF
Hourglass contraction of the gallbladder is a gallbladder with a constriction of its midpart so that it resembles an hourglass.

GALLBLADDER, INTRAHEPATIC
Intrahepatic gallbladder is a gallbladder situated within the substance of the liver.

GASTROINTESTINAL TRACT, DUPLICATION OF
Duplication of the gastrointestinal tract is manifest as a cystic area lined with intestinal mucosa and muscle lying alongside part of the gastrointestinal tract.

GROOVE, ANOVAGINAL
Anovaginal groove is a groove in the peritoneum extending from the anus to the posterior labial commissure.

HEPATIC DUCTS, ACCESSORY
Accessory hepatic ducts are extra or supernumerary hepatic ducts.

HEPATOMEGALY
Hepatomegaly is an abnormally large liver.

HERNIA, TRANSMESENTERIC
Transmesenteric hernia is a hernia caused by a loop of intestine slipping through a gap in the mesentery.

ILEOCECAL VALVE, ATRESIA OF
Atresia of the ileocecal valve is an imperforate ileocecal valve.

ILEOCECAL VALVE, STENOSIS OF
Stenosis of the ileocecal valve is a narrowed ileocecal valve.

ILEUM, AGENESIS OF
Agenesis of the ileum is failure of development of the ileum.

ILEUM, ATRESIA OF
Atresia of the ileum is an ileum without a lumen.

ILEUM, STENOSIS OF
Stenosis of the ileum is a narrowed ileum.

ILEUM, VOLVULUS OF
Volvulus of the ileum is a twisting of ileum due to incomplete mesenteric attachment.

INTESTINAL ROTATION, FAILURE OF
Failure of intestinal rotation is failure of the intestines to migrate from their fetal midline position to their adult sites.
SYNONYMS: *Incomplete Intestinal Rotation, Insufficient Intestinal Rotation.*

INTESTINE, ABSENCE OF

INTESTINE, ATRESIA OF
Atresia of the intestine is absence of a lumen in the intestines.

INTESTINE, DUPLICATIONS OF
Duplications of the intestine are the presence of parts of more than one intestinal canal.

INTESTINE, STENOSIS OF
Stenosis of the intestine is a narrowing of the intestines.

INTESTINE, TRANSPOSITION OF
Transposition of the intestine is failure of normal rotation of the intestine resulting in the bowel being on the wrong side.

INTUSSUSCEPTION
Intussusception is the infolding, or invagination, of one part of the intestine into an adjacent portion.

JEJUNUM, AGENESIS OF, ATRESIA OF, OR CONGENITAL STENOSIS OF

JEJUNUM, VOLVULUS OF
Volvulus of the jejunum is a twisting of the jejunum.

LIVER, ABSENCE OF

LIVER, ACCESSORY
Accessory liver is an extra or discrete area of liver tissue.

LIVER, CYST OF
Cyst of the liver is any dilatation or sac of the liver.

LIVER, ECTOPIC LOBE OF
Ectopic lobe of the liver is an additional area of liver tissue.

LIVER, FIBROCYSTIC DISEASE OF

Fibrocystic disease of the liver is a liver with a greatly increased number of bile ducts, which may vary from short tubular structures to developed ducts. Increase in connective tissue is quite variable. Polycystic kidneys are usually associated.

SYNONYM: *Polyductal Fibrosis.*

LIVER, GROOVES OF

Grooves of the liver are linear indentations on the surface of the liver representing scars secondary to irregularly distributed necrosis and fibrosis.

LIVER LOBULATION, ABNORMAL

Abnormal liver lobulation is the unusual lobule formation usually resulting from the pressure of adjacent organs, and ordinarily without functional significance.

LIVER, POLYCYSTIC DISEASE OF

Polycystic disease of the liver is the presence of many small cysts, or tubular structures resembling bile ducts, in the liver substance.

SYNONYM: *Congenital Cystic Disease of Liver.*

LIVER, PSEUDOLOBULATION OF

Pseudolobulation of the liver is the false appearance of lobule formation given by deep scars of the liver secondary to necrosis and fibrosis.

LOBUS LINGUIFORMIS IECORIS

Lobus linguiformis iecoris is a tonguelike process of liver tissue extending downward, usually from the right lobe.

SYNONYM: *Riedel's Lobe.*

LOWER ALIMENTARY TRACT, ABSENCE OF

LOWER ALIMENTARY TRACT, MALPOSITION OF

Malposition of the lower alimentary tract is any abnormality of normal rotational growth resulting in failure of the lower bowel to reach its normal position.

MEGALOAPPENDIX

Megaloappendix is an abnormally large appendix.

MEGALODUODENUM

Megaloduodenum is an abnormally large duodenum.

MICROCOLON

Microcolon is an abnormally small colon.

MESENTERY, DEFECT OF
Defect of the mesentery is an opening or gap in the mesentery resulting from incomplete attachment of mesentery. A loop of bowel may slip through the gap to form a transmesenteric hernia.

OBSTRUCTION, INTESTINAL
Intestinal obstruction is a blockage of the intestines due to any cause.

OMENTUM, CYST OF
Cyst of the omentum is a cyst developing in the omentum, usually due to obstructed lymphatic channels.

OMPHALOMESENTERIC DUCT, PATENT
Patent omphalomesenteric duct is a persistent and open duct from the ileum through the umbilicus.
SYNONYM: *Umbilical Fecal Fistula.*

OMPHALOMESENTERIC DUCT, PERSISTENT
Persistent omphalomesenteric duct is the persistent yolk stalk, or connection between the yolk sac and the intraembryonic gut.
SYNONYMS: *Persistent Yolk Stalk, Persistent Vitelline Duct.*

OMPHALOMESENTERIC DUCT, PERSISTENT VESSELS OF
Persistent vessels of the omphalomesenteric duct is the presence of the blood vessels of the omphalomesenteric duct.

PANCREAS, ABERRANT
Aberrant pancreas is pancreatic tissue developing in atypical sites such as the stomach or duodenum.

PANCREAS, ABSENCE OF, OR AGENESIS OF

PANCREAS, ACCESSORY
Accessory pancreas is a separate portion of the head of the pancreas.
SYNONYM: *Pancreas Accessorium* (NA).

PANCREAS, ANNULAR
Annular pancreas is a ring of pancreatic tissue surrounding the duodenum.

PANCREAS, CYSTS OF
Cysts of the pancreas are large cysts, lined with epithelium and usually occurring in the body or tail of pancreas.

PANCREAS, HYPOPLASIA OF
Hypoplasia of the pancreas is incomplete development of the pancreas.

PERICOLIC MEMBRANE SYNDROME
Pericolic membrane syndrome is a constricting band or adhesions around the colon, causing constipation and indigestion.

POLYP, UMBILICAL
Umbilical polyp is a small protrusion of tissue at the navel comprised of remnants of the yolk stalk.

RECTUM, ABSENCE OF, AGENESIS OF, ATRESIA OF, OR IMPERFORATE

RECTUM, STRICTURE OF
Stricture of the rectum is a narrowing of the rectum.
SYNONYM: *Stenosis of Rectum.*

SEPTUM, ANAL
Anal septum is a partition or wall of tissue dividing the anus into two parts.

STENOSIS, ANAL
Anal stenosis is a narrowing of the anal canal.

VOLVULUS
Volvulus is a twisting of the intestines.

Genital Organs

APLASIA, OVARIAN
Ovarian aplasia is failure of development of ovarian tissue.
SYNONYM: *Ovarian Agenesis.*

ANGIODYSTROPHIA OVARII
Angiodystrophia ovarii is an increased number of blood vessels in the ovary.

ANORCHIDISM
Anorchidism is the absence of testes.
SYNONYMS: *Anorchia, Anorchism.*

CANAL, URETHRORECTAL
Urethrorectal canal is an anomalous connection between the urethra and rectum.

CERVIX, CONGENITAL ATRESIA OF, STENOSIS OF, CONGENITAL ABSENCE OF, ACCESSORY, OR RUDIMENTARY

CLITORIS, ABSENCE OF, AGENESIS OF, OR DUPLICATION OF

CLITORIS, CLEFT OF
Cleft of the clitoris is a defect of the ventral wall often associated with epispadias or exstrophy.
SYNONYMS: *Cleavage of Clitoris, Congenital Fissure of Clitoris.*

CLITORIS, HYPERPLASIA OF
Hyperplasia of the clitoris is an abnormally large clitoris.

CLITORIS, HYPERTROPHY OF
Hypertrophy of the clitoris is a grossly enlarged clitoris. Although idiopathic clitoral hypertrophy occurs, most cases result from endocrinopathies.

CRYPTORCHISM
Cryptorchism is failure of descent of a testis.
SYNONYM: *Cryptorchidism.*

CYST, FIMBRIAL
Fimbrial cyst is a stalked vesicle attached to one of the fimbriae of the fallopian tubes and is a müllerian duct remnant.

CYST, PARAMESONEPHRIC VAGINAL
Paramesonephric vaginal cyst is a cyst developing along the course of the paramesonephric ducts.

CYSTS, PAROVARIAN
Parovarian cysts are cysts arising from mesonephric duct vestiges and lying in the mesosalpinx.

DUCTULI EPOOPHORI TRANSVERSINA
Ductuli epoophori transversina are the short tubules of the epoophoron that connect with the longitudinal duct.

DYSTOPIA TRANSVERSA EXTERNA TESTIS
Dystopia transversa externa testis is a testis transposed to the contralateral half of the scrotum, having crossed under the skin of the dorsum of the penis.

DYSTOPIA TRANSVERSA INTERNA TESTIS
Dystopia transversa interna testis is crossing of the testes through contralateral inguinal canals so that the testes lie in the scrotum on opposite sides of the body from their origin.

EJACULATORY DUCT, ABSENCE OF

EJACULATORY DUCT, ATRESIA OF
Atresia of the ejaculatory duct is an ejaculatory duct without a lumen.

ENDOCERVICAL FOLDS, HYPERTROPHY OF
Hypertrophy of the endocervical folds is the presence of unusually deep and thick transverse endocervical folds of tissue.

EPIDIDYMIS, ABSENCE OF

EPISPADIAS, MALE
Male epispadias is an opening of the urethra on the upper aspect of the penis posterior to the normal site.
SYNONYM: *Anaspadias.*

FALLOPIAN TUBE, ABSENCE OF, ACCESSORY, ATRESIA OF, OR TORTUOUS

FALLOPIAN TUBE, BLIND SAC OF
Blind sac of the fallopian tube is a diverticulum or outpouching of the fallopian tube.

FALLOPIAN TUBE, INFANTILE
Infantile fallopian tube is a hypoplastic or underdeveloped tube.

FISTULA, ABDOMINOUTERINE
Abdominouterine fistula is an abnormal communication between the uterine cavity and the peritoneal cavity.
SYNONYM: *Uteroabdominal Fistula.*

FISTULA, ENTEROVAGINAL
An enterovaginal fistula is the abnormal communication between the intestinal canal and the vagina.

FISTULA, INTESTINOVAGINAL
An intestinovaginal fistula is an abnormal communication between the intestine and the vagina.

FISTULA, RECTOPERINEAL
A rectoperineal fistula is an abnormal communication between the rectum and the perineum.

FISTULA, RECTOUTERINE
A rectouterine fistula is an abnormal communication between the rectum and the uterine cavity.
SYNONYM: *Uterorectal Fistula.*

FISTULA, RECTOVULVAL
A rectovulval fistula is an abnormal communication between the rectum and the vulvar area.

FISTULA, TUBOABDOMINAL
Tuboabdominal fistula is an abnormal communication between the tubal lumen and the peritoneal cavity.

FISTULA, UTEROINTESTINAL
Uterointestinal fistula is an abnormal communication between the uterine cavity and the intestinal canal.
SYNONYM: *Enterouterine Fistula.*

FUSION, SPLENOGONADAL
Splenogonadal fusion is a fusion of spleen and testicle.

GENITALIA, AMBIGUOUS
Ambiguous genitalia are external genital organs not clearly belonging to either sex.

GENITAL ORGANS, FEMALE, ABSENCE OF

GENITAL ORGANS, MALE, ABSENCE OF

GENITOURINARY ORGANS, ABSENCE OF

HYDROCELE
Hydrocele is a collection of fluid in the tunica vaginalis testis.
SYNONYM: *Funicular Hydrocele.*

HYDROCELE, BILOCULAR
Bilocular hydrocele is a bilateral hydrocele.
SYNONYM: *Dupuytren's Hydrocele.*

HYMEN, ABSENCE OF, OR ATRESIA OF

HYPOPLASIA, OVARIAN
Ovarian hypoplasia is inadequate or incomplete development of an ovary.

HYPOSPADIAS, MALE
Male hypospadias is an urethral opening on the inferior surface of the glans penis or scrotum.

HYPOSPADIAS, PERINEAL
Perineal hypospadias is an urethral opening in the perineal region.

HYPOSPADIAS, PSEUDOVAGINAL
Pseudovaginal hypospadias is a marked degree of perineal hypospadias.

INTERSEXUALITY
Intersexuality is the presence of both male and female sexual characteristics in one individual.

LABIA, FUSION OF
Fusion of the labia is the presence of adherent labia but does not imply anomalies of the underlying genitalia.
SYNONYM: *Synechia Vulvae.*

LABIUM, ABSENCE OF
Absence of the labium is agenesis of labia.

MACROPENIS
Macropenis is an unusually large penis.
SYNONYM: *Megalopenis.*

MESONEPHRIC DUCT, PERSISTENT
Persistent mesonephric duct is the presence of elements of the mesonephric duct system in the walls of the vagina or alongside the uterus.
SYNONYM: *Persistent Gartner's Duct.*

MICROORCHISM
Microorchism is infantile development, or hypoplasia, of both testicles.

MICROPENIS
Micropenis is an unusually small penis.
SYNONYM: *Microcaulia.*

MONORCHISM
Monorchism is the presence of a single testis.
SYNONYM: *Monorchidism.*

OVARIAN DESCENT, FAILURE OF
Failure of ovarian descent is nondescent of an ovary into its normal
pelvic fossa, so that it remains in the fetal position above the pelvic inlet.

OVARY, ABSENCE OF, UNILATERAL ABSENCE OF, ACCESSORY, OR SUPERNUMERARY

OVARY, ECTOPIC
Ectopic ovary is an ovary not in the usual place.

OVARY, INGUINAL
Inguinal ovary is an ovary located in the inguinal canal.

OVARY, TORSION OF
Torsion of the ovary is twisting of an ovary on its stalk or pedicle.

OVOTESTIS
Ovotestis is a gonad with both testicular and ovarian components.

PARADIDYMIS
Paradidymis is a group of persisting mesonephric duct tubules attached
above the head of the epididymis.

PARAMESONEPHRIC DUCT, CYST OF
Cyst of the paramesonephric duct is a cyst along the course of the
paramesonephric duct.
SYNONYM: *Müllerian Duct Cyst.*

PARAMESONEPHRIC DUCT FUSION, FAILURE OF
Failure of paramesonephric duct fusion is nonunion of the paramesonephric ducts resulting in double uteri and double cervices and perhaps
double vaginas.

PARAMESONEPHRIC DUCT REST
Paramesonephric duct rest is any remnant or persistent tissue of the
paramesonephric duct.
SYNONYM: *Müllerian Rest.*

PARASPADIAS
Paraspadias is an urethral opening on the side of the penis.

PENIS, ABSENCE OF, OR AGENESIS OF

PENIS, ADHERENT
Adherent penis is a condition in which the penis is attached to other structures, usually along the raphe and usually causing curvature.

PENIS AND SCROTUM, TRANSPOSITION OF
Transposition of the penis and scrotum is a condition in which the penis is located in perineal area, usually posterior to a partially cleft scrotum.

PENIS, CLEFT
Cleft penis is one having a dorsal groove and a ventral meatus.

PENIS, CONCEALED
Concealed penis is one hidden beneath the skin or in the pubic fat.

PENIS, MEDIAN RAPHE OF, CYSTS OF
Cysts of the median raphe of the penis are cysts along the cutaneous ridge on the inferior portion of the penis.

PENIS, DOUBLE
Double penis is a duplication or doubling of the penis.
SYNONYMS: *Diphallus, Duplication of Penis.*

PENIS, HYPOPLASIA OF
Hypoplasia of the penis is underdevelopment of the penis.
SYNONYM: *Rudimentary Penis.*

PENIS, TORSION OF
Torsion of the penis is the condition in which the penis is twisted or partially rotated.

PHALLOCAMPSIS
Phallocampsis is a bent or curved penis.

POLYORCHIDISM
Polyorchidism is the presence of more than two testes.
SYNONYMS: *Polyorchism, Supernumerary Testis.*

PREPUBERTAL CASTRATE FUNCTIONAL SYNDROME
Prepubertal castrate functional syndrome is congenital failure of gonadal development with resultant eunuchoidism.

PREPUCE, APLASIA OF
Aplasia of the prepuce is absence of the prepuce.

PROCESSUS VAGINALIS PERITONEI, PATENT
Patent processus vaginalis peritonei is a persistent and open vaginal process or extension of the peritoneal cavity down the inguinal canal.
SYNONYMS: *Nuck's Diverticulum, Patent Nuck's Canal.*

PROLAPSE, CONGENITAL CERVICAL
Congenital cervical prolapse is a dropping or downward displacement of the cervix and uterus resulting from relaxed cardinal ligaments and pelvic tissues.

PROSTATE, ABSENCE OF, OR APLASIA OF

ROUND LIGAMENT, APLASIA OF
Aplasia of the round ligament is failure of the gubernaculum testis (male) or ligamentum teres (female) to develop properly.

SCROTUM, ABSENCE OF, OR CLEFT OF

SEMINAL TRACT OR DUCT, ABSENCE OF

SPERMATIC CORD, ABSENCE OF

SPERMATOCELE
Spermatocele is a collection of semen in the tunica vaginalis.

SYNORCHIDISM
Synorchidism is fusion of the testes in the abdominal cavity.
SYNONYMS: *Synorchism, Fusion of Testes.*

TESTIS, ABSENCE OF, APLASIA OF, OR HYPOPLASIA OF

TESTIS, ECTOPIC
Ectopic testis is a testis that is not in the scrotum.

TESTIS, UNDESCENDED
Undescended testis is a testis that has failed to descend fully into the scrotum.
SYNONYMS: *Imperfectly Descended Testis, Improperly Descended Testis, Maldescent of Testis, Descensus Aberrans Testis.*

TESTIS, UNDESCENDED, WITH HYDROCELE
Undescended testis with hydrocele is failure of the normal descent of the testis with an associated hydrocele.

UROGENITAL UNION, FAILURE OF
Failure of urogenital union is failure of the cranial mesonephric tubules to join properly with the epididymis so that the testes do not unite with the efferent system.

UTERINE HORN, RUDIMENTARY
Rudimentary uterine horn is a hypoplastic uterus that has not fused with the other paramesonephric duct.

UTERUS, ABSENCE OF, OR APLASIA OF
Absence or aplasia of the uterus is complete failure of any uterine elements to develop.

UTERUS, ACCESSORY
Accessory uterus is a smaller second uterus.

UTERUS, ATRESIA OF
Atresia of the uterus is a uterus without an open canal.

UTERUS BICORNIS BICOLLIS
Uterus bicornis bicollis is a uterus with two corpora and two cervices.

UTERUS BICORNIS UNICOLLIS
Uterus bicornis unicollis is a uterus with two corpora and a single cervix.

UTERUS, BICORNUATE, WITH DOUBLE CERVIX AND DOUBLE VAGINA
Bicornuate uterus with double cervix and double vagina is a double uterus with conjoined corpora and two cervices and two vaginas.

UTERUS BILOCULARIS
Uterus bilocularis is a uterus divided into two cavities by a septum and with no external mark of separation into two organs.
SYNONYM: *Uterus Bipartitus.*

UTERUS, HYPOPLASIA OF
Hypoplasia of the uterus is an incompletely developed uterus.

UTERUS PUBESCENS
Uterus pubescens is an undeveloped uterus that is adult in type.

UTERUS, RIBBON
Ribbon uterus is a uterus represented only by a transverse band of fibromuscular tissue.

UTERUS, RUDIMENTARY
Rudimentary uterus is a uterus that has only begun to develop.

UTERUS, RUDIMENTARY, IN MALE
Rudimentary uterus in the male is the presence of a hypoplastic uterus in a male.

UTERUS, SEPTATE, WITH DOUBLE VAGINA
Septate uterus with double vagina is a uterus divided into two halves by a wall of tissue and having two cervices and two vaginas.

UTERUS, SEPTATE, WITH SINGLE VAGINA
Septate uterus with single vagina is a uterus having a thin wall dividing it into two cavities but with a single vagina.

UTERUS SIMPLEX

Uterus simplex is a uterus with a single cavity as contrasted to double uteri.

UTERUS, SINGLE-HORNED

Single-horned uterus is a uterus having only one cornu and one tube.

UTERUS, SOLID RUDIMENTARY

Solid rudimentary uterus is a solid band of fibromuscular tissue representing the uterus.

UTERUS SUBPUBESCENS

Uterus subpubescens is an incompletely developed uterus having the corpus longer than the cervix.

UTERUS SUBSEPTUS

Uterus subseptus is a uterus with an incomplete partition or wall dividing its cavities.

UTRICULUS PROSTATICUS

Utriculus prostaticus is a müllerian or paramesonephric duct remnant that may persist and form retrovesical cysts.

SYNONYMS: *Sinus Pocularis, Uterus Masculinus.*

UTERUS UNILATERALIS

Uterus unilateralis is the development of a paramesonephric duct system on one side only so that the uterus is on one side of the pelvis.

VAGINA, EMBRYONAL CYSTS OF

Embryonal cysts of the vagina are dilated sacs in the wall of the vagina, usually developing in mesonephric or paramesonephric duct remnants.

VAGINA, SEPTATE

Septate vagina is a vagina with a septum or partition of tissue, usually in the midline anteroposteriorly.

VAGINA, UNILATERAL

Unilateral vagina is a single vagina developed on one side.

VAS DEFERENS, ABSENCE OF

VULVA, ABSENCE OF, OR ATRESIA OF

VULVA, DUPLICATION OF

Duplication of the vulva is the presence of two vulvas usually associated with two vaginas and two uteri. Incomplete twinning or an included twin have been suggested as a cause.

Urinary System

AGENESIS, VESICAL
Vesical agenesis is absence of the bladder.
SYNONYM: *Bladder Agenesis.*

BLADDER, ACCESSORY
SYNONYMS: *Double Bladder, Vesica Duplex.*

BLADDER, EXTROVERSION OF
Extroversion of the bladder is a herniation of the bladder through the urethra.
SYNONYM: *Urethral Cystocele.*

BLADDER, HOURGLASS CONTRACTION OF
Hourglass contraction of the bladder is characterized by two or more compartments in the bladder, resembling an hourglass, usually due to a persistent ureteral membrane.

BLADDER, HYPOPLASIA OF
Hypoplasia of the bladder is incomplete development of the bladder.

BLADDER, PROLAPSE OF
Prolapse of the bladder is a dropping, herniation, or displacement of the bladder.

CYST, URACHAL
Urachal cyst is a cyst developing along the course of the urachus.

DUPLICATION, URETHRAL
Urethral duplication is the presence of an accessory urethra, usually associated with double penis.

EPISPADIAS, FEMALE
Female epispadias is a partial defect of the ventral wall so that the dorsal wall of the urethra becomes an open trough.

EXTERNAL MEATUS, URETHRAL CYSTS OF
Urethral cysts of the external meatus are dilatations of or near the urethra in proximity to the meatus.

591

FACIES, RENAL AGENESIS

Renal agenesis facies is a facial appearance usually associated with renal agenesis. There is a prominent epicanthic fold that forms a semicircle arising on the forehead and swinging down to cover the medial palpebral commissures and ending on the cheek. The nose is usually flattened, and the ears are flat without a formed helix and set low on the sides of the head.

SYNONYM: *Potter Syndrome.*

FISTULA, RECTOURETHRAL

Rectourethral fistula is an abnormal communication between the rectum and urethra.

FISTULA, RECTOVESICAL

Rectovesical fistula is an abnormal communication between the rectum and bladder, usually associated with imperforate anus.

FISTULA, UMBILICOURINARY

Umbilicourinary fistula is an abnormal and patent connection between the bladder and umbilical skin.

SYNONYM: *Umbilicovesical Fistula.*

FISTULA, URACHAL

Urachal fistula is an abnormal communication between a persistent urachus and the skin surface.

FISTULA, URETHRAL

Urethral fistula is an abnormal communication between the urethra and skin surface or vagina.

FISTULA, URETHRORECTAL

Urethrorectal fistula is an abnormal communication between the urethral lumen and rectal canal.

HERNIA, BLADDER

Bladder hernia is a pouching or protrusion of bladder, usually into the vagina.

HYDRONEPHROSIS

Hydronephrosis is a dilatation of the renal pelvis and calyces.

HYDROURETER

Hydroureter is a dilated ureter.

HYPOSPADIAS, FEMALE

Female hypospadias is a urethral opening along the anterior vaginal wall, posterior to the usual site.

KIDNEY, ABERRANT BLOOD VESSELS OF
Aberrant blood vessels of the kidney are renal blood vessels in an unusual or abnormal position.

KIDNEYS, ABSENCE OF
SYNONYM: *Renal Agenesis.*

KIDNEY, ACCESSORY
Accessory kidney is an extra kidney.

KIDNEY, CAKE
Cake kidney is a kidney fused into an irregular shape.
SYNONYM: *Lump Kidney.*

KIDNEY, CALCULUS OF
Calculus of the kidney is a renal stone.

KIDNEY, CONGENITAL MOVABLE
Congenital movable kidney is a kidney that changes its position easily. An ectopic kidney by contrast is fixed in an abnormal position.
SYNONYM: *Ren Mobilis.*

KIDNEY, DOUBLE
Double kidney is a second kidney on one side with duplication of the pelvis and ureter.
SYNONYMS: *Duplex Kidney, Kidney Duplication.*

KIDNEY, DOUBLE, WITH DOUBLE PELVIS
Double kidney with double pelvis is the presence of two separate kidneys with separate pelves on the same side.

KIDNEYS, DOUGHNUT
Doughnut kidneys are kidneys with polar fusion, both kidneys remaining on the same level, and resembling a doughnut or disc.
SYNONYM: *Discoid Kidney.*

KIDNEY, DYSPLASIA OF
Dysplasia of the kidney is the persistence of embryonic structures in a kidney.

KIDNEY, ECTOPY OF
Ectopy of the kidney is a misplaced kidney fixed in an abnormal position. It may be unilateral or bilateral.
SYNONYMS: *Ectopia Renis, Displaced Kidney, Dystopia of Kidney.*

KIDNEY, FETAL LOBULATION OF
Fetal lobulation of the kidney is persistence of the embryonic structure so that a multipapillary arrangement occurs.

KIDNEYS, FUSION OF
Fusion of the kidneys is the growing together of both kidneys. Various forms may result such as: cake kidney, horseshoe kidney, lump kidney, L-shaped kidney, scutiform kidney, shield kidney, sigmoid kidney, crossed ectopy, and fusion of the kidneys.

KIDNEYS, FUSION OF, CROSSED ECTOPY WITH
Crossed ectopy with fusion of the kidneys is displacement of one kidney to the other side with fusion.

KIDNEYS, FUSION OF, CROSSED ECTOPY WITHOUT
Crossed ectopy without fusion of the kidneys is displacement of one kidney to the opposite side without fusion to its mate.

KIDNEY, GIANT
Giant kidney is an abnormally large kidney.

KIDNEY, HYPERPLASIA OF
Hyperplasia of the kidney is enlargement of the kidney with the formation of new renal units.

KIDNEY, HYPERTROPHY OF
Hypertrophy of the kidney is an increase in the size and functional capacity of a kidney.

KIDNEYS, HYPOPLASIA OF
Hypoplasia of the kidneys is underdevelopment of a kidney or kidneys.
SYNONYM: *Infantile Kidney.*

KIDNEY, INTRATHORACIC
Intrathoracic kidney is an ectopic kidney located above the diaphragm.

KIDNEY, MALROTATION OF
Malrotation of the kidney is incomplete or excessive rotation of the kidney during development.

KIDNEY, MULTILOCULAR CYSTS OF
Multilocular cysts of the kidney are collections of solitary cysts, usually in one kidney (as contrasted to polycystic disease).

KIDNEY, MULTIPLE PELVES OF
Multiple pelves of the kidney are three or more major calyces in a kidney.

KIDNEY, PELVIC
Pelvic kidney is a kidney situated below the pelvic brim in the pelvis.

KIDNEYS, SIGMOID
Sigmoid kidneys are kidneys with the upper pole of one kidney fused to lower pole of the other.
SYNONYM: *Ren Sigmoideus.*

KIDNEY, SOLITARY
Solitary kidney is the complete absence of one kidney, usually with the absence of the corresponding ureter.

KIDNEY, SOLITARY CYSTS OF

KIDNEY, SPONGE
Sponge kidney is a disease of renal pyramids with multiple small cysts in medulla.
SYNONYMS: *Rein en Éponge, Cacchi-Ricci Syndrome.*

KIDNEY, SUPERNUMERARY
Supernumerary kidney is the presence of a distinct third kidney.
SYNONYM: *Triple Kidney.*

KIDNEY, UNILATERAL FUSED
Unilateral fused kidney is a displacement of one kidney to the other side and fusion with its mate.

KIDNEY PELVIS, BIFID
Bifid kidney pelvis is a kidney having a pelvis divided to form two major calyces.

KIDNEY PELVIS, EXTRARENAL
Extrarenal kidney pelvis is one in which the calyces join to form a pelvis outside the kidney. In the event of hydronephrosis, there is a large dilated sac outside the kidney.

KIDNEY PELVIS, PSEUDOSPIDER OF
Pseudospider of the kidney pelvis is a long, thin, small pelvis suggesting the spider-leg pyelogram of renal tumor.

KIDNEY PELVIS, TRIFID
Trifid kidney pelvis is a kidney with three major calyces.

MEATUS URINARIUS ATRESIUS
Meatus urinarius atresius is an imperforate external urinary meatus.

MEGALOURETER
Megaloureter is an abnormally large ureter.
SYNONYMS: *Megaureter, Primary Ureteral Atony, Ureteral Neuromuscular Dysplasia.*

MEGALOURETHRA
Megalourethra is an abnormally dilated urethra.

MEGAURETER–MEGACYSTIS SYNDROME
Megaureter-megacystis syndrome is an enlarged ureter, and an enlarged bladder, usually bilateral and without evidence of organic ureteral obstruction.

PTOSIS, RENAL
   Renal ptosis is a dropped or movable kidney.
   SYNONYM: *Kidney Ptosis.*

RENAL DISEASE, FIBROCYSTIC
   Fibrocystic renal disease is a variety of polycystic disease associated
with a marked increase in connective tissue.

RENAL DISEASE, POLYCYSTIC
   Polycystic renal disease is the presence of multiple cysts throughout
both kidneys.
   SYNONYMS: *Cystic Disease of Kidneys, Multiple Cysts of Kidneys, Poly-
             cystic Disease of Kidneys.*

RENAL PELVIS, DOUBLE, WITH DOUBLE URETER
   Double renal pelvis with double ureter is a kidney having two pelves,
each with its separate ureter.

RENUM SEXTUPLICITAS
   Renum sextuplicitas is the presence of six functioning kidneys and six
ureters. In one case, four were on the right and two on the left.

URACHUS, PERSISTENT
   Persistent urachus is the presence of a urachus.
   SYNONYM: *Patent Urachus.*

URETER, ABSENCE OF, ACCESSORY, DUPLICATION OF, OR APLASIA OF

URETERAL ORIFICES, MULTIPLE
   Multiple ureteral orifices are two or more ureteral orifices on one side
of the bladder.

URETER, BLIND–ENDING OF
   Blind-ending of the ureter is a ureter that fails to connect the bladder
with the renal pelvis.

URETER, DEVIATION OF
   Deviation of the ureter is a ureter having an abnormal course.

URETER, DISPLACED OPENING OF
   Displaced opening of the ureter is a ureter opening in an abnormal
position.

URETER, DIVERTICULUM OF
   Diverticulum of the ureter is a sacculation or blind pouch along the
course of a ureter.

URETER, ECTOPIC
   Ectopic ureter is a ureter that is abnormally situated.
   SYNONYM: *Anomalous Implantation of Ureter.*

URETER, FUSED TRIPLICATE
Fused triplicate ureter is the presence of three ureters with a single ureteral orifice in the bladder.

URETER, OCCLUSION OF
Occlusion of the ureter is an obstructed ureter.
SYNONYM: *Impervious Ureter.*

URETEROCELE
Ureterocele is a prolapse of the dilated lower end of the ureter into the bladder.

URETEROPELVIC JUNCTION, STRICTURE OF
Stricture of the ureteropelvic junction is a stenosis at the junction of the ureter with the renal pelvis.

URETEROVESICAL ORIFICE, STRICTURE OF
Stricture of the ureterovesical orifice is a narrowing of the ureter at its entrance into the bladder.

URETER, POSTCAVAL
Postcaval ureter is a ureter, always on right side, that passes behind the vena cava, owing to the persistence of the posterior cardinal vein caudal to the renal vein.
SYNONYM: *Retrocaval Ureter.*

URETER, QUADRUPLICATION OF
Quadruplication of ureter is the presence of four ureters, partial or complete, on one side.

URETER, RETROILIAC
Retroiliac ureter is a ureter passing behind the iliac artery.

URETER, STRICTURE OF
Stricture of the ureter is a narrowed ureteral lumen.

URETER, TORSION OR SPIRAL TWIST OF
Torsion or spiral twist of the ureter is a ureter that has failed to rotate with its kidney during early fetal life.

URETER, TRIFID
Trifid ureter is a ureter with a single pelvis dividing to form three ureters entering the bladder.

URETER, UNILATERAL TRIPLICATION OF
Unilateral triplication of the ureter is the presence of three ureters, each with its own renal pelvis and its own ureteral orifice in the bladder.

URETER, Y TYPE
The Y type ureter is characterized by the bifurcation of a single ureter from a single orifice producing a double ureter and pelves.

URETER, Y TYPE, INVERTED
Inverted Y type ureter is a ureter from separate vesical orifices which have united to form a single ureter and a single pelvis.

URETHRA, ATRESIA OF
Atresia of the urethra is an imperforation or absence of a urethral lumen.
SYNONYM: *Imperforate Urethra.*

URETHRA, ABSENCE OF
Absence of the urethra is agenesis or nondevelopment of a urethra.

URETHRA, ACCESSORY CHANNELS OF
Accessory channels of the urethra are variously developed urethral sinuses or tracts.

URETHRA, IMPERVIOUS
Impervious urethra is a urethra without a lumen.

URETHRA, STENOSIS OF, OR STRICTURE OF

URETHRAL MEATUS, DOUBLE
Double urethral meatus is the presence of two external urethral openings.

URETHRAL MEATUS, INTERNAL DISLOCATION OF
Internal dislocation of the urethral meatus is entrance of the prostatic urethra into the bladder to one side of the midline.

URETHRAL VALVES, POSTERIOR
Posterior urethral valves are mucous folds or fibrous bands from the verumontanum, usually causing urinary obstruction and back pressure.

URINARY MEATUS, COVERED
A covered urinary meatus is characterized by a fold of mucosa from the posterior edge of the female urethral meatus that covers the normal opening.

URINARY SPHINCTER, ABSENCE OF
Absence of the urinary sphincter is aplasia of the sphincteric muscles of the bladder and urethra.

VALVES, URETERAL
Ureteral valves are flaps of tissue resulting from the redundancy of the mucosa. They often cause obstruction and hydronephrosis.

VALVES, URETHRAL
Urethral valves are valves of fossa navicularis or of the posterior urethra. They may be redundant, causing obstruction.

Club Foot

CLAWTOE

Clawtoe is a toe that is sharply angulated in flexion.

CLUBFOOT

Clubfoot is any type of deformed or twisted foot.
SYNONYMS: *Talipes Contortus, Pes Contortus.*

METATARSUS ADDUCTOCAVUS

Metatarsus adductocavus is a combination of metatarsus adductus and talipes cavus.

METATARSUS LATUS

Metatarsus latus is flattening of the metatarsal arch resulting in a spread foot.
SYNONYM: *Talipes Transversoplanus.*

METATARSUS PRIMUS VARUS

Metatarsus primus varus is medial angulation of the first metatarsal bone away from second metatarsal bone.

METATARSUS VALGUS

Metatarsus valgus is an abnormality in which the inner border of the foot rests on the ground with a flattened arch and the outer border of the foot is relatively elevated.

METATARSUS VARUS

Metatarsus varus is medial deviation of the metatarsal bones.
SYNONYMS: *Metatarsus Adductovarus, Metatarsus Adductus, Skewfoot.*

PES SUPINATUS

Pes supinatus is an abnormality in which the inner border of the anterior portion of the foot is higher than the outer border.

TALIPES CALCANEOVALGOCAVUS

Talipes calcaneovalgocavus is a combination of talipes calcaneus, talipes valgus, and talipes cavus.

TALIPES CALCANEOVALGUS

Talipes calcaneovalgus is a combination of talipes calcaneus and talipes valgus.

TALIPES CALCANEOVARUS
Talipes calcaneovarus is the combination of talipes calcaneus and talipes varus.

TALIPES CALCANEUS
Talipes calcaneus is fixed dorsiflexion in which weight rests on the heel alone.

TALIPES CAVUS
Talipes cavus is a foot with an abnormally high arch.
SYNONYMS: *Pes Cavus, Talipes Arcuatus, Talipes Percavus, Talipes Plantaris.*

TALIPES EQUINOVALGUS
Talipes equinovalgus is the combination of talipes equinus and talipes valgus.

TALIPES EQUINOVARUS
Talipes equinovarus is a combination of talipes equinus and talipes varus.

TALIPES EQUINUS
Talipes equinus is a foot in fixed extension with weight bearing on the ball of the foot, resembling a horse's hoof.

TALIPES VALGUS
Talipes valgus is eversion of the foot with inner edge of the sole on the ground.
SYNONYMS: *Pes Abductus, Pes Pronatus, Pes Valgus, Talipes Planovalgus.*

TALIPES VARUS
Talipes varus is inversion of the foot with outer edge of sole on ground.

Limbs

ABRACHIA
Abrachia is absence of the arms.

ABSENCE OF FIBULA SYNDROME
Absence of fibula syndrome is the combination of absence of the fibula with anterior bowing of the tibia and various defects of the feet. Almost invariably, there is a dimple or pit in the skin over the middle of the tibia.

ACETABULUM, POSTERIOR ROTATION OF
Posterior rotation of the acetabulum is an acetabulum directed posteriorly instead of anterolaterally. It is usually associated with separation of the pubic rami.

ACHEIRIA
Acheiria is the absence of a hand or hands.

ANKYLODACTYLY
Ankylodactyly is adhesion of the fingers or toes to each other.

APHALANGIA
Aphalangia is the absence of toes or fingers.
SYNONYM: *Adactylia.*

ARTHROGRYPOSIS SYNDROME
Arthrogryposis syndrome is characterized by multiple joint contractures, especially of the knees and ankles, with atrophy or compensatory hypertrophy of associated muscles.
SYNONYMS: *Amyoplasia Syndrome, Kuskokwin Disease.*

ATELOPODIA
Atelopodia is imperfect foot development.

BIDACTYLY
Bidactyly is the absence of the second, third, and fourth digits leaving only the first and fifth digits.

BRACHYDACTYLY
Brachydactyly is the presence of abnormally short fingers and toes.

601

CAMPTODACTYLY
Camptodactyly is permanent flexion of one or several interphalangeal joints.

CARPAL BONES, ACCESSORY
Accessory carpal bones are supernumerary bones of the carpus or hand.

CLAVICLE, ABSENCE OF

CLAWHAND
Clawhand is an abnormal cleft between the central metacarpal bones with fusion of the soft tissue of the digits into a mass on either side of the cleft.

SYNONYMS: *Lobster Claw Hand, Main en Griffe, Main Fourché.*

CLINODACTYLY
Clinodactyly is bending or deflection of the fingers.

COXA VALGA
Coxa valga is a deformity of the hip with an increase of the angle between the shaft and the neck of the femur.

COXA VARA
Coxa vara is a deformity of the hip with a decrease of the angle between the shaft and the neck of the femur.

CUBITUS VALGUS
Cubitus valgus is a condition in which the extended forearm deviates toward the inner side of the axis of the limb.

CUBITUS VARUS
Cubitus varus is a condition in which the extended forearm deviates outward from the axis of the limb (like a gunstock).

DACTYLOGRYPOSIS
Dactylogryposis is the presence of permanently bent fingers.

DACTYLOMEGALY
Dactylomegaly is one or more abnormally large fingers.

DACTYLOSYMPHYSIS
Dactylosymphysis is a growing together or webbing of the fingers.

DIASTEMATOPYELIA
Diastematopyelia is a separation between the pubic bones.

DIGITUS POSTMINIMUM
Digitus postminimum is a pedunculated appendage to the little finger or little toe, with or without bones, but usually having a nail.

DIGITUS VALGUS
Digitus valgus is deviation of a finger toward the ulnar side.

DIGITUS VARUS
Digitus varus is deviation of a finger toward the radial side.

DIPLOPODIA
Diplopodia is partial or complete duplication of a foot.
SYNONYM: *Dipodia.*

ECTODACTYLISM
Ectodactylism is absence of a digit or digits.

ELBOW, WEBBED
Webbed elbow is the presence of taut skin between forearm and upper arm, holding the joint in flexion.

FEMUR, ANTEVERSION OF
Anteversion of the femur is anterior angulation of the femur at its neck, often associated with shortening.

FEMUR, APLASIA OF
Aplasia of the femur is shortening of the femur due to a local disturbance of bone growth.

FEMUR, UNILATERAL SHORTENING OF
Unilateral shortening of the femur is characterized by a short but otherwise normal femur on one side of the body.

FIBULA, APLASIA OF
Aplasia of the fibula is a defective or absent lower half of the fibula.

FIFTH TOE, TWO-PHALANGED
Two-phalanged fifth toe is the absence of third phalanx of the fifth toe.

FINGER, CLUBBED
Clubbed finger is a proliferation of soft tissue around the terminal phalanx without bony changes.

FINGER, MALLET
Mallet finger is a flexion deformity of a distal phalanx of a finger.

FINGER, RUDIMENTARY
Rudimentary finger is an incompletely developed finger.

FINGERS, APICAL DYSTROPHY OF
Apical dystrophy of the fingers is the absence, partial or complete, of the terminal portion of the distal phalanx of the fingers.

FOOT, ABSENCE OF
SYNONYM: *Apodia.*

GENU IMPRESSUM
Genu impressum is a knee joint that is flattened and bent to one side resulting in patellar displacement upward and on the same side.

GENU VALGUM
Genu valgum is deviation of the knees toward the midline.
SYNONYM: *Knock-knee.*

GENU VARUM
Genu varum is abnormal separation of the knees.
SYNONYM: *Bowleg, Genu Extrorsum.*

HALLUX VALGUS
Hallux valgus is deviation of the great toe away from the midline of the body.

HALLUX VARUS
Hallux varus is contracture between the first phalanx and the metatarsal bone, causing an adducted great toe.

HAMMERTOE
Hammertoe is contracture of the extensor tendon of the toe.

HEXADACTYLISM
Hexadactylism is the presence of six fingers on one hand or each hand, or six toes on one foot or each foot.

HIP, DISLOCATION OF
Dislocation of the hip is a hip with a relaxed capsule and often a shallow acetabulum so that the head of the femur is displaced.

HIP, DYSPLASIA OF
Dysplasia of the hip is abnormal development in the region of the articulation of the femur and the innominate bone.

HYPODACTYLY
Hypodactyly is the partial or complete absence of some fingers or toes.

KNEE, DISLOCATION OF
Dislocation of the knee is a knee with hyperextension, having the tibia anterior and lateral to the femur.
SYNONYM: *Genu Recurvatum.*

KNEE, WEBBED
Webbed knee is characterized by webbing or bands of skin from heel to thigh often associated with absent or cleft scrotum.
SYNONYM: *Pterygium Popliteal Syndrome.*

LEG, WEBBED
Webbed leg is characterized by skin and connective tissue between the legs binding them together.

LONG BONES, SPLAYING OF
Splaying of the long bones is the replacement of metaphyseal tissues by masses of cartilage causing interference with the formation of endochondral bone.
SYNONYMS: *Metaphyseal Dysostosis, Pyle's Disease.*

LOWER LIMB, AMELIA OF
Amelia of the lower limb is the absence of a lower limb or limbs.
SYNONYM: *Absence of Leg.*

LOWER LIMB, ECTROMELIA OF
Ectromelia of the lower limb is the absence or deformity of one or more lower limbs.

LOWER LIMB, HEMIMELIA OF
Hemimelia of the lower limb is a defective lower limb or limbs.

LOWER LIMB, MICRODACTYLIA OF
Microdactylia of the lower limb is the presence of small or short toes.

LOWER LIMB, MICROMELIA OF
Micromelia of the lower limb is an abnormally small lower limb or limbs.
SYNONYMS: *Short-Leg, Brachymelia of Lower Limb.*

LOWER LIMB, PHOCOMELIA OF
Phocomelia of the lower limb is the malformation of the legs so that they resemble the flippers of a seal.

MACRODACTYLIA
Macrodactylia is a condition in which there are abnormally large fingers.

MANUS CAVA
Manus cava is the extreme concavity of the palm.

MANUS EXTENSA
Manus extensa is the backward deviation of a clubbed hand.
SYNONYM: *Manus Superextensa.*

MANUS FLEXA
Manus flexa is the forward deviation or flexion of a clubbed hand.

MANUS PLANA
Manus plana is a flat hand lacking the normal arches.

MANUS VALGA
Manus valga is a deformed wrist due to the projecting end of the radius so that the hand deviates to the ulnar side.
SYNONYMS: *Radius Curvus, Madelung's Deformity.*

MANUS VARA
Manus vara is a deformed wrist with deviation to the radial side.

METATARSUS ATAVICUS
Metatarsus atavicus is abnormal shortening of the first metatarsal bone.
SYNONYM: *Metatarsus Brevis.*

MICROBRACHIA
Microbrachia is the presence of abnormally small arms.
SYNONYMS: *Rudimentary Arm, Micromelia of Upper Limb, Nanomelia of Upper Limb.*

MICROCHEIRIA
Microcheiria is the presence of abnormally small hands.

PATELLA, ABSENCE OF

PATELLA, RUDIMENTARY
Rudimentary patella is a hypoplastic or underdeveloped kneecap.

PELVIS, PERSISTENT INFANTILE
Persistent infantile pelvis is hypoplasia of a sacral wing or, rarely, both wings.

PEROMELIA
Peromelia are severe malformations of the limbs with absence of hands or feet.

PES GIGAS
Pes gigas are abnormally large feet.
SYNONYM: *Macropodia.*

PLATYCNEMIA
Platycnemia is an abnormally broad, flat tibia.

POLYDACTYLY
Polydactyly is the presence of extra fingers or extra toes.
SYNONYMS: *Supernumerary Digits, Hyperphalangia.*

POLYSCELIA
Polyscelia is the presence of more than two legs.

PRONATION, FOOT
Foot pronation is eversion and abduction of the foot with flattening of the longitudinal arch.

PUBIC ARCH, OPEN
Open pubic arch is characterized by the failure of fusion of the bodies of the pubic bones.

RIGIDITY, MULTIPLE ARTICULAR
Multiple articular rigidity is a stiffness of the joints, which are relatively fixed in flexion.

SACROILIAC JOINT, FUSION OF
Fusion of the sacroiliac joint is bony union between the sacrum and the ilium.

SCAPULA, HIGH
High scapula is the congenital elevation of the scapula with the lower margin turned toward the spine.
SYNONYM: *Sprengel's Deformity.*

SYNDACTYLY
Syndactyly is webbing of the fingers or toes by skin holding them together.
SYNONYM: *Symphalangy.*

SYNOSTOSES, TARSAL
Tarsal synostoses are fusions of various bones of the foot.

SYNOSTOSIS, ASTRAGALOSCAPHOID
Astragaloscaphoid synostosis is fusion of the astragalus and navicular bone in the foot.

SYNOSTOSIS, RADIOULNAR
Radioulnar synostosis is fusion of the proximal ends of the radius and ulna.

SYNOSTOSIS, RADIOULNAR–HUMERAL
Radioulnar-humeral synostosis is fusion, partial or complete, between humerus and ulna or with radius.

TALIPES PLANUS
Talipes planus is characterized by a lowered or flattened longitudinal arch of the foot.
SYNONYMS: *Pes Planus, Platypodia.*

TALIPOMANUS
Talipomanus is a deformity of the hand, which is in marked flexion and adduction.
SYNONYM: *Clubhand.*

TARSAL BONES, ACCESSORY
Accessory tarsal bones are supernumerary bones in the foot.

THUMB, ABSENCE OF

TIBIA, ANGULATION OF
Angulation of the tibia is bowing or angulation of the tibia due to an unossified segment of the lower third of the tibia.
SYNONYM: *Kyphoscoliotic Tibia.*

TIBIA, APLASIA OF
Aplasia of the tibia is partial to complete absence of the distal end of the tibia.

TIBIOTARSAL JOINT, LUXATION OF
Luxation of the tibiotarsal joint is a dislocation of the joint between the tibia and the foot.
SYNONYM: *Volkmann's Deformity.*

TOE, ABSENCE OF

TOE, CLUBBED
Clubbed toe is the proliferation of soft tissue around the terminal phalanx without bony changes.

TOES, LOCAL GIGANTISM OF
Local gigantism of the toes is characterized by abnormally large toes.

TOES, WEBBED
Webbed toes are toes with skin between the digits holding them together.
SYNONYM: *Fused Toes.*

TOXOPACHYOSTOSIS, TIBIOPERONEAL DIAPHYSIAL
Tibioperoneal diaphysial toxopachyostosis is characterized by the anteroposterior curvature and thickening of fibulae and tibiae of both legs.
SYNONYM: *Weismann-Netter Syndrome.*

UPPER LIMB, AMELIA OF
Amelia of the upper limb is the absence of an upper limb or limbs.

UPPER LIMB, ECTROMELIA OF
Ectromelia of the upper limb is absence or deformity of one or more of the upper limbs.

UPPER LIMB, HEMIMELIA OF
Hemimelia of the upper limb is the absence of the end or side of a long bone of the upper limbs.

UPPER LIMB, MICRODACTYLIA OF
Microdactylia of the upper limb is the presence of small or short fingers.

UPPER LIMB, OLIGODACTYLY OF
Oligodactyly of the upper limb is the presence of less than five digits on an extremity.

UPPER LIMB, PHOCOMELIA OF
Phocomelia of the upper limb is malformation of arms so that they resemble the flippers of a seal.

Musculoskeletal System

ACROBRACHYCEPHALY
Acrobrachycephaly is an abnormally shortened anteroposterior diameter of the skull.

ACROCEPHALY
Acrocephaly is a malformed pointed skull.

ACROMICRIA
Acromicria is the state of having a small and delicate face and extremities. Probably of pituitary origin, it is the antithesis of acromegaly.

ACROMICRIA SYNDROME
Acromicria syndrome is the combination of abnormally small hands, fetal mental retardation, and mongoloid expression.

AMYOPLASIA CONGENITA
Amyoplasia congenita is defective development of muscles during intra-uterine life.

AMYOTROPHIA CONGENITA
Amyotrophia congenita is atrophy or wasting of fetal muscles.

ANOMALIES, VERTEBRAL
Vertebral anomalies are failures of segmentation or fusion that may occur in various combinations, although the number of vertebral segments is very constant.

APLASIA, SACRAL
Sacral aplasia is defective development or absence of the sacrum.

APLEURIA, CONGENITAL
Congenital apleuria is absence of the ribs.

APPENDAGE, CAUDAL
A caudal appendage is a tail-like extension of the spinal column.

ATELOPROSOPIA
Ateloprosopia is imperfect face development.

ATELORHACHIDIA
Atelorhachidia is imperfect vertebral column development.

609

BRACHYCEPHALY
Brachycephaly is a relatively short skull, one with a cephalic index over 80.

CEBOCEPHALY
Cebocephaly is a monkey-like face with close-set eyes and small nose due to absence of the major portion of the frontonasal process.

CHEST, PYRAMID
Pyramid chest is an oblique protrusion of the sternum with the xiphoid as most prominent part.

CLINOCEPHALY
Clinocephaly is a flattened, concave, or saddle-shaped skull.

COCCYX, CONGENITAL ABSENCE OF

CRANIAL SUTURES, PREMATURE SYNOSTOSES OF
Premature synostoses of the cranial sutures are premature fusions of the bones at the base of the skull, resulting in arrested brain development.
SYNONYMS: *Craniostosis, Craniosynostosis, Tribasilar Synostosis.*

CRANIOMALACIA
Craniomalacia is softening of the skull bones.

CRANIOSCHISIS
Cranioschisis is failure of the skull to close.

CRANIOSCLEROSIS
Craniosclerosis is a thickened skull.

CRANIOSTENOSIS
Craniostenosis is contraction of the skull, or narrowing of its foramina, resulting from premature closing of the cranial sutures.

CRANIUM BIFIDUM OCCULTUM
Cranium bifidum occultum is a cleft or gap in the skull, but without abnormality of the brain or meninges.

CYMBOCEPHALY
Cymbocephaly is a depression in the skull or a bowl-shaped skull.

CYNOCEPHALY
Cynocephaly is a deformity in which the head slopes back from the orbits like the head of a dog.

DIAPHRAGM, ABSENT

DIAPHRAGM, CONGENITAL EVENTRATION OF
Congenital eventration of the diaphragm is the presence of a diaphragm with thin, defective musculature, which may stretch and protrude into the chest.
SYNONYMS: *Congenital Relaxation of the Diaphragm, Hernia of Diaphragm.*

DIASTEMATOCRANIA
Diastematocrania is a midline anteroposterior cleft or fissure of the skull.

DOLICHOCEPHALY
Dolichocephaly is an abnormally long head.

DWARFISM, ACHONDROPLASTIC
Achondroplastic dwarfism is a form of dwarfism resulting from achondroplastic changes in the cartilages of the long bones.

DYSPLASIA EPIPHYSIALIS PUNCTATA
Dysplasia epiphysialis punctata is a syndrome involving many centers of calcification that may fuse but with irregular joint surfaces. Dwarfism, anomalies of the skull and long bones, and mental retardation result.
SYNONYMS: *Chondrodystrophia Calcarea, Chondrodystrophia Calcificans Congenita, Chondrodystrophia Fetalis Calcificans, Chondrodystrophia Fetalis Hypoplastica, Chondrodystrophia Hypoplastica Calcinosa, Chondrodystrophia Punctata. Stippled Epiphyses, Conradi-Hunermann Syndrome.*

DYSPLASIA, EPIPHYSIAL
Epiphysial dysplasia is any developmental error of the epiphyses with resultant deformities.

DYSPLASIA, POLYOSTOTIC FIBROUS
Polyostotic fibrous dysplasia is replacement of the marrow and part of the cortex of one or more bones by avascular fibrous tissue.
SYNONYMS: *Fibrous Dysplasia, Osteitis Fibrosa Disseminata.*

DYSPLASIA, PROGRESSIVE DIAPHYSIAL
Progressive diaphysial dysplasia is a progressive, fusiform, symmetrical enlargement of the shafts of the long bones.
SYNONYMS: *Camurati-Engelmann Syndrome, Engelmann's Disease.*

EVENTRATION, VISCERAL
Visceral eventration is protrusion of abdominal contents through a defect in the abdominal wall.

EXOSTOSIS MULTIPLEX CARTILAGINEA
Exostosis multiplex cartilaginea is a syndrome of multiple cartilaginous exostoses with associated bone and joint deformities.
SYNONYM: *Ehrenfried's Disease.*

FIRST BRANCHIAL ARCH SYNDROME

First branchial arch syndrome is a group of anomalies resulting from inhibited development of the stapedial artery with consequent growth defects in the area it should have nourished.

FISSURE, ABDOMINAL

Abdominal fissure is failure of the ventral body wall to close.
SYNONYM: *Celosomia.*

FORAMINA, PARIETAL

Parietal foramina are soft oval defects of the parietal bones in the upper portions.

HEMIVERTEBRA

Hemivertebra is failure of one side of a vertebra to develop.

HIATUS PLEUROPERITONEALIS, HERNIA OF

Hernia of the hiatus pleuroperitonealis is the protrusion of abdominal contents into the chest cavity.
SYNONYM: *Hernia of the Foramen of Bochdalek.*

HUMPBACK, CONGENITAL

Congenital humpback is a back affected by kyphosis, scoliosis, or both.

HYPEROSTOSIS, GENERAL, WITH PACHYDERMA

General hyperostosis with pachyderma is the presence of multiple irregular centers of ossification with thickened cortices, absent striae, acromegaloid appearance, and pachyderma.
SYNONYMS: *Touraine-Solente-Golé Syndrome, Uehlinger's Syndrome.*

HYPEROSTOSIS, GENERAL, WITH STRIATIONS

General hyperostosis with striations is the presence of multiple irregular centers of ossification with thickened cortices and bony striations.
SYNONYM: *Fairbank's Disease.*

HYPEROSTOSIS, INFANTILE CORTICAL

Infantile cortical hyperostosis is the presence of multiple widespread cortical hyperostoses with immature lamellar bone and soft tissue swellings.
SYNONYMS: *Hyperplastic Periostosis, Caffey-Silverman Syndrome, Caffey's Syndrome.*

HYPERTELORISM, OCULAR

Ocular hypertelorism is a malformation of the sphenoid bone with relatively great distance between the eyes, associated with mental deficiency, depressed nasal bridge, and brachycephaly.
SYNONYMS: *Hypertelorismus Ocularis, Greig's Syndrome.*

LORDOSIS, CONGENITAL

Congenital lordosis is anteroposterior spinal curvature.

LUMBARIZATION
Lumbarization is fusion of the first sacral vertebra with the fifth lumbar vertebra.

LUMBOSACRAL JOINT, UNSTABLE
Unstable lumbosacral joint is an abnormally loose joint between the lumbar vertebra and the sacrum resulting in frequent displacement.

LÜCKENSCHÄDEL
Lückenschädel is characterized by a very thin skull with cranial fenestrations or defects.

MACROCEPHALY
Macrocephaly is a long head (dolichocephaly) or a large head (megacephaly).

MEGACEPHALY
Megacephaly is a large head.

NANOCEPHALY
Nanocephaly is a very small head.
SYNONYM: *Dwarf-head.*

OSTEOCHONDRITIS, MULTIPLE
Multiple osteochondritis consists of multiple dysplasias of bones and their cartilages.

OSTEOCHONDRODESMODYSPLASIA
Osteochondrodesmodysplasia is a syndrome of deformed bones, loose tendons, loose joints, multiple dislocations, cleft palate, pterygium colli, and cleft vertebral arches.
SYNONYM: *Rotter-Erb Syndrome.*

OSTEOCHONDROMA, MULTIPLE
Multiple osteochondroma is the presence of benign tumors of bone having a pedicle of normal bone surrounded by proliferating cartilage cells.

OSTEODYSPLASTY
Osteodysplasty consists of multiple symmetric bone abnormalities, including skull condensation, mandibular hypoplasia, deformed vertebrae, and lack of tubulation of long bones.
SYNONYM: *Melnick-Needles Syndrome.*

OSTEOGENESIS IMPERFECTA WITHOUT BLUE SCLERAE
Osteogenesis imperfecta without blue sclerae is a hereditary syndrome of brittle bones and eye defects but without bluish discoloration of the sclerae.
SYNONYM: *Vrolik's Syndrome.*

OSTEOMATOSIS
Osteomatosis is the presence of multiple bone tumors.

OSTEO–ONYCHODYSPLASIA
Osteo-onychodysplasia is a condition characterized by skeletal anomalies and dystrophy of finger and toe nails. The patella may be hypoplastic or absent.

SYNONYMS: *Ectodermal-Mesodermal Dysplasia Syndrome, Iliac Horns Syndrome, Osterreicher-Turner Syndrome, Turner's* (H.W.) *Syndrome.*

OSTEOPATHIA STRIATA
Osteopathia striata is skeletal striation, especially of the long bones.

SYNONYM: *Voorhoeve's Disease.*

OSTEOSCLEROSIS, CONGENITAL
Congenital osteosclerosis is diffuse, general hyperostosis.

SYNONYM: *Koszewski's Syndrome.*

OXYCEPHALY
Oxycephaly is an excessively high skull resulting from premature closure of the sagittal and coronal sutures.

SYNONYMS: *Tower Skull, Turricephaly.*

PECTUS CARINATUM
Pectus carinatum is the projection forward of the upper part of the sternum, causing a deformity resembling the keel of a boat.

SYNONYMS: *Chicken Breast, Keeled Breast, Pectus Gallinatum, Congenital Pigeon Breast.*

PECTUS EXCAVATUM
Pectus excavatum is a depression of the sternum, usually in the lower part.

SYNONYMS: *Congenital Funnel Breast, Chonechondrosternon, Congenital Funnel Chest, Pectus Recurvatum.*

PLAGIOCEPHALY
Plagiocephaly is an obliquely deformed skull, with one side more developed anteriorly and the other side greater posteriorly.

PLATYBASIA
Platybasia is malformation of the base of the skull; the cervical spine presses into the foramen magnum and the posterior cerebral fossae. Pressure on the medulla is frequent.

SYNONYM: *Basilar Impression.*

PLATYBASIA WITH CERVICAL SYNOSTOSIS AND ELEVATED SCAPULA
Platybasia with cervical synostosis and elevated scapula is the association of invagination of the cervical spine into the foramen magnum, fusion of the atlas with the occipital bone, and elevation of the scapulae.

SYNONYM: *Furst-Ostrum Syndrome.*

PLATYCRANIA
Platycrania is a flattened skull—one with a vertical index below 70.
SYNONYM: *Platycephalia.*

PLATYOPIA
Platyopia is a broad face.

PLATYSPONDYLIA GENERALISATA
Platyspondylia generalisata is a combination of flattened vertebrae with kyphoscoliosis, spinal ankylosis, short neck, and relative dwarfism.
SYNONYM: *Dreyfus Syndrome.*

PLATYSTENCEPHALY
Platystencephaly is a very wide skull in the occipital area with anterior narrowing.

RIB, BRANCHED
Branched rib is a rib with a divided or forked distal end.

RIB, CERVICAL
Cervical rib is a supernumerary rib in the cervical region.

RIB, CONGENITAL ABSENCE OF
SYNONYM: *Missing Rib.*

RIB, FIRST, SHORTENING OF
Shortening of the first rib is a narrowing of the upper portion of the thorax as a result of shortening of the first rib and cartilage. Deficient expansion of the lung apex results.
SYNONYM: *Freund's Anomaly.*

SACRUM, ABSENCE OF

SCAPHOCEPHALY
Scaphocephaly is a long, narrow skull with a prominent ridge resulting from premature ossification of the sagittal suture.
SYNONYM: *Scaphoid Head.*

SCHISTOCELIA
Schistocelia is an abdominal wall with a congenital cleft.

SCHISTOTHORAX
Schistothorax is a congenital cleft in the chest wall.

SCOLIOSIS, CONGENITAL
Congenital scoliosis is lateral spinal curvature.

SCOLIOSIS SCIATICA SACRALIZATION SYNDROME
Scoliosis sciatica sacralization syndrome is sacralization of the fifth lumbar vertebra, sciatica, and scoliosis.
SYNONYM: *Bertolotti's Syndrome.*

SKULL, ANTEROPOSTERIOR DYSPLASIA OF
Anteroposterior dysplasia of the skull is abnormal growth in the anteroposterior direction of the face or skull.

SKULL, CONGENITAL HYPEROSTOSIS OF
Congenital hyperostosis of the skull is cortical hyperostosis limited to the skull.

SPINE, CONGENITAL ABSENCE OF

SPONDYLOLISTHESIS
Spondylolisthesis is forward slipping or displacement of one vertebra on another.

SPONDYLOLISTHESIS, LUMBOSACRAL
Lumbosacral spondylolisthesis is loosening and slipping of a lumbar vertebra on the sacrum.
SYNONYM: *Slipped Vertebra.*

SPONDYLOLYSIS
Spondylolysis is the breaking down or dissolution of the arch of a vertebra, usually the isthmus.

SPONDYLOLYSIS, CERVICAL
Cervical spondylolysis is aplasia of the vertebral arch of a cervical vertebra.

SPONDYLOLYSIS, LUMBOSACRAL
Lumbosacral spondylolysis is aplasia of the arches of lumbosacral vertebrae.

STERNUM BIFIDUM
Sternum bifidum is a sternum cleft into two parts.

STERNUM, CLEFT
Cleft sternum is a partial or complete fissure or cleft of the sternum.
SYNONYMS: *Sternum Fissum, Sternal Fissure.*

STERNUM, CONGENITAL ABSENCE OF

STRAIGHT–BACK SYNDROME
Straight-back syndrome is an abnormally straight spine, one lacking the usual anteroposterior curves.

TAIL, PERSISTENT
Persistent tail is the presence of supernumerary vertebrae so that a small tail exists.

TEMPORAL BONE, PRIMARY CHOLESTEATOMA OF
A primary cholesteatoma of the temporal bone is an erosive tumor of the temporal bone and is formed by displaced epidermal cells.

THORACOSCHISIS
Thoracoschisis is a defect of a rib or ribs near the sternum, leaving a cleft or fissure through which a lung may herniate.

TORTICOLLIS, CONGENITAL
Congenital torticollis is a twisted neck, due to shortening of one side, usually due to a contracted and scarred sternocleidomastoid muscle.
SYNONYM: *Congenital Wryneck.*

TRIGONOCEPHALY
Trigonocephaly is a triangularly shaped skull.

VERTEBRA, CONGENITAL ABSENCE OF

VERTEBRAE, CONGENITALLY FUSED
Congenitally fused vertebrae are the abnormal union of spinal vertebrae.
SYNONYM: *Congenital Spinal Fusion.*

VERTEBRA, SUPERNUMERARY
Supernumerary vertebra is an extra vertebra.

XIPHOID PROCESS, NOTCHED
Notched xiphoid process is a cleft or notched xiphoid or ensiform process of the sternum.
SYNONYM: *Bifid Ensiform Process.*

Skin, Hair, and Nails

ACANTHOSIS, CONGENITAL
Congenital acanthosis is characterized by a thickened or hypertrophied prickle cell layer of epidermis.

ACRODERMATITIS ENTEROPATHICA
Acrodermatitis enteropathica is the association of gastrointestinal disturbances, periorificial and acral dermatitis and alopecia.
SYNONYMS: *Brandt's Syndrome, Danbolt-Closs Syndrome.*

ACROKERATOSIS VERRUCIFORMIS
Acrokeratosis verruciformis is faulty development of upper layers of epidermis with reddish papular lesions only on palms and soles.
SYNONYMS: *Acrodermatitis Verruciformis, Acrodermatosis Verruciformis, Hopf's Keratosis.*

ACROPACHYDERMA
Acropachyderma is thickening of skin of face, scalp, and extremities associated with long-bone deformities and clubbed extremities.
SYNONYMS: *Pachyacria, Brugsch's Syndrome.*

ALOPECIA, CONGENITAL
Congenital alopecia is a syndrome with partial or complete absence of hair.
SYNONYM: *Atrichia Congenita.*

ANGIOID STREAK–PSEUDOXANTHOMA ELASTICUM SYNDROME
Angioid streak-pseudoxanthoma elasticum syndrome is network of colored retinal streaks resembling large veins associated with degenerated elastic tissue in skin forming yellow plaques.
SYNONYM: *Grönblad Syndrome.*

ANONYCHIA
Anonychia is the complete or almost complete absence of nails.

APLASIA CUTIS CONGENITA
Aplasia cutis congenita is a local defect in skin due to failure of development.
SYNONYM: *Congenital Defect of Skin.*

ATHELIA
Athelia is the absence of one or more nipples.

BREAST, AXILLARY
Axillary breast is the presence of breast tissue along the anterior axillary line. It may be separate or an axillary tail of the breast itself.

BROMODERMA
Bromoderma is characterized by nodular or discoid lesions of the fetal skin resulting from bromides taken by mother during pregnancy.

CALCINOSIS CIRCUMSCRIPTA
Calcinosis circumscripta is the presence of local deposits of calcium salts in subcutaneous tissues and skin.

CALCINOSIS UNIVERSALIS
Calcinosis universalis is the presence of local deposits of calcium salts in the skin, muscles, tendon fascia, and nerves.

CLUBNAIL
Clubnail is a rounded deformed nail.

CUTIS VERTICIS GYRATA
Cutis verticis gyrata is a syndrome characterized by folds and furrows causing the face to appear corrugated or to resemble that of a bulldog.
SYNONYMS: *Bulldog Scalp, Cutis Sulcata.*

DERMATITIS, BULLOUS, KERATOGENIC
Keratogenic bullous dermatitis is the presence of blisters and the thickening of inflamed skin associated with eosinophilia in newborn girls.
SYNONYM: *Asboe-Hansen Disease.*

DERMATITIS, EXFOLIATIVE
Exfoliative dermatitis is extensive desquamation with loss of sheets of epidermis.
SYNONYM: *Ritter's Disease.*

DERMATOLYSIS
Dermatolysis is loose or pendulous skin.
SYNONYM: *Cutis Laxa.*

DISTICHIASIS
Distichiasis is the presence of two rows of eyelashes on one eyelid.

DYSKERATOSIS, BENIGN HEREDITARY INTRAEPITHELIAL
Benign hereditary intraepithelial dyskeratosis is the presence of lesions of buccal mucosa and bulbar conjunctiva.
SYNONYM: *Witkop's Disease.*

DYSKERATOSIS, CONGENITAL
Congenital dyskeratosis is hyperkeratosis palmaris et plantaris, with mental retardation, testicular hyperplasia and eye defects.
SYNONYM: *Shäfer's Syndrome.*

DYSTROPHIA PIGMENTOSA
Dystrophia pigmentosa is brownish macular skin pigmentation with hyperglycemia and asthenia.
SYNONYM: *Leschke's Syndrome.*

EYEBROWS, DUPLICATION OF
Duplication of eyebrows is the presence of two rows of hair above the eyes, sometimes with the hair growing toward the midline.

EYELASHES, CONGENITAL HYPOTRICHOSIS OF
Congenital hypotrichosis of the eyelashes is partial or complete absence of the eyelashes.

EYELASHES, TRICHOMEGALY OF
Trichomegaly of the eyelashes is the presence of abnormally long eyelashes.

EPIDERMODYSPLASIA VERRUCIFORMIS
Epidermodysplasia verruciformis is faulty development of the upper layers of the epidermis, with reddish smooth papules especially on the palms, soles, and face.

EPIDERMOLYSIS BULLOSA HEREDITARIA LETALIS
Epidermolysis bullosa hereditaria letalis are bullae, clear or hemorrhagic, that rupture, leaving denuded areas. Secondary infection and death usually occur swiftly.
SYNONYM: *Herlitz Syndrome.*

ERYTHRODERMA–ATOPY–BAMBOO HAIR SYNDROME
Erythroderma-atopy-bamboo hair syndrome is the combination of ichthyosiform erythroderma, lack of tonus, and fragmented hairs (bamboo hair).
SYNONYM: *Netherton's Syndrome.*

ERYTHRODERMA, DESQUAMATIVE
Desquamative erythroderma is characterized by reddened infiltrated areas with branny or greasy scales.
SYNONYM: *Leiner's Disease.*

ERYTHRODERMA ICHTHYOSIFORME CONGENITUM
Erythroderma ichthyosiforme congenitum is a congenital syndrome of very red, dry, scaly skin.
SYNONYM: *Epidermodysplasia Histricoides Bullosa.*

FINGERS, PSEUDOAINHUM OF
Pseudoainhum of the fingers is characterized by linear constricting bands of skin around the proximal phalanges of fingers.

HAIR, BAMBOO
Bamboo hair is characterized by regularly spaced brush fractures in hair shafts alternating with areas of relatively normal shafts, thus resembling bamboo.
SYNONYM: *Trichorrhexis Invaginata.*

HAIR, RINGED
Ringed hair is hair with alternate bands of pigment or whiteness, due to gas filled spaces in cortex and medulla of hair.
SYNONYM: *Pili Annulati.*

HAIR, TWISTED
Twisted hair is characterized by irregularly flattened and twisted hair shafts. Eyelashes are often irregular and sparse.
SYNONYM: *Pili Torti.*

HAND CREASES, ANOMALOUS
Anomalous hand creases are the abnormal or atypical number or direction of creases in the palm of the hand.

HARLEQUIN COLOR–CHANGE SYNDROME
Harlequin color-change syndrome is the transient pink discoloration of one side (half) of an infant's body, usually lasting 30 seconds to 20 minutes. It occurs several times a day, and color division is exactly at the midline of the body.

HYPERKERATOSIS PENETRANS
Hyperkeratosis penetrans is characterized by conical pegs of keratin extending downward into the corium.
SYNONYMS: *Hyperkeratosis Follicularis, Kyrle's Disease.*

HYPERTRICHOSIS, FAMILIAL
Familial hypertrichosis is excessive growth of hair, either local or general.

HYPOTRICHOSIS HEREDITARIA CONGENITA
Hypotrichosis hereditaria congenita is partial or complete failure of hair development.
SYNONYM: *Unna's Syndrome.*

ICHTHYOSIS, LAMELLAR
Lamellar ichthyosis is ichthyosis with smooth, shiny, red skin with cracks and peeling of scales.
SYNONYMS: *Ichthyosis Sebacea, Lamellar Desquamation, Carini's Syndrome.*

ICHTHYOSIS, MENTAL DEFICIENCY, AND EPILEPSY SYNDROME

Ichthyosis, mental deficiency, and epilepsy syndrome is an autosomal genetic disease characterized by mental deficiency, epilepsy, congenital ichthyosis, and other anomalies.

SYNONYM: *Rud's Syndrome.*

KERATOSIS FOLLICULARIS

Keratosis follicularis is characterized by crusting, papular, verrucous growths, usually symmetrically distributed.

SYNONYMS: *Dyskeratosis Follicularis, Keratosis Vegetans, Darier's Syndrome.*

KERATOSIS–ONYCHOGRYPOSIS SYNDROME

Keratosis-onychogryposis syndrome is keratosis palmaris et plantaris associated with onychogryposis, mental deficiency, and other anomalies.

SYNONYM: *Fischer's Syndrome.*

KERATOSIS PALMARIS ET PLANTARIS

Keratosis palmaris et plantaris is the symmetric thickening of the skin of the palms and soles.

SYNONYMS: *Ichthyosis Palmaris et Plantaris, Keratoma Palmare et Plantare Hereditarium, Tylosis of Palms and Soles, Unna-Thost Syndrome.*

KERATOSIS PALMOPLANTARIS STRIATA

Keratosis palmoplantaris striata is linear cornification of the horny layer of the epidermis of the palms and soles.

KERATOSIS PILARIS

Keratosis pilaris is keratinization of the hair follicles and the formation of follicular papules.

SYNONYMS: *Ichthyosis Follicularis, Keratosis Suprafollicularis, Lichen Pilaris, Pityriasis Pilaris.*

KERATOSIS PUNCTATA PALMARIS ET PLANTARIS

Keratosis punctata palmaris et plantaris is characterized by scattered discrete wartlike papules on the hands and feet.

SYNONYM: *Keratoderma Disseminatum Palmaris et Plantaris.*

KOILONYCHIA

Koilonychia is the concavity of the outer surface of a nail, resembling a spoon.

SYNONYMS: *Spoon Nail, Spading Nail.*

LANUGO, PERSISTENT

Persistent lanugo is the presence of an excessive amount of fine, short hair.

LENTIGO
Lentigo is increased melanin deposition causing brownish spots on the skin.

LEUKONYCHIA STRIATA
Leukonychia striata is the presence of transverse white streaks in the nails.

LEUKONYCHIA TOTALIS
Leukonychia totalis is whiteness of the entire nail.

LEUKOPATHIA UNGUIUM, CONGENITAL
Congenital leukopathia unguium is the presence of white spots or patches under the nails, resulting from air bubbles between the bed and the nail.

LIDS, PIGMENTATION OF
Pigmentation of the lids is abnormal darkening and pigmentation of the eyelids.

LYMPHEDEMA, CONGENITAL
Congenital lymphedema is a hereditary enlargement of the lower extremities due to lymphangiectasia.
SYNONYMS: *Hereditary Trophedema, Milroy's Disease.*

MADAROSIS
Madarosis is loss of the eyebrows or eyelashes.

MAL DE MELEDA
Mal de Meleda is symmetric keratodermia of the extremities endemic to the island of Meleda.

MEGALOCEROS
Megaloceros is a fetus with hornlike growths on its forehead.

MICROTHELIA
Microthelia is a small nipple.

MOLE, HAIRY
Hairy mole is a nevus covered with hair.
SYNONYM: *Nevus Pilosus.*

MULTIPLE MOLES SYNDROME
Multiple moles syndrome is a syndrome of multiple, symmetric mottling, with moles, genital hypoplasia, and mitral stenosis.
SYNONYM: *Moynahan's Syndrome.*

MONILETHRIX
Monilethrix is the presence of constrictions along shafts of hairs, resembling a string of fusiform beads. Hairs are fragile, short, and sparse.
SYNONYMS: *Beaded Hair, Moniliform Hair, Sabouraud's Syndrome.*

MONILETHRIX–CATARACT SYNDROME
Monilethrix-cataract syndrome is congenital cataract in association with beaded hair.
SYNONYM: *Prieur-Trénel Syndrome.*

NAIL, DYSTROPHY OF
Dystrophy of the nail is an abnormality of nail growth resulting from defective nutrition.
SYNONYM: *Dystrophia Unguium.*

NAIL, RACKET
Racket nail is a wide, short nail, flattened and usually affecting the thumb nails.
SYNONYM: *Nail en Raquette.*

NAILS, PITTING OF
Pitting of the nails is a dystrophy of the nails with numerous pits or depressions.

NEVUS, BLUE
Blue nevus is a dark blue discoloration caused by melanin-pigmented cells of the lower dermis.

NEVUS, BLUE RUBBER BLEB
Blue rubber bleb nevus is a syndrome of blue skin and associated intestinal hemangiomas.

NEVUS, PIGMENTED
Pigmented nevus is a pigmented skin lesion.
SYNONYM: *Pigmented Mole.*

NEVUS, WHITE SPONGE, OF MUCOSA
White sponge nevus of the mucosa is a white, elastic, porous nevus.
SYNONYMS: *Nevus Spongiosus Albus Mucosae, Cannon's Nevus.*

ONYCHATROPHY
Onychatrophy is atrophy of nails.

ONYCHAUXIS
Onychauxis is overgrowth of the nails.

ONYCHODYSTROPHY
Onychodystrophy is abnormal development of the nails.

ONYCHOGRYPOSIS
Onychogryposis is characterized by enlarged and curved nails due to overgrowth of the nail plate.

ONYCHORRHEXIS
Onychorrhexis is brittle nails.

PACHYONYCHIA
Pachyonychia is thickened nails.

PACHYONYCHIA CONGENITA SYNDROME
Pachyonychia congenita syndrome is the association of thick nails, bullae, keratoses of the palms and soles, and corneal dyskeratosis.
SYNONYMS: *Pachyonychia Ichthyosiforme, Polykeratosis Congenita, Jadassohn-Lewandowsky Syndrome.*

PHC SYNDROME
PHC syndrome consists of premolar aplasia, hyperhidrosis, and premature grayness of the hair.
SYNONYM: *Böök's Syndrome.*

PITS, SKIN
Skin pits are small depressions in the skin, usually on the face.

PLATYONYCHIA
Platyonychia is characterized by unusually flat, broad nails.

POLYONYCHIA
Polyonychia is the presence of extra or supernumerary nails.
SYNONYM: *Polyunguia.*

POROKERATOSIS
Porokeratosis is hypertrophy of the stratum corneum about the sweat gland ducts, with progressive centrifugal atrophy.
SYNONYMS: *Hyperkeratosis Excentrica, Hyperkeratosis Figurata Centrifuga Atrophica, Porokeratosis Excentrica, Mibelli's Disease.*

SCALP, GYRATE
Gyrate scalp is convoluted skin of the head with thick ridges separated by depressions.

SCALP, HYPOTRICHOSIS OF
Hypotrichosis of the scalp is an ectodermal defect often associated with dental anomalies and the absence of nails.
SYNONYM: *Jacquet's Syndrome.*

SCALP, SKIN DEFECT OF
Skin defect of the scalp is a round area of granulation tissue, usually in the midline over the vertex and about 1 to 2 cm across.

SCROTUM, PIGMENTED
Pigmented scrotum is the abnormal darkening and pigmentation of the scrotal skin.

SINUS, PILONIDAL
Pilonidal sinus is a small epithelium-lined tract leading from the skin, usually over the sacral area.

SKIN, GYRATE
Gyrate skin is convoluted skin with thick ridges separated by irregular depressions.

SKIN, HYPERELASTIC
Hyperelastic skin is skin that can be stretched a considerable amount, immediately retracting when released.

SKIN MELANOMA, BENIGN
Benign skin melanoma is a nonmalignant pigmented neoplasm resulting from the deposition of melanin in and below the skin.

SKIN TAGS, ACCESSORY
Accessory skin tags are small pedunculated outgrowths of skin.

SPOTS, MONGOLIAN
Mongolian spots are gray-blue areas over the sacral region resulting from melanoblasts in the corium. They are most frequent in dark-skinned and Oriental people.

STEATOCYSTOMA MULTIPLEX
Steatocystoma multiplex is the presence of multiple sebaceous cysts.

SYNOPHRYS
Synophrys is the growing together of the eyebrows.

TETRASTICHIASIS
Tetrastichiasis is the presence of four rows of eyelashes on one eyelid.

THELARCHE, PREMATURE
Premature thelarche is precocious growth of one or both breasts without other signs of precocious puberty.
SYNONYM: *Premature Gynarche.*

TOENAIL, ACCESSORY
Accessory toenail is an extra toenail in an abnormal place.

TRICHOEPITHELIOMA
Trichoepithelioma is a multiple, benign, basal-cell tumor, chiefly of the face, neck, or chest.
SYNONYMS: *Benign Multiple Cystic Epithelioma, Turban Tumor.*

TRICHORRHEXIS NODOSA
Trichorrhexis nodosa is the splitting and breaking of hairs, with minute nodules formed in their shafts.

SYNONYM: *Pinselhaare*.

TRISTICHIA
Tristichia is the presence of three rows of eyelashes on one eyelid.

URTICARIA PERSTANS HEMORRHAGICA
Urticaria perstans hemorrhagica is persistent purpura urticans with wheals, itching, and petechiae.

URTICARIA PIGMENTOSA
Urticaria pigmentosa is characterized by yellowish or reddish brown spots with urticaria and pruritus when traumatized.

SYNONYMS: *Mastocystosis Syndrome, Xanthelasmoidea, Nettleship's Syndrome*.

WENS
Wens are smooth nodules with lamellae of keratinized scales.

SYNONYM: *Epidermoid Cysts*.

SECTION 9: GLOSSARY OF CONGENITAL ANOMALIES

Unspecified

ABDOMINAL WALL, CALCIFICATION OVER
Calcification over the abdominal wall is the occurrence of multiple small masses of calcium, usually over the abdominal surface of the diaphragm and occasionally in other areas of the abdomen.

ADRENAL GLAND, ABERRANT
Aberrant adrenal gland is an adrenal gland in an unusual place.
SYNONYM: *Ectopic Adrenal Gland.*

ADRENAL GLAND, AGENESIS OF
Agenesis of the adrenal gland is the absence or hypoplasia of the adrenal gland.
SYNONYM: *Absent Adrenal Gland.*

ADRENAL GLAND, CONGENITAL CYST OF
Congenital cyst of the adrenal gland is an adrenal gland with one or more cysts.

ADRENAL GLAND, CYTOMEGALY OF
Cytomegaly of the adrenal gland is the presence of irregular, large cells with nuclear chromatin in large, irregular clumps in the adrenal gland.

ADRENAL GLANDS, FUSED
Fused adrenal glands are adrenal glands that have developed as one organ, usually behind the aorta.

ADRENAL GLAND, HYPOPLASIA OF
Hypoplasia of the adrenal gland is an incompletely or poorly developed adrenal gland.

ADRENAL GLAND, INCLUSION BODIES IN
Inclusion bodies in the adrenal gland are numerous vacuoles and fine, granular, acidophilic materials in the cytoplasm of the adrenal gland.

ASPLENIA
Asplenia is the absence of the spleen, usually resulting from arrested development of the truncus arteriosus.

CYST, PITUITARY DIVERTICULUM
Pituitary diverticulum cyst is a cyst arising from the lumen of the pituitary diverticulum.
SYNONYMS: *Intrapituitary Cyst, Rathke's Cleft Cyst.*

DWARF, NANOCEPHALIC
Nanocephalic dwarf is a small-headed dwarf.

HYPOPHYSIS, AGENESIS OR HYPOPLASIA OF
Agenesis or hypoplasia of the hypophysis is the partial or complete failure of development of the hypophysis.

KIDNEY, ADRENAL GLAND IN
Adrenal gland in the kidney is the incorporation of part of the adrenal gland in the cortex of the superior renal pole, often without capsular demarcation.

MIDGET
A midget is a person who is much smaller than usual.

PARATHYROID GLANDS, ABSENCE OF
Absence of the parathyroid glands is the complete failure of development of the parathyroid glands.

PITUITARY GLAND, AGENESIS OR HYPOPLASIA OF
Agenesis or hypoplasia of the pituitary gland is the partial or complete failure of development of the pituitary gland.
SYNONYM: *Absent Pituitary Gland.*

PITUITARY GLAND, INTRASPHENOIDAL
Intrasphenoidal pituitary gland is the presence of pituitary anterior-lobe tissue in the sphenoid bone.

PITUITARY GLAND, PHARYNGEAL
Pharyngeal pituitary gland is the presence of pituitary anterior-lobe tissue in the pharynx along the dorsal wall.

PSEUDOHYPOPARATHYROIDISM
Pseudohypoparathyroidism is hypoparathyroidism not responsive to parathyroid extract in the correction of hypophosphatemia and hypocalcemia.
SYNONYM: *Martin-Albright Syndrome.*

REST, ADRENOCORTICAL
Adrenocortical rest is misplaced adrenal cortical tissue.

SPLEEN, ABERRANT
Aberrant spleen is a spleen in an unusual place.

SPLEEN, ACCESSORY

Accessory spleen is one or more additional areas of splenic tissue.
SYNONYMS: *Lien Accessorius, Spleneolus.*

SPLEEN, AGENESIS OF

Agenesis of the spleen is partial or complete failure of development of the spleen.
SYNONYM: *Absent Spleen.*

SPLEEN, CYSTIC

Cystic spleen is a spleen containing cysts.

SPLEEN, ECTOPIC

Ectopic spleen is a spleen in an abnormal position.

SPLEEN, LOBULATED

Lobulated spleen is the presence of one or more grooves on the spleen, dividing it into lobes.

SPLENOMEGALY, CONGENITAL

Congenital splenomegaly is enlargement of the spleen.

SPORADIC GOITER AND CONGENITAL DEAFNESS SYNDROME

Sporadic goiter and congenital deafness syndrome is characterized by an enlarged thyroid gland with poor thyroxine synthesis and associated congenital nerve deafness.
SYNONYM: *Pendred's Syndrome.*

THYMUS GLAND, AGENESIS OR HYPOPLASIA OF

Agenesis or hypoplasia of the thymus gland is partial or complete failure of development of thymic gland tissue.
SYNONYM: *Absent Thymus Gland.*

THYROGLOSSAL DUCT, CYST OF

Cyst of the thyroglossal duct is a cyst along the path of the ductus thyroglossus between the embryonic thyroid and the posterior part of the tongue.

THYROGLOSSAL DUCT, SINUS OR FISTULA OF

Sinus or fistula of the thyroglossal duct is a sinus or fistula along the path of the embryonic ductus thyroglossus between the embryonic thyroid and the posterior part of the tongue.

THYROGLOSSAL OR THYROLINGUAL DUCT, PERSISTENT

Persistent thyroglossal or thyrolingual duct is a remnant of the thyroglossal duct that has failed to atrophy.

THYROID GLAND, ABERRANT
Aberrant thyroid gland is the presence of thyroid tissue in an abnormal place.

SYNONYM: *Ectopic Thyroid Gland.*

THYROID GLAND, AGENESIS OR HYPOPLASIA OF
Agenesis or hypoplasia of the thyroid gland is the partial or complete failure of development of the thyroid gland.

THYROID, LINGUAL
Lingual thyroid is the presence of areas of thyroid tissue in the tongue.

THYROID RESTS, ABERRANT LATERAL
Aberrant lateral thyroid rests are areas of thyroid tissue in the neck believed to arise from fourth or fifth embryonic pharyngeal pouch.

Multiple Systems

ACEPHALOBRACHIUS
Acephalobrachius is a fetus without a head or arms.
SYNONYM: *Abrachiocephalia*.

ACEPHALOCARDIA
Acephalocardia is absence of the head and heart.

ACEPHALOCHIRIA
Acephalochiria is absence of the head and hands.

ACEPHALOGASTER
Acephalogaster is one of a pair of twins that has only the lower part of its body.

ACEPHALOPODIA
Acephalopodia is absence of the head and feet.

ACEPHALORHACHIA
Acephalorhachia is absence of the head and spinal column.

ACEPHALOSTOMIA
Acephalostomia is absence of most of the head but with a mouthlike opening.

ACEPHALOTHORACIA
Acephalothoracia is a fetus without a head or thorax.

ANEMIA–OSTEODYSPLASIA SYNDROME
Anemia-osteodysplasia syndrome is a combination of hypoplastic bone deformities, growth and mental retardation, and hypochromic anemia.
SYNONYM: *Benjamin's Syndrome*.

ATAXIA–CATARACT–DWARFING–MENTAL DEFICIENCY SYNDROME
Ataxia-cataract-dwarfing-mental deficiency syndrome is a syndrome of ataxia, congenital bilateral cataracts, dwarfing, and mental retardation.

ATLODIDYMUS
Atlodidymus is a fetal monster with two heads on a single neck and single body.

BLEPHAROCHALASIS–GOITER SYNDROME
Blepharochalasis-goiter syndrome is the combination of sagging lids, double lip, and goiter.
SYNONYM: *Ascher's Syndrome.*

CALCIFICATION, PERITONEAL
Peritoneal calcification is the presence of numerous wormlike masses of calcium, chiefly over the diaphragm but also occurring elsewhere on the peritoneum.

CARDIOAUDITORY SYNDROME
Cardioauditory syndrome is a combination of syncopal attacks and congenital sensory deafness, with ventricular fibrillation and frequently sudden death.
SYNONYM: *Jervell and Lange-Nielsen Syndrome.*

CARDIOVASCULAR–DENTAL DYSPLASIA SYNDROME
Cardiovascular-dental dysplasia syndrome is a combination of multiple cardiovascular and dental deformities with mental retardation.
SYNONYM: *Beuren's Syndrome.*

CEPHALODIDYMUS
Cephalodidymus is a fetal monster with two bodies fused except for the heads.

CEPHALODIPROSOPUS
Cephalodiprosopus is a fetal monster with a partial head attached to the head of the autosite.
SYNONYM: *Diprosopus Parasiticus.*

CEREBROHEPATORENAL SYNDROME
Cerebrohepatorenal syndrome is the combination of psychomotor retardation, hypotonic liver disease, kidney anomalies, and hemosiderosis.
SYNONYM: *Zellweger's Syndrome.*

CRANIAL NERVE PARALYSIS–CLUBFOOT SYNDROME
Cranial nerve paralysis-clubfoot syndrome consists of the symmetric paralysis of the sixth and seventh cranial nerve distribution and double clubfoot.
SYNONYM: *Alajouanine's Syndrome.*

CRANIOFACIAL DYSOSTOSIS–CARDIOCUTANEOUS SYNDROME
Craniofacial dysostosis-cardiocutaneous syndrome is a combination of craniofacial dysostosis, patent ductus arteriosus, hypertrichosis, hypoplasia of labia majora, and ocular and dental anomalies.
SYNONYM: *Gorlin-Chaudry-Moss Syndrome.*

CRANIOSKELETAL DYSOSTOSIS–CORNEAL OPACITY SYNDROME

Cranioskeletal dysostosis-corneal opacity syndrome is a syndrome consisting of corneal opacities, bony abnormality, hepatosplenomegaly, and mental retardation.

SYNONYM: *Helmholz-Harrington Syndrome.*

CYCLOPIA

Cyclopia is the state of having a single or double median eye within one orbit.

SYNONYM: *Synophthalmia.*

CYCLOPS HYPOGNATHUS

Cyclops hypognathus is a cyclops with low ears, rudimentary mandible, very small mouth, and without a marked proboscis.

CYLLOSOMA

Cyllosoma is a deformity of the lower abdominal wall with ipsilateral defective development of the legs.

DOUBLE KIDNEY–CLUBBED FINGERS SYNDROME

Double kidney-clubbed fingers syndrome is a combination of clubbed fingers and double kidney, sometimes with facial asymmetry.

SYNONYM: *Alleman's Syndrome.*

DUPLICITAS ANTERIOR

Duplicitas anterior is characterized by fusion of the pelvis and lower extremities of twins but with separate thoraces and heads.

DUPLICITAS POSTERIOR

Duplicitas posterior is characterized by fusion of the heads and upper parts of the bodies of twins but with separate legs and buttocks.

DWARF, AMSTERDAM

Amsterdam dwarf is one that exhibits a syndrome of mental retardation, multiple anomalies, and bushy eyebrows.

DWARFISM–CORTICAL THICKENING SYNDROME

Dwarfism-cortical thickening syndrome is a combination of dwarfism, cortical thickening of the long bones, late closure of the anterior fontanel, and often transient hypocalcemia.

SYNONYM: *Kenny's Syndrome.*

DWARFISM–DIABETES SYNDROME

Dwarfism-diabetes syndrome consists of pituitary nanism, genital infantilism, and diabetes mellitus.

SYNONYM: *Nebecourt's Syndrome.*

DYSCEPHALIA MANDIBULO–OCULOFACIALIS
Dyscephalia mandibulo-oculofacialis is a combination of bony anomalies of the skull, with ocular anomalies and alopecia overlying the skull sutures.

DYSCRANIOPYGOPHALANGY
Dyscraniopygophalangy is a syndrome of micrognathia, ear malformation, hexadactyly, and genital malformations.
SYNONYMS: *Ullrich-Feichtiger Syndrome, Status Degenerativus, Dyscranio-Dysphalangiae.*

DYSENCEPHALIA SPLANCHNOCYSTICA
Dysencephalia splanchnocystica is a combination of skull dysostosis, microcephaly, ocular anomalies, multiple cysts of internal organs, genital dysplasias, and polydactyly.
SYNONYM: *Gruber's Syndrome.*

DYSGENESIS IRIDODENTALIS
Dysgenesis iridodentalis is characterized by abnormalities of the iris associated with dental anomalies.

DYSOSTOSIS ACROFACIALIS
Dysostosis acrofacialis is a syndrome of metacarpal synostoses, hexadactylia, mandibular cleft, and dental anomalies.

DYSOSTOSIS, OTOMANDIBULAR
Otomandibular dysostosis is a syndrome of anomalies of structures derived from first branchial arch, including colobomas of the iris, mandibular hypoplasia, and atresia and agenesis of the ear.
SYNONYM: *Francois-Haustrate Syndrome.*

DYSPLASIA, OLFACTOGENITAL
Olfactogenital dysplasia is a syndrome of cerebral malformations, hypoplastic gonads, and cranial asymmetry.
SYNONYM: *de Morsier's Syndrome.*

DYSTROPHIA PERIOSTALIS HYPERPLASTICA FAMILIARIS
Dystrophia periostalis hyperplastica familiaris is craniomandibular dysostosis with premature closure of cranial sutures, thick skull, acrocephaly and other skeletal anomalies.
SYNONYM: *Dzierzynsky's Syndrome.*

ENCEPHALOTRIGEMINAL ANGIOMATOSIS AND GLAUCOMA
Encephalotrigeminal angiomatosis and glaucoma consists of facial port wine stains of trigeminal area associated with glaucoma.
SYNONYM: *Lawford's Syndrome.*

ENCRANIUS
Encranius is a teratoid parasite that is within the cranium of the autosite.

EYE DYSPLASIA, OCULOVERTEBRAL
Oculovertebral eye dysplasia is a syndrome consisting of multiple eye anomalies and malformations of the teeth, mouth, skull, vertebrae, and ribs.
SYNONYM: *Weyers' Syndrome.*

FACIAL DIPLEGIA, CONGENITAL
Congenital facial diplegia is a complex syndrome consisting of bilateral facial paralysis and various ocular and cranial nerve anomalies.

GASTROAMORPHUS
Gastroamorphus is an amorphous twin included within the abdomen of the autosite.

GONADAL DYSGENESIS WITH MEDULLARY ELEMENT
Gonadal dysgenesis with a medullary element is the absence or aplasia of germ cells, but some medullary elements such as mesonephric remnants, rete tubules, or Leydig cells are present.

HEMIHYPERTROPHY, CONGENITAL
Congenital hemihypertrophy is the unilateral enlargement of all or part of the body.
SYNONYMS: *Curtius' Syndrome, Hemifacial Hypertrophy, Hemigigantism, Hemiocrosomia, Partial Gigantism, Steiner's Syndrome, Unilateral Hypertrophy.*

HEMIPLEGIA–PORT WINE STAIN SYNDROME
Hemiplegia-port wine stain syndrome is a syndrome of hemiplegia, contralateral port-wine stain of the face, and other anomalies.
SYNONYMS: *Nevi-Cerebral Defect-Hemiplegia Syndrome, Brushfield-Wyatt Syndrome.*

HEREDITARY EXTREMITY MALFORMATIONS SYNDROME
Hereditary extremity malformations syndrome consists of multiple symmetric abnormalities of all extremities, including dysplasia of the elbow joints with luxations, leg dysplasias, and atypical clubfoot.
SYNONYM: *Nievergeit's Syndrome.*

HOLOACARDIUS
Holoacardius is a separate twin lacking a heart and deriving its blood supply from the placental circulation of the other twin.
SYNONYMS: *Omphalosite, Placental Parasitic Twin.*

HOLOACARDIUS ACEPHALUS
Holoacardius acephalus is a separate twin lacking any heart and head.

HOLOACARDIUS ACORMUS
Holoacardius acormus is a separate twin without the lower part of its body.

HOLOACARDIUS AMORPHUS
Holoacardius amorphus is a separate twin without form or recognizable organs.

HOLOCEPHALY
Holocephaly is to have a complete head but be deficient in certain parts.

HYPOPLASTIC FINGERNAIL–TOENAIL SYNDROME
Hypoplastic fingernail-toenail syndrome is a syndrome of severe mental retardation associated with hypoplastic fingernails and toenails, attributed to a partial trisomy, probably in the C group.

INTRAUTERINE DWARFISM SYNDROME
Intrauterine dwarfism syndrome is intrauterine dwarfism with disproportionately short arms and craniofacial dysostosis, often with other anomalies.
SYNONYMS: *Russell's Dwarf, Russell's Syndrome.*

LOW BIRTH WEIGHT–DWARFISM SYNDROME
Low birth weight-dwarfism syndrome is a combination of dwarfism, low birth weight, facial anomalies, skin eruption, and mental retardation.
SYNONYM: *Dubovitz's Syndrome.*

MACROGLOSSIA–OMPHALOCELE–ADRENAL CYTOMEGALY SYNDROME
Macroglossia-omphalocele-adrenal cytomegaly syndrome is a combination of macroglossia, omphalocele, cortical cytomegaly of the fetal adrenal gland, hyperplastic visceromegaly, and other anomalies.
SYNONYM: *Beckwith's Syndrome.*

MELANOLEUKODERMA–DYSPLASIA SYNDROME
Melanoleukoderma-dysplasia syndrome is the combination of hyperpigmentation and hypopigmentation of the skin with multiple assorted anomalies.
SYNONYM: *Berlin's Syndrome.*

MICROSOMIA, HEMIFACIAL
Hemifacial microsomia is a syndrome consisting of unilateral agenesis of the mandible, microtia, and macrostomia.

MONSTER, COMPOUND
A compound monster is an infant with parts of more than one individual.

MONSTER, DOUBLE
A double monster is a fetus from a single ovum with duplication of the head, trunk, or limbs.

MONSTER, PARASITIC
A parasitic monster is the smaller of unequal conjoined twins.

MONSTER, TRIPLET
A triplet monster is one having parts of three individuals.

MYOTONY–DYSTROPHY–DYSARTHRIA SYNDROME
Myotony-dystrophy-dysarthria syndrome is a combination of muscular myotonia and dystrophy with mental deficiency and dysarthria.
SYNONYM: *Foerster's Syndrome.*

NANASOMA ESSENTIALIS
Nanasoma essentialis is abnormal smallness due to genetic factors.
SYNONYMS: *Primary Dwarfism, Pygmyism.*

NYSTAGMUS–MYOCLONUS SYNDROME
Nystagmus-myoclonus syndrome is congenital myoclonus with myoclonic nystagmus.
SYNONYM: *Lenoble-Aubineau Syndrome.*

OLIGODACTYLIA SYNDROME
Oligodactylia syndrome is ulnar aplasia with associated abnormalities of the jaws, sternum, kidney, and spleen.
SYNONYM: *Hertwig-Weyers Syndrome.*

OMACEPHALUS
Omacephalus is a fetus without upper limbs and with an imperfect or absent head.

OPHTHALMOPLEGIA–ATAXIA–AREFLEXIA SYNDROME
Ophthalmoplegia-ataxia-areflexia syndrome is a syndrome of ataxia, external ophthalmoplegia, and loss of tendon reflexes.
SYNONYM: *Fisher's Syndrome.*

OPOCEPHALUS
Opocephalus is a fetus with a single eye or close eyes and no mouth or nose.

ORBITOPAGUS
Orbitopagus is a parasitic fetus attached at an orbit of its autosite.

OROFACIAL–DWARFISM SYNDROME
Orofacial-dwarfism syndrome is an association of cleft lip and palate and lower lip fistula, often with dwarfism, infantilism, and digital and cardiac abnormalities.
SYNONYM: *Demarquay-Richet Syndrome.*

OSTEODYSPLASTIC GERODERMIA, HEREDITARY
Hereditary osteodysplastic gerodermia is progeria, nanism, and ocular, dental and osseous anomalies.
SYNONYM: *Bamatter's Syndrome.*

OSTEOHYPERTROPHIC–VARICOSE NEVUS SYNDROME
Osteohypertrophic-varicose nevus syndrome is unilateral arteriovenous malformation, overgrowth of some fingers, syndactyly, and osteohypertrophic changes in one or more extremities.
SYNONYMS: *Angioma Osteohypertrophique, Angiome Trigemene Osteohypertrophique, Angio-osteohypertrophy Syndrome, Hemangiectatic Hypertrophy, Naevus-Varicosus Osteohypertrophicus, Klippel-Trenaunay Syndrome, Klippel Trenaunay-Weber Syndrome, Weber-Klippel Syndrome.*

OSTEOPATHIA ACIDOTICA PSEUDORACHITICA SYNDROME
Osteopathia acidotica pseudorachitica syndrome is a syndrome consisting of heart and brain defects, acidosis, osteoporosis, and spontaneous fractures.
SYNONYM: *Fanconi-Albertini-Zellweger Syndrome.*

PARACEPHALUS
Paracephalus is a fetus with poorly developed head, trunk, and limbs.

PARASITE AMORPHUS
Parasite amorphus is a shapeless fetus.

POPLITEAL WEBBING–CLEFT PALATE SYNDROME
Popliteal webbing-cleft palate syndrome is a combination of cleft lip and palate, lower lip fistula, equinovarus, and popliteal webbing.
SYNONYM: *Févre-Languepin Syndrome.*

PSEUDOACEPHALUS
Pseudoacephalus is a parasitic and apparently headless twin; however, it has hidden cephalic structures.

SITUS INVERSUS
Situs inversus is visceral transposition, the organs being on the opposite side of the body from their normal sites.

SITUS INVERSUS ABDOMINALIS
Situs inversus abdominalis is the lateral transposition of the abdominal viscera.
SYNONYM: *Situs Abdominalis.*

SITUS INVERSUS THORACIS
Situs inversus thoracis is the lateral transposition of the thoracic viscera.
SYNONYM: *Situs Thoracis.*

SITUS INVERSUS VISCERUM
Situs inversus viscerum is a transposition of the viscera from one side to the other, usually in a mirror-image relationship.
SYNONYMS: *Situs Transversus, Visceral Inversion, Visceral Transposition.*

SITUS PERVERSUS
Situs perversus is abnormal location of a viscus.

SPLENIC AGENESIS SYNDROME
Splenic agenesis syndrome consists of agenesis of the spleen, heart defects, and situs inversus.
SYNONYM: *Ivemark's Syndrome.*

STRABISMUS–CLUBFOOT SYNDROME
Strabismus-clubfoot syndrome is a combination of strabismus, speech defects, clubfoot, mental deficiency, and extensor plantar reflexes.
SYNONYM: *Friedman-Roy Syndrome.*

SYMPODIA
Sympodia is fusion of the legs and feet.
SYNONYMS: *Sympus, Sirenomelia.*

TELECANTHUS
Telecanthus is an anomaly in which there is an increase in the distance between the medial canthi greater than two standard deviations above the age-adjusted mean. A variety of anomalies is often associated with telecanthus.

TERATISM
Teratism is an anomaly of fetal formation and development.

TOWER SKULL–EXOPHTHALMOS SYNDROME
Tower skull-exophthalmos syndrome is a combination of tower skull, adenoid hypertrophy, and exophthalmos.
SYNONYM: *Enslin's Triad.*

TRIPROSOPUS
Triprosopus is a fetus with three fused heads.

TWINS, CEPHALOTHORACOPAGUS
Cephalothoracopagus twins are conjoined twins in which two fetuses of equal size are fused front to front over much of the trunk region. They have a single neck and head; the face is ordinarily single; the cerebrum irregularly duplicated; the cerebellum, brainstem, and spinal cord completely duplicated.

TWINS, CRANIODIDYMUS
Craniodidymus twins are conjoined twins with two heads and partial or complete duplication of the spine. The body is usually single with two arms and two legs.

TWINS, CRANIOPAGUS
Craniopagus twins are twins with partially fused skulls; the union may be frontal, occipital, or parietal.
SYNONYM: *Cephalopagus.*

TWINS, CRANIOPAGUS OCCIPITALIS
Craniopagus occipitalis twins are twins joined in the occipital region of the skull.
SYNONYM: *Iniopagus.*

TWINS, CRYPTODIDYMUS
Cryptodidymus twins are twins of unequal size, the smaller being almost completely concealed by the larger.

TWINS, DERADELPHUS
Deradelphus twins are a variety of cephalothoracopagus twins in which there is a single face with two ears and a single, normally formed cerebrum.

TWINS, DERODIDYMUS DICEPHALUS
Derodidymus dicephalus twins are conjoined twins with separate necks and heads.

TWINS, DICEPHALUS
Dicephalus twins are conjoined twins with two heads.

TWINS, DICEPHALUS DIPUS
Dicephalus dipus twins consist of three types: (1) Dicephalus dipus dibrachius twins are conjoined twins with two heads, two arms, two legs, and partial duplication of the spine. There are varying degrees of duplication of the median shoulder; (2) dicephalus dipus tribrachius twins are conjoined twins united at the pelvis. They have a partially duplicated spine, two heads, two legs, two arms, and a median third arm or arm rudiment; (3) dicephalus dipus tetrabrachius twins are conjoined twins united at the pelvis. They have a partially duplicated spine, two heads, four arms, and two legs.

TWINS, DICEPHALUS DIPYGUS
Dicephalus dipygus twins are conjoined twins with two heads, fused bodies, and a variable reduction in the number of upper and lower extremities.

TWINS, DIPLOPAGUS
Diplopagus twins are conjoined twins, each essentially complete.

TWINS, DIPLOSOMIA
Diplosomia twins are conjoined twins, apparently functionally independent.

TWINS, DIPROSOPUS

Diprosopus twins are conjoined twins with duplication of part or all of the face.

TWINS, DIPYGUS PARASITICUS

Dipygus parasiticus twins are conjoined twins with caudal duplication, but one twin is much smaller than the other.

TWINS, ECTOPAGUS

Ectopagus twins are twins united along the sides of the chest.

TWINS, GASTROACEPHALUS

Gastroacephalus twins are unequal twins with a headless twin attached to the abdomen of the autosite.

TWINS, HEMICARDIUS

Hemicardius twins are twins in which there is partial or complete absence of one heart, the parasite depending on the heart of the autosite.

TWINS, HETERADELPHUS

Heteradelphus twins are unequal, conjoined twins; the smaller parasite is attached to the larger autosite.

TWINS, HETERALIUS

Heteralius twins are conjoined twins with one so small that it can barely be recognized.

TWINS, HETEROCEPHALUS

Heterocephalus twins are conjoined twins with heads of unequal size.

TWINS, HETERODIDYMUS

Heterodidymus twins are conjoined twins with the second head, neck, and thorax attached to the chest.

TWINS, HETEROPAGUS

Heteropagus twins are unequal and asymmetric conjoined twins with one component smaller than, and dependent on, the other. The parasite may consist of arms, or head and arms, legs and a portion of pelvis, or arms and legs. It is usually attached to the epigastrium of the autosite, less commonly to the back.

TWINS, HYPOGASTROPAGUS

Hypogastropagus twins are twins joined at the hypogastrium.

TWINS, ILIOTHORACOPAGUS

Iliothoracopagus twins are conjoined, symmetric twins, united from pelvis to thorax.
SYNONYM: *Ischiothoracopagus.*

TWINS, ISCHIOMELUS

Ischiomelus twins are conjoined twins with a parasitic limb or limbs arising from the autosite's pelvic area.

TWINS, ISCHIOPAGUS

Ischiopagus twins are twins fused in the ischial region.

TWINS, JANICEPS

Janiceps twins are anteriorly fused twins with four arms, four legs, and a single head with faces front and back.

TWINS, JANICEPS PARASITICUS

Janiceps parasiticus twins are two-faced twins but one twin (parasite) is small and attached to the larger twin (autosite).

TWINS, MONOCEPHALUS

Monocephalus twins are conjoined twins with a single head. The head may exhibit varying degrees of duplication, although the rest of the body is normal, or the entire body may be duplicated except the head.

TWINS, MONOCEPHALUS TETRAPUS DIBRACHIUS

Monocephalus tetrapus dibrachius twins are conjoined twins with a single head and trunk, two arms, partial or complete duplication of the pelvis, and four legs, the pair belonging to one member often being fused in a sirenomelous limb.

TWINS, MONOCEPHALUS TRIPUS DIBRACHIUS

Monocephalus tripus dibrachius twins are conjoined twins with a single head and trunk, two arms, partial duplication of the pelvis, and a third median leg (variably developed).

TWINS, OMPHALOPAGUS

Omphalopagus twins are conjoined twins united at the umbilicus.
SYNONYM: *Monomphalus Twins.*

TWINS, OPODIDYMUS

Opodidymus twins are conjoined twins with two heads fused posteriorly but separated and with a single body.

TWINS, POLYGNATHUS

Polygnathus twins are twins joined at the jaw of the autosite.

TWINS, PYGOAMORPHUS

Pygoamorphus twins are conjoined twins in which the parasite is attached to the buttocks of the autosite, and the parasite is reduced to a formless mass or embryoma.

TWINS, PYGODIDYMUS

Pygodidymus twins are conjoined twins fused in the cephalothoracic region but with doubled buttocks.

TWINS, PYGOMELUS
Pygomelus twins are unequal conjoined twins in which the parasite is represented by a fleshy mass or a more fully developed limb attached to the sacral or coccygeal region of the autosite.

TWINS, RACHIOPAGUS
Rachiopagus twins are twins united back to back involving the spinal column.

TWINS, STERNODYMUS
Sternodymus twins are conjoined twins attached at the sternum.
SYNONYM: *Sternopagus.*

TWINS, STERNOXIPHOPAGUS
Sternoxiphopagus twins are conjoined twins attached in the region of the sternum and xiphoid process.

TWINS, SYNCEPHALUS ASYMMETROS
Syncephalus asymmetros twins are twins with a single head, and a complete face anteriorly, but only part of a face posteriorly. Usually, above the umbilicus the body is single, but double below it.
SYNONYMS: *Iniops, Janus Asymmetros, Janiceps Asymmetros.*

Sources

Anderson, W. A. D. (ed): Pathology, ed 5. St. Louis, C. V. Mosby Co., 1966, vol 2.

Ball, Thomas L.: Gynecologic Surgery and Urology. St. Louis, C. V. Mosby Co., 1957.

Beck, Alfred C., and Rosenthal, Alexander H.: Obstetrical Practice, ed 6. Baltimore, The Williams and Wilkins Co., 1955.

Behrman, Samuel J., and Gosling, John R. G.: Fundamentals of Gynecology, ed 2. London, Oxford University Press, 1966.

Conn, Howard F., Clohecy, Robert J., and Conn, Rex B., Jr.: Current Diagnosis. Philadelphia, W. B. Saunders Co., 1966.

Danowski, T. S. (ed.): Diabetes Mellitus: Diagnosis and Treatment. New York, American Diabetes Association, Inc., 1964.

Dorland's Illustrated Medical Dictionary, ed 24. Philadelphia, W. B. Saunders Co., 1965.

Douglas, R. Gordon, and Stromme, William B.: Obstetrical Practice, ed 6. New York, Appleton-Century-Crofts, Inc., 1957.

Durham, Robert H.: Encyclopedia of Medical Syndromes. New York, Hoeber Medical Division, Harper and Row, Publishers, 1960.

Eastman, Nicholson J., and Hellman, Louis M.: Williams Obstetrics, ed 13. New York, Appleton-Century-Crofts, Inc., 1966.

Gardner, Herman L., and Kaufman, Raymond H.: Benign Diseases of the Vulva and Vagina. St. Louis, C. V. Mosby Co., 1969.

Gray, Henry: Anatomy of the Human Body, ed 27. Charles Mayo Goss (ed). Philadelphia, Lea and Febiger, 1959.

Greenhill, J. D.: Obstetrics, ed 13. Philadelphia, W. B. Saunders Co., 1965.

Hertig, Arthur T., and Gore, Hazel: Tumors of the Female Sex Organs. Part II, Tumors of the Vulva, Vagina and Uterus. Washington, D.C., Armed Forces Institute of Pathology, 1960.

Hertig, Arthur T., and Gore, Hazel: Tumors of the Female Sex Organs. Part III, Tumors of the Ovary and Fallopian Tube. Washington, D.C., Armed Forces Institute of Pathology, 1961.

Hoerr, Normand L., and Osol, Arthur (eds): Blakiston's New Gould
        Medical Dictionary, ed 2. New York, The Blakiston Division
        of McGraw Hill Book Co., Inc., 1956.

Jablonski, Stanley: Illustrated Dictionary of Eponymic Syndromes and
        Diseases and their Synonyms. Philadelphia, W. B. Saunders
        Co., 1969.

Lloyd, Charles W. (ed): Human Reproduction and Sexual Behavior.
        Philadelphia, Lea and Febiger, 1964.

Merck Manual of Diagnosis and Therapy, ed 11. Rahway, N.J., Merck
        and Co., Inc., 1966.

Netter, Frank H.: The CIBA Collection of Medical Illustration, Repro-
        ductive System, Ernst Oppenheimer (ed). Summit, N.J., CIBA
        Pharmaceutical Products, Inc., 1954, vol 2.

Nomina Anatomica. Amsterdam, Netherlands, Mouton and Co., 1966.

Novak, Edmund R., Jones, Georgeanna Seegar, and Jones, Howard W.,
        Jr.: Novak's Textbook of Gynecology, ed 7. Baltimore, The
        Williams and Wilkins Co., 1965.

Patten, Bradley M.: Human Embryology, ed 2. New York, McGraw Hill
        Book Co., Inc., 1953.

Potter, Edith L.: Rh . . . Its Relation to Congenital Hemolytic Disease
        and to Intragroup Transfusion Reactions. Chicago, Year Book
        Publishers, Inc., 1947.

Potter, Edith L.: Pathology of the Fetus and Infant, ed 2. Chicago, Year
        Book Medical Publishers, Inc., 1952.

Stedman's Medical Dictionary, ed 21. Baltimore, The Williams and
        Wilkins Co., 1966.

Taber's Cyclopedic Medical Dictionary, ed 11. Philadelphia, F. A. Davis
        Co., 1970.

Taylor, C. Stewart: Essentials of Gynecology, ed 3. Philadelphia, Lea and
        Febiger, 1964.

Tepperman, Jay: Metabolic and Endocrine Physiology. Chicago, Year
        Book Medical Publishers, Inc., 1962.

Woodruff, J. Donald, and Pauerstein, Carl J.: The Fallopian Tube.
        Baltimore, The Williams and Wilkins Co., 1969.

Abbreviation Index

Subject Index

NOTE: *Italicized* terms are synonyms.

A

ABO incompatibility, 427
Abacterial cystitis, 139
Abdomen
  pendulous, 334
  white line of, 54
Abdominal
  aorta, 15
  aortic plexus, 60
  decompression suit, 405
  hysterectomy, 211
    subtotal, 211
    total, 211
  muscle
    deficiency syndrome, 472
    external oblique, 48
    internal oblique, 48
    transverse, 48
  myomectomy, 212
  ostium, 70
    development of, 324
  pregnancy, 327, 418
    primary, 327, 418
    secondary, 327, 418
Aberrations, chromosomal, 306
Abetalipoproteinemia, 472
Abiotrophy, Marfan's, 504
Ablatio placentae, 416
Abortion, 414-416, 452
  complete, 414
  contagious, 414
  criminal, 415
  habitual, 414
  illegal, 415
  incomplete, 414
  induced, 414
  inevitable, 414
  infected, 414
  missed, 415
  nontherapeutic, 415
  rate, 415, 452
  septic, 415
  spontaneous, 415
  therapeutic, 415
  threatened, 415
Abortus, 415, 452
  brucella, 414
Abruptio placentae, 416
  syndrome, 268, 416, 447
Abruption, placental, 416

Abscess
  Bartholin, 194
  breast, 107, 397
  gland
    Bartholin's, 124
    major vestibular, 124
    vulvovaginal, 124
    paraurethral duct, 124
    Skene's duct, 124
    submammary, 107, 397
    suburethral, 137
Absolute sterility, 247
Acanthocytosis, 472
Acantholysis bullosa, 487
Acanthopelys pelvis, 355
Acanthosis
  bullosa, 487
  nigricans
    benign, 124
    malignant, 124
Acanthrocytosis, 472
Acardiac twin, 467
Acatalasia, 472
  Swiss variant, 472
  Takahara's disease, 472
Accidental hemorrhage, 416
Accommodation, 329
Acentric chromosome, 305
Acetabulum, 341
Ac-Globulin deficiency, 437, 511
Achard-Thiers syndrome, 251, 268
Acholuric jaundice, chronic, 428
Achondrodysplasia, 473
Achondroplasia, 473
  fetal, 473
  tarda, 481
Achromatin, 305
Acid
  deoxyribonucleic, 307
  desoxyribonucleic, 307
  ribonucleic, 310
Acidemia, methylmalonic, 505
Acidophil cell
  of pancreas, 3
  of pituitary, 4
Acidosis, renal tubular, 514
Aciduria
  argininosuccinic, 477
  orotic, 510
Acinar cell, 3
Acini of breast, 67

651